The Poly-Traumatized Patient with Fractures

Hans-Christoph Pape • Roy Sanders
Joseph Borrelli Jr.
(Editors)

The Poly-Traumatized Patient with Fractures

A Multi-Disciplinary Approach

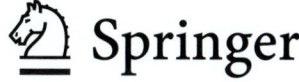

Editors
Prof. Hans-Christoph Pape
Universitätsklinikum Aachen
Klinik für Unfallchirurgie
Pauwelsstraße 30
52057 Aachen
Germany
papehc@aol.com

Dr. Joseph Borrelli Jr.
University of Texas
Southwestern Medical Center at Dallas
5323 Harry Hines Boulevard
Dallas, TX 75390
USA
joseph.borrelli@utsouthwestern.edu

Dr. Roy Sanders
Florida Orthopaedic Institute
13020 N. Telecom Parkway
Temple Terrace, FL 33637
USA
ots1@aol.com

ISBN 978-3-642-17985-3   e-ISBN 978-3-642-17986-0
DOI 10.1007/978-3-642-17986-0
Springer Heidelberg Dordrecht London New York

Library of Congress Control Number: 2011921943

© Springer-Verlag Berlin Heidelberg 2011

This work is subject to copyright. All rights are reserved, whether the whole or part of the material is concerned, specifically the rights of translation, reprinting, reuse of illustrations, recitation, broadcasting, reproduction on microfilm or in any other way, and storage in data banks. Duplication of this publication or parts thereof is permitted only under the provisions of the German Copyright Law of September 9, 1965, in its current version, and permission for use must always be obtained from Springer. Violations are liable to prosecution under the German Copyright Law.

The use of general descriptive names, registered names, trademarks, etc. in this publication does not imply, even in the absence of a specific statement, that such names are exempt from the relevant protective laws and regulations and therefore free for general use.

Product liability: The publishers cannot guarantee the accuracy of any information about dosage and application contained in this book. In every individual case the user must check such information by consulting the relevant literature.

Cover design: eStudioCalamar, Figueres/Berlin

Printed on acid-free paper

Springer is part of Springer Science+Business Media (www.springer.com)

Foreword

Standard fracture texts, primarily aimed at surgeons who deal with both simple and complex fractures, have dealt with the anatomy, pathology, diagnostics, and occasionally with the complications of musculoskeletal injury, and primarily with the techniques of fracture repair. Clinical decision making in the management of the multiply injured patient, in the light of pregnancy, extremes of age, physiology, and the extremes of associated soft tissue injury, missing bone, and the anticipation and mitigation of associated complications is the true challenge in the treatment of musculoskeletal injury. These "associated" elements of the clinical decision making process are the most difficult to teach, the most dependent on clinical experience, and have rarely been centralized and addressed in a single source.

In this comprehensive text, experts in the fields of various systems pathology, inflammatory and immune response, pediatrics, and gerontology address these issues as they effect the ultimate management of musculoskeletal injury. In fact, with the centralization of trauma care in North America and Europe, the technical fixation of the individual injury is not the primary issue in most clinical scenarios. Trauma system centralization of such patients concentrates complex, high-energy, musculoskeletal injury, frequently within the framework of the polytraumatized patient and/or extremes of age, associated injury, and physiologic conditions in a single location; patients in whom the timing and subtlety of musculoskeletal management are more important than the specific technique used.

As trauma training of the musculoskeletal surgeon evolves, he/she may be the most senior clinician on the trauma team, and need a reference to validate the opinions of those co-managing the patient, or may have to provide more than just othopaedic judgment in the absence of a full team of clinical expertise.

This compilation of issues and discussion in this single source will serve as a reference for the musculoskeletal traumatologist, whether the basis of his/her clinical training be general or orthopaedic surgery, and whether their practice is entirely trauma or they give of their time outside of their primary clinical interest to cover the call burden of an active trauma hospital.

The sections on the costs and outcomes of these injuries to the lives of our patients and the society that shares the costs of those injuries is humbling to those of us who provide care, and remind us that a good outcome is more than a good X-ray.

Houston, TX, USA   Andrew R. Burgess

Preface

This book focuses on patients with difficult fracture situations, special injury combinations or other conditions that require interdisciplinary actions.

The idea behind this book was to provide complementary information to that available in most general orthopaedic or trauma text books. Most standard text books cover classifications of specific injuries and fractures, and provide specific information for the orthopaedic attending or the one working in general surgery. In clinical practice, many patients require close interactions between multiple services involved to treat these injuries. Moreover, certain special clinical situations can occur that are difficult to standardize, such as fractures in pregnancy, fractures in osteoporotic bone and certain head and facial injuries.

The selection of authors has been twofold. First, all of them are experts in their particular field. Second, the editors have sought to include experts from all over the world, hoping that even particular problems located in certain regions can be addressed. Finally, the selection of authors was designed to hopefully provide the most global view on particular problems possible. For example, infectious complications of the bone differ according to where they are being treated. Local injury patterns and regional genetic predispositions differ and can lead to specific infections assigned to certain countries. We do hope that this book covers the vast majority of special issues and adds to the current knowledge in interdisciplinary trauma care.

Hans-Christoph Pape
Aachen

Roy Sanders
Temple Terrace

Joseph Borrelli Jr.
Dallas

Contents

1 **The Impact of Trauma on Society** 1
   Farrah Naz Hussain and Mohit Bhandari

2 **Economic Aspects of Trauma Care** 5
   Maren Walgenbach, Carsten Mand, and Edmund A.M. Neugebauer

3 **Evidence-Based Orthopaedic Trauma Care** 11
   Matthew Denkers and Richard Buckley

4 **Local Inflammatory Changes Induced by Fractures
   and Soft Tissue Injuries** 19
   Takeshi Tsukamoto

5 **Pathophysiology of Polytrauma** 33
   Theodoros Tosounidis and Peter V. Giannoudis

6 **Head Injuries: Neurosurgical and Orthopaedic Strategies** 43
   Michael A. Flierl, Kathryn M. Beauchamp, and Philip F. Stahel

7 **Nerve Injuries in Traumatic Head Injury:
   When To Explore/Suture/Transplant?** 51
   Norbert Pallua and Ahmet Bozkurt

8 **Chest Trauma: Classification and Influence
   on the General Management** 75
   Philipp Mommsen, Christian Krettek, and Frank Hildebrand

9 **Abdominal Injuries: Indications for Surgery** 89
   Clay Cothren Burlew and Ernest E. Moore

10 **Management of Pelvic Ring Injuries** 103
   David J. Hak and Sean E. Nork

11 **Urological Injuries in Polytrauma** 115
   David Pfister and Axel Heidenreich

The Impact of Trauma on Society

Farrah Naz Hussain and Mohit Bhandari

Contents

1.1	Introduction	1
1.2	The Psychological Implications of Trauma	1
1.3	Chronic Pain and Disability Due to Trauma	2
1.4	Return to Work After Trauma	3
1.5	Conclusion	3
References		4

F.N. Hussain
Orthopaedic Research Unit, Department of Surgery,
McMaster University, 293 Wellington Street North,
Suite 110, Hamilton L8L 8E7, ON, Canada
e-mail: fhussain@med.wayne.edu

M. Bhandari (✉)
Division of Orthopaedic Surgery,
McMaster University, 293 Wellington Street North,
Suite 110, Hamilton L8L 8E7, ON, Canada
e-mail: bhandam@mcmaster.ca

1.1 Introduction

Injury has become a major cause of fatality and disability in countries of all economic levels [1]. Nearly 16,000 people die from injuries each day and for each of these fatalities, several thousand individuals survive with permanently disabling injuries [2]. In the United States, trauma-related costs, such as lost wages, medical expenses, insurance administration costs, property damage, and employer costs, exceed $400 billion annually [3]. Despite this massive financial burden, the real cost can only be ascertained when one considers that trauma affects the youngest and most productive members of society [3]. Studies have shown that the functional outcome of trauma patients at 1 year or more after the injury is below that of the normal population [4]. Many continue to suffer from residual problems such as long-term physical impairments, disabilities, and handicaps that may even impact their ability to fully return to their previous work or way of life [4]. A substantial number of individuals who have suffered orthopaedic trauma may also possess less obvious forms of residual disability, such as emotional or psychosocial disabilities [5]. Strengthening trauma services for patients who have sustained musculoskeletal injuries requires a multidisciplinary approach [6]. Therefore, knowledge about the impact of trauma on society is essential to adopting such an approach to orthopaedic trauma care.

1.2 The Psychological Implications of Trauma

Trauma is sudden and unexpected in nature and can be especially frightening for victims who may have lost their ability to comprehend and adapt to the unfamiliar situation around them [7]. The management of trauma therefore requires treatment not only of the immediate physical injuries, but also the behavioural and psychological aspects associated with the event that can severely impact patient recovery [7]. Patient psychological status after orthopaedic trauma is a common source of complaints from patients and is a clinically relevant outcome [8]. As outcomes research has shifted its focus from physician-derived measures (e.g., range of motion) towards patient-derived assessments of outcome, evidence of psychological distress as a consequence of orthopaedic trauma has come to light [9]. In fact, many studies have reported high rates of psychological distress after trauma along with its strong association with outcome [9]. Starr et al. [10] surveyed 580 patients who had sustained orthopaedic trauma using the Revised Civilian Mississippi Scale for Posttraumatic Stress Disorder questionnaire. The authors reported 51% of respondents met the criteria for diagnosis of posttraumatic stress disorder (PTSD) [10]. Moreover, patients with PTSD had significantly higher Injury Severity Scores (ISS) and Extremity Abbreviated Injury Scores (EAIS) [10]. Crichlow et al. [11] interviewed 161 orthopaedic trauma patients and found that the presence of clinically relevant depression was 45%, as determined by the Beck Depression Inventory (BDIA). The authors also demonstrated a close correlation between the presence of depression and poorer scores on functional outcome measures, such as the Short Musculoskeletal Function Assessment (SMFA) [11].

Not only do psychological problems, such as PTSD and depression, pose an impact on functional outcomes, they also pose an effect on quality of life (QOL) [12]. Measures of QOL provide insight into how a disability may affect an individual's overall well-being, such as their goals, concerns, standards and expectations [12]. In an observational study investigating the extent of psychological symptoms of 215 patients following orthopaedic trauma, Bhandari et al. [8] reported that one in five met the threshold for psychological distress in all primary dimensions of the SCL-90-R. In particular, phobic anxiety and somatization (i.e., the expression of physical symptoms as a result of emotional or psychological distress) ranked high in comparison to age- and sex-matched population control subjects [8]. In terms of the relationship between psychological problems and patients' health-related quality of life, the authors found that the global severity of psychological symptoms were significantly associated with the Physical Component and Mental Component summary scores of the Medical Outcomes Study 36-item Short Form (SF-36) [8].

Although few other studies in the orthopaedic trauma literature have considered the impact of psychological distress on later QOL, studies involving patients with other injuries have come to similar conclusions concerning this relationship. O'Donnell et al. [12] examined the 12-month outcomes of 363 consecutive admissions to a Level I trauma service and found that an individual's acute psychological response (e.g., anxiety and depression) directly predicted QOL, as measured by the WHOQoL-Bref, as well as level of disability. More specifically, anxiety and depression was associated with PTSD, which in turn was associated with lower levels of QOL and functioning [12]. From this growing body of research, it is evident that the patient's psychological state is as important as injury severity and physical health to injury recovery and long-term outcomes [12]. For a complete discussion of PTSD and psychological sequelae after severe trauma, please see Chap. 28.

1.3 Chronic Pain and Disability Due to Trauma

Chronic or ongoing pain includes several symptoms and conditions, including acute post-trauma pain, depression, hostility, anxiety, sleep and rest disturbances [13, 14]. Many trauma patients suffer from long-term impairments, disabilities and handicaps, and at least half of all major trauma patients are left with one or more residual problems [4]. Therefore, knowledge about determinants of long-term functional consequences after trauma is important in order to improve the chances of a patient's recovery [4]. Trauma has been proposed as a causal factor or trigger of chronic or persistent pain [13]. Chronic pain affects as many as 50 million Americans and is one of the leading causes of disability among those under the age of 45 [13]. The overall productivity lost due to chronic pain is estimated to be four times more than productivity lost due to lost work days alone [13, 15]. In a prospective analysis of the prevalence and early predictors of chronic pain in a cohort of severe lower extremity trauma patients, Castillo et al. [13] found that more than a quarter of the study group reported that their pain highly interfered with daily activities. Pain also has other consequences for its victims, including psychological regression [14]. Those who suffer from chronic pain also use five times more health services than the general population [13, 16].

As surgeons, we know that pain is an inevitable result of traumatic injury and the accompanying healing process. However, why do patients continue to endure pain long after they have been treated? The biomedical model of health focuses on pain as the result of a physical injury [17]. This makes it difficult to clinically explain the presence of disability after the pathology related to the injury has healed [17]. Studies focusing on trauma populations suggest that factors during the course of recovery other than the injury are critical to the development of persistent pain and associated functional impairment [17]. Such factors include high initial pain intensity, PTSD, worker's compensation status, education, low recovery expectations and depression [17]. In the aforementioned study by Castillo et al. [13], several early predictors of chronic pain, including having less than a high school education, having less than a college education, low self-efficacy for return to daily activities, and high levels of alcohol consumption at baseline were identified. In addition, high reported acute pain intensity, sleep and rest dysfunction, depression and anxiety at 3 months post-discharge were found to be predictors of chronic pain at 7 years [13].

1.4 Return to Work After Trauma

Return to work is defined as a complete or almost complete return to pre-injury full-time paid employment [18]. While traumatic injury often results in psychological distress and chronic pain for its victims, another burden it poses to society is the long-term impairment of its most productive members and a subsequent loss of working days [19]. Survivors of severe injury are able to achieve a QOL comparable to the normal population once they have returned to their pre-injury occupation [20, 21]. Because it increases an individual's sense of self-worth and personal fulfilment, return to work is indicative of successful social reintegration after major trauma [18]. Return to work is therefore one of the most important methods by which to evaluate treatment outcomes [14, 19]. In the United States, more days are lost to work as a result of chronic pain than any other medical reason [13]. Road traffic injuries in particular are a major cause of trauma and have resulted in greater than 1 million deaths and 50 million injuries worldwide [22]. In 2001, 2.1 million people aged 18–65 were victims of car crashes in the United States [23]. Cumulatively, victims of these crashes lost an estimated 60.8 million days of work [23].

To realize the impact of trauma on society, it is important to consider the factors contributing to lost productivity among survivors of injury [14, 19]. Factors contributing to a delayed return to work include injury severity, pre-injury characteristics of the patient (i.e., socioeconomic status, self-efficacy, health habits, social support with respect to the home and workplace), characteristics of the pre-injury occupation (i.e., white- versus blue-collar work, physical demands, tenure, job satisfaction and flexibility), motivation to work, receipt of disability compensation, and baseline measures of physical functioning, pain, anxiety and depression [14, 17, 19]. Patients are especially delayed from returning to work if they have significant physical disabilities, psychosocial impairments, cognitive impairments or changes to their personality [18]. Recovery times can be lengthy, even taking longer than a year in certain cases [18]. Patients may also be unable to return to their pre-injury job due to the replacement of their previous roles [18]. These factors can render a return to pre-injury work status challenging for many victims of trauma and can therefore pose a significant financial and social burden to victims as well as their families [17].

1.5 Conclusion

Although much of this chapter focused on trauma victims themselves as members of society, a final thought to consider is the impact of trauma on the families of victims. Having someone close become seriously injured can be an immense source of psychological stress for family members [7]. Many may exhibit the behaviour of 'hovering', which is defined as an initial sense of confusion, distress and uncertainty prior to seeing the patient and understanding the diagnosis and prognosis [7, 24]. It can also be difficult for relatives to cope with their sudden change in role and status in the life of a loved one experiencing trauma [7]. Feelings of isolation from other family members, financial constraints and transportation concerns may also surface. Such problems are only amplified by a lack of medical knowledge [7]. Hence, comprehensive trauma services should consider providing support to family members alongside severely damaged patients.

Provision of comprehensive care of trauma patients is essential. While experiencing trauma, patients become lost in an unfamiliar and threatening situation. Many become dependent, losing control over their environment and personal well-being. During the injury, treatment and recovery procedures, and for years afterward, patients can experience immense psychological and emotional distress, chronic pain and resultant productivity loss. Although trauma can happen to anyone, its tendency to affect individuals during their youngest and most productive years poses a significant impact on society [3]. Therefore, knowledge about this impact is imperative to adopting an interdisciplinary approach to orthopaedic trauma care.

References

1. Mock C, Quansah R, Krishnan R. Strengthening the prevention and care of injuries worldwide. Lancet. 2004;363:2172–9.
2. Krug EG, Sharma GK, Lozano R. The global burden of injuries. Am J Public Health. 2000;90:523–6.
3. American College of Surgeons. The need. In: Advanced trauma life support. 7th ed. Chicago: American College of Surgeons. 2004.
4. Holtslag HR, van Beeck EF, Lindeman E, et al. Determinants of long-term functional consequences after major trauma. J Trauma. 2007;62:919–27.
5. Pensford J, Hill B, Karamitsios M, et al. Factors influencing outcome after orthopedic trauma. J Trauma. 2008;64:1001–9.
6. Spiegel DA, Gosselin RA, Coughlin RR, et al. Topics in global public health. Clin Orthop Relat Res. 2008;466:2377–84.
7. Mohta M, Sethi AK, Tyagi A, et al. Psychological care in trauma patients. Injury: Int J Care Injured. 2003;34:17–25.
8. Bhandari M, Busse JW, Hanson BP, et al. Psychological distress and quality of life after orthopedic trauma: an observational study. Can J Surg. 2008;51:15–22.
9. Starr AJ. Fracture repair: successful advances, persistent problems, and the psychological burden of trauma. J Bone Joint Surg Am. 2008;90:132–7.
10. Starr AJ, Smith WR, Frawley WH, et al. Symptoms of post-traumatic stress disorder after orthopaedic trauma. J Bone Joint Surg Am. 2004;86:1115–21.
11. Crichlow RJ, Andres PL, Morrison SM, et al. Depression in orthopaedic trauma patients. Prevalence and severity. J Bone Joint Surg Am. 2006;88:1927–33.
12. O'Donnell ML, Creamer M, Elliot P, et al. Determinants of quality of life and role-related disability after injury: impact of acute psychological responses. J Trauma. 2005;59:1328–35.
13. Castillo RC, MacKenzie EJ, Wegener ST, et al. Prevalence of chronic pain seven years following limb threatening lower extremity trauma. Pain. 2006;124:321–9.
14. MacKenzie EJ, Morris JA, Jurkovich GJ, et al. Return to work following injury: the role of economic, social, and job-related factors. Am J Public Health. 1998;88:1630–7.
15. Blyth FM, March LM, Nicholas MK, et al. Chronic pain, work performance and litigation. Pain. 2003;103:41–7.
16. von Korff M, Dworkin SF, Le Resche L. Graded chronic pain status: an epidemiologic evaluation. Pain. 1990;40:279–91.
17. Clay FJ, Newstead SV, Watson WL, et al. Bio-psychosocial determinants of persistent pain 6 months after non-life-threatening acute orthopaedic trauma. J Pain. 2010;11:420–30.
18. Holtslag HR, Post MW, van der Werken C, et al. Return to work after major trauma. Clin Rehabil. 2007;21:373–83.
19. MacKenzie EJ, Bosse MJ, Kellam JF, et al. Early predictors of long-term work disability after major limb trauma. J Trauma. 2006;61:688–94.
20. Hou W, Tsauo J, Lin C, et al. Worker's compensation and return-to-work following orthopaedic injury to extremities. J Rehabil Med. 2008;40:440–5.
21. Post RB, Sluis VD, Duis HJT. Return to work and quality of life in severely injured patients. Disabil Rehabil. 2006;28:1399–404.
22. Sharma BR. Road traffic injuries: a major global public health crisis. Public Health. 2008;122:1399–406.
23. Ebel BE, Mack C, Diehr P, et al. Lost working days, productivity, and restraint use among occupants of motor vehicles that crashed in the United States. Inj Prev. 2004;10:314–9.
24. Jamerson PA, Scheibmeir M, Bott MJ, et al. The experiences of families with a relative in the intensive care unit. Heart Lung. 1996;25:467–74.

Economic Aspects of Trauma Care

Maren Walgenbach, Carsten Mand, and Edmund A.M. Neugebauer

Contents

2.1	Introduction	5
2.2	Economic Concepts	5
2.2.1	Cost-Minimization Analysis (CMA)	6
2.2.2	Cost-Effectiveness Analysis (CEA)	6
2.2.3	Cost-Benefit Analysis (CBA)	7
2.2.4	Cost-Utility Analysis (CUA)	7
2.2.5	Cost of Illness (COI)	7
2.3	Direct and Indirect Cost of Illness	7
2.4	Road Traffic Accidents	7
2.5	Prevention	8
2.5.1	Polytrauma	8
2.5.2	Osteoporosis	8
2.6	DALY and QALY	9
References		9

M. Walgenbach and E.A.M. Neugebauer (✉)
Institute for Research in Operative Medicine (IFOM),
Private University Witten/Herdecke gGmbH,
Ostmerheimer Str. 200, 51109 Köln, Germany
e-mail: maren.walgenbach@uni-wh.de;
ifom-neugebauer-sek@uni-wh.de,
edmund.neugebauer@uni-wh.de

C. Mand
Department of Trauma, Hand and Reconstructive Surgery,
University Hospital Giessen and Marburg GmbH, Location
Marburg, Baldingerstraße, D-35043 Marburg, Germany
e-mail: mand@med.uni-marburg.de

2.1 Introduction

Trauma and injury play a major role in today's health care. The fact that over 1.2 million people die each year in road traffic accidents alone and between 20 and 50 million are injured [1] by trauma is a major health-care issue and also an important cost factor for most societies. According to the World Health Organization (WHO), trauma and injury account for 9.2% of all deaths worldwide and 10.9% of disability-adjusted life-years (DALYs – see below). Over the last few decades, the understanding of injury has gone from being regarded as random and unpredictable accidents to being seen as possibly preventable events. The WHO estimates that in the year 2020, road traffic accidents will climb to rank 6th among the 15 leading causes of death, and 3rd in causes of DALYs lost [2].

In trauma it is important not only to consider immediate consequences such as mortality, but also to take into account that for every death there are many survivors who are left with permanently disabling injuries. Another special feature of trauma care is that injuries most often affect the working populace (see Fig. 2.1) so that death or disability decreases work and spending capacities.

2.2 Economic Concepts

It is simple to present mortality and morbidity statistics of health-care systems, but it is important for societies to consider the costs and values. Economic evaluation is required for good decision making in health-care systems, in order to choose medical alternatives with both reduced costs and a higher health benefit. The aim of economic evaluation is to calculate

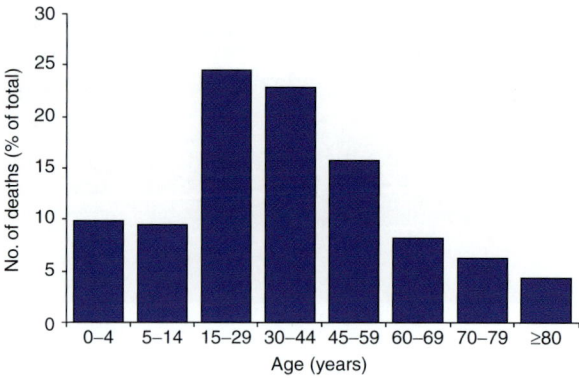

Fig. 2.1 Age distribution of global injury-related mortality, 2000 (WHO – The Injury Chart Book)

the resource costs consumed versus the health benefits provided by the practice or technology in its diverse clinical uses [3].

There are a variety of cost analysis strategies, the appropriateness of which depends upon the purpose of an assessment, as well as the availability of data and other resources. There are also different types of costs and measurements in money terms, which are similar across most efficiency evaluations [4] (see Table 2.1). More difficult is the identification and quantification of all benefits and units, which may differ between evaluations. For example, in some evaluations the value cannot be measured in monetary units and are instead expressed in different units. The main types of cost analysis are discussed below.

2.2.1 Cost-Minimization Analysis (CMA)

Cost-minimization analysis does not consider value, and this is the structural weakness of this method. A CMA calculates the least cost of alternative technologies or interventions while assuming an equal health benefit among them. Therefore, the difference between alternatives is reduced to a comparison of costs in order to estimate the treatment with the lowest cost, which is the treatment of choice [5].

In practice, it is unlikely that two different alternatives will incur the same consequences. Medical or therapeutically alternatives often differ in the number or significance of adverse effects. If the outcomes are identical, often there is no difference between the techniques.

Some authors (e.g., Drummond et al. [6]) argue that the CMA is not a complete form of economic evaluation and is only useful as an alternative for decision making [4, 5] when comparing two drugs of equal efficacy (e.g., with the same active ingredient) and equal tolerability.

2.2.2 Cost-Effectiveness Analysis (CEA)

A cost-effectiveness analysis is a more complete form of economic evaluation, in which both the costs and consequences of the alternatives being compared are examined [4]. Costs are expressed in monetary units and value in natural units, so that costs are presented per unit of effect. The effect may be years of life gained, rescued human life, reduction in prevalence, reduced duration of disease, working days gained, and also other clinical parameters such as blood pressure or cholesterol level.

Values differ for different types of issues. This is why a CEA can describe two different effects and

Table 2.1 Measurement of costs and consequences in economic evaluation

Type of study	Measurement/valuation of costs in both alternatives	Identification of consequences	Measurement/valuation of consequences
Cost analysis	Monetary units	None	None
Cost-effectiveness analysis	Monetary units	Single effect of interest, common to both alternatives, but achieved to different degrees	Natural units (e.g., life-years gained, disability-days saved, points of blood pressure reduction, etc.)
Cost-utility analysis	Monetary units	Single or multiple effects, not necessarily common to both alternatives	Healthy years (typically measured as quality-adjusted life-years)
Cost-benefit analysis	Monetary units	Single or multiple effects, not necessarily common to both alternatives	Monetary units

Source: Methods for the Economic Evaluation of Health Care Programmes

decisions. Although the chosen alternatives are similar, one effect might be measured in terms of life-years gained and the other in gained workdays. Depending on the focus, analysis of these effects may result in two different alternatives.

2.2.3 Cost-Benefit Analysis (CBA)

The cost-benefit analysis measures costs and benefits in common monetary units. The alternative to the medical or therapeutic treatment being evaluated is a do-nothing alternative entailing no costs and no benefits.

Only in cases in which the benefit is at least similar to the costs leads to an economical result and the decision in favor of the new medical or therapeutic treatment.

The challenge of this analysis is estimating an appropriate amount of money for the do-nothing alternative.

2.2.4 Cost-Utility Analysis (CUA)

A cost-utility analysis focuses on the quality of health, measures costs in monetary terms and, like the CEA, measures utility in non-monetary terms. It is different from CEA in that CEA utilizes a natural or direct measurement. The CUA measures its outcomes in terms of their utility, quality-adjusted life-years (QALYs), disability-adjusted life-years (DALYs), or a specific level of health status. This can be measured in terms of individuals or society. The results are expressed as cost per QALY gained. A CEA can only compare technologies whose outcomes are measured in the same units.

Utility is expressed on a 0–1 scale, in which 0 means death and 1 means entirely healthy. There are many questionnaires and rating scales designed to measure the health related quality of life (hrqol), which is needed in order to estimate the QALY (see Sect. 2.6).

2.2.5 Cost of Illness (COI)

This economic evaluation considers all costs of an individual disease with two approaches: prevalence cost or incidence cost.

While COI does not take different alternatives into account, this evaluation should help to estimate the burden on a social system incurred by a specific disease, and distribute resources for preventing associated treatment costs (e.g., medication to prevent osteoporosis) [6].

2.3 Direct and Indirect Cost of Illness

Every injury results in direct and indirect health-care costs. Direct costs include the immediate costs that follow an injury, such as hospital treatment, medications, prostheses, rehabilitation, and all consequential treatment and nursing costs (e.g., home care, outpatient care, and visits to health professionals). Indirect costs consist of each individual's lost productivity and ability to work, and are therefore losses in societal productivity. Other factors that potentially add to indirect costs include social isolation, economic dependence, pain, and suffering. The latter are almost impossible to quantify, but should be considered nonetheless in the calculation of indirect costs rather than underestimating the real expenses. Because trauma and injury mainly affect the working populace, indirect costs play an important role and may equal the direct costs.

Example Canada: Total direct costs from injuries in Canada in the year 2004 amounted to $10,716 million and indirect costs were $9,065 million [7]. According to the 1998 publication *The Economic Burden of Illness in Canada*, the indirect mortality cost due to injuries ranked 3rd after cancer and cardiovascular diseases, and as shown in Fig. 2.2, adults aged 15–64 years of age accounted for 91.6% of the costs [8].

2.4 Road Traffic Accidents

In 2009, the Commission for Global Road Safety from the World Health Organization issued a call for a Decade of Action for Road Safety. Nearly 90% of deaths after road traffic accidents occur in low- and middle-income countries where less than half of the world's motor vehicles are registered. Among young people (aged 5–44 years), road traffic accidents are one of the three leading causes for death, and it has been predicted that unless immediate action is taken road traffic accidents will become the fifth leading cause of death for all ages. Especially due to young

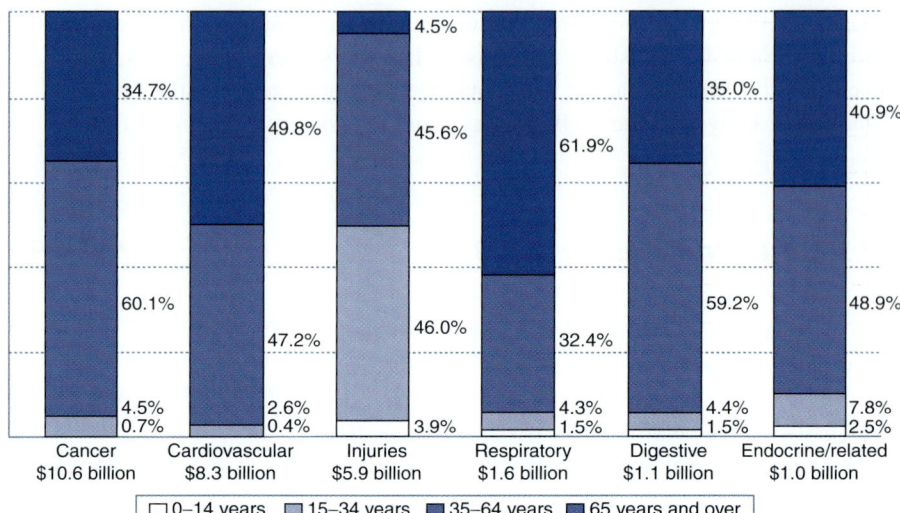

Fig. 2.2 Mortality costs by most costly diagnostic categories and age group in Canada, 1998 (*The Economic Burden of Illness in Canada*, 1998)

people dying in road traffic accidents, the economic consequences are enormous and estimates range from 1% to 3% of a country's Gross National Product (GNP), or in total about $500 billion a year.

2.5 Prevention

Injuries fall into one of two main categories:

1. Intentional injuries such as self-inflicted injuries (e.g., suicide), acts of violence, and war-related injuries
2. Unintentional injuries that including but not limited to road traffic accidents, poisoning, falls, fires, and drowning

Unintentional injuries are very responsive to prevention, and some governments have not only recognized injury as a major threat to human health and their health-care system, but have specifically founded institutions for injury prevention (e.g., the United States National Center for Injury Prevention and Control). It has also been suggested that higher income countries should turn their focus to injury prevention rather than the marginal improvement of initial trauma care, as more than half of deaths caused by unintentional injuries might be preventable with pre-injury behavioral changes [9]. Road-safety interventions (e.g., seat belts) used and established in high-income countries can be successfully translated to low- and middle-income countries where road traffic mortality and morbidity is constantly rising [10].

2.5.1 Polytrauma

As the most severely injured subgroup of trauma patients with injuries to more than one body region of which at least one or more in combination is life-threatening, polytrauma patients require complex and multidisciplinary management and still have a significantly higher mortality and morbidity than other trauma patients. The costs for this care and the provision of personnel and materials are immense, and reimbursement to hospitals among different health systems, primarily due to lack of data for an accurate cost estimation, shows a negative balance of 80–900% [11]. In the Federal Republic of Germany, a model to calculate the actual costs that a severely injured patient produces has been presented based on data derived from the national trauma registry (TraumaRegister DGU – TR-DGU). Currently a nation-wide Trauma Network is forming, and hopefully due to mandatory participation in the TR-DGU, the network will soon encompass all severely injured patients and a more correct estimation of the actual costs due to trauma will be possible [12].

2.5.2 Osteoporosis

With medical care improving people have longer life expectancies and consequently higher risk of osteoporosis. Though osteoporosis affects one-third of post-menopausal women and one-fifth of men over the age

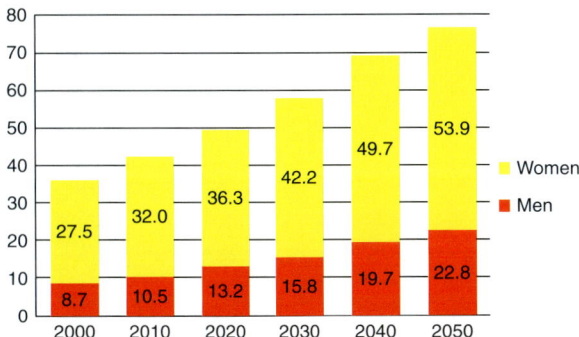

Fig. 2.3 Projected costs of osteoporosis in Europe in billion euros (Osteoporosis in Europe: Indicators of Progress)

of 50, its relevance for health-care systems is widely underestimated. Often the first symptom is a fracture after an inadequate trauma, and once a fracture has occurred, the risk of a second fracture is doubled within the year. The projected costs of osteoporosis in Europe can be seen in Fig. 2.3.

The acute hospital costs (as a part of the direct costs) of a hip fracture in Europe range from €1,000 in Estonia to €30,000 in Austria, and data suggest that total costs following a hip fracture could be 2.5 times greater. Medical treatment of established osteoporosis has proven to be cost-effective irrespective of age. However, a major problem of this "silent epidemic" is poor compliance with drug therapies that effectively reduce the risk of fractures, and thereby also reduce the overall costs and QALYs (see below) lost.

2.6 DALY and QALY

A QALY is not a measure of lost utility, but of one lost year of healthy life. DALYs are calculated by adding a society's years of life lost due to premature mortality (YLL) in the population and years of life lost due to disability (YLD) for incident cases of the health condition [13]. The latter is estimated by multiplying the number of incident cases in a given period by the average duration of the disease and a weight factor that reflects the severity of the disease. The number of deaths at each age multiplied by a global standard life expectancy for the age at which death occurs is the YLL. While DALYs include death, injury, and physical disability, they are limited in that they do not include all the health consequences (e.g., mental health) and the economic consequences stemming from a health condition.

References

1. Anonymous. Global status report on road safety: time for action. In: World Health Organization, Geneva. 2009. http://www.who.int/violence_injury_prevention/road_safety_status/2009.
2. Peden M, Mcgee K, Sharma G. The injury chart book: a graphical overview of the global burden of injuries. Geneva: World Health Organization; 2002.
3. Weinstein MC. Economic assessments of medical practices and technologies. Med Decis Making. 1981;1:309–30.
4. Drummond MF, Sculpher MJ, Torrance GW, et al. Methods for the economic evaluation of health care programmes. Oxford/New York: Oxford University Press; 2005.
5. Briggs AH, O'brien BJ. The death of cost-minimization analysis? Health Econ. 2001;10:179–84.
6. Drummond M. Cost-of-illness studies: a major headache? Pharmacoeconomics. 1992;2:1–4.
7. SMARTRISK. The economic burden of injury in Canada. 2009.
8. Anonymous. The economic burden of illness in Canada. 1998. http://www.hc-sc.gc.ca.
9. Stewart RM, Myers JG, Dent DL, et al. Seven hundred fifty-three consecutive deaths in a level I trauma center: the argument for injury prevention. J Trauma. 2003;54:66–70; discussion 70–61.
10. Stevenson M, Yu J, Hendrie D, et al. Reducing the burden of road traffic injury: translating high-income country interventions to middle-income and low-income countries. Inj Prev. 2008;14:284–9.
11. Giannoudis PV, Kanakaris NK. The unresolved issue of health economics and polytrauma: the UK perspective. Injury. 2008;39:705–9.
12. Pape HC, Grotz M, Schwermann T, et al. The development of a model to calculate the cost of care for the severely injured – an initiative of the Trauma Register of the DGU. Unfallchirurg. 2003;106:348–57.
13. Anonymous. The global burden of disease. In: World Health Organization, Geneva. Update 2004. http://www.who.int/healthinfo/global_burden_disease/GBD_report_2004update_full.pdf.

Evidence-Based Orthopaedic Trauma Care

Matthew Denkers and Richard Buckley

Contents

3.1	Origins	11
3.2	Present State	12
3.3	Evidence-Based Approach	12
3.3.1	Ask	13
3.3.2	Acquire	13
3.3.3	Appraise	13
3.3.4	Apply	14
3.3.5	Act	14
3.4	Challenges	14
3.5	Future Directions	15
3.6	Canadian Orthopaedic Trauma Society	15
3.6.1	Origins	15
3.6.2	Formalization and Funding	16
3.6.3	Commitment	16
3.6.4	Research Coordinators	16
3.6.5	Biannual Meetings	17
3.6.6	Success	18
3.7	Conclusion	18
References		18

M. Denkers
Division of Orthopaedic Surgery, Hamilton
Health Sciences, General Site – McMaster Clinic,
McMaster University, 704-237 Barton Street East,
Hamilton, ON L8L 2X2, Canada
e-mail: mattdenkers@hotmail.com

R. Buckley (✉)
Division of Orthopaedic Surgery, Foothills
Medical Centre, University of Calgary, AC 144A,
1403-29 Street NW, Calgary, AB T2N 2T9, Canada
e-mail: buckclin@ucalgary.ca

3.1 Origins

We become confident in our educated guesswork to the point where it is easy to confuse personal opinion with evidence, or personal ignorance with genuine scientific uncertainty. (Naylor [1])

Prior to existing in the orthopaedic or surgical realm, the development of evidence-based philosophy was initiated in medicine. While it would be disingenuous to contend that the inception of evidence-based medicine occurred in its entirety at any discrete time, two key points are widely recognized as holding significant importance. In 1967, Professor David L. Sackett founded Canada's first department of clinical epidemiology at McMaster University and developed the "Hierarchy of Evidence" (Fig. 3.1). In essence, this step placed greater value and emphasis on research

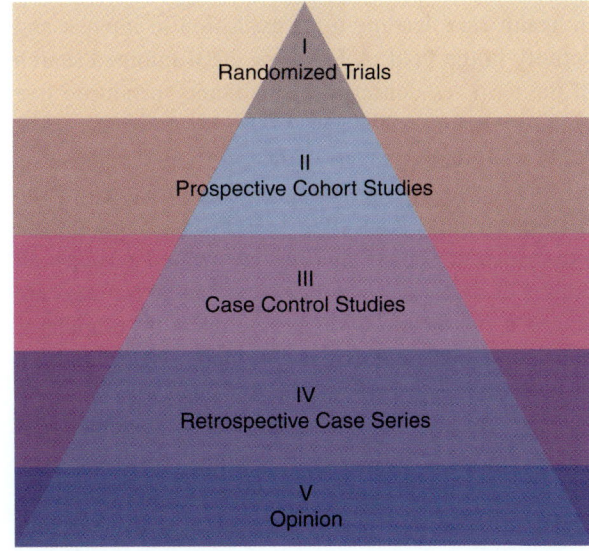

Fig. 3.1 Hierarchy of evidence

H.-C. Pape et al. (eds.), *The Poly-Traumatized Patient with Fractures*,
DOI: 10.1007/978-3-642-17986-0_3, © Springer-Verlag Berlin Heidelberg 2011

that limits bias and confounding variables through elements of study design and methodology. This model formed the foundation of evidence-based philosophy and remains one of its pillars today [2, 3].

Years later in 1990, Professor Gordon Guyatt coined the term "evidence-based medicine" (EBM) in a document for applicants to the internal medicine residency program at McMaster University. A year later, he introduced the term to the academic literature and it was defined as "an attitude of 'enlightened skepticism' towards the application of diagnostic, therapeutic, and prognostic technologies" [4]. Moving forward, the definition of EBM evolved to "the conscientious, explicit, and judicious use of the current best evidence in making decisions about the care of individual patients. The practice of evidence-based medicine means integrating individual clinical expertise with the best available external clinical evidence from systematic research" [5, 6]. From its outset, EBM sought not to blindly substitute the results of studies and trials for the accumulated expertise of the profession, but rather to offer evidence as an instrument to be wielded by those same experienced practitioners to augment and further the clinical decision-making in providing individualized care to patients.

3.2 Present State

The inherent value of EBM was recognized by many in health care, leading to an explosion in interest and activity in the field. A February 2010 Pubmed search of the term "evidence-based medicine" produced five citations before 1993 and 39,093 to date. Recently, EBM was honored as one of the top 15 medical discoveries in the past 166 years in a survey produced by the *British Medical Journal* [7]. EBM has become an axiom of our society and has permeated through all realms of medicine including orthopaedic trauma care where it has been effectively adopted by clinicians, educators, and researchers as their own paradigm "Evidence-Based Orthopaedics" [8, 9].

Many in the field have primarily attributed the advancement of orthopaedic surgery over the past decade to a more substantial emphasis on evidence-based practice in clinical decision-making. As well, many orthopaedic journals now focus on the quality of study design by assigning levels of evidence to the articles published and encouraging the pursuit of higher-level studies by their authors. Now, the question at hand has shifted from whether to implement the concepts and principles of evidence-based practice to that of determining the best and most efficient way in which to do so [8].

3.3 Evidence-Based Approach

Just as with the traditional paradigm of health care, an evidence-based approach values clinical experience. However, this experience is not valued solely for its inference of clinical acumen, but also for its ability to guide the identification of learning needs, formulation of appropriate questions, identification of relevant research, appraisal of that research, and the application of those results to clinical policy and subsequently individual patients' circumstances and needs [8, 10]. As evidence-based skills have been refined over time, an approach has been produced that allows a clear and concise framework from which to work [2, 10–12]. This approach has come to be known as the "Evidence Cycle" and consists of the five As (Fig. 3.2):

- Ask (formulate a clearly delineated and relevant clinical question)
- Acquire (conduct a comprehensive and efficient literature search)
- Appraise (critically appraise the available evidence)

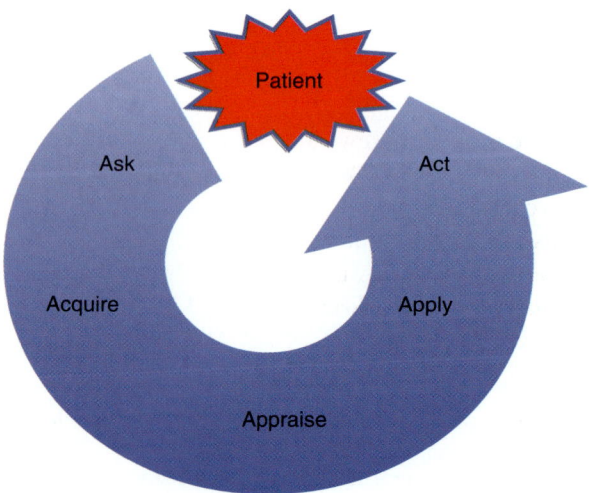

Fig. 3.2 Evidence cycle

- Apply (determine applicability of best evidence to the clinical situation)
- Act (using clinical expertise to integrate the best available research evidence with the clinical circumstance and the patients' values)

3.3.1 Ask

A prudent question is one-half of wisdom. (Francis Bacon [1561–1626])

If you want a wise answer, ask a reasonable question. (Johann Wolfgang Von Goethe [1749–1832])

In order to obtain a relevant answer, it is necessary to begin with an appropriate question. Conceptually, as health-care practitioners we ask two types of questions – background and foreground [2]. When the objective of the question is to gain an understanding of a condition's pathophysiology, epidemiology, and general treatment options, background questions are asked. Once practitioners have a thorough understanding of the background information, they should then begin to ask foreground questions, the answers to which will direct them in the management of specific aspects of patient care. Whereas background questions have the potential to lead to a broad spectrum of answers, foreground questions narrow down the possible answers and directly impact clinical decision-making [2, 13]. This is accomplished by clearly delineating a relevant question and to this end, the PICO approach is useful [2, 8, 11, 14]:

- *Population*
- *Intervention*
- *Comparison*
- *Outcomes*

So, the question "How should femoral shaft fractures be treated?" could be developed through the PICO approach to become, "In middle-aged adults with a midshaft femoral fracture (*Population*) does reamed (*Intervention*) versus unreamed intramedullary femoral nailing (*Comparison*) reduce the risk of nonunion (*Outcome*)?"

3.3.2 Acquire

The ability to thoroughly and efficiently search for literature pertaining to the question is necessary to make well-informed clinical decisions. Armed with a skillfully constructed question required to conduct a focused and successful literature search, the practitioner must now decide where to look. There are presently numerous electronic databases with powerful search engines necessary to deal with the ever-expanding volume of studies and trials. Pubmed (www.pubmed.gov) and Google Scholar (www.scholar.google.com) are two quality and free search engines. As well, most academic institutions and many professional organizations have made available medical librarian services that can greatly increase in the ease and efficiency of searching the literature.

Conceptually, evidence sources can be considered to fall into one of the following groups:

- Preappraised: abstracts or guidelines
- Summarized: systematic reviews or meta-analysis
- Primary studies: individual studies [8]

Preappraised sources may be useful to busy practicing clinicians interested in guidelines that are usually the product of local or regional professional associations. These recommendations are the result of consensus meetings and although not all guidelines are evidence based, most are based on systematic reviews or randomized trials. Guidelines should demonstrate diligence by assigning levels of recommendation based on the quality of the founding evidence. It is often valuable then to review the founding studies identified in order to appraise it personally. Summarized sources in the form of systematic reviews or meta-analyses are also valuable in addressing specific questions. When summarized evidence is not available, clinicians may then turn to a search of primary studies. Those conducting a systematic review will also need to perform searches casting a broader net intended to capture all of the relevant primary studies addressing the subject.

3.3.3 Appraise

An evidence-based approach to a clinician's practice relies on an awareness of the evidence upon which the practice is based as well as the strength of inference and the degree of certainty permitted by that evidence [12]. A critical appraisal of the available evidence determines its significance and applicability to the clinical situation in question. Assigning levels of evidence can be a rapid approach to evaluating study quality, by determining the following:

- Primary question of the study
- Study type (therapeutic, prognostic, diagnostic, economic, or decision analysis)
- Level of evidence I–IV [15]

When assigning levels of evidence, greater agreement exists between reviewers trained in epidemiology; however, those without training still demonstrate high levels of agreement [16]. Studies that limit bias to greater extents are assigned higher levels of evidence. Caveats exist in that a poor quality study with methodological limitations is downgraded a level (e.g., A randomized controlled trial with less than 80% follow-up is downgraded from level 1 to level 2). To meet specific needs, gradation schemes founded on the original levels of evidence have been created. The GRADE System is an example of a thorough and validated model being widely adopted as a standard [17].

3.3.4 Apply

> Good doctors use both individual clinical expertise and the best available external evidence, and neither alone is enough. Without clinical expertise, practice risks becoming tyrannized by evidence, for even excellent external evidence may be inapplicable to or inappropriate for an individual patient. (Sackett [6])

For conceptual purposes, evidence-based practice has been refined to the *conscientious* use of *current best evidence* in making *health-care decisions* given the *clinical circumstances*. Implicit in this are the following components (Fig. 3.3):

- *Conscientious* – requires clinical expertise
- *Current best evidence* – hierarchy of evidence
- *Health-care decisions* – patient values
- *Clinical circumstances* – factors pertinent to the situation [8]

In essence, clinical judgment must be exercised in deciding how to apply the evidence in a balanced fashion to individual patients given their circumstances and preferences.

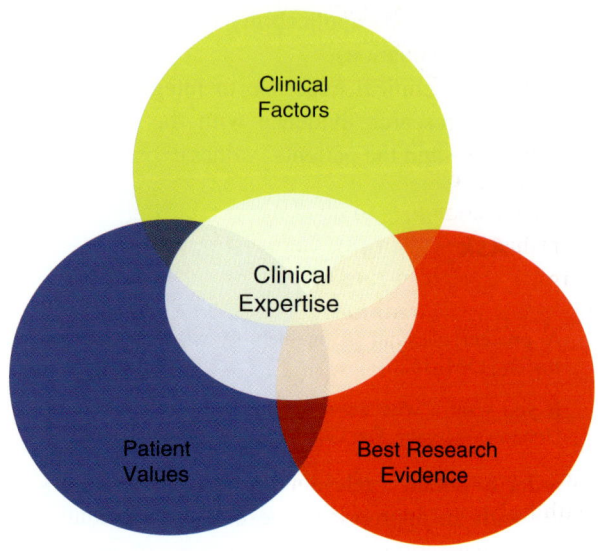

Fig. 3.3 Model of evidence-based practice

3.3.5 Act

In actuality, the evidence cycle begins and ends with the patient. A patient issue induces a question thereby initiating the cycle that concludes with acting on that patient issue.

3.4 Challenges

Many misconceptions of evidence-based practice exist. Detractors have mistakenly contended evidence-based practice equates evidence with results from randomized clinical trials, statistical significance with clinical relevance, evidence with decisions, and lack of evidence of efficacy with evidence for the lack of efficacy [8, 9, 18]. As described above, evidence-based practice is not the blind transference of study results into clinical applications, but an integration of the results from best evidence with the clinical circumstances and patient values as guided by clinical expertise.

Another challenge resides in the vast and expanding amount of literature and publications available with >3,800 biomedical journals present in Medline and >7,300 citations of varying quality added weekly. As evidence-based practice relies upon awareness and a subsequent critical appraisal of the available evidence, this can be a daunting task.

Surgery lags behind medicine in embracing and employing evidence-based practice in part because of some inherent challenges specific to surgery. There are a lack of advanced trained evidence-based practitioners leading to a limitation in role-modeling and the mentorship of colleagues and trainees. As increased emphasis continues to be placed here, some improvement has been seen [8]. Challenges also exist during surgical training where demands on trainees' time are high and the traditional pedagogical infrastructure does not always lend itself to adopting evidence-based philosophy. Strategies to correct this include hiring staff surgeons with training in evidence-based practice, instituting critical appraisal as part of the curriculum, and maximizing interdepartmental communication with research and epidemiology colleagues [19].

3.5 Future Directions

It is recognized that many questions related to orthopaedic trauma surgery will never be subjected to randomized clinical trials because of the rarity of the condition or unique ethical or logistical limitations of the clinical circumstances. Most of these situations, though, can be addressed with level 2 and 3 studies with acceptance as the highest level of available evidence. However, historically, the majority of orthopaedic literature on most conditions has been in the form of nondefinitive case series on a variety of treatment options. The number of published randomized clinical trials in orthopaedics is relatively low [20]. This circumstance provides ample opportunities for the pursuit of randomized clinical trials to address these questions in situations where a position of reasonable equipoise is afforded. As the world becomes functionally smaller, multicenter and international trials are becoming increasingly feasible and will strengthen our foundation of literature and body of knowledge.

3.6 Canadian Orthopaedic Trauma Society

Beyond understanding, valuing and utilizing evidence-based principles while studying and practicing orthopaedic trauma surgery is the advanced act of contributing to the available body of knowledge in the field [21]. Evidence-based principles must reside at the core here as well, so that the field is on solid ground as it is advanced by its researchers and thought leaders. This of course may be accomplished in many ways, but important lessons may be learned by exploring one model of success where the whole has been recognized as greater than the sum of its parts.

3.6.1 Origins

The Canadian Orthopaedic Trauma Society (COTS) [21] has been successful in producing a number of multicenter randomized trials in the field of orthopaedic trauma surgery. The humble beginnings of this pioneering group can be traced back to a social meeting in 1990 between three collegial academic orthopaedic trauma surgeons from different centers discussing a clinical problem. Although this initial meeting did not produce a study of merit, it more importantly produced an appreciation for the potential held by the collaboration and communication between centers. From its point of inception, COTS has now grown to consist of over 50 members from different academic centers meeting at least biannually and contributing to randomized trials.

The functional basis of the group began with meetings for a study on the management of intra-articular fractures of the calcaneus [21]. The surgeons hailing from coast to coast were involved not merely in contributing patients, but also in the development of the study design and protocol. The merits of this early venture lead to the acquisition of funding. As success begets success, interested colleagues from other Canadian academic centers were invited to discuss clinical issues and to consider the prospect of creating a group to conduct randomized clinical trials.

At least 13 publications have been written in journals discussing difficult topics like:

1. Operative versus nonoperative treatment of calcaneal fractures
2. Nailing versus plating of midshaft humeral fractures
3. Complications around calcaneal fractures
4. Nonunion following nailing of femur fractures with and without reaming
5. Reaming versus not reaming intramedullary nails of the femur with comparison of the rates of ARDS in multi-injured patients

6. ORIF versus circular fixator treatment for bicondylar tibial plateau fractures
7. Operative versus nonoperative treatment of midshaft clavicle fractures

Other studies that have also been done with the help of COTS include:

1. SPRINT study – reamed versus unreamed tibial nail study, which is the definitive study on whether or not to ream a tibia with nailing
2. Low molecular weight Heparin versus nothing when treating patients with lower extremity fractures distal to the knee
3. Os calcis study – to fill the void or not using calcium phosphate cement
4. ORIF versus total elbow arthroplasty in severe distal humeral fractures in the osteoporotic age group

New studies just initiated include:

1. ORIF versus nonoperative care of ulnar shaft study
2. ORIF versus nonspanning external fixation versus closed reduction with percutaneous fixation for distal radial fractures
3. ORIF versus nonoperative treatment for Weber B unstable isolated fibular fractures
4. ORIF versus primary subtalar fusion for displaced Sanders IV intra-articular calcaneal fractures
5. Operative versus nonoperative treatment of humeral shaft fractures

COTS has continued to deal with the toughest fracture problems that have not been answered. This group has been progressive and aggressive in trying to answer the questions that have been difficult to answer with single center studies. Multicenter, randomized collaborative teamwork has been essential.

3.6.2 Formalization and Funding

Moving forward, decisions regarding how to formalize and legitimize the group were required. It was necessary to choose either an independent existence or one under the umbrella of a preexisting association. It was decided for both legal and funding reasons to stay within the Canadian Orthopaedic Association (COA) and use the Canadian Orthopaedic Fund as the research fund depot. In essence, preexisting infrastructure was utilized in keeping with its mandate and to the mutual benefit of both COTS and the COA. This was not only efficient and cost-effective, but its legitimacy allowed a more aggressive approach to pursuing grants and research funding from various sources (i.e., peer reviewed, association, community, industry).

3.6.3 Commitment

Similar goals and interests of the involved members are not enough in and of themselves to ensure the functional success of such a group. A group of "alpha" individuals coming together with strong personal biases and ideas requires another key ingredient for successful group dynamics. A running internal joke is that COTS stands for "Compromising Orthopaedic Trauma Surgeons." Individual flexibility is required in the development of standardized protocols integral to the design and success of the trials. Asking surgeons to alter or leave behind their previous treatment methods is no small task, but easier to achieve when done as a group for a greater purpose. Empowering this acceptance is the involvement of every group member in establishing each study protocol. This effectively leads to "buy-in" and motivation for as many centers as possible to be involved in each and every study while embracing an "all for one, one for all" philosophy. Furthermore, seeing trials through to completion with adherence to protocol and avoiding the temptation to abandon or change methods because of contemporary technical developments (albeit without confirmed evidence) lead to the successful conclusion of trials. Unquestionably, the universal acceptance of a negotiated protocol followed by dedication to the protocol for the length of the study are the keys to the success of the group in producing practice-changing trials.

In addition, a proactive approach has been taken toward the future membership of the group. To facilitate the recruitment and mentorship of subsequent generations of active members, COTS annually makes available a Young Investigator Grant for principal investigators less than 40 years of age in an effort to enthuse and motivate the next generation of COTS investigators.

3.6.4 Research Coordinators

As of June 2010, there were 60 surgeons across Canada involved in the COTS group. As important has been the collaboration with research coordinators from across the country with the development of a very strong coordinated research coordinators study group. Twenty research coordinators now help coordinate and collaborate study patients, results, and statistics from across the country.

The respect and collaboration between the COTS surgeons and research coordinators is another key to the group's success. These team members play important roles in the group at the local sites, but COTS also supports the travel of coordinators to biannual national meetings. Here the contribution to the development of protocols by those who will implement them aids in the completion and success of those protocols. There is reciprocity between their recognition and involvement as "Associate Members" of COTS and the pride and accountability they have with respect to their roles and contributions. This inherently leads to increased enthusiasm and commitment to the production and completion of trials as well as decreased turnover and attrition of personnel. Indeed, their increased autonomy and ownership in their roles is reflected by their initiation of an independent Trauma Coordinator Group with biannual meetings at both the COA and Orthopaedic Trauma Association (OTA) meetings. Their duties are many and are essential to the success of the group:

- Data collection, analysis, monitoring
- Recruitment and enrolment of subjects
- Protection of subjects and their rights in conjunction with institutional review boards
- Development of informed consent forms
- Reporting of adverse events
- Development of case report forms
- Grant and budget development
- Report preparation
- Education of other health-care professionals, patients, or families about studies and protocol requirements
- Dissemination of study results

3.6.5 Biannual Meetings

COTS provides funding for one surgeon and one coordinator from each center to attend the biannual meetings. Attendance is promoted by scheduling the meetings at national (i.e., COA) and international orthopaedic meetings (i.e., OTA). The regularity of the meetings is required to maintain team rapport and the enthusiasm required to complete medium- and long-term protocols. The COTS biannual meetings focus on the ongoing protocol refinement and the presentation of new protocols.

As mentioned, the development of a research protocol is a collaborative effort hinging on compromise. To this end, all centers participate in protocol development, despite the fact that some may not contribute patients to each study depending on local resources, manpower, or technical limitations. New protocols presented to the group can differ in their stage of development from that of an idea or question to that of a completed pilot study. Typically, a "champion" presents the protocol at its question stage and seeks feedback from the group. The proposed protocol question is then appraised on its merits of suitability and feasibility in the following manner:

- Is it a question worth answering?
- Is there controversy or debate?
- Is there sufficient interest among surgeons?
- Does a large enough study population exist in combined centers to allow completion?
- Study design – is RCT the best choice?

If the protocol question passes the group screen, the champion then completes the requisite literature search, study design, inclusion and exclusion criteria, outcomes to be measured, power analysis, and estimation of time of completion. Following this, the champion then submits the protocol to the group for review of the appropriateness of its:

- Study design
- Primary outcome (time to healing, functional outcome, quality of life?)
- Outcome measures (validated and sensitive enough to provide an answer)
- Subject selection (age limits, fracture classifications, exclusion criteria)
- Follow-up schedule (frequency and duration required)
- Standardization – how much is possible between centers?
- Budget – feasibility?

As a result of this process, the protocol is a product of compromise and collaboration. The principal investigator then standardizes the format of the protocol and prepares supporting documentation and the forms to

Table 4.1 Diagnostic criteria for systemic inflammatory response syndrome (SIRS)

Body temperature > 38°C or < 36°C
Heart rate > 90/min
Respiratory rate > 20 breaths/min or paCo$_2$ < 32 mmHg
White blood cell count > 12,000/mm^3 or < 4,000/mm^3 or the presence of >10% immature neutrophils (band forms)

SIRS can be diagnosed when two or more of these criteria are present

may protract recovery, but no organ dysfunction develops in this stage. Inflammatory mediators contribute to wound repair and recruitment of immune cells at the local site. In stage 2, a mild form of SIRS develops. Patients demonstrate dysfunction of one or two organ systems early in the clinical course of trauma but this resolves rapidly within 2 days. This stage is not a pathological state. Host defense is activated, and the balance of pro- and anti- inflammatory mediators is in equilibrium. In stage 3, a massive systemic inflammatory response (SIRS) develops rapidly after the initial trauma. These patients are at risk of death in the first few days. In stage 4, the early course of SIRS is less severe, but secondary insults such as additional surgery and infection deteriorate the state of disease markedly. Patients progress from one to two organ system dysfunction to MOF, often leading to death.

The steps of an inflammatory reaction to trauma involve mediators (cytokines, chemokines, complement, oxygen radicals, eicosanoid, and nitric oxide (NO)) and effectors (neutrophils, monocytes/macrophages, and endothelial cells). These factors are interrelated and interconnected by upregulatory and downregulatory mechanisms. The combination of these factors develop into severe SIRS, acute respiratory distress syndrome (ARDS) and sepsis, progressing to MOF depending on the type of injured tissue, the procedures of treatment after injury, age, gender, and physical condition (exogenous and endogenous factors) (Fig. 4.1).

4.2 Acute-Phase Reaction

During this phase, inflammation resulting from tissue injury induces an increase in plasma concentration of a number of liver-derived proteins (the acute-phase proteins; APP). These proteins are observed within an hour after trauma. Pro-inflammatory cytokines (TNF-α, IL-1β, IL-6) released locally by Kupffer-cells can systematically influence other cell types such as hepatocytes to synthesize more APPs. Positive APPs such as C-reactive protein (CRP), procalcitonin (PCT), serum amyloid A(SAA), complement proteins,

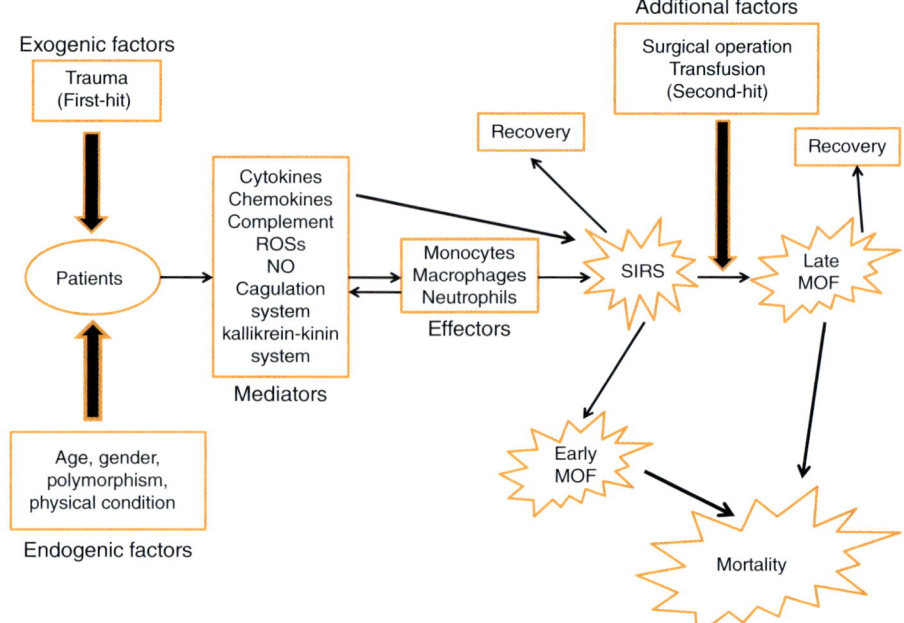

Fig. 4.1 Factors (exogenous, endogenous, additional factors), mediators, and effectors participated in the development of MOF

coagulation proteins, proteinase inhibitors, and metal-binding proteins are increased during this phase [3], whereas the production of negative APPs, such as albumin, high-density lipoproteins (HDL), protein C, protein S, and ATIII are decreased [4, 5].

Plasma concentrations of CRP are normally below 10 mg/L [6], but may increase over several hours depending on the severity of trauma [7, 8]. Hepatic synthesis of CRP is regulated mainly by IL-6. Serum levels of CRP can be detected about 12 h after systemic detection of IL-6. Clinically, the plasma levels of CRP are relatively nonspecific and may not have a positive correlation between severity of injury, and is not predictive of posttraumatic complications such as infections [9].

PCT is physiologically produced in the thyroid gland as the precursor molecule of calcitonin [5]. During sepsis, stimulation by endotoxins or proinflammatory cytokines such as interleukin-1β or tumor necrosis factor dramatically increases the serum levels of PCT up to 1,000-fold [7]. Recent studies have shown that PCT may be a practical biomarker for predicting posttraumatic complications such as severe SIRS, MOF, and sepsis [7, 10–12].

4.3 Immune Response After Trauma

The biological immune response after trauma is divided into an early innate phase, and a later adaptive response. These immune mechanisms are responsible for recognition, activation, discrimination, regulation, and eradication of invading pathogen-derived signals [13]. The innate immune response is the first line of defense, consisting of an epithelial barrier against exogenous non-self antigens and microorganisms. This includes the integrity of epithelial and mucosal cells: skin, respiratory tract, alimentary tract, urogenital tract, and conjunctiva. Exogenous pathogens that escape the first barrier are rapidly recognized and removed by the multiple components of innate immune cells such as monocytes/macrophages, natural killer cells, dendritic cells, and neutrophils [14]. Following the innate immune response, the specific acquired immune response occurs. The adaptive immune response is conducted by the interaction of antigen-presenting cells (APCs; dendritic cells, monocytes/macrophages), T lymphocytes, and B lymphocytes. The APCs capture invading pathogens and create peptide-MHC (major histocompatibility complex) protein complexes. T lymphocytes recognize the peptide-MHC protein complex via T cells expressing antigen-binding receptors (TCRs) and are activated. Activated T lymphocytes release cytokines to activate and amplify the cells of the immune system. T-helper lymphocytes (CD4+ T cells) differentiate into two phenotypes according to the cytokines they release, the Th1 and Th2 lymphocytes. Th1 cells promote the pro-inflammatory response through the release of IL-2, TNF, and interferon-γ (INF-γ), while Th2 cells produce anti-inflammatory cytokines (IL-4, IL-5, and IL-10), which suppress macrophage activity [5]. Recently, attention has been focused on the Th1/Th2 ratio. IL-12 secreted from monocytes/macrophages promotes the differentiation of Th1 cells by increasing the production of INF-γ [15, 16]. Several studies have shown that a suppressed IL-12, IL-2, and INF-γ, and elevated IL-4 are observed after major trauma, which correlated with a shift of the Th1/Th2 ratio toward the Th2-type pattern [17–19]. This imbalance in Th1/Th2-type cytokine response (from pro-inflammatory response to anti-inflammatory response) is not only a compensatory response but also increases the risk of infection by immunosuppression [20]. However, most recent reports do not support this view and the clinical relevance of the pathomechanism of Th1/Th2 shift after major trauma remains unclear [21, 22].

4.4 Mediators After Trauma

4.4.1 Plasma Protein–Derived Mediators

The inflammatory response is also mediated by plasma proteins in three interrelated systems: the complement, kallikrein-kinin, and clotting systems. Pro-inflammatory mediators, toxins, and direct tissue damage activate these cascade systems. The complement system consists of more than 30 proteins. In the resting state, complement proteins circulate as inactive forms in plasma. The activation of the complement system can occur through three established pathways (alternative, classical, and lectin). The classical pathway of complement is activated by antigen–antibody complexes (immunoglobulin M or G [IgM, IgG]), or activated coagulation factor XII (FXII). The alternative pathway is activated by bacterial products such as lipopolysaccharide (LPS).

Complement system activation results in the generation of biologically active peptides. The cleavage of C3 and C5 by their respective convertases (C3 C3a and C3b, C5 C5a and C5b) induces the formation of opsonins, anaphylatoxins, and membrane attack complexes (MACs) [23, 24]. The anaphylatoxins C3a and C5a have pro-inflammatory roles, which include the recruitment and activation of phagocytic cells (polymorphonuclear cells (PMNs), monocytes, and macrophages), the enhancement of the hepatic acute-phase reaction, stimulation of the release of vasoactive mediators such as histamine, and promoting the adhesion of leukocytes to endothelial cells. C5b forms a complex by the consecutive binding of proteins C6–C9, culminating in the formation of MACs (C5b–9), which leads to the disruption and formation of pores in the cellular membrane causing lysis (death) of the target cells at the end stage of the complement cascade [25]. Furthermore, the inflammatory response of complement activation leads to the production of free oxygen radicals and arachidonic acid metabolites and cytokines. The complement system is key to innate and adaptive immunity for defense against microbial pathogens. However, excessive consumption of complement proteins causes tissue damage after trauma. Clinically, complement activation occurs immediately after trauma and the plasma levels of C3 and C3a in traumatized patients are related to the severity of the injury, septic complications, and mortality [26–28].

The kallikrein-kinin system involves a system of plasma proteases, and is related to the complement and clotting cascades (the intrinsic coagulation cascade) [29]. This contact system consists of plasma proteins factor XII (Hageman factor; FXII), prekallikrein, high molecular weight kininogen (HMWK), and FXI. Contact with a negatively charged surface such as a foreign body or the membrane of an activated platelet activates FXII [29]. The active protein FXIIa converts prekallikrein into the proteolytic enzyme kallikrein, which in turn cleaves the plasma glycoprotein precursor HMWK to form bradykinin [30]. Bradykinin increases vascular permeability and causes dilation of blood vessels by its action on smooth muscle. In turn, as a positive feedback, kallikrein itself accelerates the conversion of FXII to FXIIa. Kallikrein can also activate fibrinolysis to counterbalance the clotting cascade activated by FXIIa. Furthermore, kallikrein has also been shown to have chemotactic activity, converting C5 into the chemoattractant product C5a.

The major mechanism of activation of the coagulation cascade following trauma is via the extrinsic coagulation system [31]. The extrinsic cascade mediates inflammation by tissue factor (TF). Exposure of the FVII to TF results in the conversion of FVII to FVIIa. The FVIIa-TF complex activates FX to FXa, and FXa converts prothrombin to thrombin (FIIa). Thrombin activates FV, FVIII, and FXI, which result in enhanced thrombin formation. Thrombin also cleaves fibrinogen, and the fibrin clot is formed following polymerization and stabilization. In normal conditions, small amounts of TF are exposed to the circulating blood. However, under pathophysiologic conditions, TF is upregulated on the surface of neutrophils, macrophages, and endothelial cells. Endotoxin, activated complement, and cytokines (TNF-α and IL-1 β) also express TF. TF is highly thrombogenic, and upregulation often results in hypercoagulability, leading to an increased tendency of thrombosis [32, 33]. In addition, coagulation mediators (FVIIa, FXa, and FIIa) elicit inflammation with the expression of TNF, cytokines, adhesion molecules (MCP-1, ICAM-1, VCAM-1, selectines, etc.), and growth factors (VEGF, etc.) [33]. Inhibitors to prevent a hypercoagulable state include antithrombin III (AT III), protein C, Protein S, and tissue factor pathway inhibitor (TFPI). ATIII inhibits FIXa, Xa, and thrombin. TFPI suppresses the activity of TF/VIIa/Xa complexes [34]. Protein C is activated by the thrombin–thrombomodulin complex on endothelial cells, and activated protein C, in combination with free protein S cleaves and inactivates FV and FVIII [35]. Therapeutically intervening with the production or activity of inhibitors could help improve outcome by mitigating complications such as sepsis and ARDS.

4.5 Cytokines

4.5.1 Pro-inflammatory Cytokines

Pro-inflammatory cytokines play key local and systemic roles as intercellular messengers to initiate, amplify, and perpetuate an inflammatory response after trauma (Table 4.2). The bioactivity of cytokines is complex. Cytokines are produced by many cell types (principally activated lymphocytes and macrophages, but also endothelial, epithelial, and connective tissue cells). They have multiple targets and act in

Table 4.2 Features of the major pro-inflammatory cytokines

Pro-inflammatory cytokines	Cellular sources	Function in inflammation
TNF	Monocytes/macrophages, mast cells, T lymphocytes, epithelial cells	Stimulates upregulation of endothelial adhesion molecules. Induction of their cytokines, chemokines, and no secretion. The inducer of acute-phase response. Induce fever. Short half-life, not useful marker of the inflammatory response after trauma
IL-1	Monocytes/macrophages, T lymphocytes endothelial cells, some epithelial cells	Stimulate to TNF
IL-6	Monocytes/macrophages, T lymphocytes endothelial cells	Inducer of acute-phase response. Stimulate proliferation of T and B lymphocytes. Long half-life, the best prognostic marker of complications after trauma (SIRS, sepsis, MOF)
Chemokines (IL-8)	Macrophages, endothelial cells, T lymphocytes, mast cells	The function of chemoattractant, leukocytes activation. Useful for diagnostic markers of AIDS

a pleiotropic manner. After trauma, production of pro-inflammatory cytokines such as TNF-α, IL-1β, IL-6, and IL-8 is initiated by monocytes and macrophages. TNF-α, IL-1β are released within 1–2 h after trauma, and are the main pro-inflammatory mediators of an acute-phase response [36]. IL-6 and IL-8 are released secondary in a subacute fashion.

TNF-α and IL-1β have a similar functions, and may act alone or in conjunction with each other [37]. The release of TNF-α and IL-1β is stimulated by bacterial endotoxins or other microbial products, immune complexes, and a variety of inflammatory stimuli. They are important early mediators of inflammation and fundamentally function to repair damaged tissue. As stated, TNF-α and IL-1β are released within 1–2 h of stimulation and usually return to baseline levels within 4 h. TNF-α increases the activity of neutrophils and monocytes by activating the underlying endothelium. TNF-α promotes the expression and release of adhesion molecules such as ICAM1 or E-selectin, and increases the permeability of endothelial cells, which mediates neutrophil migration into the damaged tissue [36]. This then further promotes the synthesis of other cytokines (IL-2, 4, 6, 8), chemokines, growth factors, eicosanoids, and NO [36, 37]. Several studies have shown the validity of TNF-α as a serum marker for complications after trauma. However, the results are inconsistent and to date, no data is available indicating whether TNF-α correlates to the severity of trauma or trauma outcome [38–43].

Many different cell types produce IL-6. In addition to immune cells such as monocytes, macrophages, neutrophils, T cells, and B cells, IL-6 is also produced by endothelial cells, smooth muscle cells, and fibroblasts. IL-6 upregulates the hepatic acute-phase response, stimulating the production of C-reactive protein (CRP), procalcitonin, serum amyloid A, fibrinogen, α1-antitrypsin, and complement factors, which then promote neutrophil activation. There is evidence that serum IL-6 level correlates with the severity of trauma and the risk of subsequent ARDS and MOF [44, 45]. IL-6 is a clinically relevant and feasible parameter to estimate the severity of injury and prognosis after trauma [46, 47]. In addition, for patients requiring second or subsequent surgeries following trauma, IL-6 may prove to be an important biological marker in deciding the correct timing of surgery. Patients with high initial levels of IL-6 (>500 pg/dL) after trauma are recommended to delay secondary procedures for more than 4 days [48]. The chemokine IL-8 is secreted by monocytes/macrophages, neutrophils, and endothelial cells. After trauma, serum levels of IL-8 are elevated within 24 h. Its production following trauma stimulates leukocyte recruitment to the inflammation site and stimulate neutrophils to migrate to the injured tissue. Plasma levels of IL-8 correlate with the subsequent development of ARDS and MOF [47, 49–51].

4.5.2 Anti-inflammatory Cytokines

IL-10 is synthesized by T lymphocytes and monocytes/macrophages. The pivotal role of IL-10 is to inhibit the

Table 4.3 Features of the major anti-inflammatory cytokines

Anti-inflammatory cytokines	Cellular sources	Function in inflammation
IL-10	Monocytes/macrophages, T lymphocytes	Inhibit pro-inflammatory cytokines secretion, oxygen radical production, adhesion molecule expression, and Th-1 lymphocyte proliferation. Enhance B lymphocyte survival, proliferation, and antibody production. IL-10 levels are correlated with severity of injury and the risk of development of sepsis, ARDS, and MOF
IL-6	See the table of anti-inflammatory cytokines	Reduction of TNF and IL-1 synthesis. Regulate the release of IL-1 Ra and sTNF-Rs

production of monocyte/macrophage-derived TNF-α, IL-6, and IL-8, and free oxygen radicals [52]. IL-10 plasma levels are proportional to the severity of trauma and to posttraumatic complications [53–57] (Table 4.3).

In addition to its pro-inflammatory role, IL-6 also has anti-inflammatory properties. As an immunoregulatory cytokine, IL-6 stimulates macrophages to release anti-inflammatory cytokines such as IL-1 receptor antagonists and soluble TNF receptors [3]. Moreover, IL-6 induces macrophages to release prostaglandin E_2 (PGE_2), the most powerful endogenous immune suppressant. PGE2 regulates the synthesis of TNF-α and IL-1β from macrophages and induces the release of IL-10 [58–60].

4.6 Reactive Oxygen Species (ROSs)

Reactive oxygen species are released by leukocytes after exposure to pro-inflammatory cytokines, chemokines, complement factors, and bacterial products. There are several mechanisms of ROS production: mitochondrial oxidation, metabolism of arachidonic acid, activation of nicotinamide-adenine dinucleotide phosphate (NADPH) oxidase, and activation of xanthine oxidase. With ischemia and subsequent reperfusion, reintroduced molecular oxygen reacts with hypoxanthine and xanthine oxidase generated as the result of ATP consumption during the ischemia phase, to generate superoxide anions. Superoxide anions are further reduced to hydrogen peroxide (H_2O_2) by super oxide dismutase (SOD). The initial ROSs (superoxide anion and hydrogen peroxide) are relatively low-energy oxygen radicals and are not considered to cause high levels of cytotoxicity [61]. The most detrimental of the reactive oxygen species are hydroxyl radicals (·OH⁻), which are generated from superoxide anions and hydrogen peroxide by the Haber–Weiss reaction (·O_2^- + H_2O_2 ·OH⁻ + O_2) or from hydrogen peroxide by the Fenton reaction in the presence of iron (Fig. 4.2). ROSs cause lipid peroxidation, cell membrane disintegration, and DNA damage to endothelial and parenchymal cells [62, 63]. Furthermore, ROSs secreted from polymorphonuclear leukocytes (PMNs) induce

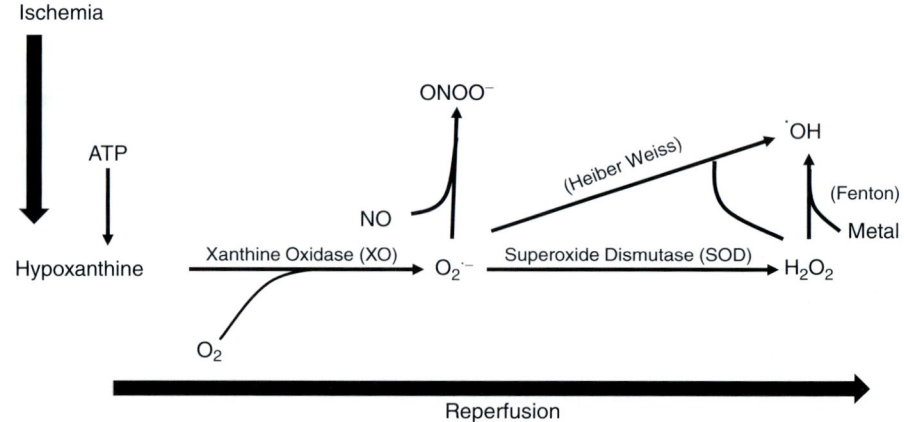

Fig. 4.2 Reactive oxygen species (ROSs)

cytokine, chemokines [64], heat shock protein (HSP) [65], and adhesion molecules (P-selectinem ICAM-1) [66] leading to cell and tissue damage.

4.7 Nitric Oxide (NO)

Nitric oxide (NO) is generated from the amino acid L-arginine by three isoforms of nitric oxidase synthases (NOSs). The isoforms are neuronal NOS (nNOS or NOS-1), endothelial NOS (eNOS or NOS-3), and inducible NOS [iNOS or NOS-2]). The isoforms nNOS and eNOS are expressed constitutively by neurons in the brain and enteric nervous system (nNOS), and endothelial cells (eNOSs), while iNOS is expressed for the most part by stimulation of pro-inflammatory cytokines (TNF-α, IL-1β) and toxins (LPS) [67]. Low levels of NO synthesized by nNOS and eNOS are beneficial to control smooth muscle relaxation and microbial killing, whereas large amounts of NO synthesized by iNOS are harmful and contribute to tissue damage. It acts by causing vasodilation, increase in vascular permeability, and inhibition of platelet aggregation [68, 69]. In addition, NO interacts with superoxide anion to form peroxinitrite anion (ONOO$^-$), which is a cytotoxin. ONOO$^-$ causes lipid peroxidation, cell membrane disintegration, and DNA damage of endothelial and parenchymal cells as well as the generation of hydroxyradicals. It is thought to be responsible for many of the toxic effects of NO [69].

4.8 Damage-Associated Molecular Patterns (DAMPs)

The innate immune system provides the first line of defense against infection and trauma. The cells of the innate immune system, including T cells (CD4+ and CD8+), neutrophils, monocytes, macrophages, natural killer (NK) cells, and dendritic cells (DC), are activated by endogenous danger signals such as pathogen-associated molecular patterns (PAMPs; exogenous danger cells) and alarmins (endogenous danger cells) [70]. PAMPs (LPS, bacterial DNA, viral RNA) and alarmins including high mobility group box 1 (HMGB1), heat shock proteins (HSPs), S100, hyaluronan, and oxygen free radicals are recognized by pattern recognition receptors (PRRs). PRRs include toll-like receptors (TLRs) and the receptor for advanced glycation end products (RAGE) [71]. These signaling molecules are normal cell constituents. However, they can either be passively released from necrotic cells or actively secreted in response to cellular injury. The exogenous PAMPs and endogenous alarmins are subgroups of damage-associated molecular patterns (DAMPs) [72].

HMGB1 is the most pro-inflammatory of all DAMPs. HMGB1 is released actively by immune cells such as monocytes, macrophages, and dendritic cells. HMGB1 may signal through RAGE, or via toll-like receptors, TLR2 and TLR4. Activation of these receptors results in the activation of NFkB, which increases the expression of ICAM-1and VCAM-1 on the surface of endothelial cells, and stimulates the production of pro-inflammatory cytokines [73–77]. After trauma, excessive tissue damage increases the intercellular signaling of DAMPs, which further upregulate the expression of PPRs and inflammatory mediators. Recently, the interaction of HMGB1 and TLR4 received attention as key mediators in the initial inflammatory response in various clinical and experimental models, such as in hemorrhagic shock, bilateral femur fractures, and hepatic ischemia/reperfusion injury [78–85].

4.9 Cells Implicated in Trauma

4.9.1 Neutrophils

After trauma, neutrophils migrate to the site of tissue damage and to remote organ tissue. Local neutrophil migration is important for wound healing and for protection against invading organisms, and remote organ tissue migration induces SIRS [86]. The migration is composed of three steps. The first step, production of leukocyte selectins (L-selectins) and E and P selectins on the endothelium is induced by pro-inflammatory cytokines and toxins [87]. These adhesion molecules are responsible for the rolling of neutrophils. The second step involves expression of integrins on neutrophils such as CD11 and CD18, and intercellular adhesion molecules (ICAM-1) and vascular cell adhesion molecules (VCAM-1) on the surface of endothelial cells [88–90]. The interaction of these upregulated molecules activate neutrophils to reinforce the contact between neutrophils and endothelial cells ("sticking" of neutrophils to endothelial cells). In the final step, the migration, accumulation, and activation ("priming") of neutrophils into tissues are mediated by chemokines and complement anaphylatoxins (C5a and C3a). Usually, primed neutrophils stimulated by the inciting trauma are not harmful to the host (intermediate state: the state of between resting and full activating state). Massive initial trauma or additional insult elicits a more powerful neutrophil response [91]. In this state, neutrophils are attracted and activated further to degranulate. This is the so-called respiratory burst, which induces secondary organ tissue injury. The active substances released from degranulated neutrophils include neutral protease (elastase and capthesin G), oxygen radicals, myeloperoxidase (MPO), NO, leukotrienes, and platelet-activating factor (PAF). In trauma patients, increased levels of soluble ICAM-1 correlate with the development of complications after trauma (sepsis, MOF) [88, 92].

4.9.2 Monocytes/Macrophages

Monocytes/macrophages and neutrophils have a central and essential role for the innate host defense, tissue repair and remodeling, and for the intermediaries to the antigen-specific adaptive immune response. Monocytes are circulating precursors of macrophages. Monocytes migrate into the different tissues (liver, spleen, lung, etc.) in the absence of local inflammation and become tissue macrophages. When monocytes/macrophages are activated by phagocytosis in response to trauma, they regulate the activation of T and B lymphocytes, which induce antigen presentation by the major histocompatibility complex II (MHC II). Monocytes/macrophages also release chemokines, cytokines (TNF, IL-6, IL-10, IL-12, TGF-β), and various growth factors (fibroblast growth factor [FGF], epidermal growth factor [EGF], and platelet-derived growth factor [PDGF]) to form new extracellular matrix and to promote angiogenesis and generation of new tissue at the site of injury. Additionally, activated monocytes/macrophages produce NO, adhesion molecules, eicosanoides, and PAF. The monocyte/macrophage cellular response after trauma has beneficial effect to the host. However, severe trauma induces massive monocyte/macrophage activation. In this state, the effect of the monocyte/macrophage response is systemic with detrimental effects. Systemically, it influences the immune response microcirculation and metabolism of remote organ systems. The deactivation of monocytes and decreased expression of MHC II on the surface of monocytes are observed after major trauma and these correlate with the severity of injury [93].

4.10 Mechanisms of the Development of Organ Dysfunction

4.10.1 Severity of Initial Injury (First-Hit)

An initial traumatic insult activates an inflammatory cascade that stimulates the host's immune system. If the initial traumatic insult is massive, this causes severe SIRS. In this situation, the production and release of pro-inflammatory mediators overwhelms the anti-inflammatory response resulting in rapid MOF and early death.

An initial traumatic insult that is not as severe induces a moderate state of SIRS. In this instance, inflammatory and immune cells are in a "primed" state. However, some patients go on to develop posttraumatic complications (sepsis, ARDS, and MOF). The development of these complications is regulated by various exogenous and endogenous factors. Among these factors, it is important to understand the relationship between the biological changes and the anatomical region of initial injury. The central nervous system is a rich source of inflammatory mediators. Traumatic brain injuries with the disruption of the blood brain barrier (BBB) allow immune cells to migrate into the subarachnoid space, leading to an accumulation of leukocytes from the systemic circulation. These cells release inflammatory mediators, which can damage brain tissue and induce systemic inflammation [5, 94–96]. Trauma to the chest area, particularly lung contusions, leads to an early increase in plasma cytokine mediators, which has been shown to be associated with systematic inflammatory reactions such as pneumonia, ARDS, and MOF [97–99]. Patients with severe soft tissue injuries to the extremities, with resulting hemorrhagic shock or severe muscle crush syndrome are at risk of developing more serious injury. Ischemia/reperfusion injury (I/R) leads to the production of large quantities of reactive oxygen species (ROSs). Femoral fractures with soft tissue injuries results in an alteration of biological parameters such as increased cardiac output, decreased systemic vascular resistance, tachycardia, and decreased hepatic blood flow [100]. Long bone fractures and unstable pelvic fractures are characterized by a high blood loss and are associated with severe soft tissue injury, which initiate a local inflammatory response and generate inflammatory mediators [55, 101–105]. This body of evidence suggests that the initial trauma itself predisposes trauma patients to posttraumatic complications.

4.10.2 Two-Hit Theory

Traumatized patients who survive the initial injury may still be at risk of death from sepsis and multiple organ failure. Secondary insults following the initial injury exaggerate the systemic inflammatory response and upset the balance of pro- and anti-inflammatory mediators. Secondary insults are compounded by endogenous and exogenous factors. Endogenous secondary insults include respiratory distress, cardiovascular instability, I/R injury, and infection. Exogenous secondary insults include surgical interventions [106–108], blood transfusions, and missed injuries.

Clinical studies have revealed that orthopaedic surgical intervention can also cause major changes to the inflammatory response, and these changes are in proportion to the magnitude of surgery. For instance, femoral nailing induces plasma levels of IL-6 and IL-10 to increase and human leukocyte antigen-DR on monocytes have been shown to reduce significantly [109, 110]. Furthermore, reamed femoral nailing appears to be associated with greater impairment of immune reactivity than unreamed nailing [110].

Blood transfusions are a paramount therapy in the management of trauma/hemorrhagic shock patients. However, various studies have demonstrated that blood transfusions are associated with infection, SIRS, ARDS, and MOF after trauma [111–116].

4.10.3 Ischemia/Reperfusion Injury

Ischemia/reperfusion (I/R) injury is a common and important event in clinical situations such as trauma, hemorrhagic shock, transplantation, cardiac arrest (hypoxemia, hypotension of systemic tissue), contusions, lacerations, vascular injuries, and compartment syndrome (hypoxemia, hypotension of local tissue). Inadequate microvascular flow results in the activation of leukocytes, and converts local endothelial cells into a proinflammatory and prothrombotic phenotype. I/R injury consists of two specific stages. First is the ischemia and hypoxemia stage. During this period, oxygen and nutrients to tissues are deprived temporarily by the disruption of blood supply. The second is the reperfusion stage. This stage is the revascularization or return of supply of oxygen to the ischemic tissue. During the ischemic phase, the lack of oxygen leads to the decreased production as well as the consumption of adenosine triphosphate (ATP). As consumption of ATP continues, it is degraded into adenosine diphosphate (ADP) and adenosine monophosphate (AMP), which is further degraded to inosine and hypoxanthine [117]. ATP depletion leads to an alteration in intercellular calcium and sodium concentration. It also results in the activation of cytotoxic enzymes such as proteases or phospholipases, all culminating to reversible or irreversible cellular damage. The hallmark of the reperfusion phase is the generation of by-products of neutrophil activation, which induces secondary tissue damage and organ dysfunction. On reperfusion with the reintroduction of molecular oxygen into the ischemic tissue, molecular oxygen reacts with leukocytes and endothelial cells to promote the generation of reactive oxygen species and platelet-activation factor. The interactions of neutrophils and endothelial cells have been shown to contribute to massive interstitial edema caused by microvascular capillary leakage after reperfusion injury.

4.10.4 Bacterial Translocation

Bacterial translocation (BT) is defined as the phenomenon that both viable and nonviable bacteria, as well as their products (bacterial cell wall components, LPS, and peptidogycan) cross the intestinal barrier to external sites such as the mesenteric lymph nodes, liver, and spleen. BT occurs as a result of a loss of integrity of the gut barrier function after trauma, hemorrhagic shock, and burns [118]. BT may be associated with posttraumatic complications [119, 120]. Although most data on BT and its complications have shown consistent results in animal models of hemorrhagic shock, trauma, and severe burns, its importance in humans is questionable, with variable results in clinical studies. In addition, it is still debatable whether BT is an important pathophysiologic event or simply an epi-phenomenon of severe disease [121].

4.11 Conclusion

Following trauma, acute inflammatory reactions may be triggered by infections (bacterial, viral, fungal, parasitic) and microbial toxins, or by any of several molecules released from necrotic tissue (HMGB1, hyaluronum, etc.). Pattern recognition receptors (PRRs) referred as to toll-like receptors can detect these stimuli, and trigger a signaling pathway that leads to the production of various mediators. In the acute phase of trauma, vasodilatation is induced by vasodilatatory mediators (NO, prostaglandins), quickly followed by increased permeability of the microvasculature. Vasodilatation and extravasation of plasma result in hemoconcentration, which facilitates the peripheral migration of neutrophils. Neutrophil migration from the blood stream into the interstitial tissue is divided into several steps, which are mediated by endothelial cell adhesion molecules, cytokines produced from monocytes/macrophages and various other cells, chemokines, the complement system, and arachidonic acid. Migrated neutrophils produce several mediators such as neutral protease, reactive oxygen species (ROSs), lipids (leukotriene, PAF), and NO. These mediators act as secondary tissue damage factors depending on the degree of initial injury as well as additional insults. During inflammation, the plasmaic cascade, consisting of the complement cascade, the kallikrein-kinin system, and the coagulation cascade are activated by toxins and pro-inflammatory mediators such as cytokines and arachidonic acid metabolites. Activation of the complement system induces the production of complement proteins, causing an increase in vascular permeability, chemotaxis, and opsonization. Excessive activation of the coagulation system results in a hypercoagulable state, which leads to disseminated intravascular coagulation (DIC). The kallikrein-kinin system results in kinins, which have vasoactive properties. In addition to its role in stimulating inflammation, the immune system (innate and adaptive) has a vital role involving the biological response after trauma.

References

1. Bone RC, Balk RA, Cerra FB, et al. Definitions for sepsis and organ failure and guidelines for the use of innovative therapies in sepsis. The ACCP/SCCM Consensus Conference Committee. American College of Chest Physicians/Society of Critical Care Medicine. Chest. 1992;101:1644–55.
2. Bone RC. Toward a theory regarding the pathogenesis of the systemic inflammatory response syndrome: what we do and do not know about cytokine regulation. Crit Care Med. 1996;24:163–72.
3. Lin E, Calvano SE, Lowry SF. Inflammatory cytokines and cell response in surgery. Surgery. 2000;127:117–26.
4. Gruys E, Toussaint MJ, Niewold TA, et al. Acute phase reaction and acute phase proteins. J Zhejiang Univ Sci B. 2005;6:1045–56.
5. Keel M, Trentz O. Pathophysiology of polytrauma. Injury. 2005;36:691–709.
6. el Hassan BS, Peak JD, Whicher JT, et al. Acute phase protein levels as an index of severity of physical injury. Int J Oral Maxillofac Surg. 1990;19:346–9.
7. Castelli GP, Pognani C, Cita M, et al. Procalcitonin as a prognostic and diagnostic tool for septic complications after major trauma. Crit Care Med. 2009;37:1845–9.
8. Du Clos TW. Function of C-reactive protein. Ann Med. 2000;32:274–8.
9. Gosling P, Dickson GR. Serum c-reactive protein in patients with serious trauma. Injury. 1992;23:483–6.
10. Mimoz O, Benoist JF, Edouard AR, et al. Procalcitonin and C-reactive protein during the early posttraumatic systemic inflammatory response syndrome. Intensive Care Med. 1998;24:185–8.
11. Uzzan B, Cohen R, Nicolas P, et al. Procalcitonin as a diagnostic test for sepsis in critically ill adults and after surgery or trauma: a systematic review and meta-analysis. Crit Care Med. 2006;34:1996–2003.
12. Wanner GA, Keel M, Steckholzer U, et al. Relationship between procalcitonin plasma levels and severity of injury, sepsis, organ failure, and mortality in injured patients. Crit Care Med. 2000;28:950–7.
13. Lenz A, Franklin GA, Cheadle WG. Systemic inflammation after trauma. Injury. 2007;38:1336–45.
14. Pillay J, Hietbrink F, Koenderman L, et al. The systemic inflammatory response induced by trauma is reflected by multiple phenotypes of blood neutrophils. Injury. 2007;38:1365–72.
15. Trinchieri G. Interleukin-12 and the regulation of innate resistance and adaptive immunity. Nat Rev Immunol. 2003;3:133–46.
16. Watford WT, Moriguchi M, Morinobu A, et al. The biology of IL-12: coordinating innate and adaptive immune responses. Cytokine Growth Factor Rev. 2003;14:361–8.
17. Decker D, Schondorf M, Bidlingmaier F, et al. Surgical stress induces a shift in the type-1/type-2 T-helper cell

balance, suggesting down-regulation of cell-mediated and up-regulation of antibody-mediated immunity commensurate to the trauma. Surgery. 1996;119:316–25.
18. O'Sullivan ST, Lederer JA, Horgan AF, et al. Major injury leads to predominance of the T helper-2 lymphocyte phenotype and diminished interleukin-12 production associated with decreased resistance to infection. Ann Surg. 1995;222: 482–90; discussion 90–2.
19. Spolarics Z, Siddiqi M, Siegel JH, et al. Depressed interleukin-12-producing activity by monocytes correlates with adverse clinical course and a shift toward Th2-type lymphocyte pattern in severely injured male trauma patients. Crit Care Med. 2003;31:1722–9.
20. Miller AC, Rashid RM, Elamin EM. The "T" in trauma: the helper T-cell response and the role of immunomodulation in trauma and burn patients. J Trauma. 2007;63:1407–17.
21. Heizmann O, Koeller M, Muhr G, et al. Th1- and Th2-type cytokines in plasma after major trauma. J Trauma. 2008; 65:1374–8.
22. Wick M, Kollig E, Muhr G, et al. The potential pattern of circulating lymphocytes TH1/TH2 is not altered after multiple injuries. Arch Surg. 2000;135:1309–14.
23. Fosse E, Pillgram-Larsen J, Svennevig JL, et al. Complement activation in injured patients occurs immediately and is dependent on the severity of the trauma. Injury. 1998;29: 509–14.
24. Mollnes TE, Fosse E. The complement system in trauma-related and ischemic tissue damage: a brief review. Shock. 1994;2:301–10.
25. Mastellos D, Lambris JD. Complement: more than a 'guard' against invading pathogens? Trends Immunol. 2002;23: 485–91.
26. Hecke F, Schmidt U, Kola A, et al. Circulating complement proteins in multiple trauma patients – correlation with injury severity, development of sepsis, and outcome. Crit Care Med. 1997;25:2015–24.
27. Kapur MM, Jain P, Gidh M. The effect of trauma on serum C3 activation and its correlation with injury severity score in man. J Trauma. 1986;26:464–6.
28. Sharma DK, Sarda AK, Bhalla SA, et al. The effect of recent trauma on serum complement activation and serum C3 levels correlated with the injury severity score. Indian J Med Microbiol. 2004;22:147–52.
29. Sugimoto K, Hirata M, Majima M, et al. Evidence for a role of kallikrein-P6nin system in patients with shock after blunt trauma. Am J Physiol. 1998;274:R1556–60.
30. Joseph K, Kaplan AP. Formation of bradykinin: a major contributor to the innate inflammatory response. Adv Immunol. 2005;86:159–208.
31. Chu AJ. Blood coagulation as an intrinsic pathway for proinflammation: a mini review. Inflamm Allergy Drug Targets. 2009;9(1):32–44.
32. Abraham E. Coagulation abnormalities in acute lung injury and sepsis. Am J Respir Cell Mol Biol. 2000;22:401–4.
33. Chu AJ. Tissue factor mediates inflammation. Arch Biochem Biophys. 2005;440:123–32.
34. Riddel Jr JP, Aouizerat BE, Miaskowski C, et al. Theories of blood coagulation. J Pediatr Oncol Nurs. 2007;24:123–31.
35. Rigby AC, Grant MA. Protein S: a conduit between anticoagulation and inflammation. Crit Care Med. 2004;32: S336–41.
36. Dinarello CA. Proinflammatory cytokines. Chest. 2000; 118:503–8.
37. Kim PK, Deutschman CS. Inflammatory responses and mediators. Surg Clin North Am. 2000;80:885–94.
38. Ayala A, Perrin MM, Meldrum DR, et al. Hemorrhage induces an increase in serum TNF which is not associated with elevated levels of endotoxin. Cytokine. 1990;2:170–4.
39. Rabinovici R, John R, Esser KM, et al. Serum tumor necrosis factor-alpha profile in trauma patients. J Trauma. 1993;35: 698–702.
40. Rhee P, Waxman K, Clark L, et al. Tumor necrosis factor and monocytes are released during hemorrhagic shock. Resuscitation. 1993;25:249–55.
41. Roumen RM, Hendriks T, van der Ven-Jongekrijg J, et al. Cytokine patterns in patients after major vascular surgery, hemorrhagic shock, and severe blunt trauma. Relation with subsequent adult respiratory distress syndrome and multiple organ failure. Ann Surg. 1993;218:769–76.
42. Stylianos S, Wakabayashi G, Gelfand JA, et al. Experimental hemorrhage and blunt trauma do not increase circulating tumor necrosis factor. J Trauma. 1991;31:1063–7.
43. Zingarelli B, Squadrito F, Altavilla D, et al. Role of tumor necrosis factor-alpha in acute hypovolemic hemorrhagic shock in rats. Am J Physiol. 1994;266:H1512–5.
44. Biffl WL, Moore EE, Moore FA, et al. Interleukin-6 in the injured patient. Marker of injury or mediator of inflammation? Ann Surg. 1996;224:647–64.
45. Gebhard F, Pfetsch H, Steinbach G, et al. Is interleukin 6 an early marker of injury severity following major trauma in humans? Arch Surg. 2000;135:291–5.
46. Pape HC, Tsukamoto T, Kobbe P, et al. Assessment of the clinical course with inflammatory parameters. Injury. 2007; 38:1358–64.
47. Partrick DA, Moore FA, Moore EE, et al. Jack A. Barney Resident Research Award winner. The inflammatory profile of interleukin-6, interleukin-8, and soluble intercellular adhesion molecule-1 in postinjury multiple organ failure. Am J Surg. 1996;172:425–9; discussion 9–31.
48. Pape HC, van Griensven M, Rice J, et al. Major secondary surgery in blunt trauma patients and perioperative cytokine liberation: determination of the clinical relevance of biochemical markers. J Trauma. 2001;50:989–1000.
49. DeLong Jr WG, Born CT. Cytokines in patients with polytrauma. Clin Orthop Relat Res. 2004;422:57–65.
50. Donnelly SC, Strieter RM, Kunkel SL, et al. Interleukin-8 and development of adult respiratory distress syndrome in at-risk patient groups. Lancet. 1993;341:643–7.
51. Pallister I, Dent C, Topley N. Increased neutrophil migratory activity after major trauma: a factor in the etiology of acute respiratory distress syndrome? Crit Care Med. 2002;30: 1717–21.
52. Oswald IP, Wynn TA, Sher A, et al. Interleukin 10 inhibits macrophage microbicidal activity by blocking the endogenous production of tumor necrosis factor alpha required as a costimulatory factor for interferon gamma-induced activation. Proc Natl Acad Sci USA. 1992;89:8676–80.
53. Armstrong L, Millar AB. Relative production of tumour necrosis factor alpha and interleukin 10 in adult respiratory distress syndrome. Thorax. 1997;52:442–6.
54. Donnelly SC, Strieter RM, Reid PT, et al. The association between mortality rates and decreased concentrations of

54. interleukin-10 and interleukin-1 receptor antagonist in the lung fluids of patients with the adult respiratory distress syndrome. Ann Intern Med. 1996;125:191–6.
55. Giannoudis PV, Smith RM, Perry SL, et al. Immediate IL-10 expression following major orthopaedic trauma: relationship to anti-inflammatory response and subsequent development of sepsis. Intensive Care Med. 2000;26:1076–81.
56. Neidhardt R, Keel M, Steckholzer U, et al. Relationship of interleukin-10 plasma levels to severity of injury and clinical outcome in injured patients. J Trauma. 1997;42:863–70; discussion 70–1.
57. Pajkrt D, Camoglio L, Tiel-van Buul MC, et al. Attenuation of proinflammatory response by recombinant human IL-10 in human endotoxemia: effect of timing of recombinant human IL-10 administration. J Immunol. 1997;158:3971–7.
58. Opal SM, DePalo VA. Anti-inflammatory cytokines. Chest. 2000;117:1162–72.
59. Phipps RP, Stein SH, Roper RL. A new view of prostaglandin E regulation of the immune response. Immunol Today. 1991;12:349–52.
60. Tilg H, Trehu E, Atkins MB, et al. Interleukin-6 (IL-6) as an anti-inflammatory cytokine: induction of circulating IL-1 receptor antagonist and soluble tumor necrosis factor receptor p55. Blood. 1994;83:113–8.
61. Sasaki M, Joh T. Oxidative stress and ischemia-reperfusion injury in gastrointestinal tract and antioxidant, protective agents. J Clin Biochem Nutr. 2007;40:1–12.
62. Cristofori L, Tavazzi B, Gambin R, et al. Early onset of lipid peroxidation after human traumatic brain injury: a fatal limitation for the free radical scavenger pharmacological therapy? J Investig Med. 2001;49:450–8.
63. Kong SE, Blennerhassett LR, Heel KA, et al. Ischaemia-reperfusion injury to the intestine. Aust N Z J Surg. 1998; 68:554–61.
64. Remick DG, Villarete L. Regulation of cytokine gene expression by reactive oxygen and reactive nitrogen intermediates. J Leukoc Biol. 1996;59:471–5.
65. Schreck R, Rieber P, Baeuerle PA. Reactive oxygen intermediates as apparently widely used messengers in the activation of the NF-kappa B transcription factor and HIV-1. EMBO J. 1991;10:2247–58.
66. Gasic AC, McGuire G, Krater S, et al. Hydrogen peroxide pretreatment of perfused canine vessels induces ICAM-1 and CD18-dependent neutrophil adherence. Circulation. 1991;84:2154–66.
67. Villarete LH, Remick DG. Nitric oxide regulation of interleukin-8 gene expression. Shock. 1997;7:29–35.
68. Cirino G, Distrutti E, Wallace JL. Nitric oxide and inflammation. Inflamm Allergy Drug Targets. 2006;5:115–9.
69. Laroux FS, Pavlick KP, Hines IN, et al. Role of nitric oxide in inflammation. Acta Physiol Scand. 2001;173:113–8.
70. Srikrishna G, Freeze HH. Endogenous damage-associated molecular pattern molecules at the crossroads of inflammation and cancer. Neoplasia. 2009;11:615–28.
71. Delneste Y, Beauvillain C, Jeannin P. Innate immunity: structure and function of TLRs. Med Sci (Paris). 2007;23:67–73.
72. Bianchi ME. DAMPs, PAMPs and alarmins: all we need to know about danger. J Leukoc Biol. 2007;81:1–5.
73. Andersson U, Wang H, Palmblad K, et al. High mobility group 1 protein (HMG-1) stimulates proinflammatory cytokine synthesis in human monocytes. J Exp Med. 2000; 192:565–70.
74. Fiuza C, Bustin M, Talwar S, et al. Inflammation-promoting activity of HMGB1 on human microvascular endothelial cells. Blood. 2003;101:2652–60.
75. Treutiger CJ, Mullins GE, Johansson AS, et al. High mobility group 1 B-box mediates activation of human endothelium. J Intern Med. 2003;254:375–85.
76. Wang H, Bloom O, Zhang M, et al. HMG-1 as a late mediator of endotoxin lethality in mice. Science. 1999;285:248–51.
77. Wang H, Vishnubhakat JM, Bloom O, et al. Proinflammatory cytokines (tumor necrosis factor and interleukin 1) stimulate release of high mobility group protein-1 by pituicytes. Surgery. 1999;126:389–92.
78. Fan J, Li Y, Levy RM, et al. Hemorrhagic shock induces NAD(P)H oxidase activation in neutrophils: role of HMGB1-TLR4 signaling. J Immunol. 2007;178:6573–80.
79. Goldstein RS, Gallowitsch-Puerta M, Yang L, et al. Elevated high-mobility group box 1 levels in patients with cerebral and myocardial ischemia. Shock. 2006;25:571–4.
80. Kim JY, Park JS, Strassheim D, et al. HMGB1 contributes to the development of acute lung injury after hemorrhage. Am J Physiol Lung Cell Mol Physiol. 2005;288:L958–65.
81. Klune JR, Dhupar R, Cardinal J, et al. HMGB1: endogenous danger signaling. Mol Med. 2008;14:476–84.
82. Levy RM, Mollen KP, Prince JM, et al. Systemic inflammation and remote organ injury following trauma require HMGB1. Am J Physiol Regul Integr Comp Physiol. 2007; 293:R1538–44.
83. Ombrellino M, Wang H, Ajemian MS, et al. Increased serum concentrations of high-mobility-group protein 1 in haemorrhagic shock. Lancet. 1999;354:1446–7.
84. Tsung A, Sahai R, Tanaka H, et al. The nuclear factor HMGB1 mediates hepatic injury after murine liver ischemia-reperfusion. J Exp Med. 2005;201:1135–43.
85. Yang R, Harada T, Mollen KP, et al. Anti-HMGB1 neutralizing antibody ameliorates gut barrier dysfunction and improves survival after hemorrhagic shock. Mol Med. 2006;12:105–14.
86. Botha AJ, Moore FA, Moore EE, et al. Postinjury neutrophil priming and activation: an early vulnerable window. Surgery. 1995;118:358–64; discussion 64–5.
87. Zallen G, Moore EE, Johnson JL, et al. Circulating postinjury neutrophils are primed for the release of proinflammatory cytokines. J Trauma. 1999;46:42–8.
88. Law MM, Cryer HG, Abraham E. Elevated levels of soluble ICAM-1 correlate with the development of multiple organ failure in severely injured trauma patients. J Trauma. 1994;37:100–9; discussion 9–10.
89. Seekamp A, Jochum M, Ziegler M, et al. Cytokines and adhesion molecules in elective and accidental trauma-related ischemia/reperfusion. J Trauma. 1998;44:874–82.
90. Simon SI, Green CE. Molecular mechanics and dynamics of leukocyte recruitment during inflammation. Annu Rev Biomed Eng. 2005;7:151–85.
91. Brochner AC, Toft P. Pathophysiology of the systemic inflammatory response after major accidental trauma. Scand J Trauma Resusc Emerg Med. 2009;17:43.
92. Endo S, Inada K, Kasai T, et al. Levels of soluble adhesion molecules and cytokines in patients with septic multiple organ failure. J Inflamm. 1995;46:212–9.
93. Ayala A, Ertel W, Chaudry IH. Trauma-induced suppression of antigen presentation and expression of major histocompatibility class II antigen complex in leukocytes. Shock. 1996;5:79–90.

94. Ghirnikar RS, Lee YL, Eng LF. Inflammation in traumatic brain injury: role of cytokines and chemokines. Neurochem Res. 1998;23:329–40.
95. Morganti-Kossmann MC, Satgunaseelan L, Bye N, Kossmann T. Modulation of immune response by head injury. Injury. 2007;38:1392–400.
96. Schmidt OI, Heyde CE, Ertel W, et al. Closed head injury – an inflammatory disease? Brain Res Brain Res Rev. 2005; 48:388–99.
97. Knoferl MW, Liener UC, Perl M, et al. Blunt chest trauma induces delayed splenic immunosuppression. Shock. 2004; 22:51–6.
98. Perl M, Gebhard F, Bruckner UB, et al. Pulmonary contusion causes impairment of macrophage and lymphocyte immune functions and increases mortality associated with a subsequent septic challenge. Crit Care Med. 2005;33:1351–8.
99. Strecker W, Gebhard F, Perl M, et al. Biochemical characterization of individual injury pattern and injury severity. Injury. 2003;34:879–87.
100. Schirmer WJ, Schirmer JM, Townsend MC, Fry DE. Femur fracture with associated soft-tissue injury produces hepatic ischemia. Possible cause of hepatic dysfunction. Arch Surg. 1988;123:412–5.
101. Giannoudis PV, Pape HC, Cohen AP, et al. Review: systemic effects of femoral nailing: from Kuntscher to the immune reactivity era. Clin Orthop Relat Res. 2002; 404:378–86.
102. Hauser CJ, Joshi P, Zhou X, et al. Production of interleukin-10 in human fracture soft-tissue hematomas. Shock. 1996;6:3–6.
103. Hauser CJ, Zhou X, Joshi P, et al. The immune microenvironment of human fracture/soft-tissue hematomas and its relationship to systemic immunity. J Trauma. 1997;42:895–903; discussion 4.
104. Pape HC, Schmidt RE, Rice J, et al. Biochemical changes after trauma and skeletal surgery of the lower extremity: quantification of the operative burden. Crit Care Med. 2000;28:3441–8.
105. Perl M, Gebhard F, Knoferl MW, et al. The pattern of preformed cytokines in tissues frequently affected by blunt trauma. Shock. 2003;19:299–304.
106. Angele MK, Chaudry IH. Surgical trauma and immunosuppression: pathophysiology and potential immunomodulatory approaches. Langenbecks Arch Surg. 2005;390: 333–41.
107. Flohe S, Flohe SB, Schade FU, et al. Immune response of severely injured patients – influence of surgical intervention and therapeutic impact. Langenbecks Arch Surg. 2007;392:639–48.
108. Ni Choileain N, Redmond HP. Cell response to surgery. Arch Surg. 2006;141:1132–40.
109. Giannoudis PV, Smith RM, Bellamy MC, et al. Stimulation of the inflammatory system by reamed and unreamed nailing of femoral fractures. An analysis of the second hit. J Bone Joint Surg Br. 1999;81:356–61.
110. Smith RM, Giannoudis PV, Bellamy MC, et al. Interleukin-10 release and monocyte human leukocyte antigen-DR expression during femoral nailing. Clin Orthop Relat Res. 2000;373:233–40.
111. Malone DL, Dunne J, Tracy JK, et al. Blood transfusion, independent of shock severity, is associated with worse outcome in trauma. J Trauma. 2003;54:898–905; discussion 7.
112. Moore EE, Johnson JL, Cheng AM, et al. Insights from studies of blood substitutes in trauma. Shock. 2005;24: 197–205.
113. Moore FA, Moore EE, Sauaia A. Blood transfusion. An independent risk factor for postinjury multiple organ failure. Arch Surg. 1997;132:620–4; discussion 4–5.
114. Sauaia A, Moore FA, Moore EE, et al. Early predictors of postinjury multiple organ failure. Arch Surg. 1994; 129:39–45.
115. Shander A. Emerging risks and outcomes of blood transfusion in surgery. Semin Hematol. 2004;41:117–24.
116. Silliman CC, Moore EE, Johnson JL, et al. Transfusion of the injured patient: proceed with caution. Shock. 2004;21:291–9.
117. Nakao A, Kaczorowski DJ, Sugimoto R, et al. Application of heme oxygenase-1, carbon monoxide and biliverdin for the prevention of intestinal ischemia/reperfusion injury. J Clin Biochem Nutr. 2008;42:78–88.
118. Macintire DK, Bellhorn TL. Bacterial translocation: clinical implications and prevention. Vet Clin North Am Small Anim Pract. 2002;32:1165–78.
119. Fukushima R, Kobayashi S, Okinaga K. Bacterial translocation in multiple organ failure. Nippon Geka Gakkai Zasshi. 1998;99:497–503.
120. Nieuwenhuijzen GA, Goris RJ. The gut: the 'motor' of multiple organ dysfunction syndrome? Curr Opin Clin Nutr Metab Care. 1999;2:399–404.
121. Lichtman SM. Bacterial [correction of baterial] translocation in humans. J Pediatr Gastroenterol Nutr. 2001;33:1–10.

Pathophysiology of Polytrauma

Theodoros Tosounidis and Peter V. Giannoudis

Contents

5.1	Introduction	33
5.2	Initial Response	34
5.3	Inflammatory Response	34
5.4	Clinical Course and Appropriate Actions	36
5.5	Clinical Course and Immunomarkers	37
References		39

T. Tosounidis
Orthopaedic Trauma Fellow, Leeds General Infirmary, Leeds, UK

P.V. Giannoudis (✉)
Professor of Trauma and Orthopaedic Surgery,
Leeds General Infirmary, Leeds, UK and
A Floor Clarendon Wing, Leeds General Infirmary,
Great George Street, Leeds, LS1 3EX, UK
e-mail: pgiannoudi@aol.com

5.1 Introduction

The pathophysiology of the multiply injured patient is dominated by the rapid onset of a shock state (hypovolemia) and the subsequent effort of the organism to maintain survival and to eventually return to its pre-injury state. Even though there is no international consensus to the definition of polytrauma and the description of shock [1], it is nowadays clear that the homeostastatic mechanisms of the injured patient are activated at multiple levels in an effort to overcome the stress reactions and to preserve the function of vital organs. Due to the advances made in every discipline of medicine, our understanding of the sequence of events that follow severe trauma has greatly expanded.

Traditionally the response to major trauma had been conceptualized as a three phase physiological process being divided into the hypodynamic flow phase, the hyperdynamic flow phase, and the recovery phase to the pre-injury level [2, 3]. This sequence of phases reflected our perception of stress responses through vascular adaptation and circulating volume regulation. Lately, however, it has become clear that the stress response to trauma consists of more composite reactions. Multiple trauma triggers the activation of different pathways, which contribute to the development of the so-called Systemic Inflammatory Response Syndrome (SIRS), while simultaneously as part of the homeostatic mechanisms, a Counter Anti-inflammatory Response Syndrome (CARS) is initiated so that a fine balance of regulatory events could prevail [4, 5]. "Shock generates shock" and the cascade of events that follow a severe injury may be modified from actions and interventions that are irrelevant to the initial injury. The basis of response to injury is conceptualized as an immune mediated phenomenon with systemic implications to the organism. The evolution of Early Total Care (ETC) to Damage Control Orthopaedics (DCO) represents a shift paradigm of treatment based on the understanding of the pathophysiology of the polytrauma patient [6–8].

5.2 Initial Response

The initial injury poses a certain trauma load to the organism. Local tissue destruction (fractures, soft tissue damage), primary organ injury (lung, head), acidosis, hypoxia, and pain perception trigger the activation of local and systematic reactions in order to control hemorrhage and the function of vital organs [9].

Shock due to hemorrhage, hypoxia due to lung injury and low circulatory volume, brain injury, and hypothermia constitute the major threats to patient's survival. During the initial phase of resuscitation attention should be drawn only to life saving procedures and interventions. Classification of the patient into one of the four categories of shock is of paramount importance as it provides a reliable guidance for further action [6, 10]. One should bear in mind that there are specific groups of patients, for instance very young children and athletes, that require special attention. These patients can compensate shock for a prolonged period of time before they rapidly collapse.

Resuscitation begins at the scene of injury and continues in the emergency room. "Scoop and run" policy is the current recommendation for pre-hospital care [11] and aims to secure airway, control major bleeding, and support circulation until the patient arrives at the hospital. In addition to ATLS, standardized lifesaving procedures and protocols have been established over the years assisting the clinicians with the decision making process.

Achieving the end points of resuscitation is an indication that the circulating volume has been restored. These end points include stable hemodynamics, stable oxygen saturation, lactate level less than 2 mmol/L, no coagulation disturbances, normal temperature, urinary output greater than 1 mL/kg/h, and no requirement for inotropic support [6].

If shock remains untreated it will lead to dilutional coagulopathy and the so-called acute coagulopathy of trauma and shock [12, 13]. The latter is probably due to the activation of the protein C pathway and represents an independent parameter that could predict the outcome [14]. The endothelial damage due to systemic inflammation and trauma-induced complementopathy seems also to play a significant role in the development of coagulation disturbances [15]. Almost one-fourth of patients that suffer major trauma develop trauma-induced coagulopathy that is related to hypothermia and acidosis and constitute the "lethal triad" [14, 16]. This triad of symptoms (triangle of death) has been recognized as a significant cause of mortality. Consequently, in order to prevent the lethal triad two factors are essential, early control of bleeding and prevention of further heat loss [17].

The immediate central nervous system response after major trauma is mainly driven by the activation of the neuroendocrine axis. Pain, fear, by-products of metabolism that cross the blood–brain barrier, and brain injury itself are the basic stimuli for the activation of this axis. The hypothalamus and subsequently the sympathetic-adrenal system are activated. In addition, stimuli from aortic and carotid receptors trigger the renin-angiotensin system in an effort to control blood pressure through vasoconstriction and increased heart rate [9, 18]. At the same time the organism enters a reduced metabolic state in order to minimize the energy expenditure [9, 18, 19].

5.3 Inflammatory Response

Nowadays, it is well recognized that major trauma induces an intense immuno-inflammatory response. The magnitude of this response depends on the initial trauma load sustained, pain stimuli, the systemic and local release of pro-inflammatory cytokines, the age, sex, as well as the genetic makeup of the patient. The activation of various cells such as polymorphonuclear leukocytes (PMNL), monocytes, lymphocytes, natural killer (NK), and parenchymal cells leads to dysfunction of the endothelial membrane of almost every vital organ and the development of SIRS [9, 20, 21]. The microenvironment theory describes the interactions between PMNL and endothelial cells facilitated by the expression of adhesion molecules. When firm adhesion is established then the PMNL can extravasate and induce remote organ injury [22]. This injury affects not only the tissues at the site of injury but the endothelium of vital organs and especially the lungs. Activated neutrophils migrate to the site of injury. Vascular endothelial damage and increased endothelial permeability may occur leading to generalized hypoxemia causing further sequestration and priming of neutrophils and macrophages, facilitating activation of the coagulation, complement, and the prostaglandin system [23].

Apart from the aforementioned systemic early innate response, paracrine action of locally produced inflammatory mediators plays a significant role. Prostaglandins and thromboxanes from damaged endothelial membranes, as well as histamine, bradykinin, and kallidin from interstitial mast cells are locally produced and can magnify capillary permeability and local tissue edema. At the same time the cascade of these events can be amplified from the dissemination of these mediators to the peripheral bloodstream [23].

In the early phase, major trauma also triggers the release of signaling molecules called alarmins that mainly play a role in the activation of innate immune response without the presence of a bacterial focus. Alarmins are also chemoattractants and activators of antigen presenting cells (APCs) [24]. They belong to the so-called Damage Associate Molecular Patterns (DAMPS) [25] that include the alarmins and the Pathogen Associated Molecular Patterns (PAMPs). PAMPs represent inflammatory molecules of microbial origin recognized by the immune system as foreign due to their peculiar molecular patterns. Alarmins act as "danger molecules" and are actively secreted from the dead cells in the site of injury and passively released from cells that are in the process of imminent cellular death or apoptosis (Fig. 5.1) [26, 27]. Antibacterial peptides, S100, heat-shock proteins, and high-mobility group box 1 (HMGB1), with the latter being the most important, are some of the molecules included in the family of alarmins [28]. Our knowledge about these molecules has substantiated over the last years and their role in the development of the "aseptic SIRS" and the pathogenesis of Multiple Organ Dysfunction Syndrome (MODS) is under ongoing investigation. In fact blockade of HMGB1 in animal models of trauma has been shown to decrease the inflammatory response and to improve outcomes [29, 30].

Cytokines are polypeptides that are produced from a variety of cells such as monocytes/macrophages and T-helper lymphocytes. Interleukin-1 (IL-1), IL-6, IL-8, IL-10, and Tumor Necrosis Factor (TNF) are cytokines that transmit signals between cells, thus enhancing their communication and playing an important role in the development of SIRS and MODS. In particular, TNF activates cells such as NK-cell and macrophages and induces apoptosis [31]. It leads to thromboxane A2, prostaglandin, selectin, platelet activation factor, and intracellular adhesion molecules production. It exerts its effects via remote and local action. Up to date effective inhibition of TNF has not been successful although blocking it might work in septic patients [32]. Interleukin 1 (IL-1) is another cytokine involved in signaling during major trauma. Its secretion pathway has not been fully understood so far. It induces T-cell and macrophage application and activates a cascade that leads to transcription of many different pro-inflammatory cytokines [23]. Interleukin 6 (IL-6) is the most extensively studied cytokine that is promptly detectable after major trauma (within hours). Its plasma half-life and the consistent pattern of expression have established it as the most widely studied pro-inflammatory molecule [33]. It regulates growth and differentiation of lymphocytes, and activates NK-cells and neutrophils. At the same time it inhibits the apoptosis of neutrophils having therefore a role both as a pro-inflammatory and anti-inflammatory protein [34, 35]. In animal models it has been shown that blockade of IL-6 increases survival [36]. It has also been proved that a certain cut-off of 200 pg/dL could effectively be used as a diagnostic and predictive means of SIRS and later complications in the clinical setting [33]. IL-8 belongs to chemotactic cytokines which are called chemokines and act as chemoattractants. Depending on its concentration gradient IL-8 can acts as an angiogenic factor and a very effective chemmoattractant. It activates the neutrophills as well as lymphocytes, monocytes, endothelial cells, and fibroblasts [37].

The physiologic response to trauma is a multifaceted phenomenon that can be influenced and modified by several different variables. It has been shown to be gender dependent and the role of sex hormones in the course of post-injury immune response is now accepted. In animal models, males and ovariectomised females exhibit a more intense alteration in immune function following hemorrhage after trauma [38]. Furthermore, there is evidence that posttraumatic complications could be influenced by the genetic background (genotype) of each patient [21, 39–41].

Fig. 5.1 Danger sensing mechanisms at trauma. *DAMPs* danger associated molecular patterns, *PAMPs* pathogen associated molecular patterns

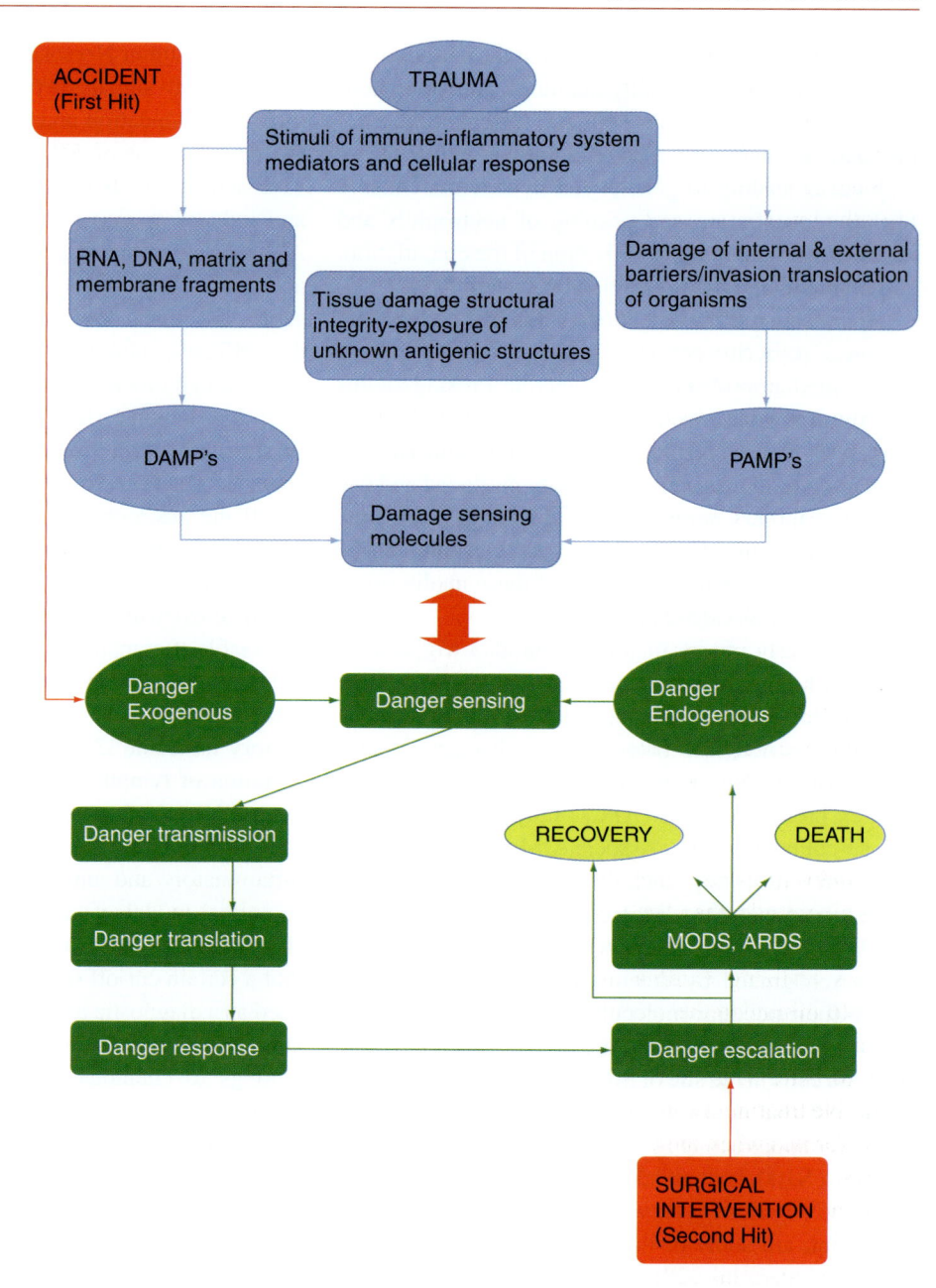

5.4 Clinical Course and Appropriate Actions

The magnitude of the inflammatory response is mainly dependent on the magnitude of the traumatic load during injury. This response (SIRS) can be very intense due to the initial injury (first hit) or can be exaggerated from actions and intervention during treatment (second hit) [42, 43]. Any additional interventional (e.g., massive transfusions) or surgical (e.g., prolonged operations, operations with severe tissue damage) load represents an exogenous hit. Furthermore antigenic load from infections, ischaemia/reperfusion injuries, acidosis, respiratory or cardiovascular distress add an endogenous hit. An uncontrolled inflammatory response may lead to remote organ damage primarily in the lung leading to the development of adult respiratory distress syndrome (ARDS), MODS, and potentially death. At the same time CARS is evolving. If this hypoinflammation is overwhelming, it may lead to immune-suppression that is responsible for the subsequent septic complications [44, 45]. An uneventful clinical course indicates that a fine balance between these extreme reactions of the immune system has prevailed.

Staging of the physiological status of the patient after the initial assessment and life saving procedures dictates the sequence and priorities of any further actions. The patient may be classified in one of four categories: stable, borderline, unstable, and extremis [6, 10]. Stable patients have no immediate life-threatening injuries and do not need inotropic support to become hemodynamically stable. Borderline patients have been stabilized during the initial period but the type of their injuries makes them vulnerable to further rapid deterioration. Unstable patients have not achieved the end points of resuscitation and are hemodynamically unstable. Extremis patients usually suffer from the lethal triad and require inotropic support. These patients are very "sick" and usually they succumb as a result of their injuries. The clinical condition of the patient in any given time reflects a stage in ongoing evolving immune inflammatory reactions. If the magnitude of the initial trauma is well tolerated and physiological markers of stress are not abnormal, early implementation of definite care can be performed with uneventful recovery. If the initial injury is of great magnitude, then hemorrhage control takes priority and temporary stabilization of musculoskeletal injuries utilizing external fixators is performed, in order to minimize the second hit insult and to protect the organism from an exaggerated SIRS, which might lead to ARDS, MODS, or even death. Secondary definitive treatment and reconstruction procedures can be performed when the clinical condition of the patient allows. The rationale behind any intervention is to eliminate the extent of the "second hit" whenever possible [8, 10, 42]. This staged approach minimizes the degree of surgical insult to the patient who is in an unstable equilibrium after major trauma. The management of these patients can be divided into four stages. During the acute phase only the resuscitation and life saving procedures are performed. After the initial resuscitation and during the primary stabilization period major extremity injuries, arterial injuries, and compartment syndromes are managed with DCO. In the secondary period the patient is reassessed constantly and appropriate actions are taken. Major procedures are not justified due to the additional burden that may exert to the already compromised patient's immunological status (second hit). Subsequently, between days 5 and 10 the so-called period of "window of opportunity" definite fracture treatment can be performed [16]. Thereafter, any complex reconstruction procedures can be performed [6] (Fig. 5.2). Although concerns about longer hospital stays and cost implications are still present, this approach has definitely modified the perceptions and daily practice of the Trauma Orthopaedic Surgeons [7].

5.5 Clinical Course and Immunomarkers

From the above described theory of "two" or "multiple hits," it is becoming evident that monitoring the patient's status and clinical course via a scoring system of inflammation would be useful in both guiding our clinical decisions with regard to therapeutic intervention and predicting the possible outcome and complications in the setting of polytrauma. Various attempts have been made and are ongoing to describe the degree of the inflammatory response [46–53].

Immunomonitoring is a term used to describe the value of monitoring the inflammatory markers that are released and can be clinically measured in the setting of polytrauma. The necessity of "immunovigilance" and its possible clinical implications became clearer during the last few years. Until recently we could only draw indirect information regarding the inflammatory status of the patient mainly from clinical markers such as fluid balance [21, 51], lactate, and base deficit [54]. However, as our understanding of the complex mechanisms involved in the immune response after trauma has expanded and as our technical ability to measure various molecular mediators has improved, a new era in documenting the evolving physiological status of the traumatized patient at the molecular level has been established.

The markers of immune reactivity that may have clinical utility are the acute phase reactants (liposaccharide-binding protein, C-reactive protein, precalcitonin), the markers of mediator activity (TNF-a, IL-1, IL-10, IL-6, IL-8), and the markers of cellular activity (Human Leukocyte Antigen) [55]. Whilst the first category has been proven to be nonspecific for trauma, there is evidence that molecules from the other two categories may have some predictive value.

More specifically, TNF-a was one from the first markers that was studied. It has been correlated with

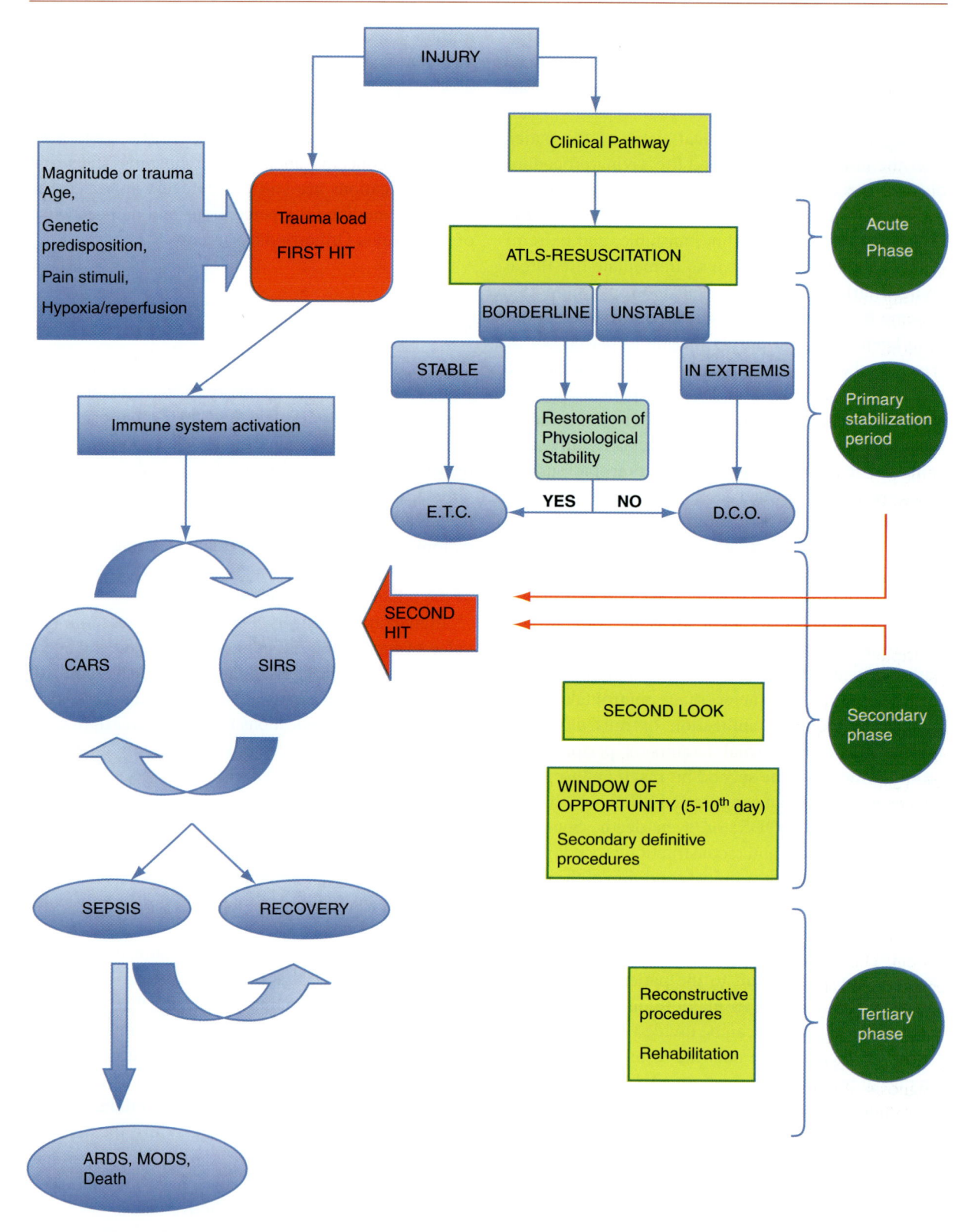

Fig. 5.2 The immune response after trauma, its correlation to clinical status of the patient and the appropriate management in any given phase. *ETC* early total care, *DCO* damage control orthopaedics, *ARDS* adult respiratory distress syndrome, *MODS* multiple organ dysfunction syndrome, *ATLS* advanced trauma life support, *SIRS* systemic inflammatory response syndrome, *CARS* counter anti-inflammatory response syndrome

poorer outcome in multiple traumatized patients in the intensive care unit but nowadays is not considered a reliable predictive index for the clinical course of inflammation in trauma unless sepsis is present [56]. The clinical utility of IL-1 and IL-10 has not been effectively supported so far [21]. The expression of Major Histocompatibility Complex antigens (MHC class II) at the mononuclear cells of the peripheral blood has also been attempted to be associated to morbidity due to sepsis after trauma [57]. Many other circulating molecules have been described as potential predictors of the clinical course including the serum amyloid A, procalcitonin, C3 complement, and haptoglobin [58–60]. It appears that a continuously high level or a second rise in their values is correlated with complications and MODS, respectively [51].

Continuous monitoring is more reliable in the case of the pro-inflammatory cytokines and especially in the case of IL-6. The relatively persistent pattern of expression and the long plasma half-life have established IL-6 as the most clinically useful molecule [33]. High values have been correlated to adverse outcome after early surgery [61, 62]. IL-6 is considered to be of prognostic value for Systemic Inflammatory Response, sepsis, and Multiple Organ Failure [51]. IL-6 and SIRS have been correlated to New Injury Severity Score (NISS) and to each other. A numerical value of 200 pg/dL has been proven to be of diagnostic documentation of a SIRS state [63]. The relatively recent discovery of the alarmins (danger signaling molecules subcategorized as DAMPs and PAMPs) seems to be promising for their use as a predictive marker, but up to date there are no powerful studies to support that. On the other hand, the characterization and quantification of endothelial injury after trauma has been attempted to be correlated with the inflammatory and clinical status of the traumatized patient. The molecules that are released from the injured endothelium and are measurable in plasma are mainly the selectins (L-, P-, E- selectin), the vascular adhesion molecules, the thrombomodulin, and the vW-factor. L-selectin has been shown to be positively related to the prognosis of potential complication after major trauma but definite conclusion can be drawn as yet [64].

Finally, the completion of the human genome project has open other avenues in the clinical setting for the investigation of the genetic makeup of the patient and how this could influence the physiological responses and outcome [65]. Currently there is evidence to support the involvement of various polymorphic variants of genes in determining the post-traumatic course [66]. Although such as approach appears to be promising, results from different studies have not been reproducible because of the ethnic admixture, variable linkage disequilibrium, and genotype misclassification [66–68]. Further studies in the future would provide more evidence about the contribution of genes in determining the clinical outcome of patients.

References

1. Butcher N, Balogh ZJ. The definition of polytrauma: the need for international consensus. Injury. 2009;40 Suppl 4:S12–22.
2. Giannoudis PV, Dinopoulos H, Chalidis B, Hall GM. Surgical stress response. Injury. 2006;37 Suppl 5:S3–9.
3. Smith RM, Giannoudis PV. Trauma and the immune response. J R Soc Med. 1998;91:417–20.
4. Aosasa S, Ono S, Mochizuki H, et al. Activation of monocytes and endothelial cells depends on the severity of surgical stress. World J Surg. 2000;24:10–6.
5. Ono S, Aosasa S, Tsujimoto H, et al. Increased monocyte activation in elderly patients after surgical stress. Eur Surg Res. 2001;33:33–8.
6. Giannoudis PV. Surgical priorities in damage control in polytrauma. J Bone Joint Surg Br. 2003;85:478–83.
7. Giannoudis PV, Giannoudi M, Stavlas P. Damage control orthopaedics: lessons learned. Injury. 2009;40 Suppl 4:S47–52.
8. Roberts CS, Pape HC, Jones AL, et al. Damage control orthopaedics: evolving concepts in the treatment of patients who have sustained orthopaedic trauma. Instr Course Lect. 2005;54:447–62.
9. Keel M, Trentz O. Pathophysiology of polytrauma. Injury. 2005;36:691–709.
10. Pape HC, Tornetta III P, Tarkin I, et al. Timing of fracture fixation in multitrauma patients: the role of early total care and damage control surgery. J Am Acad Orthop Surg. 2009;17:541–9.
11. Smith RM, Conn AK. Prehospital care – scoop and run or stay and play? Injury. 2009;40 Suppl 4:S23–6.
12. Cosgriff N, Moore EE, Sauaia A, et al. Predicting life-threatening coagulopathy in the massively transfused trauma patient: hypothermia and acidoses revisited. J Trauma. 1997;42:857–61; discussion 61–62.
13. Siegel JH, Rivkind AI, Dalal S, Goodarzi S. Early physiologic predictors of injury severity and death in blunt multiple trauma. Arch Surg. 1990;125:498–508.
14. Brohi K, Singh J, Heron M, Coats T. Acute traumatic coagulopathy. J Trauma. 2003;54:1127–30.
15. Gebhard F, Huber-Lang M. Polytrauma – pathophysiology and management principles. Langenbecks Arch Surg. 2008; 393:825–31.
16. Stahel PF, Heyde CE, Wyrwich W, Ertel W. Current concepts of polytrauma management: from ATLS to "damage control". Orthopade. 2005;34:823–36.
17. Cirocchi R, Abraha I, Montedori A, et al. Damage control surgery for abdominal trauma. Cochrane Database Syst Rev. 2010;1:CD007438.
18. Hill AG, Hill GL. Metabolic response to severe injury. Br J Surg. 1998;85:884–90.

19. Plank LD, Hill GL. Sequential metabolic changes following induction of systemic inflammatory response in patients with severe sepsis or major blunt trauma. World J Surg. 2000;24:630–8.
20. Cipolle MD, Pasquale MD, Cerra FB. Secondary organ dysfunction. From clinical perspectives to molecular mediators. Crit Care Clin. 1993;9:261–98.
21. Giannoudis PV. Current concepts of the inflammatory response after major trauma: an update. Injury. 2003;34:397–404.
22. Hietbrink F, Koenderman L, Rijkers G, Leenen L. Trauma: the role of the innate immune system. World J Emerg Surg. 2006;1:15.
23. Lenz A, Franklin GA, Cheadle WG. Systemic inflammation after trauma. Injury. 2007;38:1336–45.
24. Oppenheim JJ, Yang D. Alarmins: chemotactic activators of immune responses. Curr Opin Immunol. 2005;17:359–65.
25. Bianchi ME. DAMPs, PAMPs and alarmins: all we need to know about danger. J Leukoc Biol. 2007;81:1–5.
26. El Mezayen R, El Gazzar M, Seeds MC, et al. Endogenous signals released from necrotic cells augment inflammatory responses to bacterial endotoxin. Immunol Lett. 2007;111:36–44.
27. Raucci A, Palumbo R, Bianchi ME. HMGB1: a signal of necrosis. Autoimmunity. 2007;40:285–9.
28. Pugin J. Dear SIRS, the concept of "alarmins" makes a lot of sense! Intensive Care Med. 2008;34:218–21.
29. Levy RM, Mollen KP, Prince JM, et al. Systemic inflammation and remote organ injury following trauma require HMGB1. Am J Physiol Regul Integr Comp Physiol. 2007;293:R1538–44.
30. Sawa H, Ueda T, Takeyama Y, et al. Blockade of high mobility group box-1 protein attenuates experimental severe acute pancreatitis. World J Gastroenterol. 2006;12:7666–70.
31. DeLong Jr WG, Born CT. Cytokines in patients with polytrauma. Clin Orthop Relat Res. 2004;422:57–65.
32. Abraham E. Why immunomodulatory therapies have not worked in sepsis. Intensive Care Med. 1999;25:556–66.
33. Giannoudis PV, Harwood PJ, Loughenbury P, et al. Correlation between IL-6 levels and the systemic inflammatory response score: can an IL-6 cutoff predict a SIRS state? J Trauma. 2008;65:646–52.
34. Lin E, Calvano SE, Lowry SF. Inflammatory cytokines and cell response in surgery. Surgery. 2000;127:117–26.
35. Xing Z, Gauldie J, Cox G, et al. IL-6 is an antiinflammatory cytokine required for controlling local or systemic acute inflammatory responses. J Clin Invest. 1998;101:311–20.
36. Riedemann NC, Neff TA, Guo RF, et al. Protective effects of IL-6 blockade in sepsis are linked to reduced C5a receptor expression. J Immunol. 2003;170:503–7.
37. Keane MP, Strieter RM. Chemokine signaling in inflammation. Crit Care Med. 2000;28:N13–26.
38. Choudhry MA, Bland KI, Chaudry IH. Trauma and immune response – effect of gender differences. Injury. 2007;38:1382–91.
39. Bogner V, Kirchhoff C, Baker HV, et al. Gene expression profiles are influenced by ISS, MOF, and clinical outcome in multiple injured patients: a genome-wide comparative analysis. Langenbecks Arch Surg. 2007;392:255–65.
40. Gundersen Y, Vaagenes P, Thrane I, et al. Response of circulating immune cells to major gunshot injury, haemorrhage, and acute surgery. Injury. 2005;36:949–55.
41. Liese AM, Siddiqi MQ, Siegel JH, et al. Attenuated monocyte IL-10 production in glucose-6-phosphate dehydrogenase-deficient trauma patients. Shock. 2002;18:18–23.
42. Giannoudis PV, Smith RM, Bellamy MC, et al. Stimulation of the inflammatory system by reamed and unreamed nailing of femoral fractures. An analysis of the second hit. J Bone Joint Surg Br. 1999;81:356–61.
43. Morley JR, Smith RM, Pape HC, et al. Stimulation of the local femoral inflammatory response to fracture and intramedullary reaming: a preliminary study of the source of the second hit phenomenon. J Bone Joint Surg Br. 2008;90:393–9.
44. Bone RC. Sir Isaac Newton, sepsis, SIRS, and CARS. Crit Care Med. 1996;24:1125–8.
45. Schroder O, Laun RA, Held B, et al. Association of interleukin-10 promoter polymorphism with the incidence of multiple organ dysfunction following major trauma: results of a prospective pilot study. Shock. 2004;21:306–10.
46. Bochicchio GV, Napolitano LM, Joshi M, et al. Systemic inflammatory response syndrome score at admission independently predicts infection in blunt trauma patients. J Trauma. 2001;50:817–20.
47. Donnelly SC, MacGregor I, Zamani A, et al. Plasma elastase levels and the development of the adult respiratory distress syndrome. Am J Respir Crit Care Med. 1995;151:1428–33.
48. Giannoudis PV, Smith RM, Windsor AC, et al. Monocyte human leukocyte antigen-DR expression correlates with intrapulmonary shunting after major trauma. Am J Surg. 1999;177:454–9.
49. Harwood PJ, Giannoudis PV, van Griensven M, et al. Alterations in the systemic inflammatory response after early total care and damage control procedures for femoral shaft fracture in severely injured patients. J Trauma. 2005;58:446–52; discussion 52–54.
50. Nast-Kolb D, Waydhas C, Gippner-Steppert C, et al. Indicators of the posttraumatic inflammatory response correlate with organ failure in patients with multiple injuries. J Trauma. 1997;42:446–54; discussion 54–55.
51. Pape HC, Tsukamoto T, Kobbe P, et al. Assessment of the clinical course with inflammatory parameters. Injury. 2007;38:1358–64.
52. Partrick DA, Moore EE, Moore FA, et al. Release of anti-inflammatory mediators after major torso trauma correlates with the development of postinjury multiple organ failure. Am J Surg. 1999;178:564–9.
53. Wanner GA, Keel M, Steckholzer U, et al. Relationship between procalcitonin plasma levels and severity of injury, sepsis, organ failure, and mortality in injured patients. Crit Care Med. 2000;28:950–7.
54. Rossaint R, Cerny V, Coats TJ, et al. Key issues in advanced bleeding care in trauma. Shock. 2006;26:322–31.
55. Sears BW, Stover MD, Callaci J. Pathoanatomy and clinical correlates of the immunoinflammatory response following orthopaedic trauma. J Am Acad Orthop Surg. 2009;17:255–65.
56. Riche F, Panis Y, Laisne MJ, et al. High tumor necrosis factor serum level is associated with increased survival in patients with abdominal septic shock: a prospective study in 59 patients. Surgery. 1996;120:801–7.
57. Ayala A, Ertel W, Chaudry IH. Trauma-induced suppression of antigen presentation and expression of major histocompatibility class II antigen complex in leukocytes. Shock. 1996;5:79–90.

58. Casl MT, Coen D, Simic D. Serum amyloid A protein in the prediction of postburn complications and fatal outcome in patients with severe burns. Eur J Clin Chem Clin Biochem. 1996;34:31–5.
59. Dehne MG, Sablotzki A, Hoffmann A, et al. Alterations of acute phase reaction and cytokine production in patients following severe burn injury. Burns. 2002;28:535–42.
60. Spies M, Wolf SE, Barrow RE, et al. Modulation of types I and II acute phase reactants with insulin-like growth factor-1/binding protein-3 complex in severely burned children. Crit Care Med. 2002;30:83–8.
61. Guillou PJ. Biological variation in the development of sepsis after surgery or trauma. Lancet. 1993;342:217–20.
62. Pape HC, van Griensven M, Rice J, et al. Major secondary surgery in blunt trauma patients and perioperative cytokine liberation: determination of the clinical relevance of biochemical markers. J Trauma. 2001;50:989–1000.
63. Barber RC, Chang LY, Purdue GF, et al. Detecting genetic predisposition for complicated clinical outcomes after burn injury. Burns. 2006;32:821–7.
64. Giannoudis PV, Tosounidis TI, Kanakaris NK, Kontakis G. Quantification and characterisation of endothelial injury after trauma. Injury. 2007;38:1373–81.
65. Hildebrand F, Pape HC, van Griensven M, et al. Genetic predisposition for a compromised immune system after multiple trauma. Shock. 2005;24:518–22.
66. Giannoudis PV, van Griensven M, Tsiridis E, Pape HC. The genetic predisposition to adverse outcome after trauma. J Bone Joint Surg Br. 2007;89:1273–9.
67. Abraham E. Host defense abnormalities after hemorrhage, trauma, and burns. Crit Care Med. 1989;17:934–9.
68. Nadel S. Helping to understand studies examining genetic susceptibility to sepsis. Clin Exp Immunol. 2002;127:191–2.

Head Injuries: Neurosurgical and Orthopaedic Strategies

Michael A. Flierl, Kathryn M. Beauchamp, and Philip F. Stahel

Contents

6.1	Pathophysiology of TBI	43
6.2	Clinical Assessment of TBI	44
6.3	Strategies of Fracture Fixation in TBI Patients	45
6.4	Conclusion	47
References		47

M.A. Flierl
Department of Orthopaedic Surgery,
Denver Health Medical Center,
University of Colorado Denver School of Medicine,
777 Bannock Street, Denver, CO 80204, USA

K.M. Beauchamp
Department of Neurosurgery, Denver Health Medical Center,
University of Colorado Denver School of Medicine,
777 Bannock Street, Denver, CO 80204, USA

P.F. Stahel (✉)
Department of Orthopaedic Surgery and Department of Neurosurgery, Denver Health Medical Center,
University of Colorado Denver School of Medicine,
777 Bannock Street, Denver, CO 80204, USA
e-mail: philip.stahel@dhha.org

6.1 Pathophysiology of TBI

Despite modern intensive care strategies, the clinical outcome of severely head-injured patients remains poor [1–3]. The high mortality rates in this patient population are often attributed to the development of secondary insults to the injured brain [4–6]. While *primary brain injury* is a result of the mechanical forces applied to the skull at the time of impact, *secondary brain injury* evolves over time and thus cannot be detected on initial CT imaging studies [7, 8]. Evidence of secondary brain injury has been found on autopsy in 70–90% of all fatally head-injured patients [7, 9]. Secondary brain injury is initiated by a trauma-induced, host-mediated inflammatory response within the intracranial compartment [10–14], and is aggravated by hypoxia, metabolic acidosis, cerebral fat emboli from the fracture site, injury-triggered activation of the coagulation system, and development of cerebral edema [9, 15–19].

The immuno-patho physiological sequelae of Traumatic Brain Injury (TBI) are highly complex, and involve numerous brain-derived pro-inflammatory mediators, such as cytokines, chemokines, complement anaphylatoxins, excitatory molecules, electrolyte disturbances, and blood-derived leukocytes which are migrating across the blood–brain barrier [11, 20–24]. The resulting complex neuro-inflammatory network leads to a pro-inflammatory environment with brain edema and brain tissue destruction by leukocyte-released proteases, lipases, and reactive oxygen species. In addition, these events culminate in the breakdown of the blood–brain barrier and allow neurotoxic circulating molecules to enter the brain. As a result, the traumatized brain is highly susceptible to secondary injuries caused by intracerebral inflammation, as well as systemic neurotoxic molecules, which are normally "blocked" under physiological conditions (Fig. 6.1).

H.-C. Pape et al. (eds.), *The Poly-Traumatized Patient with Fractures*,
DOI: 10.1007/978-3-642-17986-0_6, © Springer-Verlag Berlin Heidelberg 2011

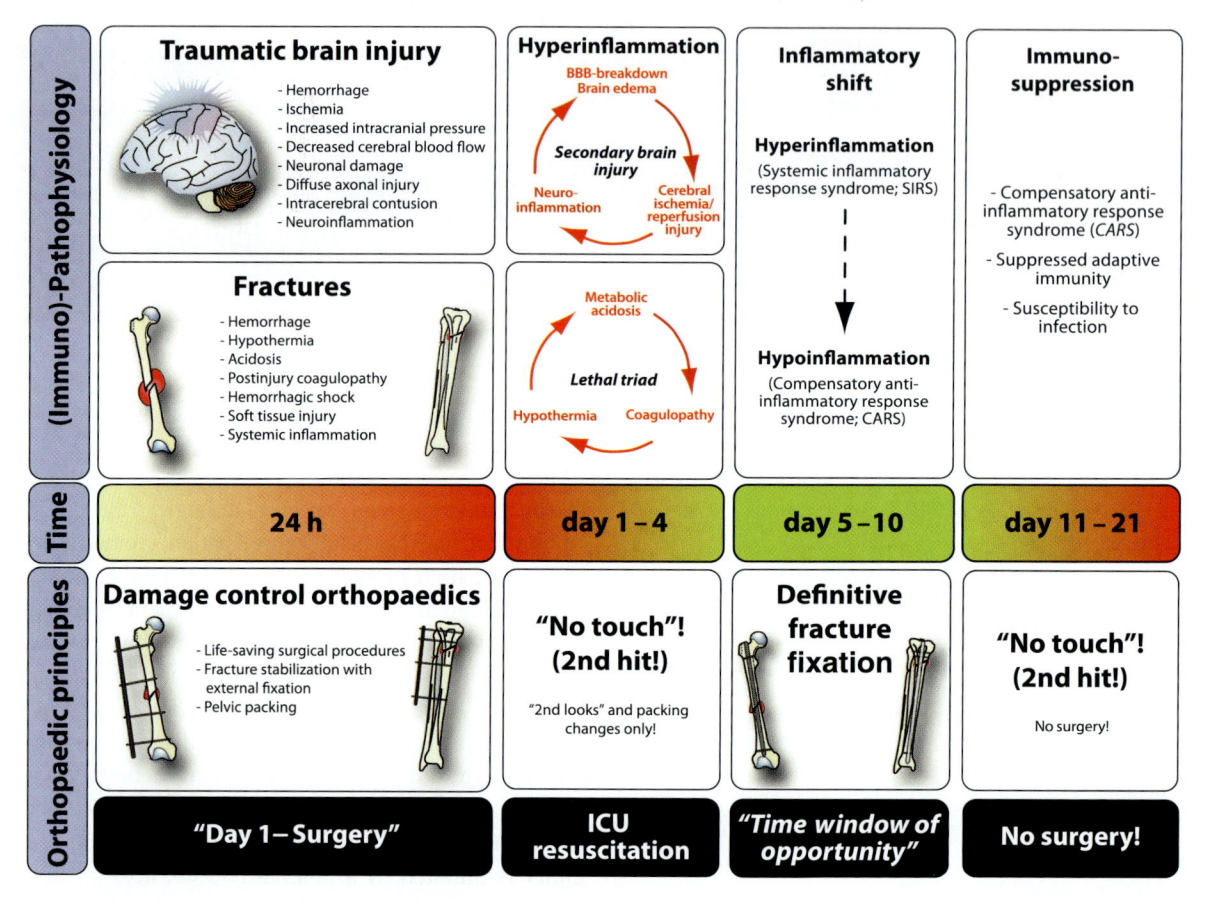

Fig. 6.1 Schematic of priorities in the management of associated orthopedic injuries in patients with severe head injuries, based on the understanding of the underlying immunological pathophysiology

In TBI patients who have sustained concomitant major trauma to the musculoskeletal system, a profound *systemic* inflammatory response is also triggered in parallel, involving cytokines/chemokines, complement activation products, the coagulation system, stress hormones, neuronal signaling, and numerous inflammatory cells [25–30]. To date, we have an incomplete understanding of how the cerebral and systemic inflammatory responses interact and inter-communicate with each other, and whether there is "spill-over" from the intracerebral into the systemic "compartment" and vice versa, exacerbating the inflammatory response.

Consequently, the treating surgeon must be aware of the neuropathology of TBI as well as the systemic inflammatory events when deciding on the optimal management approach in this vulnerable patient population, as inappropriate treatment may result in an iatrogenic secondary insult to the brain [14, 31].

6.2 Clinical Assessment of TBI

On hospital admission, all head-injured patients are systemically assessed and resuscitated according to the American College of Surgeons' *Advanced Trauma Life Support* (ATLS®) protocol. Closed head injury is typically diagnosed by (1) the history of trauma, (2) the clinical status, and (3) computed tomography (CT) scan. The neurologic status is assessed after stabilization of vital functions [17]. The level of consciousness is rapidly evaluated by the Glasgow Coma Scale

(GCS), which grades the severity of TBI as mild (GCS 14/15), moderate (GCS 9–13), and severe (GCS 3–8) [17]. The post-resuscitation GCS score is of clinical importance due to the significant correlation with patient outcome [32]. A head CT should be obtained under the following circumstances: (1) altered level of consciousness with GCS <14 (moderate or severe brain injury), (2) abnormal neurological status, (3) differences in pupil size or reactivity, (4) suspected skull fracture, (5) intoxicated patients. The CT should be repeated whenever the patient's neurologic status deteriorates [17]. During the initial management of TBI, hypoxemia, hypotension, hypercarbia, and hypoglycemia must be avoided or rapidly corrected to minimize the development of secondary brain damage [17]. Hemodynamic stability should be maintained using an isotonic electrolyte solution [33]. Maintenance of an adequate cerebral perfusion pressure (CPP=mean arterial pressure [MAP] – intracranial pressure [ICP]) above 70–80 mmHg is recommended in the early phase post trauma [17, 34, 35]. Cerebral edema should be rapidly addressed using osmotic drugs, and intracranial volume may be reduced by draining cerebrospinal fluid (CSF) via intra-ventricular catheters, or surgical hematoma evacuation.

Augmentation of the intravascular volume with osmotic therapeutics, such as mannitol, results in a transient increase in MAP and CPP and induces cerebral vasoconstriction, reducing the intracranial volume [17]. Osmotic therapy using mannitol or hypertonic saline is currently recommended if the patient displays clinical signs of trans-tentorial herniation, progressive neurological deterioration, or bilaterally dilated and nonreactive pupils [17]. Results of the Corticosteroid Randomization after Significant Head Injury (CRASH) trial have made the use of gluco-corticoids obsolete and contrast indicated in severely head-injured patients [36, 37].

Intra-ventricular catheters are used to monitor intracranial pressures and allow CSF drainage to decrease the ICP [35]. Current guidelines recommend continuous ICP monitoring in patients (1) with *severe* head injury (GCS<9) and abnormal admission CT scan; (2) with *severe* head injury (GCS<9) and normal initial CT scan, but with a prolonged coma >6 h; (3) requiring evacuation of intracranial hematomas; (4) with neurological deterioration (GCS<9) in patients with initially mild or moderate head injury; and (5) head-injured patients requiring prolonged mechanical ventilation, unless the initial CT scan is normal [17, 34, 38, 39].

Craniotomy with evacuation of intracranial mass lesion must be undertaken as soon as possible in patients with clinically relevant and surgically accessible hematomas [92]. Elevated intracranial pressure is one of the most common causes of death and disability in the severely brain-injured patient. When intracranial hypertension is refractory to medical treatment, many patients undergo decompressive craniectomy. However, the indication, timing, and method of decompressive craniectomy are not well defined [40, 41]. Recent literature suggests that hinge craniectomy achieves similar outcomes with respect to ICP control and early outcomes when compared to standard decompressive craniectomy [40]. An additional benefit of this modality is that patients will not have to undergo a delayed cranioplasty for skull defect closure.

6.3 Strategies of Fracture Fixation in TBI Patients

Choosing the ideal timing and modality of fracture fixation in head-injured patients is of paramount importance to avoid a detrimental "second hit" injury to the brain [14, 42]. However, selecting a "safe" treatment modality of the multiply injured patient with concomitant TBI can be difficult.

The initial assessment and management of any trauma patient with TBI should follow the ATLS® algorithm [25, 43]. Hypoxemia and hypotension, the "lethal duo of TBI" [44], need to be avoided at all times, as both will exacerbate post-traumatic edema with potentially detrimental consequences [33]. Adequate oxygenation, appropriate fluid resuscitation, and maintenance of the CCP above 70 mmHg are of paramount importance [33, 45].

To best achieve these goals in multiply injured patients with TBI, modern ventilation strategies and damage control resuscitation principles have been developed, aiming to avoid overly aggressive fluid management exacerbating cerebral edema, respectively [46–50]. Glucose-containing crystalloid fluids should be avoided in TBI patients, as hyperglycemia induces local acidosis and oxidative stress, promotes edema formation, impairs nitric oxide-mediated vasodilation, and

10. Baethmann A, Lehr D, Wirth A. Prospective analysis of patient management in severe head injury. Acta Neurochir Suppl. 1998;71:107–10.
11. Ghirnikar RS, Lee YL, Eng LF. Inflammation in traumatic brain injury: role of cytokines and chemokines. Neurochem Res. 1998;23:329–40.
12. Morganti-Kossman MC, Rancan M, Stahel P, et al. Inflammatory responses to traumatic brain injury: an overview for the new millennium. In: Rothwell NJ, Loddick S, editors. Immune and inflammatory responses in the nervous system. 2nd ed. Oxford: Oxford University Press; 2002. pp. 106–26.
13. Neugebauer E, Hensler T, Rose S, et al. Severe craniocerebral trauma in multiple trauma. An assessment of the interaction of local and systemic mediator responses. Unfallchirurg. 2000;103:122–31.
14. Elf K, Nilsson P, Enblad P. Prevention of secondary insults in neurointensive care of traumatic brain injury. Eur J Trauma. 2003;29:74–80.
15. Golding EM. Sequelae following traumatic brain injury. The cerebrovascular perspective. Brain Res Brain Res Rev. 2002;38:377–88.
16. Rosomoff HL, Kochanek PM, Clark R, et al. Resuscitation from severe brain trauma. Crit Care Med. 1996;24:S48–56.
17. Stahel PF, Smith WR. Closed head injury. In: Bland KI, Büchler MW, Csendes A, et al., editors. General surgery: principles and international practice. 2nd ed. London: Springer; 2009. p. 131–42.
18. Jeremitsky E, Omert L, Dunham CM, et al. Harbingers of poor outcome the day after severe brain injury: hypothermia, hypoxia, and hypoperfusion. J Trauma. 2003;54:312–9.
19. Wu XH, Shi XY, Gan JX, et al. Dynamically monitoring tissue factor and tissue factor pathway inhibitor following secondary brain injury. Chin J Traumatol. 2003;6:114–7.
20. Ransohoff RM. Chemokines in neurological trauma models. Ann NY Acad Sci. 2002;961:346–9.
21. Ransohoff RM. The chemokine system in neuroinflammation: an update. J Infect Dis. 2002;186 Suppl 2:S152–6.
22. Stahel PF, Morganti-Kossmann MC, Kossmann T. The role of the complement system in traumatic brain injury. Brain Res Rev. 1998;27:243–56.
23. Zhuang J, Shackford SR, Schmoker JD, et al. The association of leukocytes with secondary brain injury. J Trauma. 1993;35:415–22.
24. Schoettle RJ, Kochanek PM, Magargee MJ, et al. Early polymorphonuclear leukocyte accumulation correlates with the development of posttraumatic cerebral edema in rats. J Neurotrauma. 1990;7:207–17.
25. Gebhard F, Huber-Lang M. Polytrauma-pathophysiology and management principles. Langenbecks Arch Surg. 2008; 393(6):825–31.
26. Stahel PF, Smith WR, Moore EE. Role of biological modifiers regulating the immune response after trauma. Injury. 2007;38:1409–22.
27. Woolf PD. Hormonal responses to trauma. Crit Care Med. 1992;20:216–26.
28. Tracey KJ. The inflammatory reflex. Nature. 2002;420: 853–9.
29. Tracey KJ, Czura CJ, Ivanova S. Mind over immunity. FASEB J. 2001;15:1575–6.
30. Arand M, Melzner H, Kinzl L, et al. Early inflammatory mediator response following isolated traumatic brain injury and other major trauma in humans. Langenbecks Arch Surg. 2001;386:241–8.
31. Grotz MR, Giannoudis PV, Pape HC, et al. Traumatic brain injury and stabilisation of long bone fractures: an update. Injury. 2004;35:1077–86.
32. Davis DP, Serrano JA, Vilke GM, et al. The predictive value of field versus arrival Glasgow Coma Scale score and TRISS calculations in moderate-to-severe traumatic brain injury. J Trauma. 2006;60:985–90.
33. Bratton SL, Chestnut RM, Ghajar J, et al. Guidelines for the management of severe traumatic brain injury. I. Blood pressure and oxygenation. J Neurotrauma. 2007;24 Suppl 1: S7–13.
34. Bratton SL, Chestnut RM, Ghajar J, et al. Guidelines for the management of severe traumatic brain injury. VIII. Intracranial pressure thresholds. J Neurotrauma. 2007;24 Suppl 1:S55–8.
35. Bratton SL, Chestnut RM, Ghajar J, et al. Guidelines for the management of severe traumatic brain injury. VI. Indications for intracranial pressure monitoring. J Neurotrauma. 2007;24 Suppl 1:S37–44.
36. Edwards P, Arango M, Balica L, et al. Final results of MRC CRASH, a randomised placebo-controlled trial of intravenous corticosteroid in adults with head injury-outcomes at 6 months. Lancet. 2005;365:1957–9.
37. Roberts I, Yates D, Sandercock P, et al. Effect of intravenous corticosteroids on death within 14 days in 10008 adults with clinically significant head injury (MRC CRASH trial): randomised placebo-controlled trial. Lancet. 2004;364: 1321–8.
38. Bratton SL, Chestnut RM, Ghajar J, et al. Guidelines for the management of severe traumatic brain injury. IX. Cerebral perfusion thresholds. J Neurotrauma. 2007;24 Suppl 1: S59–64.
39. Bratton SL, Chestnut RM, Ghajar J, et al. Guidelines for the management of severe traumatic brain injury. VII. Intracranial pressure monitoring technology. J Neurotrauma. 2007;24 Suppl 1:S45–54.
40. Kenning TJ, Gandhi RH, German JW. A comparison of hinge craniotomy and decompressive craniectomy for the treatment of malignant intracranial hypertension: early clinical and radiographic analysis. Neurosurg Focus. 2009; 26:E6.
41. Paci GM, Sise MJ, Sise CB, et al. Preemptive craniectomy with craniotomy: what role in the management of severe traumatic brain injury? J Trauma. 2009;67:531–6.
42. Leker RR, Shohami E. Cerebral ischemia and trauma-different etiologies yet similar mechanisms: neuroprotective opportunities. Brain Res Rev. 2002;39:55–73.
43. Stahel PF, Smith WR, Moore EE. Current trends in resuscitation strategy for the multiply injured patient. Injury. 2009;40 Suppl 4:S27–35.
44. Stahel PF, Smith WR, Moore EE. Hypoxia and hypotension, the "lethal duo" in traumatic brain injury: implications for prehospital care. Intensive Care Med. 2008;34:402–4.
45. Stiefel MF, Udoetuk JD, Storm PB, et al. Brain tissue oxygen monitoring in pediatric patients with severe traumatic brain injury. J Neurosurg. 2006;105:281–6.

46. Sagraves SG, Toschlog EA, Rotondo MF. Damage control surgery – the intensivist's role. J Intensive Care Med. 2006;21:5–16.
47. Spinella PC, Priestley MA. Damage control mechanical ventilation: ventilator induced lung injury and lung protective strategies in children. J Trauma. 2007;62:S82–3.
48. Holcomb JB. Damage control resuscitation. J Trauma. 2007;62:S36–7.
49. Holcomb JB, Jenkins D, Rhee P, et al. Damage control resuscitation: directly addressing the early coagulopathy of trauma. J Trauma. 2007;62:307–10.
50. Spahn DR, Cerny V, Coats TJ, et al. Management of bleeding following major trauma: a European guideline. Crit Care. 2007;11:R17.
51. Diaz-Parejo P, Stahl N, Xu W, et al. Cerebral energy metabolism during transient hyperglycemia in patients with severe brain trauma. Intensive Care Med. 2003;29:544–50.
52. Garg R, Chaudhuri A, Munschauer F, et al. Hyperglycemia, insulin, and acute ischemic stroke: a mechanistic justification for a trial of insulin infusion therapy. Stroke. 2006;37:267–73.
53. Kinoshita K, Kraydieh S, Alonso O, et al. Effect of posttraumatic hyperglycemia on contusion volume and neutrophil accumulation after moderate fluid-percussion brain injury in rats. J Neurotrauma. 2002;19:681–92.
54. Holbein M, Bechir M, Ludwig S, et al. Differential influence of arterial blood glucose on cerebral metabolism following severe traumatic brain injury. Crit Care. 2009;13:R13.
55. Stahel PF, Ertel W, Heyde CE. Traumatic brain injury: impact on timing and modality of fracture care. Orthopade. 2005;34:852–64.
56. Keel M, Trentz O. Pathophysiology of polytrauma. Injury. 2005;36:691–709.
57. Rose S, Marzi I. Mediators in polytrauma – pathophysiological significance and clinical relevance. Langenbecks Arch Surg. 1998;383:199–208.
58. Bone LB, Johnson KD, Weigelt J, et al. Early versus delayed stabilization of femoral fractures. A prospective randomized study. J Bone Joint Surg Am. 1989;71:336–40.
59. Bose D, Tejwani NC. Evolving trends in the care of polytrauma patients. Injury. 2006;37:20–8.
60. Giannoudis PV, Veysi VT, Pape HC, et al. When should we operate on major fractures in patients with severe head injuries? Am J Surg. 2002;183:261–7.
61. Kalb DC, Ney AL, Rodriguez JL, et al. Assessment of the relationship between timing of fixation of the fracture and secondary brain injury in patients with multiple trauma. Surgery. 1998;124:739–44; discussion 744-735.
62. Velmahos GC, Arroyo H, Ramicone E, et al. Timing of fracture fixation in blunt trauma patients with severe head injuries. Am J Surg. 1998;176:324–9; discussion 329–330.
63. Wang MC, Temkin NR, Deyo RA, et al. Timing of surgery after multisystem injury with traumatic brain injury: effect on neuropsychological and functional outcome. J Trauma. 2007;62:1250–8.
64. Bhandari M, Guyatt GH, Khera V, et al. Operative management of lower extremity fractures in patients with head injuries. Clin Orthop Relat Res. 2003;407:187–98.
65. Kotwica Z, Balcewicz L, Jagodzinski Z. Head injuries coexistent with pelvic or lower extremity fractures – early or delayed osteosynthesis. Acta Neurochir (Wien). 1990;102: 19–21.
66. Poole GV, Miller JD, Agnew SG, et al. Lower extremity fracture fixation in head-injured patients. J Trauma. 1992;32:654–9.
67. Reynolds MA, Richardson JD, Spain DA, et al. Is the timing of fracture fixation important for the patient with multiple trauma? Ann Surg. 1995;222:470–8; discussion 478–481.
68. Hofman PA, Goris RJ. Timing of osteosynthesis of major fractures in patients with severe brain injury. J Trauma. 1991;31:261–3.
69. Nau T, Aldrian S, Koenig F, et al. Fixation of femoral fractures in multiple-injury patients with combined chest and head injuries. ANZ J Surg. 2003;73:1018–21.
70. Brundage SI, McGhan R, Jurkovich GJ, et al. Timing of femur fracture fixation: effect on outcome in patients with thoracic and head injuries. J Trauma. 2002;52:299–307.
71. Seibel R, LaDuca J, Hassett JM, et al. Blunt multiple trauma (ISS 36), femur traction, and the pulmonary failure-septic state. Ann Surg. 1985;202:283–95.
72. Johnson KD, Cadambi A, Seibert GB. Incidence of adult respiratory distress syndrome in patients with multiple musculoskeletal injuries: effect of early operative stabilization of fractures. J Trauma. 1985;25:375–84.
73. Charash WE, Fabian TC, Croce MA. Delayed surgical fixation of femur fractures is a risk factor for pulmonary failure independent of thoracic trauma. J Trauma. 1994;37:667–72.
74. Starr AJ. Timing fracture repair in patients with severe brain injury (Glasgow Coma Scale score <9). J Trauma. 1998; 45:980.
75. Stahel PF, Moore EE, Schreier SL, et al. Transfusion strategies in postinjury coagulopathy. Curr Opin Anaesthesiol. 2009;22:289–98.
76. Lehmann U, Rickels E, Krettek C. Multiple trauma with craniocerebral trauma. Early definitive surgical management of long bone fractures? Unfallchirurg. 2001;104:196–209.
77. Mousavi M, Kolonja A, Schaden E, et al. Intracranial pressure-alterations during controlled intramedullary reaming of femoral fractures: an animal study. Injury. 2001;32:679–82.
78. Lehmann U, Reif W, Hobbensiefken G, et al. Effect of primary fracture management on craniocerebral trauma in polytrauma. An animal experiment study. Unfallchirurg. 1995;98:437–41.
79. Anglen JO, Luber K, Park T. The effect of femoral nailing on cerebral perfusion pressure in head-injured patients. J Trauma. 2003;54:1166–70.
80. Townsend RN, Lheureau T, Protech J, et al. Timing fracture repair in patients with severe brain injury (Glasgow Coma Scale score <9). J Trauma. 1998;44:977–82; discussion 982-973.
81. Jaicks RR, Cohn SM, Moller BA. Early fracture fixation may be deleterious after head injury. J Trauma. 1997;42:1–5; discussion 5-6.
82. Forteza AM, Koch S, Romano JG, et al. Transcranial Doppler detection of fat emboli. Stroke. 1999;30:2687–91.
83. Giannoudis PV, Pape HC, Cohen AP, et al. Review: systemic effects of femoral nailing: from Kuntscher to the immune reactivity era. Clin Orthop Relat Res. 2002;404:378–86.
84. Harwood PJ, Giannoudis PV, van Griensven M, et al. Alterations in the systemic inflammatory response after early total care and damage control procedures for femoral

85. Gray AC, White TO, Clutton E, et al. The stress response to bilateral femoral fractures: a comparison of primary intramedullary nailing and external fixation. J Orthop Trauma. 2009;23:90–7; discussion 98–99.
86. Pape HC. Effects of changing strategies of fracture fixation on immunologic changes and systemic complications after multiple trauma: damage control orthopedic surgery. J Orthop Res. 2008;26:1478–84.
87. Pape HC, Rixen D, Morley J, et al. Impact of the method of initial stabilization for femoral shaft fractures in patients with multiple injuries at risk for complications (borderline patients). Ann Surg. 2007;246:491–9; discussion 499–501.
88. Nowotarski PJ, Turen CH, Brumback RJ, et al. Conversion of external fixation to intramedullary nailing for fractures of the shaft of the femur in multiply injured patients. J Bone Joint Surg Am. 2000;82:781–8.
89. Scalea TM. Optimal timing of fracture fixation: have we learned anything in the past 20 years? J Trauma. 2008;65:253–60.
90. Rixen D, Grass G, Sauerland S, et al. Evaluation of criteria for temporary external fixation in risk-adapted damage control orthopedic surgery of femur shaft fractures in multiple trauma patients: "evidence-based medicine" versus "reality" in the trauma registry of the German Trauma Society. J Trauma. 2005;59:1375–94; discussion 1394-1375.
91. Flierl MA, Stoneback JW, Beauchamp KM, et al. Femur shaft fracture fixation in head-injured patients – when is the right time? J Orthop Trauma. 2010;24:107–14.
92. Marinkovic I, Strbian D, Pedrono E, et al. Decompressive craniectomy for intracerebral hemorrhage. Neurosurgery. 2009;65:780–86; 781 p following 786; discussion 786.

(Continued from previous page: shaft fracture in severely injured patients. J Trauma. 2005;58:446–52; discussion 452-444.)

Nerve Injuries in Traumatic Head Injury: When To Explore/Suture/Transplant?

Norbert Pallua and Ahmet Bozkurt

Contents

7.1	Introduction	51
7.2	**General Aspects of Peripheral Lesions**	**52**
7.2.1	Classification of Peripheral Nerve Injuries	52
7.2.2	Principles of Peripheral Nerve Repair	53
7.2.3	Algorithms for Open and Closed Injuries: Timing of Nerve Repairs	55
7.3	**Specific Aspects of Facial Nerve Lesions**	**56**
7.3.1	Anatomy	56
7.3.2	Etiology, Classification, Diagnostic Assessment	58
7.3.3	Non-surgical Management	61
7.3.4	Surgical Management	61
References		**73**

N. Pallua (✉) and A. Bozkurt
Department of Plastic Surgery,
Hand Surgery – Burns Unit, RWTH Aachen
University, Pauwelsstraße 30, 52074 Aachen,
Germany
e-mail: npallua@ukaachen.de; abozkurt77@gmx.de

7.1 Introduction

Fractures in the head region represent a major challenge in the field of reconstructive surgery. Craniofacial injuries may lead to a number of nerve lesions. For example, the abducens nerve may suffer lesions after a transverse fracture of the middle cranial fossa leading to oculomotor palsies [1].

Maxillofacial fractures are mostly observed along facial bone sutures and foramina (i.e., mental, infraorbital and supraorbital). This leads to peripheral trigeminal nerve injuries (e.g., sensory deficit in the face, pain) due to nerve compression caused by displaced bone fragments, soft tissue edema and secondary ischemia, laceration from fracture edges or displaced bone fragments, traction from a displaced fracture, crushing, avulsion, and partial or complete nerve transection. For example, in a recent retrospective study, the most commonly injured nerve was the inferior alveolar nerve caused by a mandibular angle fracture, followed by the mental nerve due to a mandibular parasymphysis fracture, the infraorbital nerve from a zygomaticomaxillary complex fracture, and the lingual as well as the long buccal nerve from a mandibular body fracture [2]. Most frequent surgical procedures are external decompression and neurolysis, as well as end-to end neurorrhaphy and autologous nerve grafting [2].

Temporal bone fractures (Fig. 7.1) following head trauma are a well-known cause of facial nerve paralysis. Approximately 22% of skull fractures are temporal bone fractures [3, 4]. It has been shown that between 25% and 70% of temporal bone fractures are associated with facial nerve paralysis, and that transverse fractures of the petrous portion are more commonly

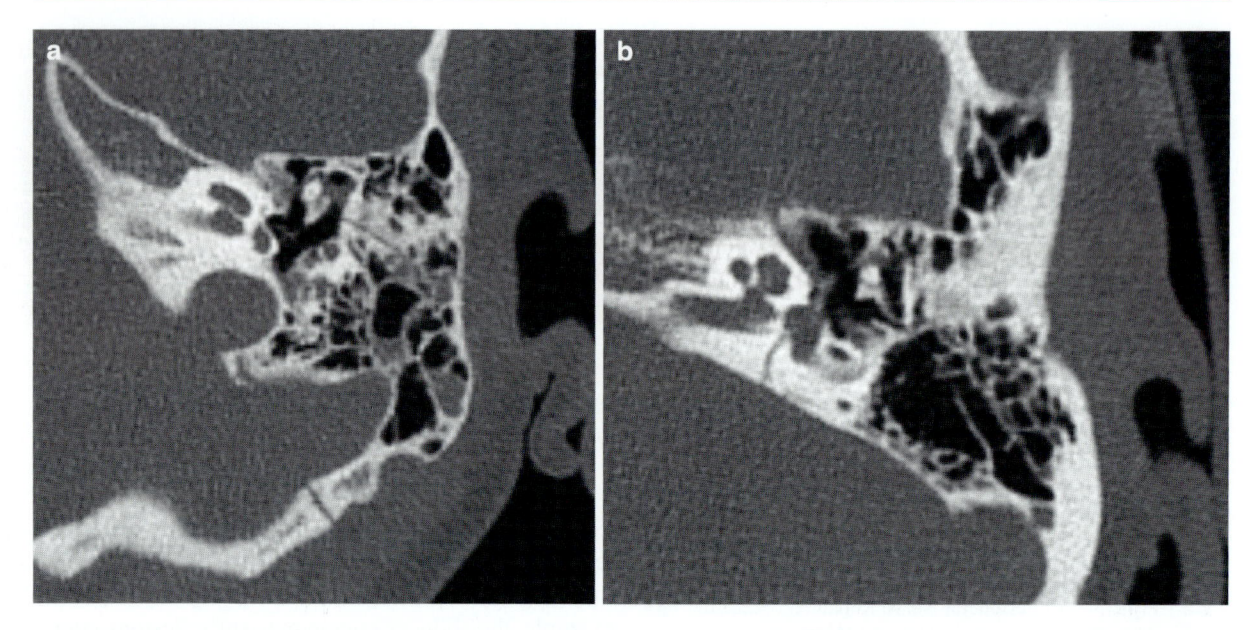

Fig. 7.1 High-resolution computer tomography demonstrating a longitudinal (**a**) and a transverse (**b**) temporal bone fracture (Kindly provided by Prof. Dr. Günther and Dr. Keil, Department of Radiology, RWTH Aachen University Hospital)

associated with facial nerve paralysis although longitudinal fractures are more prevalent [5, 6].

Furthermore, strong posteriorly directed force applied to the mandible can lead to a mandibular fracture followed by displacement of the mandibular condyle toward the external auditory canal or superiorly against the mandibular fossa, causing it to penetrate into the middle cranial fossa or even fracture the temporal bone. High-energy mechanisms, e.g., those due to motor vehicle accidents, are the most common reasons for temporal bone fractures [7].

Since facial nerve paralysis is the most challenging peripheral nerve injury, we describe exemplarily the evaluation and surgical management of posttraumatic facial nerve paralysis in detail. This includes information on *general* aspects which can be applied for the management of other nerve lesions, i.e., (a) classification of peripheral nerve lesions, (b) principles of peripheral nerve repair, (c) algorithms for open and closed injuries (timing of nerve repairs). Subsequent sections deal with *specific* characteristics of facial nerve injuries, i.e., (d) anatomy, (e) etiology, classification, and diagnostic assessment, (f) nonsurgical management, and (g) surgical management.

7.2 General Aspects of Peripheral Lesions

7.2.1 Classification of Peripheral Nerve Injuries

The most prevalent classifications of peripheral nerve lesions can be traced back to Seddon [8] and Sunderland [9]. The classification by Seddon [8] consists of three different types of injuries, i.e., neurapraxia, axonotmesis, and neurotmesis. This classification was further expanded for clinical use by Sunderland [9] to include five separate degrees of injury. Finally, Mackinnon further expanded Sunderland's classification [10] with the addition of a sixth-degree injury. This is a neuroma-in-continuity with a mixed nerve injury, composed of fascicles of varying degrees of nerve injury [11].

The first-degree nerve injury (I) or neurapraxia is a local transient conduction block at the site of trauma, mostly due to compression. In contrast to other nerve injuries, it is characterized by the absence of any degenerative changes (no Wallerian degeneration) without axonal discontinuity, and thus, without a

Tinel's sign. Recovery may vary from a few days to several weeks.

In axonotmesis or second-degree injury (II), axonal disruption with preservation of the endoneurium may be caused by a stretch or crush injury, followed by Wallerian degeneration. The internal architecture of the nerve is completely preserved. The diagnosis of a second-degree injury (II) is made during a period of several weeks or months. A Tinel's sign will be detectable, which will advance along the course of the nerve according to the rate of regenerating axons by 1–3 mm/day. This is important for clinical decision making. In the management of a closed injury, a patient who recovers within 3 months is diagnosed retrospectively with a neurapraxia, whereas a patient with an advancing Tinel's sign, whose gradual progression of recovery advances to complete, is diagnosed with an axonotmetic injury. However, if the recovery is not complete but demonstrates the characteristics of axonotmesis, a third-degree injury (III) is present. As one can see from these clinical scenarios, significant time may elapse before neurapraxia, second- and third-degree injuries, and (see below) fourth- and fifth-degree injuries can be distinguished.

A third-degree injury (III) is also axonotmetic, but in addition to the second-degree injury (II), also involves a disruption of the endoneurial sheath. Fascicles remain grossly intact, but mismatch of fibers from proximal to distal can occur. Some of the fibers fail to progress from proximal to distal and may form a disorganized conglomeration of nerve fibers and scar tissue within the perineurium (i.e., the endoneurial sheaths). Clinical recovery depends on the degree of intrafascicular scarring and the fascicular topography at the site of injury. Nerve conduction studies are not always discriminating as the electrical activity of only few axons can give a false-positive impression of effective regeneration. Furthermore, topographic mismatch can inhibit successful clinical recovery. Therefore, microsurgical repair offers a poorer outcome than spontaneous recovery of a third-degree lesion. This is especially important regarding the change in nerve fiber topography over the proximal course of the facial nerve (e.g., fibers to the stapedius, chorda tympani, motor fibers to the facial muscles of the eye, midface, forehead, lower face, lower lip). The more proximal the lesion is, the higher the likelihood of syn- and dyskinesis [12] (see below).

A fourth-degree injury (IV) is equivalent to a neurotmesis with anatomic continuity characterized by an intact epineurium, but with complete disruption of subepineurial layers and replacement with scar formations. At the site of injury a neuroma is formed; a Tinel sign is detectable, but without progress from proximal to distal. A lengthy period of observation is required for reliable diagnosis, but a surgical intervention with scar excision and microsurgical repair is usually required. A fifth-degree injury (V) or neurotmesis without anatomic continuity is a complete transection of the nerve. Spontaneous recovery is not possible.

7.2.2 Principles of Peripheral Nerve Repair

There are a variety of circumstances and variables which influence the outcome of a nerve reconstruction. This includes (a) the timing of repair, (b) the level of injury, (c) the type of the nerve lesion, (d) general and specific comorbidities, (e) the fascicular anatomy of the injury, (f) the surgeon's experience, skills, and strategy, and (g) the appropriate equipment, such as an operating microscope with proper magnification or surgical loupe, instrumentation, and microsutures (8–0 to 11–0 nylon sutures) [11].

The field of peripheral nerve surgery progressed greatly with the introduction of microsurgery and the early works of Millesi and coworkers [13], who propagated tension-free repair ideas regarding nerve grafting techniques [14]. Since then, the central dogma of peripheral nerve surgery is a tension-free coaptation of nerve to nerve (end-to-end neurorrhaphy) or nerve to graft. Tension will invariably lead to an increased and detrimental fibrotic reaction at the coaptation site and ischemia. End-to-end nerve coaptation is commonly performed with 10–0 monofilament in an epineurial (Fig. 7.2) or perineural (fascicular) fashion [15, 16].

Neurolysis is an additional surgical technique. Chronic nerve injuries secondary to compression or traction may lead to fibrosis of the connective tissue elements of a peripheral nerve. External neurolysis is defined as the release of the nerve or the scarred (outer, epifascicular) epineurium from surrounding nonneural

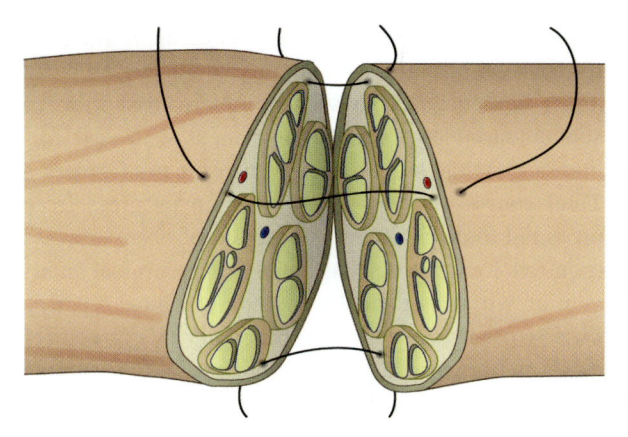

Fig. 7.2 Epineural nerve repair is performed under the operating microscope using microsurgical instruments and 10–0 monofilament nylon with a tapered needle. The nerve edges are freshened using a sharp microscissor, and a blue or green square of silicone sheeting is used beneath the nerve ends to improve visibility while suturing. For perineural (fascicular) repair (not shown), both adventitia and epineurium are dissected back several millimeters for exposure of the fascicles. Removal of adventitia (blood supply!) and epineurium (orientation!) should be performed sparingly.

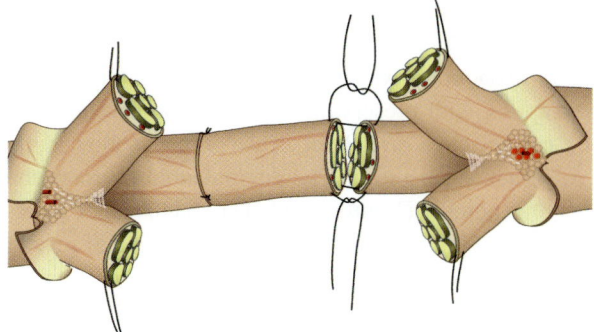

Fig. 7.3 Interfascicular autologous nerve transplantation

soft tissues. In contrast, internal neurolysis is the release of fascicles encapsulated in scarred (inner, interfascicular) epineurium. Millesi introduced a classification on the basis of fibrosis (type A–C fibrosis; [17]) differentiating between involvement of the epifascicular epineurium (fibrosis type A) or the interfascicular tissue (fibrosis type B), or the presence of a complete fibrosis of fascicles (fibrosis type C). Surgical options include epifascicular epineurotomy, epifascicular epineurectomy, interfascicular epineurectomy and, if neurolysis will not help, nerve resection and nerve grafting [17]. However, it must be noted that any manipulation of interfascicular anatomy has been shown to result in reactive fibrosis, and the caveat to any internal neurolysis is a careful consideration of risk-to-benefit ratios [18].

In the case of fourth to fifth-degree injuries (IV–V) or a sixth-degree injury (VI) with a neuroma-in-continuity, nerve grafting may be necessary if tension-free end-to-end neurorrhaphy is not possible. After both the length of the nerve deficit and the number of required fascicles for interfascicular autologous nerve transplantation (Fig. 7.3) are determined, nerve grafts are harvested. The autologous nerve graft should be oriented in a reverse fashion from its native position in order to prevent regenerating fibers diverting through small branches from the distal neurorrhaphy site and the distal stump. Nerve coaptations can be performed either in an epineurial or fascicular (perineural) fashion. Corresponding proximal and distal fascicles must be identified to avoid misalignment. Typical donor nerves are sensible nerves such as the medial and lateral antebrachial cutaneous nerve, saphenous nerve, greater auricle nerve, and the sural nerve. Harvesting results in a loss of sensibility at the respective site of innervation. The sural nerve is the most frequently used donor nerve (Fig. 7.4). It is located through a short longitudinal incision posterior to the lateral malleolus (Fig. 7.5). After identification, it is followed proximally either through a continuous incision or a series of transverse step cuts (preferred option) placed after palpation of the path of the nerve with gentle traction on the distal end. The nerve can be traced into the popliteal fossa and the gastrocnemius. Atraumatic harvesting of the nerve grafts avoiding stretch, strain, or compression is essential and prevents the disconnection of the endoneural tubes and damage to the axons (Fig. 7.5).

End-to-side neurorrhaphy allows for target-muscle reinnervation with simultaneous preservation of donor-nerve function. End-to-side nerve repair is the technique of coapting the distal end of an injured (transected) nerve (e.g., facial nerve trunk; see below [Fig. 7.11]) to the side of an uninjured donor nerve (e.g., hypoglossus nerve; see below), either by simple microsurgical coaptation without alteration of the donor nerve, or in conjunction with a surgical incision

7 Nerve Injuries in Traumatic Head Injury: When To Explore/Suture/Transplant?

within the donor nerve (preferred option). It has been suggested as a technique for repair of peripheral nerve injuries, where the proximal nerve stump is unavailable or a significant nerve gap exists.

7.2.3 Algorithms for Open and Closed Injuries: Timing of Nerve Repairs

In open nerve injuries, an open wound with an anatomically appropriate neurologic deficit requires exploration and possible microsurgical nerve reconstruction. If the transection was not sharp and involves a larger gap that cannot be coapted without tension, proximal and distal nerve stumps are marked and approximated with non-resporbables sutures to prevent larger gaps. Approximately at 3 weeks débridement of the scarred nerve and nerve reconstruction must be performed [11].

Closed nerve injuries may be caused by direct pressure to or stretching of the peripheral nerves. Many closed nerve injuries are first-degree injuries (I) that result in recovery within 12 weeks. According to Mackinnon [10], an initial detailed clinical examination is followed by a nerve conduction study and electromyography at 2 weeks and again at 4–6 weeks after injury. The patient undergoes monthly clinical and electrodiagnostic evaluations for evidence of recovery for a total of 3 months. At 3 months, if there is no

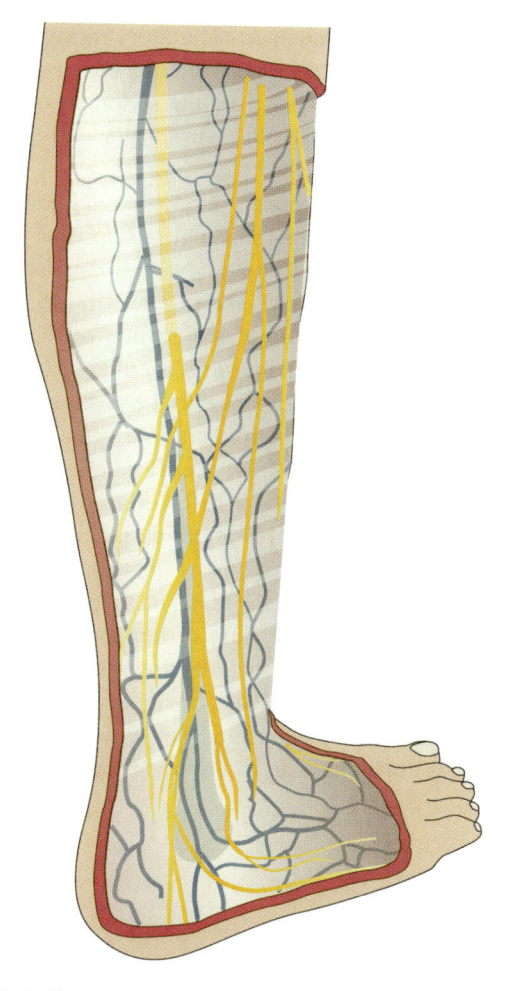

Fig. 7.4 The sural nerve is located posterior to the lateral malleolus and anterior to the Achilles' tendon

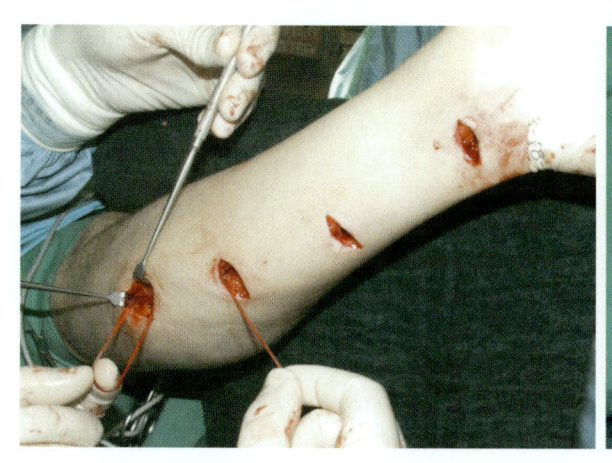

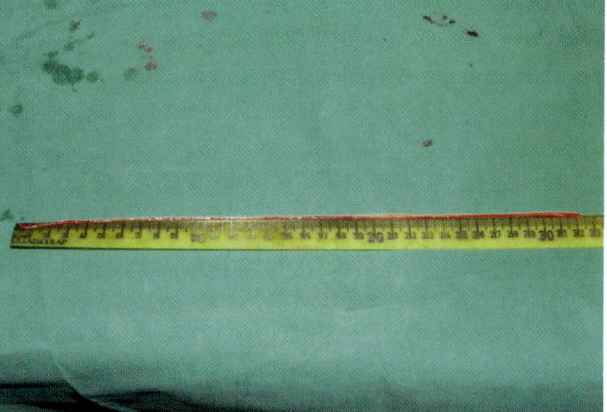

Fig. 7.5 After identification of the sural nerve in its distal part, it can be traced proximally for the required length

evidence of recovery either clinically or in nerve conduction studies, surgical intervention (decompression/ neurolysis/ direct nerve repair/ nerve grafting) is required [11].

7.3 Specific Aspects of Facial Nerve Lesions

7.3.1 Anatomy

The facial nerve is the 7th of 12 paired cranial nerves. It is a mixed nerve with motor and motor-sensory division (intermedius nerve) with extracranial, intratemporal, and extratemporal relationships [19]. The motor division with its extratemporal cervicotemporal and cervicofacial division is responsible for the innervation of facial mimetic muscles. The motor-sensory division provides neuropathways for general as well as special sensory transmission of taste, proprioception, and lacrimation. The facial nerve enters the petrous temporal bone into the internal auditory meatus (close to the inner ear) then runs a meandering course through the facial canal, emerges from the stylomastoid foramen and passes through the parotid gland (Figs. 7.6 and 7.7) [20].

There are three main intratemporal branches: greater petrosal (parasympathetic), stapedius nerve (branchial motor), and chorda tympani (parasympathetic and taste from the anterior two-thirds of the tongue) [21]. The extratemporal portion of the facial nerve begins at the stylomastoid foramen. There are three main preparotid branches: to the posterior auricular muscle, posterior belly of digastric muscle, and stylohyoid muscle. Initially, the facial nerve trunk begins in a deep position below the earlobe and becomes more superficial before it passes between the superficial and deep portions of the parotid gland. Within the parotid gland, the facial nerve trunk usually divides into two main trunks (temporofacial and cervicofacial division [19] with five main branches (temporal, zygomatic, buccal, marginal mandibular, and cervical). These main branches leave the parotid gland at its upper, medial, and inferior border. There is

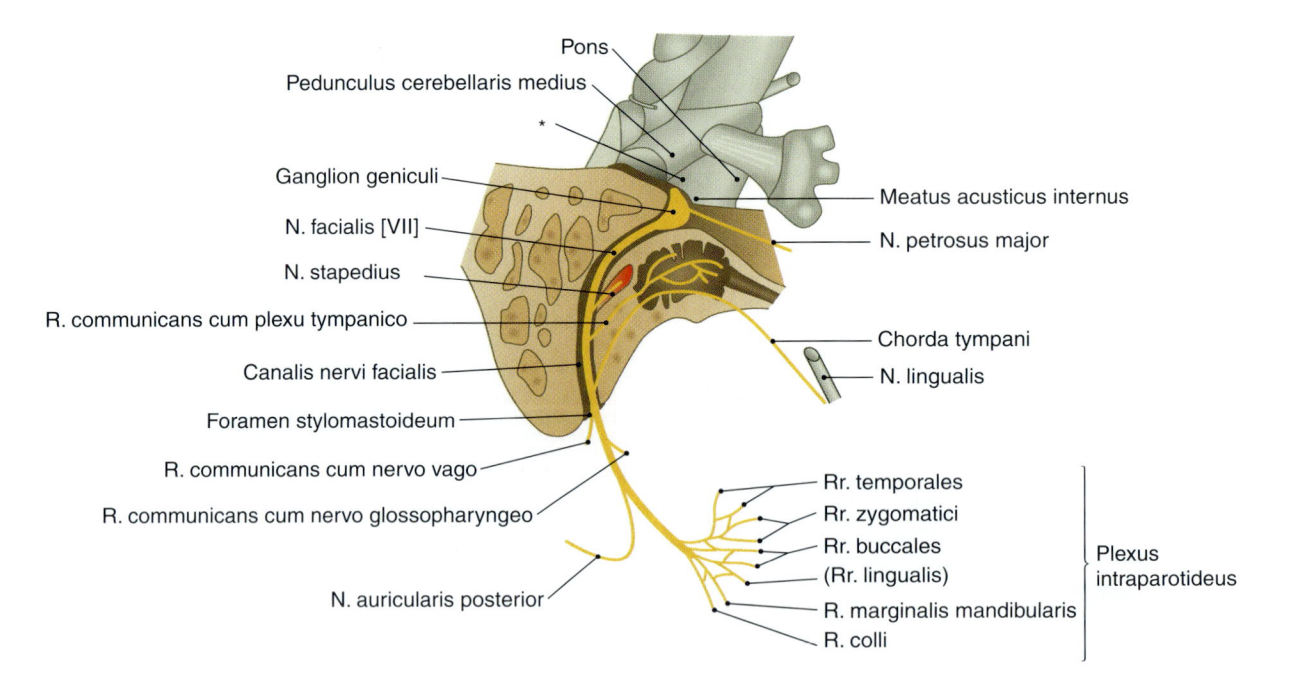

Fig. 7.6 Intratemporal course of the facial nerve

Fig. 7.7 Extratemporal course of the facial nerve and mimic muscles

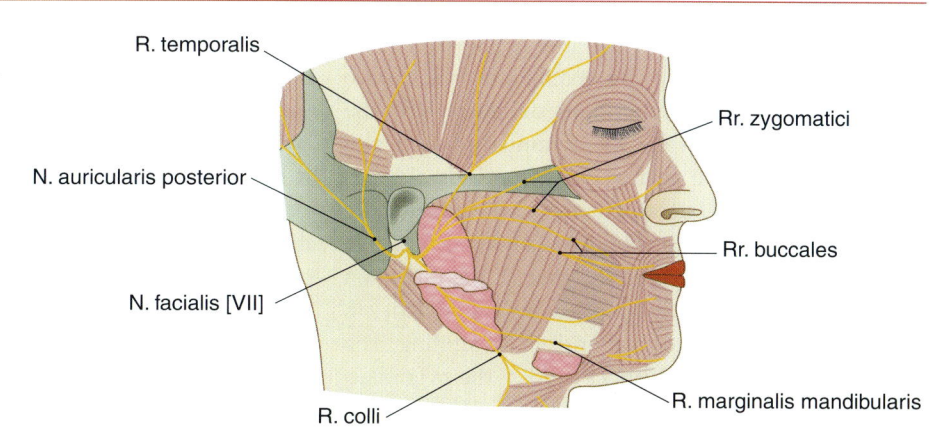

further arborization and interchange further distally. It is important for the surgeon to know that there is a wide variation in peripheral branching and interconnection between the temporal, zygomatic and buccal branches. Likewise, it is important to know that there is almost no interconnection between these branches and the mandibular branches. This is the reason for the low incidence of spontaneous reinnervation after transection of the mandibular branch [19]. At the medial margin of the parotid gland, the nerve branches lie approximately 10 mm from the skin surface, becoming progressively more superficial, especially in the temporal region where the facial nerve branches lie only a few millimeters deep to the surface [22]. These branches supply the mimetic musculature with 17 paired muscles and one unpaired muscle (the orbicularis oris muscle).

The temporal branch appears at the upper border of the gland [19]. The temporal branches cross the zygomatic arch and run within or just deep to the superficial layer of the superficial temporal fascia [23]. A useful landmark for plotting the course is a line connecting a point from 1.5 cm lateral to the lateral border of the eyebrow and the intertragal notch of the ear [23]. Another practical landmark is the palpable frontal branch of the superficial temporal artery, which is usually superior and lateral to the temporal branches of the facial nerve [24–26]. The temporal branches supply the frontalis, procerus, corrugator supercilii, and superior portion of the orbicularis oculi. The lower branches follow a submuscular course for the innervation of the superior portion of the orbicularis oculi muscle [27]. For the innervation of the frontalis muscle, the upper branches enter the lateral border of the muscle at the level of the supraorbital ridge approximately 3 cm above the lateral canthus and 1.6 cm below the superficial temporal artery [28]. The frontalis muscle has two main functions: brow elevation (during movement) and brow suspension (at rest). Impaired muscle function leads to brow ptosis on the ipsilateral side. The orbicularis oculi muscle acts as a sphincter to close the eyelids. In contrast, upper eyelid opening is mainly performed by the levator palpebrae superioris muscle innervated by the third cranial nerve (oculomotor nerve). The orbicularis oculi muscle is one continuous muscle, but has three subdivisions: (a) pretarsal, covering the tarsal plate; (b) preseptal, overlying the orbital septum; and (c) orbital, forming a ring over the orbital margin. The pretarsal and preseptal portions act together when a patient blinks, whereas the orbital portion is recruited for forceful eye closure and to lower the eyebrows. The motor nerve branches enter the upper and lower portions of the orbicularis oculi just medial to its lateral edge.

The zygomaticobuccal branches consist of five to eight branches lying deep near the parotid-masseteric fascia in the same plane as the parotid duct. There is an extensive functional overlap. A lesion of one or more branches does not necessarily lead to a functional deficit. As landmark, the zygomatic branches are usually under an oblique line between the tragus and the lateral palpebral commissure with a close relationship to the buccal branches [29]. Anatomical studies have shown that the mean horizontal distance between the tragus of the ear and the emergence of the most upper zygomatic branches from the ventral border of the parotid gland is approximately 3 cm [29]. The zygomaticobuccal branches supply the lip elevators (zygomaticus major and minor, levator labii superioris, levator anguli oris), the lower portion of the orbicularis oculi, orbicularis oris, and buccinator. The zygomaticus muscles move the commissure at an angle of approximately 45°, the levator anguli oris elevates the commissure vertically and medially, and the levator labii superioris elevates the lip vertically and laterally to expose the upper teeth. Functional facial nerve mapping and cross-facial nerve grafting (see below) require the precise identification and stimulation of these zygomaticobuccal branches to isolate the exact branches responsible for smiling. The motor branches reach the upper third of the zygomaticus major at the deep surface. The nerve fibers to the levator labii superioris first pass underneath the zygomaticus major muscle and also reach its deep surface. In contrast, the levator anguli oris, belonging to the deepest layer, is innervated on its superficial surface by the same branch that supplies innervation to the buccinator. Anatomically and functionally, the orbicularis oris muscle consists of a superficial and deep part. The deep layers of the muscle encircle the mouth orifice and function as its sphincter. The superficial component also brings the lips together, but its fibers can contract independently to provide expression.

One to three marginal mandibular branches emerge from the inferior border of the parotid gland approximately 4 cm beneath the base of the earlobe near the angle of the mandible. In 81% of patients, these nerve branches lie above the mandibular border and in 19% of patients, inferior to the mandibular border [30]. These branches supply the lower lip depressors (dep-ressor anguli oris and depressor labii inferioris), the mentalis muscle, as well as upper platysma and lower orbicularis oris.

The cervical branches leave the parotid gland below the angle of the mandible and runs on the deep surface of its target muscle, i.e., the platysma muscle.

7.3.2 Etiology, Classification, Diagnostic Assessment

Facial paralysis can be classified anatomically as congenital (syndromic and isolated non-syndromic) or acquired (traumatic including iatrogenic) as a consequence of tumors or inflammatory diseases and idiopathic. Facial nerve paralysis can be unilateral or bilateral. In addition, the degree of muscle involvement varies from total to partial paralysis [19–21, 31].

The three most frequent causes of facial nerve paralysis are Bell's palsy, trauma, and intra- or extracranial neoplasm. Physical trauma, especially fractures of the temporal bone, may cause acute facial nerve paralysis. The likelihood of facial nerve paralysis depends on the location of the trauma (Fig. 7.8). In most cases, facial

Fig. 7.8 Schematic illustration depicting the long and convoluted course of the facial nerve. Depending on the site or level of injury (sites 1–6 with *red bars*), facial nerve lesions lead to characteristic symptoms: site (1) paresis of mimetic muscles; site (2) in addition: loss of taste at the anterior two-third of the tongue and salivation (chorda tympani↓); site (3) in addition: hyperacusis (nerve to stapedius↓); site (4) in addition: impaired lacrimation (greater petrosal nerve↓); site (5) cerebellopontine angle; site (6) central paralysis (corticobulbaris tract↓)

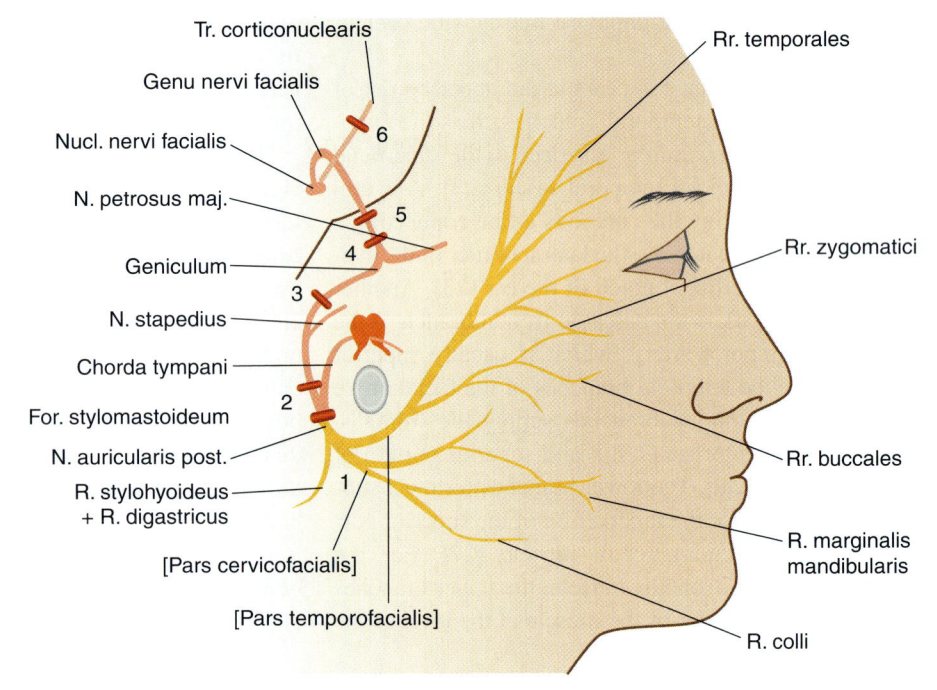

paralysis results from temporal bone fractures. The highest frequency occurs in cases with transverse fractures in the horizontal plane followed by longitudinal fracture in the vertical plane. Patients may show symptoms like hemotympanum (blood behind the tympanic membrane), hematorrhea out of the external auditory meatus, but also sensory deafness and vertigo due to involvement to the vestibulocochlear nerve.

A neuroanatomical classification divides facial nerve paralysis into three categories: central, intratemporal, and extratemporal. Central paralysis of the supranuclear type is characterized by a paralysis of the lower face, sparing the forehead due to cross-innervation of the upper portion of the face and forehead. The anatomical course of the facial nerve is long and convoluted. Therefore, depending on the site or level of injury, intratemporal facial paralysis can lead to facial paralysis with hyperacusis (nerve to stapedius↓), loss of taste at the anterior two-third of the tongue (chorda tympani↓), lacrimation (greater petrosal nerve↓), and salivation (chorda tympani↓) (Fig. 7.8). Extratemporal paralysis is a pure motor deficit of one or more branches of the facial nerve and their innervation of the muscles for facial innervation (Fig. 7.7).

The clinical presentation of the degree of facial nerve paralysis may vary. Complete paralysis (either unilateral or bilateral) is defined by the loss of all motor activity to mimetic muscles. In contrast, partial facial paralysis implies the lesion of one or more peripheral facial nerve branches. Clinical assessment of facial paralysis documents the following findings: (a) volitional and involuntary movement, (b) symmetry at rest, (c) degree, strength, and quality of muscle movements related to each facial nerve branch [19].

Examination of the face begins with the brow (temporal branches: frontalis forehead contraction, brow elevation). The discrepancy between the eyebrow height at the position of the brow at rest and during movement must be noted. The superior visual field may be diminished by the ptotic brow [21].

The eye closure must be thoroughly assessed, including a test of the function of the orbicularis oculi muscle (temporal and zygomatic branches). This includes documentation of the height of the palpebral aperture in the open and closed position (degree of lagophthalmus), testing Bell's phenomenon (an upward and outward movement of the globe during eye closure, while the eyelid on the paralyzed side of the face remains open), measuring scleral show at the lower lid margin, presence of the corneal reflex, assessment of lower lid ectropium (snap test, position of inferior canalicular punctum), and documentation of corneal ulcerations with desiccation and reactive excessive tear flow.

The nasal airway is examined next; forced inspiration may reveal a collapse of upper and lower nasal muscles as well as drooping of the cheek (zygomatic and buccal branches). Then, the mouth and surrounding structures are examined. Documentation should provide information on the inability to smile, the amount of philtral deviation, the presence or absence of a nasolabial fold, commissural of depression and deviation, upper lip drooping, vermilion inversion, as well as evaluation of lower lip depressor function at rest and during movement. Furthermore, speech should be tested and an intraoral examination should be performed to check dental hygiene and to look for evidence of cheek biting. Patients should be asked about their ability to speak, eat, and drink properly due to the inability to control their lips.

In all facial regions, it is essential to document any presence of synkinesis or dyskinesis. Dyskinesis are abnormal involuntary movements, such as spasms and tics, while synkinesis is a simultaneous contraction of two or more groups of muscles that normally do not contract together, or performing an unintended movement while making a voluntary movement [20]. Synkinesis is thought to occur from a misdirected sprouting of axons. The most common types of synkinesis are eye closure with smiling [32], brow wrinkling when the mouth is moved [33], and mouth grimacing when the eyes are closed.

An assessment of the other cranial nerves, particularly the trigeminal, accessory, and hypoglossus, is also performed. Additional cranial nerve involvement may exacerbate the morbidity of facial nerve paralysis. These nerves should also be assessed as possible donor motor nerves.

In addition to a clinical assessment of facial paralysis, further diagnostic tests may be performed including: (a) salivary flow tests, (b) taste tests, (c) stapedius muscle reflex, (d) lacrimation tests (Schirmer-test), (e) needle electromyography (EMG) and nerve conduction studies, as well (f) computer tomography (CT) and magnetic resonance imaging (MRI) [19].

The most widely used grading system is the House–Brackmann score, which evaluates the upward (superior) movement of the mid-portion of the top of the brow as well as the outward (lateral) movement of the

Table 7.1 Facial nerve grading system according to House and Brackmann [34] – facial nerve grading system I

Grade	Description	Characteristics
I	Normal	Normal facial function in all areas

II	Mild dysfunction	• Gross: slight weakness noticeable only on close inspection; may have very slight synkinesis.
		• At rest: normal symmetry and tone.
		• Motion
		  – Forehead: moderate to good function
		  – Eye: complete closure with minimum effort
		  – Mouth: slight asymmetry

III	Moderate dysfunction	• Gross: obvious but not disfiguring difference between two sides; noticeable but not severe synkinesis, contracture, and/or hemifacial spasm
		• At rest: normal symmetry and tone
		• Motion
		  – Forehead: slight to moderate movement
		  – Eye: complete closure with effort
		  – Mouth: slightly weak with maximum effort

IV	Moderately severe dysfunction	• Gross: obvious weakness and/or disfiguring asymmetry
		• At rest: normal symmetry and tone
		• Motion
		  – Forehead: none
		  – Eye: incomplete closure
		  – Mouth: asymmetric with maximum effort

V	Severe dysfunction	• Gross: only barely perceptible motion
		• At rest: asymmetry
		• Motion
		  – Forehead: none
		  – Eye: incomplete closure
		  – Mouth: slight movement

VI	Total paralysis	No movement

Table 7.2 Correlation between other grading systems and the six-point grading scale by House and Brackmann [34] – facial nerve grading system II

Grade	Description	Measurement	Function (%)	Estimated function (%)
I	Normal	8/8	100	100
II	Mild	7/8	76–99	80
III	Moderate	5/8–6/8	51–75	60
IV	Moderately severe	3/8–4/8	26–50	40
V	Severe	1/8–2/8	1–25	20
VI	Total	0/8	0	0

angle of the mouth. Each area of reference scores 1 point for each 0.25 cm movement, up to a maximum of 1 cm. The scores are then added together totalling a maximum number of eight (Tables 7.1 and 7.2) [34]. Similarly, Terzis and coworkers introduced a functional grading systems in order to provide a quantitative comparison between pre-and postoperative clinical findings (Table 7.3) [35, 36]. This helps to assess the effectiveness and quality of the neuromuscular reconstruction of the face. Furthermore, to provide an exact and objective estimation, Frey and coworkers introduced a three-dimensional video system for standardized pre- and postoperative functional assessment of their neuromuscular reconstruction of the face [37–39]. Movement analyses quantify changes in the amplitude of movements caused by surgery on the reconstructed

Table 7.3 Grading system according to Terzis and coworkers [35, 36] – facial nerve grading system III

Terzis functional and esthetic grading system (used for the grading of smile and overall esthetic outcome)			
Group	Grading	Description	Result
I	1	Deformity, no contraction	Poor
II	2	No symmetry, minimal contraction	Fair
III	3	Moderate symmetry and contraction	Moderate
IV	4	Symmetry, nearly full contraction	Good
V	5	Symmetrical smile with full contraction	Excellent

Terzis grading for assessment of eye closure	
Grade	Description
1	No eye closure
2	Poor eye closure
3	Incomplete eye closure
4	Nearly complete eye closure
5	Complete eye closure

Terzis grading for assessment of lip depressors	
Grade	Description
0	Total paralysis
0.5	Trace contraction
1	Observable movement but no symmetry
1.5	Almost complete excursion of lower lip
2	Normal symmetrical movement of lower lip

side in comparison to the non-paralyzed side, and changes in static and dynamic symmetry.

7.3.3 Non-surgical Management

Nonsurgical management is an important and integral part in the treatment of patients with facial nerve paralysis [21]. An interdisciplinary plan of therapy management should be designed preoperatively and in concert with upcoming surgical interventions. Depending on individual deficits and symptoms, this may include consultation with an ophthalmologist (e.g., due to limited eye closure, tear transport, conjunctivitis, corneal ulceration, etc.), an otolaryngologist (e.g., due to intranasal airway problems, hearing loss, stapedial malfunction, etc.), a dentist (e.g., due to oral hygiene), a nutritionist (e.g., due to feeding problems), a physiotherapist, a speech therapist (e.g., due to speech problems, articulation errors), and/or a psychologist or psychiatrist (e.g., due to psychosocial problems).

In particular, the eye requires careful attention either before or in concert with surgical interventions. Therapeutic strategies focus on both protection of the eye and maintenance of lubrication with the goal of enabling comfortable eyes free of pain. This can be achieved by the lid taping, particularly while sleeping, as well as soft contact lenses, moisture chambers, modified eyeglasses with a lateral shield, forced blinking exercises, eye patches, etc.

Furthermore, especially after surgery, neuromuscular training is important to assure and improve the surgical results. This training includes transcutaneous electrical nerve stimulation (TENS), biofeedback and self-directed mirror exercises etc. [40].

7.3.4 Surgical Management

Over the decades, a multitude of surgical procedures have been developed. A trusting physician–patient relationship is important for the selection of the most appropriate and effective surgical interventions to match the patient's requirements. The surgeon and patient must have clearly defined goals with a clear priority list. The upper lip and cheek region may serve as an example. Although paralysis of the oral musculature results in significant functional problems (speech difficulties, problems chewing food, cheek biting, etc.), most patients ask for corrections of facial asymmetry at rest or smile reconstruction. If the patient asks only for symmetry at rest, static procedures may be sufficient. If the patient asks for restoration of smile, static and dynamic procedures with regional muscle transfer (e.g., temporalis and/or masseter muscle) can provide excellent results. If the patient is willing to accept more complex and time-consuming procedures (e.g., cross-facial nerve grafting and free muscle transfer; see below), this may restore both voluntary and involuntary facial movements plus symmetry. Usually most patients require a combination of surgical procedures (static and dynamic) tailored to their needs, motivation, and general physical status. A well-planned and elaborated static procedure may yield a better esthetic and functional outcome than a poorly planned and poorly executed complex microsurgical procedure [20].

7.3.4.1 General Considerations

Specific surgical procedures for the functional restoration of the facial nerve and/or mimetic muscles include direct neurorrhaphy (end-to-end epineural or perineural nerve coaptation), entubation nerve repair, autologous nerve grafting, nerve transfer, cross-facial nerve grafting (CFNG), regional and microneurovascular free muscle transfer. Normally, these specific techniques are combined with traditional plastic surgical techniques (ancillary procedures) in order to augment the functional outcome [20].

This variety of surgical options can, therefore, be divided into (a) static versus dynamic, (b) single-stage versus Multi-stage or (c) regional (forehead, eye region, midface, mouth) procedures.

The first attempt for facial nerve reconstruction is primary repair by tension-free nerve coaption of the proximal and distal nerve stump. Mobilization or external neurolysis may help to approximate the nerve stumps and to avoid detrimental tension on the nerve sutures. As a secondary step, if the nerve deficit is too long autologous nerve transplantation is required. The sural nerve is the typical donor nerve. However, as alternative, the great auricular nerve has been used in a one-stage procedure to serve as a pedicled vascularized donor nerve [41]. A second alternative to autologous nerve grafting is entubation neurorrhaphy by means of using autologous veins or bioartificial nerve conduits. A variety of bioartificial nerve grafts has been developed over the last decades. There exist sophisticated nerve guide concepts with longitudinal microstructure for orientated axonal growth, but these are still in the preclinical (experimental) testing phase [42–44]. Simpler concepts are based on hollow conduits, which already have FDA and CE approval supporting nerve regeneration to a limited degree [45]. However, recently, a resorbable nerve conduit has been used for facial nerve repair [45].

For further reconstructive options, it is important to know that the quality of facial muscle reinnervation is inversely proportional with the denervation time. Over time (generally after 12 months), there is a decrease of acetylcholinesterase receptor activity in the muscle fibers, and muscle fiber volume shows increased intramuscular fibrosis. These pathophysiologic findings define the (individual) time frame for functional muscle reinnervation [20]. Many authors, therefore, make their reconstructive algorithm dependent on the denervation time. A widely accepted reconstructive algorithm has been recommended by Terzis [46] in case of traumatic facial nerve paralysis:

1. Denervation time ≤ 6 months: CFNG
2. Denervation time between 6 months to 2 years and 3 months: "Baby-sitter procedure" (mini-hypoglossus & CFNG) ± muscle transfers
3. Denervation time > 2 years and 3 months: CFNG + muscle transfers

7.3.4.2 Specific Considerations Regarding Facial Nerve Paralysis in Temporal Bone Fractures

Since the fascicular topography of the facial nerve is poor in its proximal part, primary repair or nerve grafting proximal to the stylomastoid foramen can result in significant dyskinesis and synkinesis [47]. In addition to the technical and surgical complexity involved, some authors recommend against performing an ipsilateral nerve graft for complete facial main trunk lesions because the possibility of mass facial movements after regeneration may be significant. This typically refers to patients with a complete facial palsy at or proximal to the stylomastoid foramen. In contrast, nerve grafting is recommended for the reconstruction of fascicles of the partial lesioned facial nerve distal to the stylomastoid foramen to prevent syn- or dyskinesis [48]. In contrast, other authors do perform nerve grafting proximal to the stylomastoid foramen not only after cranial tumors, but also after skull base trauma with petrous bone fractures. Samii and Matthies [49] presented a large number of patients ($n = 160$) with the reconstruction (by means of end-to-end neurorrhaphy, autologous nerve grafting or fibrin glue) of the facial nerve in the face, but also more proximal (at the brainstem, within the mastoid, and at the stylomastoid foramen) leading to satisfactory functional and cosmetic results.

Furthermore, there is some controversy concerning the indications, timing, and choice of approach in the management of traumatic facial nerve paralysis [4]. Despite all arguments, it should be always kept in mind that many patients with temporal bone fractures (Fig. 7.1) have suffered multiple traumas and are unstable for a period of time. Some authors recommend decompression for patients with acute facial nerve paralysis secondary to head trauma if electroneurography shows more than 90% degeneration within the first 3 weeks of the onset of facial nerve paralysis. If the patients are admitted more than 3 weeks after the onset, decompression should be considered when electromyography shows total denervation potentials. Middle cranial fossa approach allows for the management of most cases. In patients where early intervention was not possible, decompression up to 4 months after onset can still have beneficial effects [4].

7.3.4.3 Cross-facial Nerve Grafting (CFNG)

The major surgical goal of facial reanimation is not only symmetry at rest, but also voluntary and emotional animation with synchronized coordinated facial expression. The concept of alternative motor donor nerves includes the use of the accessory, hypoglossal, trigeminal, and phrenic nerves [20, 46]. In addition to donor site morbidity with possible loss of function, the major drawback is insufficient functional outcome with uncoordinated mass facial movements. Movements appear exaggerated and disproportionate without spontaneous emotional expression in comparison with the non-paralyzed side.

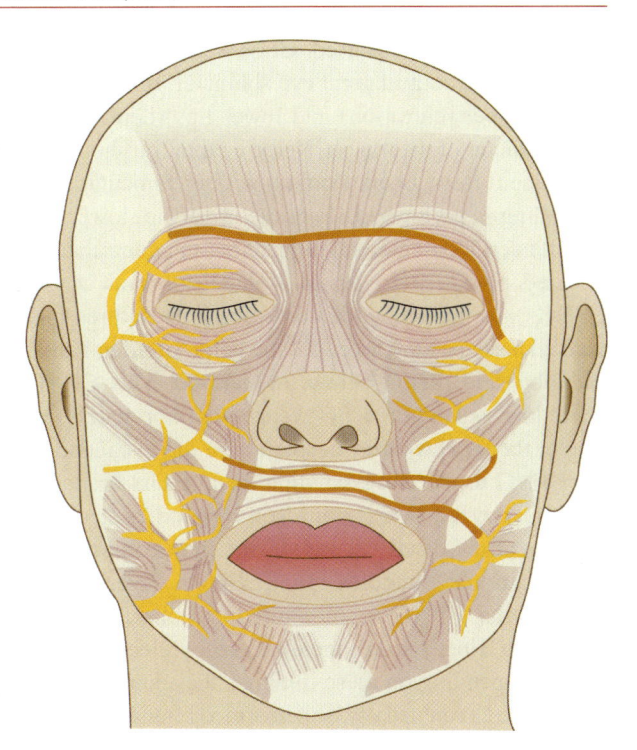

Fig. 7.9 Cross-facial nerve grafting (CFNG) [50]

To achieve coordinated animation and emotional expression, the concept of cross-facial nerve grafting (CFNG) (Fig. 7.9) was introduced in the 1970s [51]. The basic idea is to use redundant facial nerve branches with motor axons from the non-paralyzed side for the specific innervation of the appropriate mimetic muscles in the paralyzed side. As strikingly expressed by Terzis and coworkers, the facial nerve nucleus of the non-paralyzed side acts as a "pacemaker" forwarding signals through CFNGs to the paralyzed side. It is essential that the donor nerve branches are similar and correspond to the recipient branches in order to provide coordinated and symmetrical facial movements [46].

After a preauricular modified facelift incision, all branches of the non-affected extratemporal facial nerve trunk at the level of the anterior parotid margin are identified and mapped using a low intensity nerve microstimulator. As surgical landmark, a vertical line between the lateral canthus and the midbody of the mandible serves as anterior border. After selection and transection of redundant distal ends of the zygomaticus, buccal, and/or marginalis mandibulae branches, these are coapted to a sural nerve graft [46, 51] or, additionally, a saphenous nerve graft. Depending on the preoperative clinical findings and loss of function, up to four CFNGs are used. CFNGs are dedicated for the respective contralateral eye sphincter, lip retractors for the upper (elevation) and lower lips (depression), and sphincter of the mouth. Nerve coaptation should be performed after subcutaneous tunnelling. Subcutaneous tunnelling is performed along the upper lip, lower lip, and the cervicomental angle reaching the contralateral affected preauricular region [46]. Distal ends of the CFNGs are marked with non-resorbable sutures and banked near the attachment of the helix, pretragal area, ear lobe, and region below the earlobe. This CFNG procedure usually does not weaken the non-paralyzed side of the face. A direct coaptation of the distal end of the CFNG to the corresponding distal facial branches of the paralyzed side is not recommended as scar formations at the distal coaptation site may compromise the functional outcome [12]. Nerve regeneration through the CFNG is monitored by observing the advancing Tinel's sign supplemented by electromyography. Depending on these findings, the second operation (stage 2) can usually be performed after an interval of 9–12 months. The second operation may be either nerve coaptation of the CFNGs to the corresponding contralateral distal facial nerve branches (Fig. 7.9) or coaptation to the motor nerve branch of a free neurovascular muscle transplant (see below; Fig. 7.12).

Disadvantages of the CFNG procedure include (a) donor site morbidity (e.g. sensory deficit), (b) long time interval for reinnervation of the target muscles, (c) limited axonal growth for efficient reinnervation, and (d) possible functional deficits at the non-paralyzed site (motor deficit). Recently, Terzis and coworkers summarized a number of important recommendations [46]. First, nerve branches should never be manipulated before microstimulation. Second, only redundant nerve branches should be used. The usage of both neighboring and branches to the frontalis muscle are contraindicated. Third, for contralateral eye reanimation, the respective branch of the upper zygomatic division, which only supplies the upper and lower orbicularis oculi, should be used. Fourth, for contralateral smile restoration, only branches of the zygomatic division should be used, which supply lip elevators and the commissure, but not the eye sphincter.

According to Terzis and coworkers [46], the CFNG procedure alone achieves a synchronous and coordinated functional outcome for patients with a denervation period less than 6 months. If the facial nerve lesion is present for longer than 6 months, a strong motor

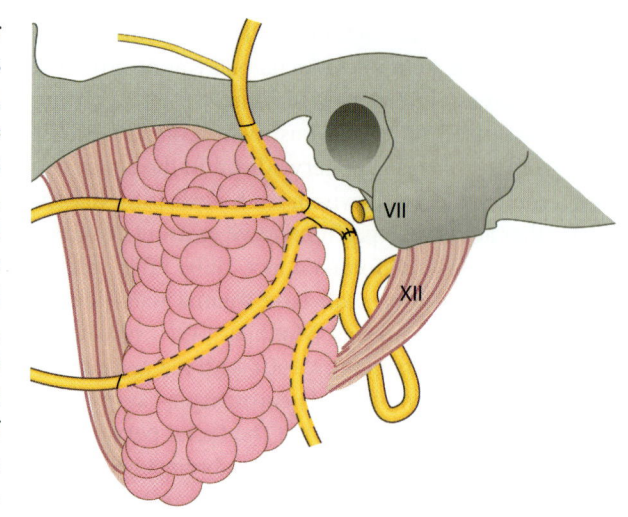

Fig. 7.10 Conventional hypoglossus transfer (end-to-end nerve coaptation). The hypoglossus is traced distally, transected, and rotated to the stump of the facial nerve [50]. In the mini-hypoglossus transfer (not shown) as popularized by Terzis [46], only 40% of the oligofascicular hypoglossus nerve cross-section is coapted either in an end-to-end or end-to-side manner to the facial nerve or trunk of the paralyzed side

donor nerve is required for the preservation of facial muscle viability, while the regenerating motor fibers grow across the CFNG from the contralateral facial nerve. This is accomplished by using the ipsilateral hypoglossus nerve (Figs. 7.10 and 7.11). When there is a prolonged denervation time (>2 years), facial muscles are usually irreversibly atrophied and fibrotic. For smile restoration in these cases, CFNG should be combined with a free microneurovascular muscle flap [52] (Fig. 7.12).

To prevent postoperative lesions of freshly coaptated nerves, mouth and jaw movements must be limited. This is accomplished by special bandages. Furthermore, a soft diet is administered and speaking is only allowed with teeth in occlusion for the first 4 weeks. After 6 weeks, ultrasound and massage therapy is applied to prevent scar formation at the coaptation sites.

7.3.4.4 Minihypoglossal to Facial Nerve Transfer ("Babysitter Procedure")

The concept of muscle reinnervation using the contralateral non-injured facial nerve by means of CFNGs has two major drawbacks. First, the distance for axonal growth within the CFNG is relatively

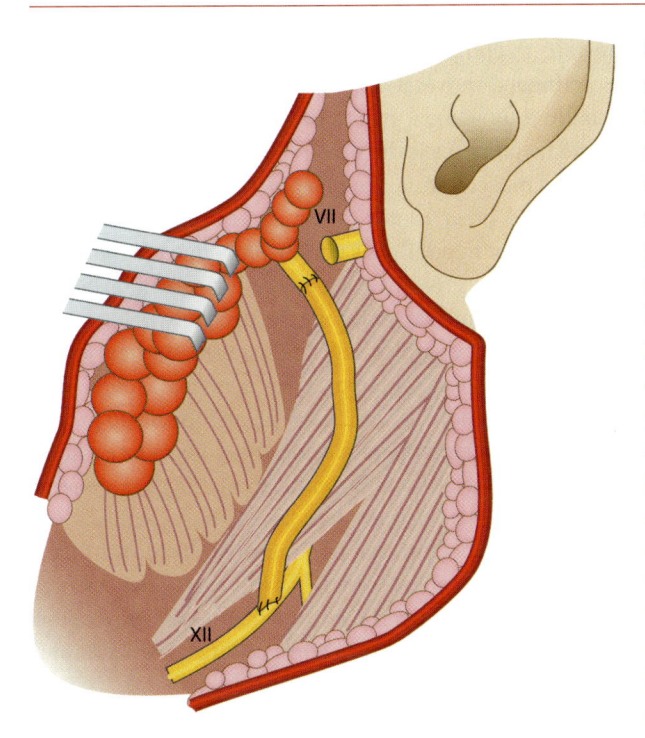

Fig. 7.11 Autologous nerve graft between the hypoglossus and facial nerve (so-called jump graft; end-to-side nerve coaptation) [50]

extensive and takes a long time (~1 mm/day). This regeneration time must be added to the time interval between onset of facial nerve injury and cross-facial grafting. This creates a long denervation time compromising the reversibility of muscular atrophy. A general rule states that reversibility of muscular atrophy is generally warranted if the time between onset of facial nerve paralysis and cross-facial grafting is less than 6 months. If the time period is longer than 6 months, the facial muscles of the paralyzed side could be irreversibly atrophied before reinnervation begins. Second, the contralateral facial nerve is optimal to provide voluntary and synchronized coordinated movements, but the axonal input can sometimes be too weak to achieve a strong muscle tone. One reason could be that the two coaptation sites lead to additional loss of axons [53]. According to others [54], a CFNG-procedure without further motor nerve input may be beneficial for eyelid control, but not for the movement of the mouth.

In 1984, Terzis introduced a sophisticated concept called the "babysitter procedure" [35, 36, 46]. The main item of this two-staged concept is the use of an ipsilateral strong motor donor nerve like the hypoglossus nerve. Such a nerve crossover helps to preserve facial muscle viability; the facial muscles are preserved while the regenerating motor fibers grow across the cross-facial nerve graft. Due to both the short distance and strong motor input, a rapid reinnervation of the paretic facial muscle takes place, while axons from the contralateral facial nerve regenerate through the CFNG. In the first stage, approximately 40% of the ipsilateral hypoglossus nerve is coapted either in an end-to-end or end-to-side manner to the facial nerve or trunk of the paralyzed side. The hypoglossus nerve is explored by means of a curved inframandibular incision followed by retraction of the posterior belly of the digastric muscle. For both procedures (end-to-end and end-to-side), 40% of the oligofascicular hypoglossus nerve cross-section is lesioned under microscopical magnification. More detailed fibers from the superior aspect without contribution to the ansa cervicales should be selected. In case of an end-to-side coaptation, the stump of the mobilized facial trunk is coapted to the site of neurectomy of the partially neurectomized hypoglossus nerve. According to Terzis [46], partial neurectomy with transection of the perineurium is the most effective method. If this is not possible, the hypoglossus nerve is dissected longitudinally using the distal end superolaterally for end-to-end coaptation with the facial nerve trunk. An autologous nerve transplantation may be performed to bridge the coaption sites. At the same time, the CFNGs are placed (step 1). Approximately 9–12 months later, depending on the advancing Tinel's sign along the CFNGs, the second operation is performed (step 2). At this time, distal ends of the CFNGs are coapted to selected branches of the affected facial nerve in an end-to-end fashion. According to Terzis, the coaptation between the so-called mini-hypoglossus and facial trunk remains intact, resulting in a duplicity of innervation (CFNG: reanimation, "pacemaking," synchronizing; mini-hypoglossus: no reanimation, salvage of paretic muscle) [35, 36, 46].

In cases with insufficient functional outcome or prolonged denervation periods, a regional or microneurovascular free muscle transfer can be performed. Therefore, Terzis and coworkers developed an algorithm with precise inclusion criteria [46], in which needle electromyography is essential for decision making. If clinically denervated or paretic facial muscles reveal fibrillations, the babysitter procedure with the CFNG procedure (step 1) may be performed. In contrast, the absence of fibrillations represents a contraindication for this procedure. Approximately 6 months after step 1, reevaluations should be done using clinical tests and EMG. The patient is asked to push his tongue against the teeth. If this leads to strong facial muscle contractions, the second step (approximately after 9–12 months after step1) with microcoaptations of the CFNGs to contralateral distal facial nerve branches may be performed. In cases of absent or inadequate facial muscle contractions (e.g., late cases), a regional (at step 2 or 3) or free muscle transfer (step 2) may be necessary [46].

In contrast to the conventional (100% of the hypoglossus nerve cross section; Fig. 7.10) hypoglossus to facial nerve transfer [55], the mini-hypoglossus transfer (40% of the hypoglossus nerve cross section) has two advantages [56]. First, this procedure minimizes postoperative complications like hemiglossal atrophy, as well as problems with speech, mastication, or swallowing. Second, the conventional hypoglossus transfer results in only uncoordinated movements. In contrast, the babysitting procedure in combination with CFNGs results in synchronous movements between affected and non-affected site.

For the mini-hypoglossus transfer, preoperative clinical and electrophysiological tests are inevitably necessary to both ensure that the hypoglossus nerve is intact and to evaluate any postoperative paretic lesions (e.g., hemitongue atrophy). In patients with a lesioned hypoglossus nerve, alternative motor donors are required, e.g., ipsilateral trigeminal nerve, accessory nerve, or the C7 root.

An integral part of the surgical procedure is an optimized rehabilitation program. According to the specifications of Terzis [46], patients should perform exercises in front of a mirror. To recruit the non-affected facial nerve, patients should smile on the non-paralyzed side followed by the paralyzed side. For recruitment of the mini-hypoglossus, patients should press their tongue while smiling. In addition patients are instructed to use a slow pulse muscle stimulator to generate muscle contraction.

7.3.4.5 Free Microneurovascular Muscle Transfer

It is necessary to avoid or minimize frustrations due to unrealistic expectations. In particular, this applies to patients with a long denervation period and the necessity for free muscle transfer for smile reconstruction. Due to the complexity with 18 muscles involved in facial expression (7 for upper lip elevation and 2 for lower lip depression), it is not feasible and almost impossible to restore a complete symmetry with synchronous and coordinated movements. One transplanted muscle will lead to a movement in one direction with one function. If the facial nerve is the motor donor nerve for the transplanted muscle, smile, and laughter will be spontaneous. In case of other motor donor nerves (e.g., trigeminal, accessory or hypoglossus nerve), other movements (e.g., teeth clenching) will be necessary for activation of the transplanted muscle and smile, respectively [21].

For such a complex and multistaged surgical intervention (e.g., CFNG [step 1], microneurovascular free muscle transfer [Fig. 7.12; step 2], and touch-up procedures [step 3]), preoperative consultations must exclude absolute or relative contraindications against general anesthesia (preexisting diseases). Many authors are hesitant with performing free muscle transfer for facial reanimation in patients older than 60 years. Furthermore, patients must be clearly informed and educated about the tediousness of multistage procedures. For example, after free muscle transplantation, it can take up to 18 months before full movement can be achieved.

Preoperative counselation also includes analysis of the individual smile. This helps to estimate the size of the muscle, point of origin, tension, and direction of movement.

Single-Stage Free Microneurovascular Muscle Transfer (Presence of Contralateral Facial Nerve)

Free microneurovascular transplantation of a muscle flap with a long nerve segment, such as the latissimus dorsi or rectus abdominis [57] or even the gracilis [58], have been reported as single-stage procedure. The motor nerve is tunnelled across the lip and coapted to contralateral non-affected facial nerve branches. Advantages of this single-stage procedure is that patients only need one operation (no CFNG procedure), and that only one nerve coaptation site is necessary minimizing risk of axonal loss at a second coaption site. Denervation atrophy of the transplanted muscle was not described as significant until axonal regeneration and reinnervation occur. After reinnervation, the transplanted muscle contracts with observable facial movement. However, in many cases, the muscle does not always contract when the patient smiles. This is due to the fact that the nerve segment of the free muscle is coapted to contralateral facial branches which are close to the mouth after performing a nasolabial incision. This approach does not allow a facial nerve mapping (see above) to recruit the most appropriate nerve branches [21].

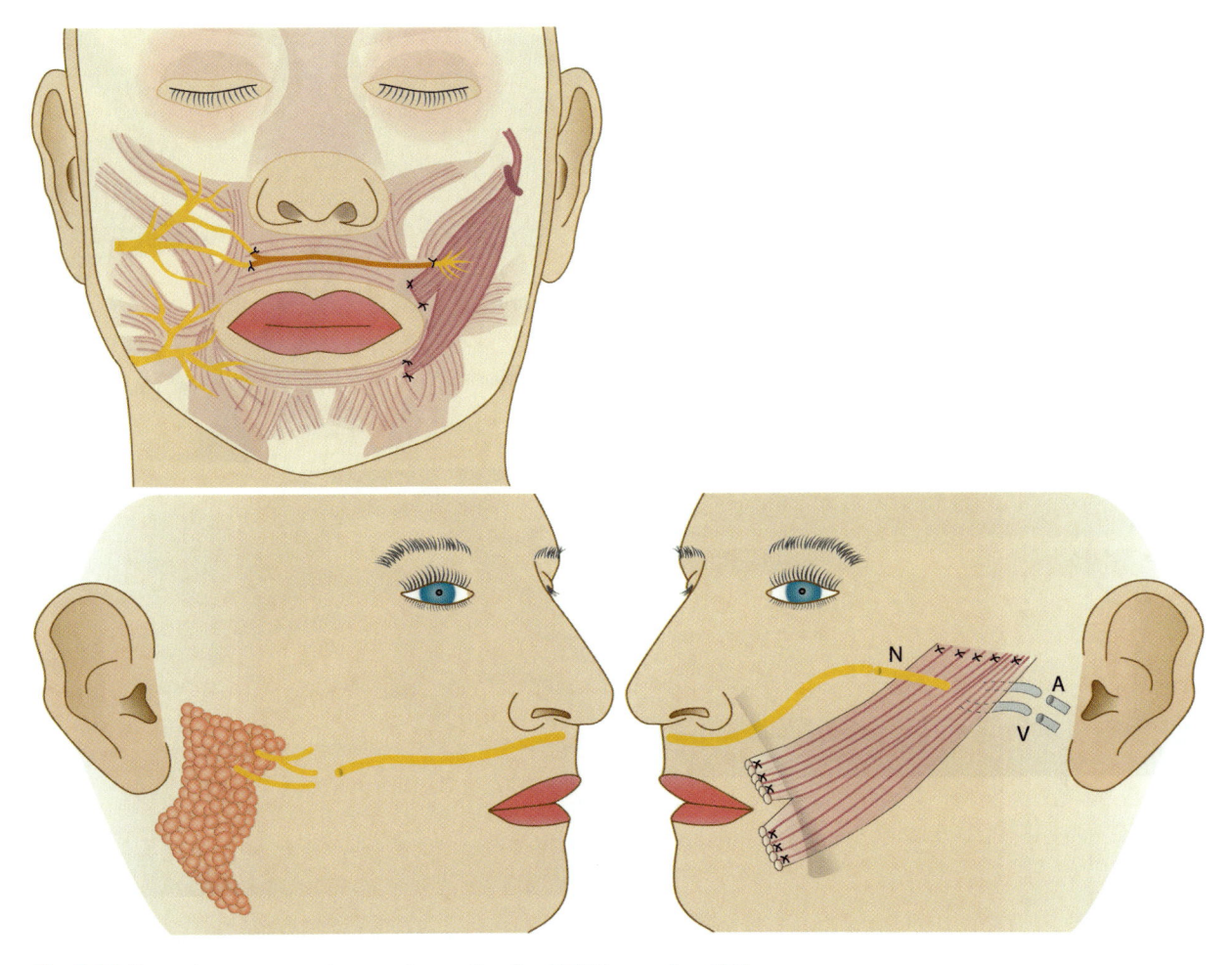

7 Nerve Injuries in Traumatic Head Injury: When To Explore/Suture/Transplant?

Fig. 7.12 Free microneurovascular muscle transfer after CFNG-procedure [50]

Another single-stage muscle flap has been presented by Zuker and coworkers. In cases of bilateral facial nerve paralysis (see below), they coapted the nerve segment of the free muscle to a trigeminal branch which supplies the masseter muscle [58]. In children, this procedure provided a symmetric smile with adequate muscle excursion, while performing a smile motion, although not voluntary or truly spontaneous.

Two-Staged Free Microneurovascular Muscle Transfer (Presence of Contralateral Facial Nerve)

In patients with unilateral facial nerve paralysis, the preferred option is to perform a two-stage reconstruction consisting of facial nerve mapping and CFNG procedure (Fig. 7.13) (stage 1; with or without "babysitter") followed by a microneurovascular muscle transplantation (stage 2) (Figs. 7.12 and 7.14) [21]. For functional microneurovascular transplantation, these muscles require both an adequate pedicle for vascular anastomoses and an adequate motor nerve for nerve coaptation. Regarding dimensions of the muscle flap, the original size of the muscle flap either matches the dimensions in the lower face, or a more suitable approach is to pare down a muscle to the desired size before transplantation [59]. Thus, many different muscles can be used and can be customized to fit the functional requirements of the face and individual physiognomy respectively. In addition to the gracilis muscle [52, 58], the latissimus dorsi muscle [60, 61] and the pectoralis minor [62–64] have been used with satisfying results.

However, the gracilis muscle is the preferred muscle for transplantation. The anatomy of this versatile muscle flap is well known, and its preparation is a well-described standard procedure in plastic surgery. It has a safe and reliable neurovascular pedicle. There

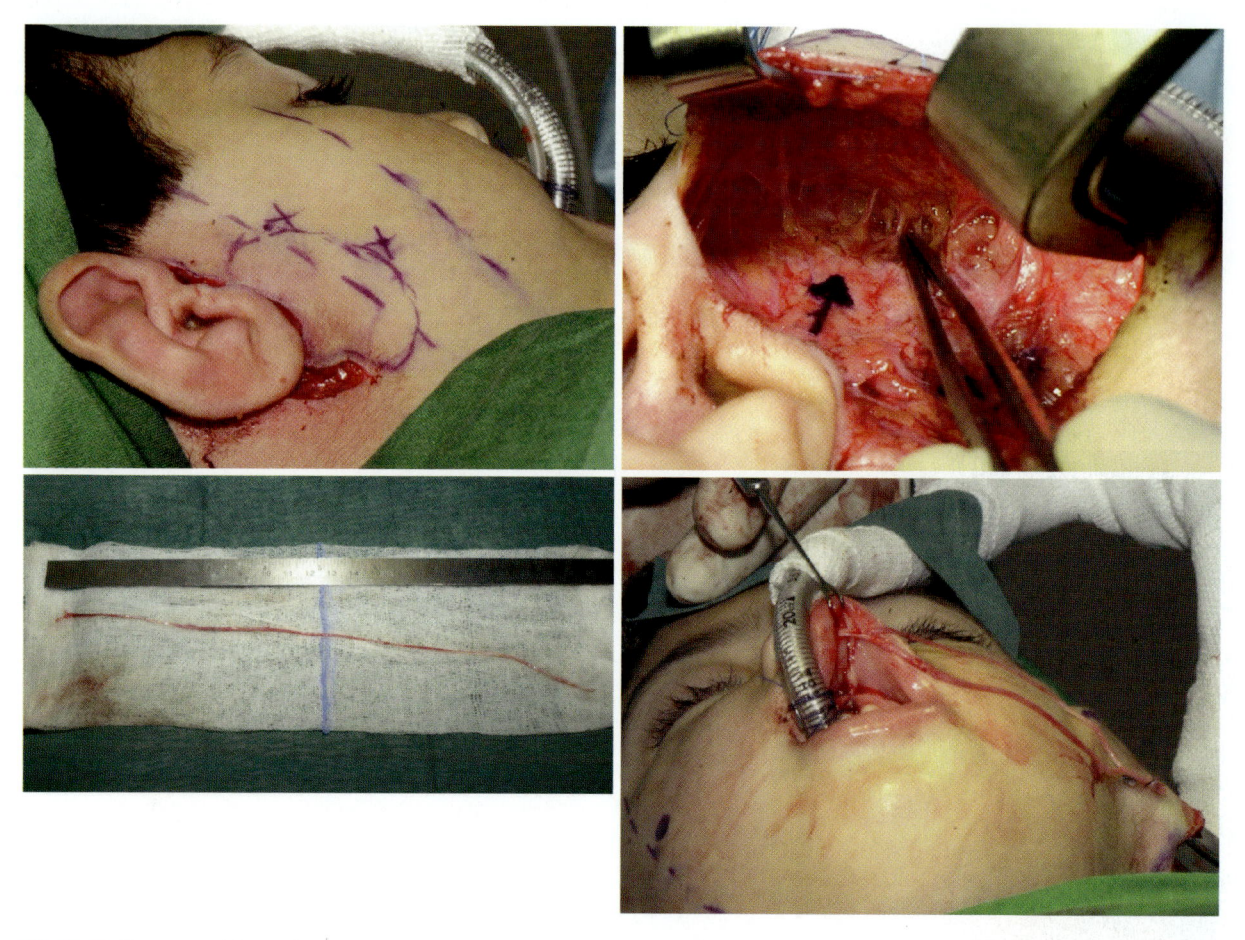

Fig. 7.13 Two-staged free microneurovascular muscle transfer in the presence of contralateral facial nerve. Intraoperative view of step 1: CFNG-procedure

is no significant functional loss in the leg, and the patient is left with a well-hidden scar in the medial aspect of the thigh. Two teams of surgeons can easily work simultaneously; one team prepares the recipient site in the face, while the second team harvests the muscle flap at the donor site. The muscle can usually be split longitudinally and then cut down or debulked to the required size for the patient's anatomical requirements; usually 30–70% of the cross section of the muscle. The muscle flap is removed with short extra length, and both ends of the muscle are supported with mattress sutures. The hilus of the gracilis muscle is positioned close to the mouth, and the obturator nerve can be tunnelled into the upper lip for nerve coaptation. The attachment of the muscle flap at the mouth (site of insertion) is a critical part of the procedure with possible insertion into the fibers of the paralyzed orbicularis oris muscle at, above, and below the commissure. However, in each case, the preoperative smile analysis helps to identify the points of insertion. Likewise, the preoperative smile analysis is essential for determining the point of origin of the muscle, which can be the zygomatic body, zygomatic arch, temporal fascia, or preauricular fascia, etc. After muscle placement, the vascular pedicle (gracilis muscle: medial circumflex femoral artery and vein) is usually anastomosed to the facial vessels followed by the nerve coaptations. As an alternative, the superficial temporal vessel can also be used. Movement of the muscle is usually not observable until 6 months after the operation, and reaching maximal movement generally takes up to 18 months. At this stage, an assessment is made of resting tension in the muscle and its excursion with smiling. Touch-up procedures (e.g., tightening, loosening, debulking, etc.) are often required [21].

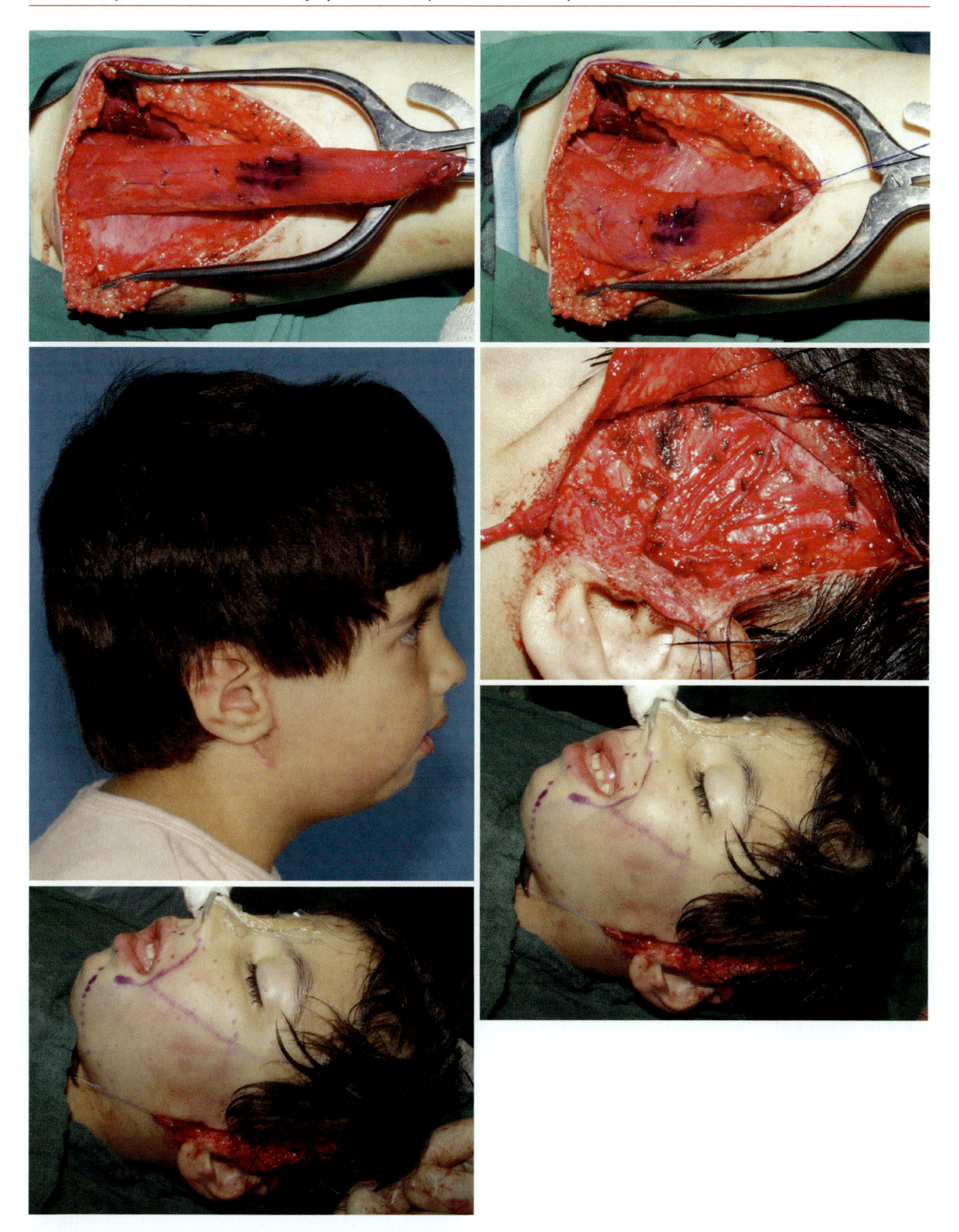

Fig. 7.14 Two-staged free microneurovascular muscle transfer in the presence of contralateral facial nerve. Intraoperative view of step 2: Free (gracilis) muscle transfer

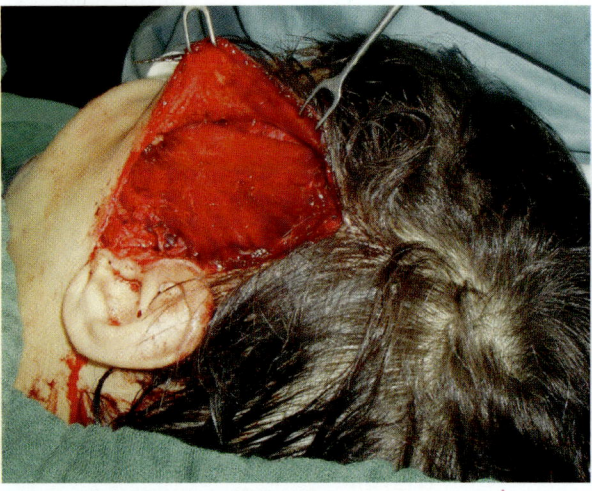

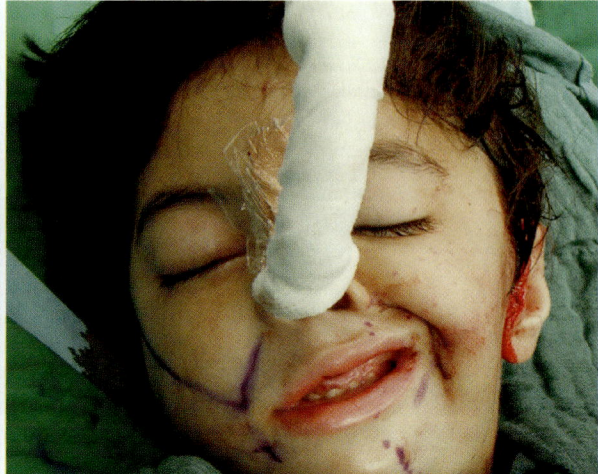

Fig. 7.14 (continued)

Two-Stage Muscle Flaps: Free Microneurovascular Muscle Transplantation (Absence of Facial Nerve)

In cases of bilateral facial nerve paralysis, alternative effective motor nerves are required. The masseteric nerve is a branch of the anterior division of the mandibular nerve (trigeminal nerve). In contrast to the spontaneous expression resulting from use of the contralateral facial nerve via CFNG, use of the masseteric nerve does not result in spontaneity of activity, but does allow for conscious activity. Although this transfer does not produce emotional movements, however, patients do learn to smile with some degree of coordination because mastication (trigeminal nerve) and smiling (facial nerve) are not opposing functions [20]. Initially, the patients are instructed to bite down for muscle activation. With time and training, the smile can become spontaneous, especially in younger patients. Terzis and coworkers recommend an end-to-side nerve coaptation in order to minimize complete paralysis of the masseteric muscle [46]. In cases with bilateral nerve paralysis, surgery on the contralateral side is performed at least 2 months later [21].

7.3.4.6 Regional Muscle Transfer

If free muscle transplantation is not feasible, regional muscle transfer of the muscles of mastication such as the temporalis and/or masseter muscle (supplied by the trigeminal nerve) is an effective alternative for dynamic restoration. Patients have to relearn how to perform movements like smiling or closure of the eye because they have to clench their teeth for muscle activation. Since the first description by Gillies [21, 39], a variety of modifications and combinations have helped to popularize these techniques [50, 65–68]. As there are a vast number of techniques and further refinements, we can only give a short overview of the most widely used procedures.

The temporalis muscle can provide both a certain degree of static suspension at rest (e.g., oblique lift of the mouth) and voluntary movement (e.g., smiling), but without control of the direction of movement. The temporalis muscle can be transferred in an anterograde (Figs. 7.15 and 7.16) and/or retrograde fashion. For retrograde transfer [69], the temporalis muscle can be released from its origin, turned over the zygomatic arch, and extended to the eye and/or mouth. To gain length, especially in order to reach the mouth, the temporalis muscle may be elongated with fascial or tendon grafts. For the treatment of the lagopthalmus (upper lid) and ectropium (lower lid), a strip of temporalis muscle with its overlying fascia is elevated from its origin, turned over, and passed to the lateral canthus. The fascia is partially elevated from the muscle flap and tunnelled along the upper and lower lid to the medial canthal ligament for fixation. With activation of the temporalis muscle, the fascial strips are pulled tight, thereby closing the eyes. An unwanted side effect of this procedure is movement of the eyelids while chewing. A further disadvantage of this procedure is a visible hollow in the temporal region and, more importantly, a prominent bulge of muscle over the zygomatic arch. To avoid these disadvantages, the anterograde

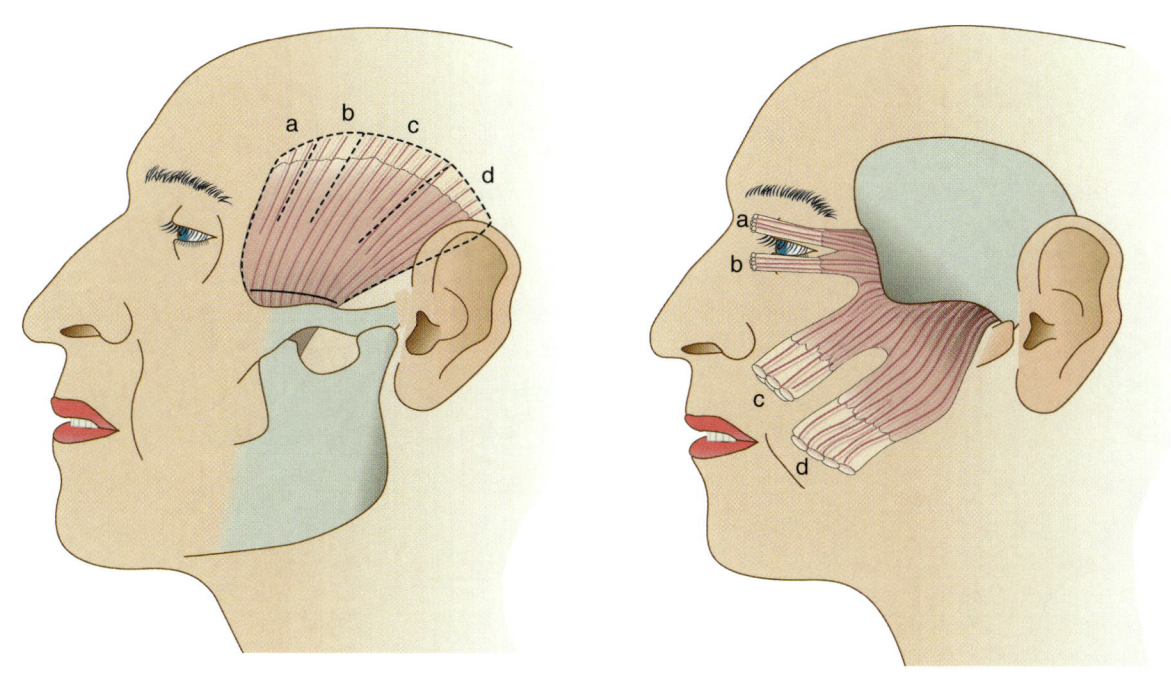

7 Nerve Injuries in Traumatic Head Injury: When To Explore/Suture/Transplant?

Fig. 7.15 Temporalis transfer according to Rubin [50, 66, 67]

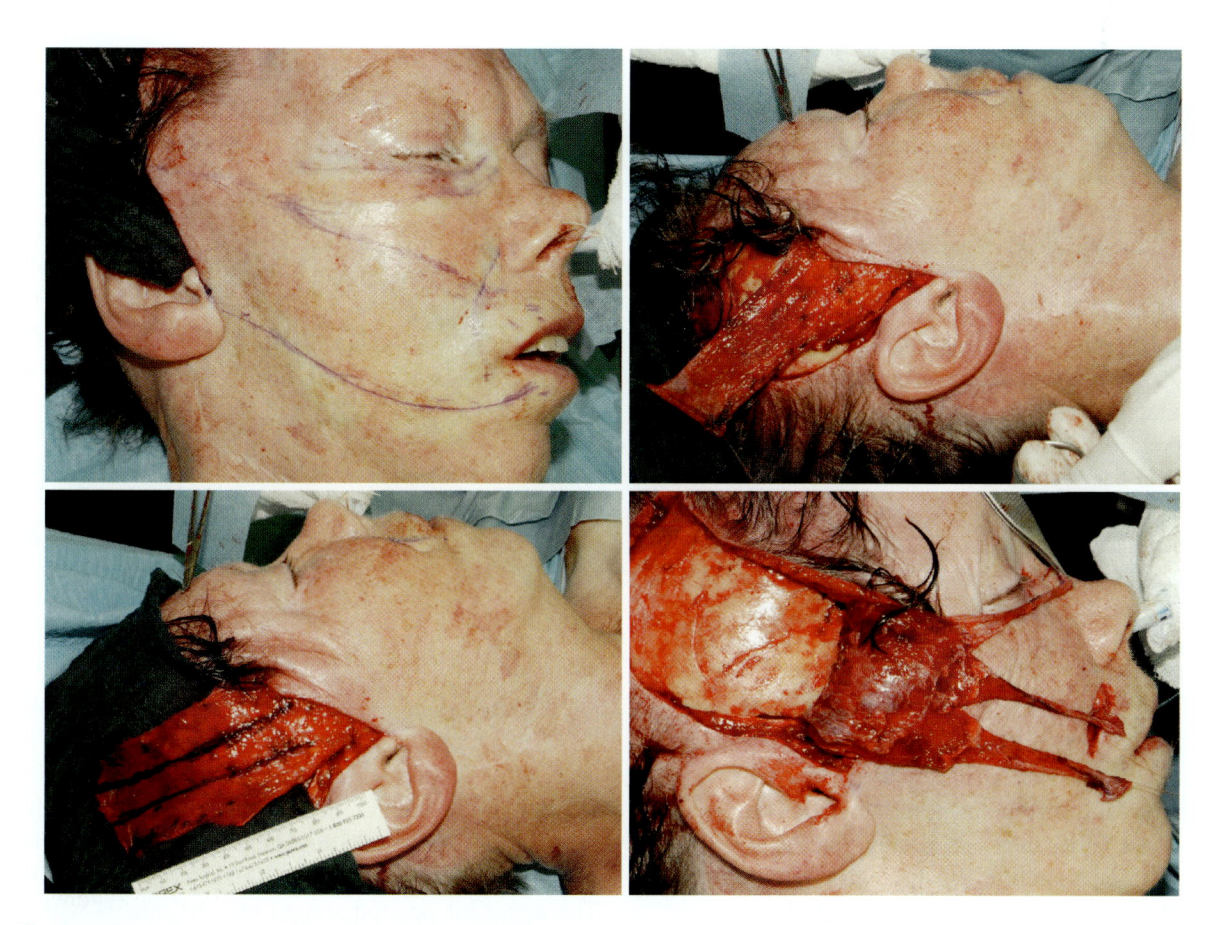

Fig. 7.16 Intraoperative examples of temporalis transfer

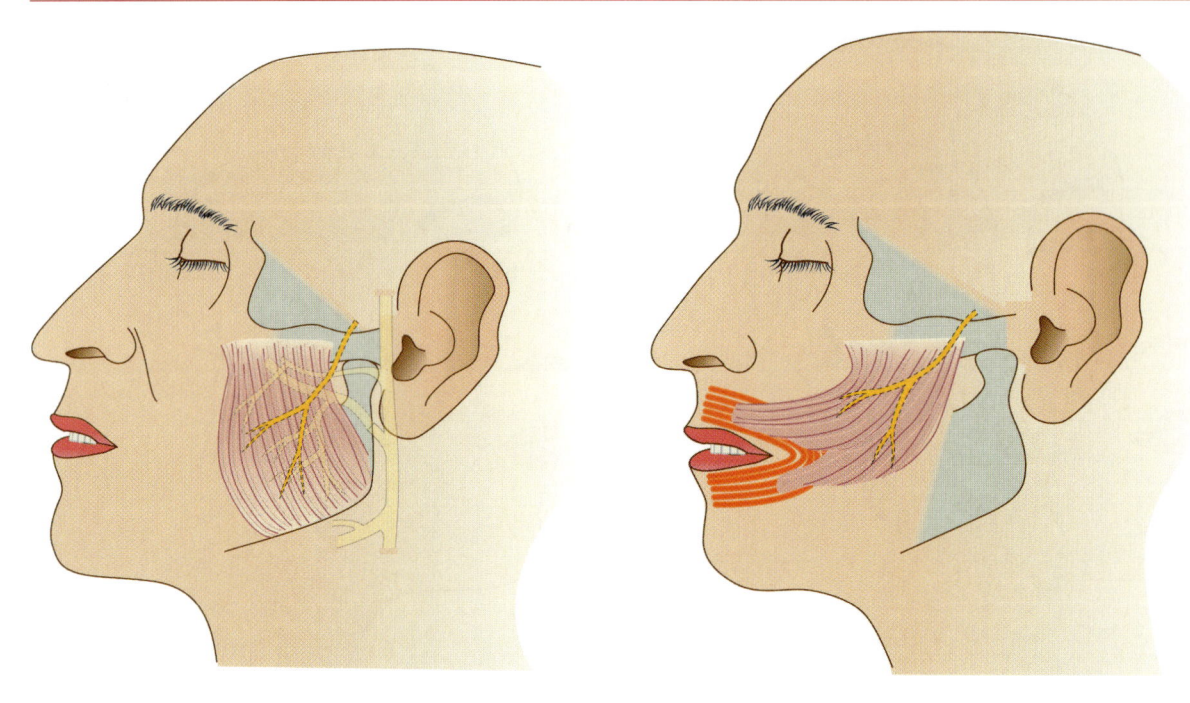

Fig. 7.17 Masseter muscle transposition according to Baker and Conley [50, 71]

temporalis muscle transfer [70] is an alternative. In this case, the muscle is detached from its insertion point at the coronoid process of the mandible.

The masseter muscle can be rotated and transferred to the mouth, either completely (Fig. 7.17) or partially, with its anterior portion from the insertion point on the mandible [71]. Adequate static suspension of the mouth can be achieved. Regarding dynamic aspects, the masseter muscle transfer can provide a full smile to only a limited degree due to lack of force and excursion. Therefore, a combination of the temporalis and masseter muscle has been described with the temporalis muscle transferred to the upper lip and the nasolabial fold, while the masseter muscle is rotated to the commissure and lower lip (Fig. 7.18) [67]. A further modification of the muscle transfer procedure has been advocated by Olivari combining both dynamic and static procedures [65].

7.3.4.7 Further Static Procedures

For the sake of completeness, there are a huge number of static procedures, especially for the eye and lip region. We, therefore, mention these in note form and refer to the respective literature [50, 65].

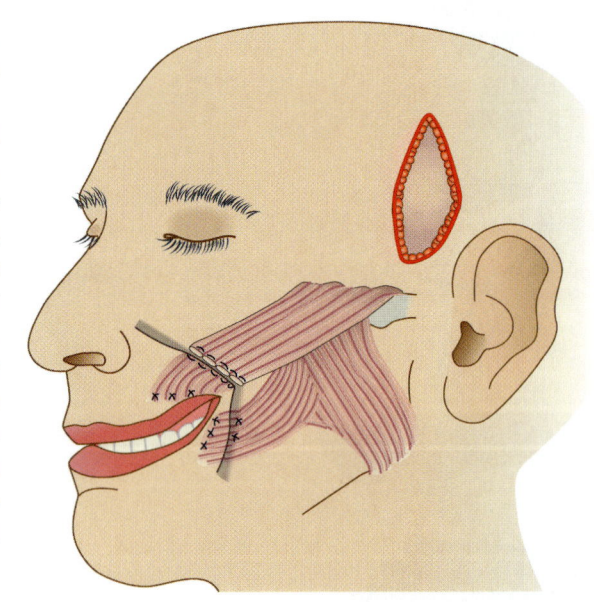

Fig. 7.18 Temporalis with masseter transfer according to Rubin [50, 66]

Static surgical corrections of the brow (brow ptosis) include direct brow lift (direct excision), coronal brow lift with static suspension, or endoscopic brow lift. The upper lid (lagopthalmus) may be treated with a tarsorrhaphy, fascial, or tendon slings, as well as the implantation of gold or platinum weights or special springs. Procedures for the lower lid (ectropion) treatment may include a lateral canthoplasty or horizontal lid shortening. Static slings, alar base elevation, and septoplasty can be helpful regarding the nasal airway. Regarding the oral commissures and the upper lip, static slings as well as soft tissue balancing procedures (facelift, midfacelift, mucosal excision or advancement) may be used. Procedures for the lower lip include depressor labii inferioris resection, muscle transplantation (digastric, platysma), as well as wedge excision.

References

1. Antoniades K, Karakasis D, Taskos N. Abducent nerve palsy following transverse fracture of the middle cranial fossa. J Craniomaxillofac Surg. 1993;21(4):172–5.
2. Bagheri SC, Meyer RA, Khan HA, Steed MB. Microsurgical repair of peripheral trigeminal nerve injuries from maxillofacial trauma. J Oral Maxillofac Surg. 2009;67:1791–9.
3. Cannon CR, Jahrsdoefer RA. Temporal bone fractures: review of 90 cases. Arch Otolaryngol. 1983;109:285–8.
4. Sanus GZ, Tanriöver N, Tanriverdi T, Uzan M, Akar Z. Late decompression in patients with acute facial nerve paralysis after temporal bone fracture. Turk Neurosurg. 2007;17:7–12.
5. Chan EH, Tan HM, Tan TY. Facial palsy from temporal bone lesions. Ann Acad Med Singapore. 2009;34:322–9.
6. Lambert PR, Brackmann DE. Facial paralysis in longitudinal temporal bone fractures: a review of 26 cases. Laryngoscope. 1984;94:1022–6.
7. Johnson F, Semaan MT, Megerian CA. Temporal bone fracture: evaluation and management in the modern era. Otolaryngol Clin North Am. 2008;41:597–618.
8. Seddon HJ, Medawar PB, Smith H. Rate of regeneration of peripheral nerves in man. J Physiol. 1943;102:191–215.
9. Sunderland S. A classification of peripheral nerve injuries producing loss of function. Brain. 1951;74:491–516.
10. Mackinnon SE. Closed nerve injury. In: Marsh JL, editor. Current therapy in plastic and reconstructive surgery. Philadelphia: BC Decker; 1989.
11. Winograd JM, Mackinnon SE. Peripheral nerve injuries: repair and reconstruction. In: Mathes SJ, editor. Plastic surgery, 2nd ed., Volume VII: The hand and upper limb, Part 1. Philadelphia: Elsevier; 2006.
12. Frey M. Fazialisparese. In: Berger A, Hierner R, editors. Plastische Chirurgie- Band II: Kopf und Hals. Berlin-Heidelberg: Springer; 2005.
13. Millesi H, Meissl G, Berger A. The interfascicular nerve-grafting of the median and ulnar nerves. J Bone Joint Surg Am. 1972;54:727–50.
14. Shenaq SM, Kim JYS. Repair and grafting of peripheral nerve. In: Mathes SJ, editor. Plastic surgery, 2nd ed., Volume I: General principles. Philadelphia: Elsevier; 2006.
15. Tupper JW. Fascicular repair. In: Gelberman RH, editor. Operative nerve repair and reconstruction, vol. I. Philadelphia: J.B. Lippincott; 1991.
16. Wilgis EFS. Techniques of epineural and group fascicular repair. In: Gelberman RH, editor. Operative nerve repair and reconstruction, vol. I. Philadelphia: J.B. Lippincott; 1991.
17. Millesi H. Brachial plexus injury in adults: operative repair. In: Gelberman RH, editor. Operative nerve repair and reconstruction, vol. II. Philadelphia: J.B. Lippincott; 1991.
18. Birch R, Bonney G, Parry CB. Principles of nerve repair. In: Birch R, Bonney G, Parry CB, editors. Surgical disorders of the peripheral nerves. New York: Churchill Livingstone; 1998.
19. Fabian RL. Facial nerve paralysis. In: Gelberman RH, editor. Operative nerve repair and reconstruction, vol. I. Philadelphia: J.B. Lippincott; 1991.
20. Rosson GD, Redett RJ. Facial palsy: anatomy, etiology, grading, and surgical treatment. J Reconstr Microsurg. 2008;24(6):379–89.
21. Zuker RM, Manktelow RT, Hussain G. Facial paralysis. In: Mathes SJ, editor. Plastic surgery, 2nd ed., Volume III: The head and neck, Part 2. Philadelphia: Elsevier; 2006.
22. Rudolph R. Depth of the facial nerve in facelift dissection. Plast Reconstr Surg. 1990;85:537–44.
23. Day C, Nahai F. Forehead correction of aging. In: Mathes SJ editor. Plastic surgery, 2nd ed., Volume II: The head and neck, Part 1. Philadelphia: Elsevier; 2006.
24. Lei T, Xu DC, Gao JH, Zhong SZ, Chen B, Yang DY, et al. Using the frontal branch of the superficial temporal artery as a landmark for locating the course of the temporal branch of the facial nerve during rhytidectomy: an anatomical study. Plast Reconstr Surg. 2005;116(2):623–9.
25. Lei T, Gao JH, Xu DC, Zhong SZ, Li XJ, Chen B, et al. The frontal-temporal nerve triangle: a new concept of locating the motor and sensory nerves in upper third of the face rhytidectomy. Plast Reconstr Surg. 2006;117(2):385–94.
26. Stuzin JM, Baker TJ. Aging face and neck. In: Mathes SJ, editor. Plastic surgery, 2nd ed., Volume II: The head and neck, Part 1. Philadelphia: Elsevier; 2006.
27. Freilinger G, Gruber H, Happak W, Pechmann U. Surgical anatomy of the mimic muscle system and the facial nerve: importance for reconstructive and aesthetic surgery. Plast Reconstr Surg. 1987;80:686–90.
28. Ishikawa Y. An anatomical study of the distribution of the temporal branch of the facial nerve. J Craniomaxillofac Surg. 1990;18:287–92.
29. Saylam C, Ucerler H, Orhan M, Ozek C. Anatomic guides to precisely localize the zygomatic branches of the facial nerve. J Craniofac Surg. 2006;17(1):50–3.
30. Dingman RO, Grabb WC. Surgical anatomy of the mandibular ramus of the facial nerve based on the dissection of 100 facial halves. Plast Reconstr Surg. 1962;29:266–72.
31. Westin LM, Zuker R. A new classification system for facial paralysis in the clinical setting. J Craniofac Surg. 2003;14:672–9.
32. Guerrissi JO. Selective myectomy for postparetic facial synkinesis. Plast Reconstr Surg. 1991;87:459–66.
33. Neely JG. Computerized quantitative dynamic analysis of facial motion in the paralyzed and synkinetic face. Am J Otol. 1992;13:97–107.
34. House JW, Brackmann DE. Facial nerve grading system. Otolaryngol Head Neck Surg. 1985;93:146–7.

35. Terzis JK, Tzafetta K. The "babysitter" procedure: minihypoglossal to facial nerve transfer and cross-facial nerve grafting. Plast Reconstr Surg. 2009;123(3):865–76.
36. Terzis JK, Tzafetta K. "Babysitter" procedure with concomitant muscle transfer in facial paralysis. Plast Reconstr Surg. 2009;124(4):1142–56.
37. Frey M, Jenny A, Giovanoli P, Stüssi E. Development of a new documentation system for facial movements as a basis for the international registry for neuromuscular reconstruction in the face. Plast Reconstr Surg. 1994;93(7):1334–49.
38. Frey M, Giovanoli P, Gerber H, Slameczka M, Stüssi E. Three-dimensional video analysis of facial movements: a new method to assess the quantity and quality of the smile. Plast Reconstr Surg. 1999;104(7):2032–9.
39. Frey M, Michaelidou M, Tzou CH, Pona I, Mittlböck M, Gerber H, et al. Three-dimensional video analysis of the paralyzed face reanimated by cross-face nerve grafting and free gracilis muscle transplantation: quantification of the functional outcome. Plast Reconstr Surg. 2008;122(6):1709–22.
40. Diels HJ. Neuromuscular retraining for facial paralysis. Otolaryngol Clin North Am. 1997;30:727–43.
41. Koshima I, Nanba Y, Tsutsui T, Takahashi Y, Itoh S. New one-stage nerve pedicle grafting technique using the great auricular nerve for reconstruction of facial nerve defects. J Reconstr Microsurg. 2004;20:357–61.
42. Bozkurt A, Brook GA, Moellers S, Lassner F, Sellhaus B, Weis J, et al. In vitro assessment of axonal growth using dorsal root ganglia explants in a novel three-dimensional collagen matrix. Tissue Eng. 2007;13(12):2971–9.
43. Bozkurt A, Deumens R, Beckmann C, Olde Damink L, Schügner F, Heschel I, et al. In vitro cell alignment obtained with a Schwann cell enriched microstructured nerve guide with longitudinal guidance channels. Biomaterials. 2009;30(2):169–79.
44. Bozkurt A, Brook GA, Heschel I, Lassner F, Möllers S, Olde Damink L, et al. Peripheral nervous system: neuro-tissue engineering using a microstructured collagen matrix. In: Schumpelick V, Schackert HK, Bruch HP, editors. Chirurgisches Forum und DGAV 2009: für experimentelle und klinische Forschung. Berlin-Heidelberg: Springer; 2009. p. 289–91.
45. Meek MF, Coert JH. US Food and Drug Administration / Conformit Europe-approved absorbable nerve conduits for clinical repair of peripheral and cranial nerves. Ann Plast Surg. 2008;60(4):466–72.
46. Terzis JK, Konofaos P. Nerve transfers in facial palsy. Facial Plast Surg. 2008;24(2):177–93.
47. Myckatyn TM, Mackinnon SE. The surgical management of facial nerve injury. Clin Plast Surg. 2003;30:307–18.
48. Dellon AL. Restoration of facial nerve function: an approach for the twenty-first century. Neurosurg Q. 1992;2:199–222.
49. Samii M, Matthies C. Indication, technique and results of facial nerve reconstruction. Acta Neurochir Wien. 1994; 130:125–39.
50. Burgess LPA, Goode RL. Reanimation of the paralyzed face. New York/Stuttgart: Thieme Medical Publishers; 1994.
51. Anderl H. Cross-face nerve transplantation in facial palsy. Proc R Soc Med. 1976;69:781–3.
52. Harii K, Ohmori K, Torii S. Free gracilis muscle transplantation, with microneurovascular anastomoses for the treatment of facial paralysis. A preliminary report. Plast Reconstr Surg. 1976;57:133–43.
53. Frey M, Koller R, Liegl C, Happak W, Gruber H. Role of a muscle target organ on the regeneration of motor nerve fibres in long nerve grafts: a synopsis of experimental and clinical data. Microsurgery. 1996;17:80–8.
54. Manktelow RT, Zuker RM. Cross-facial nerve graft—the long and short graft: the first stage for microneurovascular muscle transfer. Oper Tech Plast Reconstr Surg. 1999;6(3): 151–209.
55. Conley J, Baker DC. Hypoglossal-facial nerve anastomosis for reinnervation of the paralyzed face. Plast Reconstr Surg. 1979;63:63–72.
56. Mersa B, Tiangco DA, Terzis JK. Efficacy of the "babysitter" procedure after prolonged denervation. J Reconstr Microsurg. 2000;16:27–35.
57. Koshima I, Tsuda K, Hamanaka T, Moriguchi T. One-stage reconstruction of established paralysis using a rectus abdominis muscle transfer. Plast Reconstr Surg. 1997;99: 234–8.
58. Zuker RM, Goldberg CS, Manktelow RT. Facial animation in children with Moebius syndrome after segmental gracilis muscle transplant. Plast Reconstr Surg. 2000;106:1–8.
59. Manktelow RT, Zuker RM. Muscle transplantation by fascicular territory. Plast Reconstr Surg. 1984;73:751–7.
60. Dellon AL, Mackinnon SE. Segmentally innervated latissimus dorsi muscle. Microsurgical transfer for facial reanimation. J Reconstr Microsurg. 1985;2:7–12.
61. Mackinnon SE, Dellon AL. Technical considerations of the latissimus dorsi muscle flap: a segmentally innervated muscle transfer for facial reanimation. Microsurgery. 1988;9: 36–45.
62. Harrison DH. The pectoralis minor vascularized muscle graft for the treatment of unilateral facial palsy. Plast Reconstr Surg. 1985;75:206–16.
63. Scevola S, Cowan J, Harrison DH. Does the removal of pectoralis minor impair the function of pectoralis major? Plast Reconstr Surg. 2003;112:1266–73.
64. Terzis JK. Pectoralis minor: a unique muscle for correction of facial palsy. Plast Reconstr Surg. 1989;83:767–76.
65. Olivari N. Practical plastic and reconstructive surgery: an atlas of operations and techniques. Heidelberg: Kaden Publishing; 2008.
66. Rubin L. Temporalis and masseter muscle transposition. In: May M, editor. The facial nerve. New York: Thieme; 1986.
67. Rubin L. Reanimation of total unilateral facial paralysis by the contiguous facial muscle technique. In: Rubin L, editor. The paralyzed face. St. Louis: Mosby-Year Book; 1991.
68. Salimbeni G. Eyelid reanimation in facial paralysis by temporalis muscle transfer. Oper Tech Plast Reconstr Surg. 1999; 6:159.
69. Gillies H. Experiences with fascia lata grafts in the operative treatment of facial paralysis. Proceedings of the Royal Society of Medicine, London; 1935.
70. McLaughlin CR. Surgical support in permanent facial paralysis. Plast Reconstr Surg. 1953;11:302–14.
71. Baker DC, Conley J. Regional muscle transposition for rehabilitation of the paralyzed face. Clin Plast Surg. 1979;6: 317–31.

Chest Trauma: Classification and Influence on the General Management

8

Philipp Mommsen, Christian Krettek, and Frank Hildebrand

Contents

8.1	Introduction	75
8.1.1	Chest Wall Injuries	76
8.1.2	Injuries to Intrathoracic Organs	76
8.2	Diagnostics	78
8.2.1	Chest Radiography	78
8.2.2	Computed Tomography (CT) of the Chest	79
8.2.3	Thoracic Ultrasonography	79
8.2.4	Bronchoscopy	79
8.3	Classification	79
8.3.1	Abbreviated Injury Scale	80
8.3.2	Pulmonary Contusion Score According to Tyburski	80
8.3.3	CT-Dependent Score According to Wagner and Jamieson	80
8.3.4	Thoracic Trauma Severity Score	80
8.4	Treatment	81
8.4.1	Airway Management	82
8.4.2	Ventilation	82
8.4.3	Positioning Therapy	82
8.4.4	Fracture Treatment in Multiple Trauma Patients with Thoracic Trauma	83
8.4.5	Surgical Chest Wall Stabilization	84
	References	84

P. Mommsen, C. Krettek, and F. Hildebrand (✉)
Trauma Department, Hannover Medical School,
Carl-Neuberg-Strasse 1, 30625 Hanover, Germany
e-mail: mommsen.philipp@mh-hannover.de;
krettek.christian@mh-hannover.de;
hildebrand.frank@mh-hannover.de

8.1 Introduction

Depending on the mechanism of injury, thoracic trauma occurs as blunt chest trauma or penetrating injuries.

Isolated chest injuries mostly occur as minor blunt trauma with mild injuries (e.g., thoracic bruises, rib fractures). The majority of these isolated blunt thoracic injuries can be treated conservatively. The mortality rate in young adults amounts to 0–5%. Mortality associated with these injuries increases to 10–15% in the elderly [1–3]. Age ≥ 85, initial blood pressure < 90 mmHg, hemothorax, pneumothorax, serial rib fracture, and pulmonary contusion have been identified as risk factors for posttraumatic complications/adverse events and poor outcome [4].

Severe thoracic trauma occurs in 80–90% of multiple trauma patients [5]. In Europe, most of these injuries are caused by blunt trauma, whereas penetrating injury mechanism only accounts for 8–9% of these cases [5]. Severe thoracic trauma is the second most common diagnosis in patients with multiple trauma [6]. The incidence of acute respiratory distress syndrome (ARDS), systemic inflammatory response syndrome (SIRS), multiple organ dysfunction syndrome (MODS), and infectious complications (pneumonia) is substantially higher in multiple trauma patients with severe thoracic trauma [3, 7–9]. Severe thoracic trauma also causes a significant increase in ventilation time and length of stay on intensive care unit in these patients [6]. Moreover, thoracic injuries are associated with a mortality of 30–40% in multiple trauma patients [1–3, 8, 10, 11] and trauma associated fatalities of 20–25%. Between 50% and 75% of deceased polytraumatized patients had a thoracic injury [1–3, 8, 10–12].

Thoracic injuries can affect the chest wall and intrathoracic organs including pleura, diaphragm, lungs, mediastinum, and the great blood vessels.

8.1.1 Chest Wall Injuries

Rib fractures account for the majority of thoracic injuries and are found in 60% of blunt chest trauma, typically involving the ribs IV–X. In cases of fractures to the first two ribs, a severe thoracic trauma must be assumed as these ribs provide protection to vital structures. Therefore, lesions of the brachial plexus and vessels (e.g., subclavian artery and vein) may occur and lung contusions are likely. Lower rib fractures are mainly caused by direct local trauma and may involve abdominal organs such as the liver, spleen, and kidneys. In the elderly, minor trauma often results in rib fractures due to decreased bone elasticity and osteoporosis. Chest wall pain associated with rib fractures is likely to lead to reduced ventilation with possible fluid retention and subsequent complications such as pneumonia and atelectasis. In older patients, each additional rib fracture increases the probability of death by 19% and the incidence of pneumonia by 27% [13, 14]. Furthermore, pleural or pulmonary lacerations with the development of pulmonary hematoma, hemothorax, and pneumothorax may also be caused by fractured ribs.

Serial rib fractures are defined as the fracture of at least three ribs and occur in almost one-third of all rib fractures. In addition to the usual risks of single rib fractures, an increasing number of rib fractures leads to reduced chest wall stability with the risk for developing a flail chest.

A *flail chest* occurs in approximately 15% of patients with blunt chest trauma [15] and is characterized by at least five contiguous single fractures or three adjacent segmental rib fractures. This results in an unstable flail segment with a paradoxical respiratory motion (inward motion during inspiration and outward motion during expiration). Posterior flail segments are stabilized by overlying muscles as well as the scapula and therefore may not cause severe complications. In contrast, anterior and lateral flail segments are mobile and can seriously impair respiratory function. Additionally, a flail chest is frequently associated with lung contusions [12].

Sternum fractures are seen in about 5% of patients with thoracic trauma [16]. Most fractures involve the upper or mid body of the sternum. Accompanying injuries are lung and myocardial contusions as well as fractures of the thoracic spine.

Sternoclavicular dislocations may be either anterior or posterior. Posterior dislocations are more severe, as they can cause injuries to the mediastinal blood vessels, trachea and esophagus [17]. Anterior dislocations, which are more common, can be treated conservatively, whereas posterior dislocation requires closed or surgical reduction.

Fractures of the scapula are uncommon, with a prevalence of approximately 4% in patients with multiple injuries [18], and are associated with concomitant lesions including pneumothorax, hemothorax, pulmonary injuries and spinal injuries in 35–98% [19]. Most fractures occur in the body and neck of the scapula and can be treated conservatively. In contrast, displaced glenoid intraarticular fractures and displaced juxtaarticular fractures require a surgical intervention [19, 20].

8.1.2 Injuries to Intrathoracic Organs

8.1.2.1 Pleural Injuries

A *pneumothorax* is defined as the air entrapment into the pleural cavity either from within the body after blunt trauma, usually due to pleural laceration by fractured ribs (closed pneumothorax), or from the outside environment associated with penetrating injuries (open pneumothorax) [16]. Lesions of the tracheobronchial tree are a further cause for a pneumothorax. A pneumothorax occurs in 15–40% of patients with blunt chest trauma [21–23]. The most frequent complication of a pneumothorax is the development of tension pneumothorax.

A *tension pneumothorax* occurs when a pneumothorax permits entry into but not exit of air from the thoracic cavity. This results in a collapse of the ipsilateral lung followed by compression of mediastinum and contralateral lung. Suspected tension should be immediately decompressed by needle thoracostomy or a chest tube.

A *hemothorax* results from vascular lesions after blunt or penetrating trauma. It is present in 40% of blunt thoracic trauma. Various bleeding sources can contribute to a hemothorax including intercostal arteries, internal mammary arteries, lung parenchyma, heart, hilar, and great vessels. The therapy for a hemothorax is the placement of a chest tube. An undrained, massive hemothorax can lead to a *tension hemothorax* with an ipsilateral lung compression and a resulting mediastinum displacement [16]. A chronic hemothorax can be complicated by pleural empyema or a fibrothorax, resulting in a restrictive pulmonary disease [12].

A *chylothorax* is caused by damage to the thoracic duct. A left-sided chylothorax is found in case of ruptures of the upper part of the thoracic duct, whereas a right-sided chylothorax is seen in injury of the lower levels, when the thoracic duct has already crossed the midline.

8.1.2.2 Diaphragm Injuries

A diaphragmatic rupture can be caused by blunt or penetrating injuries, and occurs in 0.2–5% of patients with blunt chest trauma [24, 25]. Ruptures on the left side are three to four times more common than lesions on the right side. In 5–10% of the cases a bilateral rupture is found [12]. A high proportion of diaphragmatic ruptures go primarily undiagnosed [12]. The mortality of missed diaphragm ruptures has been reported to be as high as 30% [26]. Therefore, a CT scan should be performed if there is any suspicion.

8.1.2.3 Lung Injuries

Parenchymal lung injuries appear as pulmonary contusions and lacerations. *Pulmonary contusions* are the second most frequent injuries in thoracic trauma and are found in 30–50% of multiple trauma patients with blunt chest trauma [12]. Pulmonary contusions are caused by direct trauma on lung parenchyma or by indirect mechanisms such as deceleration and shear forces. Lesions usually occur in peripheral lung sections adjacent to bony structures [26]. Pulmonary contusions become apparent 3–6 h after trauma and generally resolve within 5–7 days [26, 27]. Histopathologically, these injuries are characterized by an extravasation of blood and edema into the interstitial and alveolar space. Especially in younger patients, pulmonary contusions could be found without accompanying osseous lesions. The lack of rib fractures does not exclude the presence of substantial lung contusion in these patients [12, 16] as severe thoracic injuries occur in 25% without concomitant bony injuries [28, 29]. However, serial rib fractures and a flail chest are commonly associated with pulmonary contusions [30]. *Pulmonary lacerations* are characterized by a disruption of the parenchymal architecture. With the exception of stab wounds, lung lacerations are always accompanied by pulmonary contusions [31]. Pulmonary contusions and lacerations can be complicated by the development of *acute respiratory distress syndrome* (*ARDS*). ARDS is the consequence of a systemic inflammatory response following thoracic or general trauma within 24–48 h. Pathophysiologically, ARDS is caused by the damage of the alveolar-capillary barrier by activated neutrophils, resulting in an extravasation of fluid into the alveolar space [32, 33]. This systemic inflammatory reaction can also affect uninjured pulmonary sections [28, 34] and manifests radiographically as a diffuse bilateral pulmonary infiltration [27].

8.1.2.4 Injuries to the Mediastinum

A *pneumomediastinum* (*mediastinal emphysema*) occurs in pharyngeal, tracheobronchial, and esophageal lesions due to penetrating or blunt trauma. Besides chest radiography, esophageal and tracheobronchial endoscopy should be considered for diagnostics. A *mediastinal hematoma* results from vascular injuries, possibly resulting in an enlargement of the mediastinum due to significant hematoma. The criteria for the diagnosis of mediastinal widening are a diameter of greater than 8 cm and a mediastinum to chest ratio greater than 0.25.

Tracheobronchial injuries include lacerations due to penetrating trauma and ruptures from blunt trauma. Tracheobronchial trauma occurs in 0.2–8% of all patients with blunt chest trauma, and a high coincidence of accompanying pulmonary or vascular injuries has been reported [35, 36]. Tracheal lesions usually appear as transverse tears between cartilaginous tracheal rings or longitudinal tears in the posterior tracheal membrane. In tracheal injuries, surgical repair is required in order to ensure airway continuity.

Esophageal injuries are extremely rare after blunt chest trauma. Most esophageal lesions are located in the cervical and upper thoracic sections and may occur after penetrating as well as blunt thoracic trauma. Depending on their location, esophageal lesions can result in right- or left-sided pleural effusion. In order to

Several scoring systems for the classification of blunt chest trauma have been developed. Most of the thoracic trauma scores are based on pathological–anatomical changes. One of the most commonly used scoring system is the Thoracic Abbreviated Injury Scale (AIS$_{chest}$). Further anatomic scoring systems are the Wagner-Score [74] and Pulmonary Contusion Score (PCS) by Tyburski [75]. Other scoring systems, such as the Thoracic Trauma Severity Score, have additionally included physiological parameters [76].

8.3.1 Abbreviated Injury Scale

The Abbreviated Injury Scale (AIS), first described in 1969 (John D. States) and revised in 1998 is a prognostic scoring system that allocates a severity score to every injury to each of the different body regions (head, face, neck, thorax, abdomen, spine, upper extremity, lower extremity, external and other trauma). The score value ranges from 0 to 6, and higher severity scores are associated with a lower probability of survival. The AIS is an anatomical scoring system for injury severity assessment of different body regions. It is the basis for calculation of the Injury Severity Score (ISS). In general, the AIS correlates with mortality [77, 78] and the AIS$_{chest}$ has been demonstrated to be an independent predictor for prolonged hospitalization [79, 80] and duration of mechanical ventilation [81], and a risk factor for the development of posttraumatic MODS [82].

8.3.2 Pulmonary Contusion Score According to Tyburski

The Pulmonary Contusion Score (PCS) was developed in 1999 by Tyburski and colleagues [75]. This score is based on plain radiograph of the chest at the time of admission and 24 h after trauma. After division of the lung into an upper, middle, and lower third, the pulmonary contusion in every third is assessed by a value of 1–3 and added afterwards. A score value of 1–2 is classified as mild, a value of 3–9 as moderate, and a value of 10–18 as severe pulmonary contusion (Table 8.1). A higher mortality and prolonged duration of mechanical ventilation was reported in cases of an increase in the severity of lung contusion during the first 24 h [75]. The usefulness of this score is limited due to the fact that the assessment of pulmonary contusion is difficult in chest radiography.

8.3.3 CT-Dependent Score According to Wagner and Jamieson

Wagner and Jamieson developed a thoracic trauma score based on CT scan [74]. As shown in Fig. 8.1, the severity of thoracic trauma is divided into different sections depending on the extension of pulmonary lesions. Pulmonary lesions of ≥28% of total air space are classified as grade 1, 19–27% as grade 2, and <19% as grade 3. The authors showed an association between the size and type of parenchymal injuries and the need for mechanical ventilation [74].

8.3.4 Thoracic Trauma Severity Score

The Thoracic Trauma Severity Score (TTS) is a CT-independent scoring system based on five anatomical and physiological parameters at the time of admission: extension of pulmonary contusion, rib fractures, pleural lesion, age and Horrowitz ratio PaO$_2$/FiO$_2$ [76]. Each parameter is assigned a value of 0–5 (Table 8.2). The TTS score ranges from 0 to 25.

Table 8.1 Pulmonary contusion score according to Tyburski et al. [75]

Calculation of the pulmonary contusion score (PCS)		
• Dividing the lung fields into upper, middle and lower third		
• Assigning a score of 1–3 to each region on the basis of the amount of radiologic parenchymal changes		
Mild pulmonary contusion	Moderate pulmonary contusion	Severe pulmonary contusion
PCS 1–2	PCS 3–9	PCS 10–18

Fig. 8.1 CT-dependent score according to Wagner and Jamieson [74]

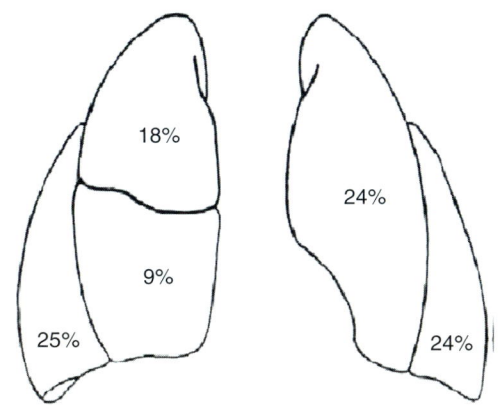

(Lung diagram with percentages: 18%, 24%, 9%, 25%, 24%)

Grade 1
- ≥28% of total air space consolidated or lacerated
- All patients require mechanical ventilation for pulmonary insufficiency

Grade 2
- 19–27% of total air space consolidated or lacerated
- 60% of these patients require mechanical ventilation for pulmonary insufficiency

Grade 3
- <19% of total air space consolidated or lacerated
- No mechanical ventilation required for pulmonary insufficiency

Table 8.2 Thoracic trauma severity score according to Pape et al. [76]

Grade	PO$_2$/FiO$_2$	Rib fractures	Pulmonary contusion	Pleural lesion	Age (years)	Points
0	>400	0	None	None	<30	0
I	300–400	1–3 unilateral	1 lobe unilateral	Pneumothorax	30–40	1
II	200–300	4–6 unilateral	1 lobe bilateral or 2 lobes unilateral	Hemothorax/hemopneumothorax unilateral	41–54	2
III	150–200	>3 bilateral	<2 lobes bilateral	Hemothorax/hemopneumothorax bilateral	55–70	3
IV	<150	Flail chest	≥2 lobes bilateral	Tension pneumothorax	>70	5

The sensitivity and specificity of the different scoring systems for predicting posttraumatic complications and outcome has not been fully elucidated. In general, CT-dependent scores are thought to be more reliable for the assessment of trauma severity and susceptibility to posttraumatic complications, such as ARDS. However, CT-independent scoring systems might be helpful for an early evaluation of the risk profile after thoracic trauma, but should be based on anatomical and physiological parameters due to the limited diagnostic value of conventional radiography of the chest.

8.4 Treatment

Severe chest trauma represents the second most common diagnosis in multiple trauma [5, 6]. There is a high coincidence of thoracic injuries and extremity trauma (e.g., femoral fractures). Timing and type of fracture care substantially influence the pulmonary function and the development of posttraumatic complications in patients with accompanying thoracic trauma.

Besides general aspects for the treatment of chest trauma, this chapter also focuses on the significance of adequate treatment strategies for fracture stabilization in multiple trauma patients with severe chest trauma in order to avoid pulmonary dysfunction.

8.4.1 Airway Management

Usually, oral intubation has already been performed at the scene of accident or in the emergency department. If not, it must be considered in the initial posttraumatic period as early intubation has been shown to reduce morbidity and mortality. Indications for intubation include traumatic brain injury (Glasgow Coma Scale<9), impairment of consciousness with expired adverse-effects reflex, thoracic trauma with impaired respiratory function, respiratory insufficiency (SaO_2<90%, breathing rate<10/min or>30/min), hemorrhagic shock, and substantial airway trauma. In case of suspected ventilation time of more than 7–10 days, tracheotomy is recommended. Tracheotomy seems to be favored due to improvements in respiratory mechanics and the reduction of infectious complications. However, the effects of tracheotomy on the total ventilation time and the duration of intensive care treatment are the subject of controversy.

8.4.2 Ventilation

In the anaesthesized, ventilated patient, a reduction of pulmonary functional residual capacity due to supine positioning has been observed. Furthermore, reduced thoracic compliance aggravated by thoracic trauma results in a hypoventilation of dorsobasal lung sections with an increased risk for developing atelectases. As these lung sections show the best pulmonary perfusion, a ventilation-perfusion-mismatch with increased intrapulmonary shunting is commonly observed. Additionally, the increased intrathoracic pressure during mechanical ventilation exerts circulatory effects with a decreased cardiac output. Besides traumatic pulmonary injuries, mechanical ventilation with a high inspiratory pressure can cause additional direct damage to lung parenchyma. Therefore, lung protective ventilation with low tidal volume (5–6 mL/kg), high positive endexspiratory pressure (PEEP) and limited inspiratory peak pressure (<35 cm H_2O) should be used in case of severe thoracic trauma.

8.4.3 Positioning Therapy

Positioning therapy is supposed to be important in the prevention and treatment of pulmonary functional disorders. There are a variety of positioning procedures including the semi recumbent position, the lateral position, the prone position and the continuous axial rotational therapy. Mechanically ventilated patients should always be positioned in *semi recumbent position* (45°) in order to avoid pulmonary aspiration and ventilator-associated pneumonia. In patients with unilateral lung injuries, a *lateral position* of nearly 90° ("good lung down") is recommended.

Complete *prone position* is defined as patient's transfer by 180° from supine position. Incomplete prone position is a transfer between 130° and <180°. Prone positioning is used in patients suffering from severe ARDS with life-threatening hypoxemia (PaO_2/FiO_2<100). Contraindications for the application of the prone position include open abdomen, unstable spinal injuries, head trauma with increased intracerebral pressure, severe arrhythmia, acute shock syndrome and substantial facial trauma [83–85]. Prone positioning is recommended for at least 12 h. This results in an increased pulmonary gas exchange due to an improvement of the ventilation-perfusion ratio [86–88] and recruitment of alveolar space with reduced atelectases [89–93]. These effects occur either immediately (≤30 min) or up to 12 h after retransfer into supine position [94–96]. Incomplete prone position is less effective [97]. Compared to continuous axial rotational therapy, therapeutic effects are stronger and occur faster in prone position. After 72 h, no differences are evident between both positioning procedures [98]. A substantial increase in the intraabdominal pressure is not caused by the prone position in patients without abdominal injuries [99, 100]. Despite the improvement of arterial oxygenation, prone positioning has not resulted in a significant reduction in morbidity, ventilation time and length of stay in the intensive care unit in patients with ARDS (PaO_2/FiO_2<300) [101, 102]. In contrast, a decrease of ventilator-associated pneumonia after prone positioning has been described [101, 102]. Prone position may be complicated by facial edema (20–30%), pressure ulcera (20%), patient incompliance (20%), arrhythmia (5%), as well as tube and catheter dislocation (1–2%) [101].

Continuous axial rotational therapy consists of the continuous rotation of the patient about the longitudinal axis in a self-rotating bed. Depending on the different bed systems a rotation up to 62° to each side can be achieved. This kinetic therapy has potential indications for the prevention of pulmonary complications (e.g., atelectases, pneumonia) in patients with thoracic trauma [103–105]. Furthermore, it is therapeutically used for the treatment of ARDS without severe hypoxemia. In case of contraindications for prone positioning, continuous axial rotational therapy may also be performed in case of ARDS with life-threatening hypoxemia. Kinetic therapy is recommended for at least 3–5 days [103–105]. The positive effects of the axial rotation therapy [103, 105–109] are described for axial rotation of more than 40° to each side. Contraindications are unstable spine injuries, acute shock syndrome, and adiposity (≥160 kg). Complications associated with kinetic therapy include pressure ulcera, hemodynamic instability, kinetosis, and catheter dislocation.

In the literature, the use of continuous axial rotational therapy is discussed controversially. Clinical trials have failed to show a significant effect on morbidity, ventilation time and length of stay in the intensive care unit [110–114]. Furthermore, recent studies have not found a beneficial effect from mechanical ventilation with prophylactic kinetic therapy as compared to early extubation and aggressive weaning in patients with severe thoracic trauma [115, 116]. Due to small and inhomogeneous study populations, the generalized application of these results to the treatment of severe blunt chest trauma patients is questionable. Nevertheless, the role of prophylactic ventilation including kinetic therapy and its prognostic relevance must be clarified in further studies. Furthermore, reliable parameters for the indication of kinetic therapy should be validated.

8.4.4 Fracture Treatment in Multiple Trauma Patients with Thoracic Trauma

It has been long recognized that in patients with severe abdominal injuries initial management should avoid complex operative procedures. Performed under emergency conditions, such interventions should be rapid and minimally traumatic to the patient. The primary focus is hemorrhage control and other life saving measures. Complex reconstructive work is delayed until the patient is better able to withstand the additional surgical trauma. This approach was adopted in patients with extremity or pelvic injuries as it became apparent that patients undergoing drawn out operations following major trauma suffered an excess of complications. Homeostatic anomalies, the systemic inflammatory response, multiple organ dysfunction and an increased mortality were observed.

In general, there are two treatment strategies for fracture care in multiple trauma patients. Primary definitive fracture fixation is performed within the concept of "Early Total Care" (ETC), whereas "Damage Control Orthopaedics" (DCO) suggests temporary external fracture fixation with secondary definitive osteosynthesis after stabilization of the patient's physiological and immunological status on intensive care unit [117–122]. Although early fracture fixation has been described as essential to avoid pulmonary complications after multiple trauma [123, 124], the optimal treatment strategy (ETC versus DCO) for fracture care remains the focus of intensive research [117–125]. This is particularly true for multiple trauma patients with severe chest trauma [125]. Several investigations demonstrated a decreased risk for infection and pulmonary dysfunction after ETC treatment in these patients [119, 122, 126, 127], while other studies have reported an increase in pulmonary failure after ETC [121, 125, 128]. In a prospective randomized, clinical study it has been demonstrated that patients in an uncertain clinical situation develop "Acute Lung Injury" (ALI) significantly more often after ETC treatment as compared to fracture stabilization according to the DCO concept [121]. An analysis of the trauma registry of the German Trauma Society has also shown a very inconsistent application of ETC and DCO in patients with chest trauma [129]. Pape et al. [130] introduced the concept of the borderline patient (Table 8.3), which is distinguishable from stable, unstable, and "in extremis" patients (Fig. 8.2).

Table 8.3 Borderline patients according to Pape et al. [130]

- ISS>40
- Hypothermia<35°C
- Multiple trauma with ISS>20 and AIS_{chest}>2
- Multiple trauma with abdominal/pelvic injury (AIS>2) and shock (RR_{systol}<90 mmHg)
- Bilateral lung contusion in chest radiography or CT
- Pulmonary artery pressure (PAP)>24 mmHg
- Increase of PAP>6 mmHg during femoral nailing

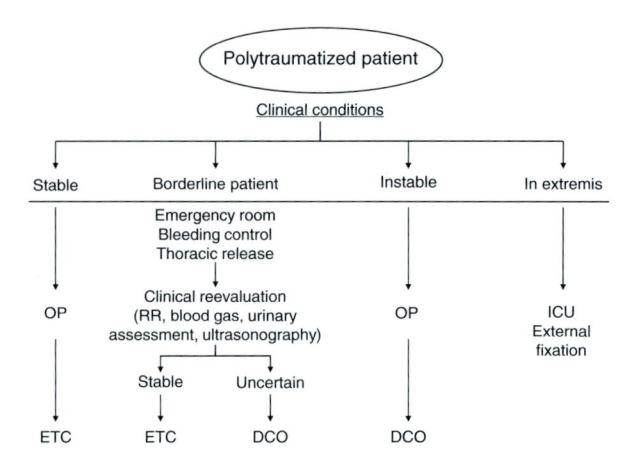

Fig. 8.2 Treatment algorithm according to Pape et al. [130]

For the identification of these patients, the severity of thoracic trauma and physiological pulmonary parameters are of central importance. This emphasizes the significance of chest trauma for the development of posttraumatic complications after fracture stabilization in multiple trauma patients. According to Pape et al. [130], ETC can be performed in stable patients, while DCO is recommended in unstable and "in extremis" patients. The timing of secondary definitive osteosynthesis in patients who have undergone temporary external fixation does not seem to be advantageous before day 5 after trauma [121, 131]. Giannoudis also recommended secondary fracture fixation based on defined parameters (Table 8.4) [131].

In conclusion, early definitive fracture stabilization seems to increase the risk for adverse outcome in multiple trauma patients with severe chest trauma. However, further prospective randomized studies are needed to increase the sensitivity and specificity of parameters to identify those patients who might benefit from DCO concept of fracture care.

Table 8.4 Signs of stabilization according to Giannoudis [131]

- Hemodynamic stability
- Stable arterial oxygenation
- Lactate < 2 mmol/L
- Absence of coagulopathy
- Normothermia
- Urine production > 1 mL/kg/h
- No need for catecholamines

8.4.5 Surgical Chest Wall Stabilization

Operative stabilization of the chest may become necessary in case of a flail chest. The vast majority of patients with a flail chest can be treated conservatively with sufficient pain relief, supplemental oxygen, mask continuous positive airway pressure (CPAP), and tracheobronchial toilet [132, 133]. In case of respiratory insufficiency under supplemental oxygen, mechanical ventilation for internal pneumatic stabilization is indicated. However, long-term ventilation could be complicated by ventilator-associated pneumonia. Therefore, the aim of surgical stabilization is to achieve a mechanically stable chest wall in order to reduce duration of ventilation and to avoid ventilator-associated complications. Indications for surgical intervention are still controversially discussed as most of the published studies are case reports or lacking detailed information on injury severity. Operative chest wall stabilization seems to be indicated in patients with a flail chest and respiratory insufficiency, but without pulmonary contusions and concomitant severe head injury [133]. In these patients, operative stabilization should be performed within the first 48 h after trauma. There seems to be no role for surgical stabilization in patients with accompanying pulmonary contusions, as the underlying pulmonary injury rather than chest wall instability is thought to be responsible for the respiratory failure. Therefore, primary operative stabilization should be avoided in these patients [132]. Further possible indications for an operative stabilization of the chest are an unsuccessful weaning from the ventilator due to paradoxical segment movement, a severe chest wall deformity (impression >5 cm) and a flail chest with indication for thoracotomy due to intrathoracic injury [133].

References

1. Hoff SJ, Shotts SD, Eddy VA, et al. Outcome of isolated pulmonary contusion in blunt trauma patients. Am Surg. 1994;60:138–42.
2. Richardson JD, Adams L, Flint LM. Selective management of flail chest and pulmonary contusion. Ann Surg. 1982;196:481–7.
3. Stellin G. Survival in trauma victims with pulmonary contusion. Am Surg. 1991;57:780–4.
4. Lotfipour S, Kaku SK, Vaca FE, et al. Factors associated with complications in older adults with isolated blunt chest trauma. West J Emerg Med. 2009;10:79–84.

5. Pinilla JC. Acute respiratory failure in severe blunt chest trauma. J Trauma. 1982;22:221–6.
6. Bardenheuer M, Obertacke U, Waydhas C, et al. Epidemiology of the severely injured patient. A prospective assessment of preclinical and clinical management. AG Polytrauma of DGU. Unfallchirurg. 2000;103:355–63.
7. Clark GC, Schecter WP, Trunkey DD. Variables affecting outcome in blunt chest trauma: flail chest vs. pulmonary contusion. J Trauma. 1988;28:298–304.
8. Johnson JA, Cogbill TH, Winga ER. Determinants of outcome after pulmonary contusion. J Trauma. 1986;26:695–7.
9. Pape HC, Auf'm'kolk M, Paffrath T, et al. Primary intramedullary femur fixation in multiple trauma patients with associated lung contusion – a cause of posttraumatic ARDS? J Trauma. 1993;34:540–7; discussion 547–8.
10. Gaillard M, Herve C, Mandin L, et al. Mortality prognostic factors in chest injury. J Trauma. 1990;30:93–6.
11. Inthorn D, Huf R. Thoracic trauma in multiple trauma. Anästhesiol Intensivmed Notfallmed Schmerzther. 1992;27:498–501.
12. Trupka A, Nast-Kolb D, Schweiberer L. Thoracic trauma. Unfallchirurg. 1998;101:244–58.
13. Bulger EM, Arneson MA, Mock CN, et al. Rib fractures in the elderly. J Trauma. 2000;48:1040–6; discussion 1046–7.
14. Shorr RM, Rodriguez A, Indeck MC, et al. Blunt chest trauma in the elderly. J Trauma. 1989;29:234–7.
15. Locicero III J, Mattox KI. Epidemiology of chest trauma. Surg Clin North Am. 1989;69:15–9.
16. Waydhas C. Thoracic trauma. Unfallchirurg. 2000;103:871–89; quiz 890, 910.
17. Buckley BJ, Hayden SR. Posterior sternoclavicular dislocation. J Emerg Med. 2008;34:331–2.
18. Weening B, Walton C, Cole PA, et al. Lower mortality in patients with scapular fractures. J Trauma. 2005;59:1477–81.
19. Butters KP. Fractures of the scapula. In: Buchholz RW, Heckmann JD, Court-Brown C, editors. Rockwood and Green's fractures in adults. 6th ed. Philadelphia: Lippincott Williams & Wilkins; 2006. p. 1257–84.
20. Zlowodzki M, Bhandari M, Zelle BA, et al. Treatment of scapula fractures: systematic review of 520 fractures in 22 case series. J Orthop Trauma. 2006;20:230–3.
21. Livingston DH, Haurer CJ. Trauma to the chest wall and lung. In: Moore EE, Feliciano DV, Mattox KL, editors. Trauma. Philadelphia: McGraw-Hill; 2004. p. 507–37.
22. Mayberry JC. Imaging in thoracic trauma: the trauma surgeon's perspective. J Thorac Imaging. 2000;15:76–86.
23. Miller LA. Chest wall, lung, and pleural space trauma. Radiol Clin North Am. 2006;44:213–4, viii.
24. Mirvis SE, Shanmuganagthan K. Imaging hemidiaphragmatic injury. Eur Radiol. 2007;17:1411–21.
25. Sliker CW. Imaging of diaphragm injuries. Radiol Clin North Am. 2006;44:199–211, vii
26. Gavelli G, Canini R, Bertaccini P, et al. Traumatic injuries: imaging of thoracic injuries. Eur Radiol. 2002;12:1273–94.
27. HO MI, Gutierrez FR. Chest radiography in thoracic polytrauma. AJR Am J Roentgenol. 2009;192:599–612.
28. Obertacke U, Neudeck F, Hellinger A, Schmit-Neuburg KP. Pathophysiologie, Diagnostik und Therapie der Lungenkontusion. Akt Chir. 1997;32:32–48.
29. Shorr RM, Crittenden M, Indeck M, et al. Blunt thoracic trauma. Analysis of 515 patients. Ann Surg. 1987;206:200–5.
30. Miller HAB, Taylor GA. Flail chest and pulmonary contusion. In: McMutry RY, McLellan BA, editors. Management of blunt trauma. Baltimore: Williams & Wilkins; 1990. p. 186–98.
31. Gams E, Kalweit G. Thoraxverletzungen. In: Mutschler W, Haas N, editors. Praxis der Unfallchirurgie. Stuttgart/New York: Thieme; 1998.
32. Donnelly SC, Haslett C, Dransfield I, et al. Role of selectins in development of adult respiratory distress syndrome. Lancet. 1994;344:215–9.
33. Windsor AC, Mullen PG, Fowler AA, et al. Role of the neutrophil in adult respiratory distress syndrome. Br J Surg. 1993;80:10–7.
34. Allen GS, Coates NE. Pulmonary contusion: a collective review. Am Surg. 1996;62:895–900.
35. Euathrongchit J, Thoongsuwan N, Stern EJ. Nonvascular mediastinal trauma. Radiol Clin North Am. 2006;44:251–8, viii.
36. Riley RD, Miller PR, Meredith JW. Injury to the esophagus, trachea and bronchus. In: Moore EE, Feliciano DV, Mattox KL, editors. Trauma. Philadelphia: McGraw-Hill; 2004. p. 539–52.
37. Marshall GB, Farnquist BA, Macgregor JH, et al. Signs in thoracic imaging. J Thorac Imaging. 2006;21:76–90.
38. Salehian O, Teoh K, Mulji A. Blunt and penetrating cardiac trauma: a review. Can J Cardiol. 2003;19:1054–9.
39. Bertinchant JP, Polge A, Mohty D, et al. Evaluation of incidence, clinical significance, and prognostic value of circulating cardiac troponin I and T elevation in hemodynamically stable patients with suspected myocardial contusion after blunt chest trauma. J Trauma. 2000;48:924–31.
40. Bayer MJ, Burdick D. Diagnosis of myocardial contusion in blunt chest trauma. JACEP. 1977;6:238–42.
41. Uffmann M, Fuchs M, Herold CJ. Radiologic imaging of thoracic trauma. Radiologe. 1998;38:683–92.
42. Dorr F. Differential diagnosis and treatment control of blunt chest trauma with computed tomography. Anästhesiol Intensivmed Notfallmed Schmerzther. 1999;34 Suppl 1:S41–4.
43. Ball CG, Kirkpatrick AW, Laupland KB, et al. Incidence, risk factors, and outcomes for occult pneumothoraces in victims of major trauma. J Trauma. 2005;59:917–24; discussion 924-915.
44. De Moya MA, Seaver C, Spaniolas K, et al. Occult pneumothorax in trauma patients: development of an objective scoring system. J Trauma. 2007;63:13–7.
45. Misthos P, Kakaris S, Sepsas E, et al. A prospective analysis of occult pneumothorax, delayed pneumothorax and delayed hemothorax after minor blunt thoracic trauma. Eur J Cardiothorac Surg. 2004;25:859–64.
46. Ball CG, Ranson K, Dente CJ, et al. Clinical predictors of occult pneumothoraces in severely injured blunt polytrauma patients: a prospective observational study. Injury. 2009;40:44–7.
47. Fulton RI, Peter ET. The progressive nature of pulmonary contusion. Surgery. 1970;67:499–506.
48. Greene R. Lung alterations in thoracic trauma. J Thorac Imaging. 1987;2:1–11.
49. Marts B, Durham R, Shapiro M, et al. Computed tomography in the diagnosis of blunt thoracic injury. Am J Surg. 1994;168:688–92.

50. Perry Jr JF, Galway CF. Chest injury due to blunt trauma. J Thorac Cardiovasc Surg. 1965;49:684–93.
51. Regel G, Sturm JA, Neumann C, et al. Bronchoscopy of lung contusion in severe thoracic trauma. Unfallchirurg. 1987;90:20–6.
52. Schild HH, Strunk H, Weber W, et al. Pulmonary contusion: CT vs plain radiograms. J Comput Assist Tomogr. 1989;13:417–20.
53. Traub M, Stevenson M, Mcevoy S, et al. The use of chest computed tomography versus chest X-ray in patients with major blunt trauma. Injury. 2007;38:43–7.
54. Blostein PA, Hodgman CG. Computed tomography of the chest in blunt thoracic trauma: results of a prospective study. J Trauma. 1997;43:13–8.
55. Rizzo AG, Steinberg SM, Flint LM. Prospective assessment of the value of computed tomography for trauma. J Trauma. 1995;38:338–42; discussion 342-333.
56. Omert L, Yeaney WW, Protetch J. Efficacy of thoracic computerized tomography in blunt chest trauma. Am Surg. 2001;67:660–4.
57. Guerrero-Lopez F, Vazquez-Mata G, Alcazar-Romero PP, et al. Evaluation of the utility of computed tomography in the initial assessment of the critical care patient with chest trauma. Crit Care Med. 2000;28:1370–5.
58. Mcgonigal MD, Schwab CW, Kauder DR, et al. Supplemental emergent chest computed tomography in the management of blunt torso trauma. J Trauma. 1990;30:1431–4; discussion 1434–5.
59. Trupka A, Kierse R, Waydhas C, et al. Shock room diagnosis in polytrauma. Value of thoracic CT. Unfallchirurg. 1997;100:469–76.
60. Brink M, Deunk J, Dekker HM. Criteria for the selective use of chest computed tomography in blunt trauma patients. Eur Radiol. 2010;20:818–28.
61. Brink M, Kool DR, Dekker HM, et al. Predictors of abnormal chest CT after blunt trauma: a critical appraisal of the literature. Clin Radiol. 2009;64:272–83.
62. Ivatury RR, Sugerman HJ. Chest radiograph or computed tomography in the intensive care unit? Crit Care Med. 2000;28:1234–5.
63. Karaaslan T, Meuli R, Androux R, et al. Traumatic chest lesions in patients with severe head trauma: a comparative study with computed tomography and conventional chest roentgenograms. J Trauma. 1995;39:1081–6.
64. Soldati G, Testa A, Sher S, et al. Occult traumatic pneumothorax: diagnostic accuracy of lung ultrasonography in the emergency department. Chest. 2008;133:204–11.
65. Zhang M, Liu Zh, Yang JX, et al. Rapid detection of pneumothorax by ultrasonography in patients with multiple trauma. Crit Care. 2006;10:R112.
66. Rothlin MA, Naf R, Amgwerd M, et al. Ultrasound in blunt abdominal and thoracic trauma. J Trauma. 1993;34:488–95.
67. Walz M, Muhr G. Sonographic diagnosis in blunt thoracic trauma. Unfallchirurg. 1990;93:359–63.
68. Blaivas M, Lyon M, Duggal S. A prospective comparison of supine chest radiography and bedside ultrasound for the diagnosis of traumatic pneumothorax. Acad Emerg Med. 2005;12:844–9.
69. Lichtenstein DA, Meziere G, Lascols N, et al. Ultrasound diagnosis of occult pneumothorax. Crit Care Med. 2005;33:1231–8.
70. Soldati G, Testa A, Pignataro G, et al. The ultrasonographic deep sulcus sign in traumatic pneumothorax. Ultrasound Med Biol. 2006;32:1157–63.
71. Hara KS, Prakash UB. Fiberoptic bronchoscopy in the evaluation of acute chest and upper airway trauma. Chest. 1989;96:627–30.
72. Regel G, Seekamp A, Aebert H, et al. Bronchoscopy in severe blunt chest trauma. Surg Endosc. 1990;4:31–5.
73. Hoffmann P, Gahr R. Comment on the contribution by Th. Joka et al.: Early diagnosis of lung contusion by bronchoscopy. Unfallchirurg (1987) 90:286. Unfallchirurg. 1989;92:92–6.
74. Wagner RB, Jamieson PM. Pulmonary contusion. Evaluation and classification by computed tomography. Surg Clin North Am. 1989;69:31–40.
75. Tyburski JG, Collinge JD, Wilson RF, et al. Pulmonary contusions: quantifying the lesions on chest X-ray films and the factors affecting prognosis. J Trauma. 1999;46:833–8.
76. Pape HC, Remmers D, Rice J, et al. Appraisal of early evaluation of blunt chest trauma: development of a standardized scoring system for initial clinical decision making. J Trauma. 2000;49:496–504.
77. Eren S, Balci AE, Ulku R, et al. Thoracic firearm injuries in children: management and analysis of prognostic factors. Eur J Cardiothorac Surg. 2003;23:888–93.
78. Oestern HJ, Kabus K. The classification of the severely and multiply injured – what has been established? Chirurg. 1997;68:1059–65.
79. Athanassiadi K, Gerazounis M, Theakos N. Management of 150 flail chest injuries: analysis of risk factors affecting outcome. Eur J Cardiothorac Surg. 2004;26:373–6.
80. Esme H, Solak O, Yurumez Y, et al. The prognostic importance of trauma scoring systems for blunt thoracic trauma. Thorac Cardiovasc Surg. 2007;55:190–5.
81. Joosse P, Soedarmo S, Luitse JS, et al. Trauma outcome analysis of a Jakarta University Hospital using the TRISS method: validation and limitation in comparison with the major trauma outcome study. Trauma and Injury Severity Score. J Trauma. 2001;51:134–40.
82. Sharma BR. The injury scale – a valuable tool for forensic documentation of trauma. J Clin Forensic Med. 2005;12:21–8.
83. Bein T. Patient positioning-kinetic therapy in intensive medicine. Anaesthesist. 1998;47:74–80.
84. Leonet S, Fontaine C, Moraine JJ, et al. Prone positioning in acute respiratory failure: survey of Belgian ICU nurses. Intensive Care Med. 2002;28:576–80.
85. Muhl E, Hansen M, Bruch HP. Kinetic therapy within the scope of treating septic surgical patients. Anästhesiol Intensivmed Notfallmed Schmerzther. 1997;32:249–52.
86. Lamm WJ, Graham MM, Albert RK. Mechanism by which the prone position improves oxygenation in acute lung injury. Am J Respir Crit Care Med. 1994;150:184–93.
87. Mure M, Domino KB, Lindahl SG, et al. Regional ventilation-perfusion distribution is more uniform in the prone position. J Appl Physiol. 2000;88:1076–83.
88. Pappert D, Rossaint R, Slama K, et al. Influence of positioning on ventilation-perfusion relationships in severe adult respiratory distress syndrome. Chest. 1994;106:1511–6.
89. Albert RK, Hubmayr RD. The prone position eliminates compression of the lungs by the heart. Am J Respir Crit Care Med. 2000;161:1660–5.

90. Gattinoni L, Pelosi P, Vitale G, et al. Body position changes redistribute lung computed-tomographic density in patients with acute respiratory failure. Anesthesiology. 1991;74:15–23.
91. Guerin C, Badet M, Rosselli S, et al. Effects of prone position on alveolar recruitment and oxygenation in acute lung injury. Intensive Care Med. 1999;25:1222–30.
92. Marini JJ. How to recruit the injured lung. Minerva Anestesiol. 2003;69:193–200.
93. Walz M, Muhr G. Continuously alternating prone and supine positioning in acute lung failure. Chirurg. 1992;63:931–7.
94. Lee DI, Chiang HT, Lin SI, et al. Prone-position ventilation induces sustained improvement in oxygenation in patients with acute respiratory distress syndrome who have a large shunt. Crit Care Med. 2002;30:1446–52.
95. Mcauley DF, Giles S, Fichter H, et al. What is the optimal duration of ventilation in the prone position in acute lung injury and acute respiratory distress syndrome? Intensive Care Med. 2002;28:414–8.
96. Reutershan J, Schmitt A, Dietz K, et al. Alveolar recruitment during prone position: time matters. Clin Sci (Lond). 2006;110:655–63.
97. Bein T, Sabel K, Scherer A, et al. Comparison of incomplete (135 degrees) and complete prone position (180 degrees) in patients with acute respiratory distress syndrome. Results of a prospective, randomised trial. Anaesthesist. 2004;53:1054–60.
98. Staudinger T, Kofler J, Mullner M, et al. Comparison of prone positioning and continuous rotation of patients with adult respiratory distress syndrome: results of a pilot study. Crit Care Med. 2001;29:51–6.
99. Hering R, Vorwerk R, Wrigge H, et al. Prone positioning, systemic hemodynamics, hepatic indocyanine green kinetics, and gastric intramucosal energy balance in patients with acute lung injury. Intensive Care Med. 2002;28:53–8.
100. Hering R, Wrigge H, Vorwerk R, et al. The effects of prone positioning on intraabdominal pressure and cardiovascular and renal function in patients with acute lung injury. Anesth Analg. 2001;92:1226–31.
101. Gattinoni L, Tognoni G, Pesenti A, et al. Effect of prone positioning on the survival of patients with acute respiratory failure. N Engl J Med. 2001;345:568–73.
102. Guerin C, Gaillard S, Lemasson S, et al. Effects of systematic prone positioning in hypoxemic acute respiratory failure: a randomized controlled trial. JAMA. 2004;292:2379–87.
103. Fink MP, Helsmoortel CM, Stein KI, et al. The efficacy of an oscillating bed in the prevention of lower respiratory tract infection in critically ill victims of blunt trauma. A prospective study. Chest. 1990;97:132–7.
104. Pape HC, Remmers D, Weinberg A, et al. Is early kinetic positioning beneficial for pulmonary function in multiple trauma patients? Injury. 1998;29:219–25.
105. Stiletto R, Gotzen L, Goubeaud S. Kinetic therapy for therapy and prevention of post-traumatic lung failure. Results of a prospective study of 111 polytrauma patients. Unfallchirurg. 2000;103:1057–64.
106. Bein T, Reber A, Metz C, et al. Acute effects of continuous rotational therapy on ventilation-perfusion inequality in lung injury. Intensive Care Med. 1998;24:132–7.
107. Mullins CD, Philbeck Jr TE, Schroeder WJ, et al. Cost effectiveness of kinetic therapy in preventing nosocomial lower respiratory tract infections in patients suffering from trauma. Manag Care Interface. 2002;15:35–40.
108. Pape HC, Regel G, Borgmann W, et al. The effect of kinetic positioning on lung function and pulmonary haemodynamics in posttraumatic ARDS: a clinical study. Injury. 1994;25:51–7.
109. Pape HC, Weinberg A, Graf B, et al. Continuous axial position change in post-traumatic lung failure – preventive or therapeutic indications? Anästhesiol Intensivmed Notfallmed Schmerzther. 1997;32:245–9.
110. Clemmer TP, Green S, Ziegler B, et al. Effectiveness of the kinetic treatment table for preventing and treating pulmonary complications in severely head-injured patients. Crit Care Med. 1990;18:614–7.
111. Deboisblanc BP, Castro M, Everret B, et al. Effect of air-supported, continuous, postural oscillation on the risk of early ICU pneumonia in nontraumatic critical illness. Chest. 1993;103:1543–7.
112. Delaney A, Gray H, Laupland KB, et al. Kinetic bed therapy to prevent nosocomial pneumonia in mechanically ventilated patients: a systematic review and meta-analysis. Crit Care. 2006;10:R70.
113. Goldhill DR, Imhoff M, Mclean B, et al. Rotational bed therapy to prevent and treat respiratory complications: a review and meta-analysis. Am J Crit Care. 2007;16:50–61; quiz 62.
114. Traver GA, Tyler MI, Hudson LD, et al. Continuous oscillation: outcome in critically ill patients. J Crit Care. 1995;10:97–103.
115. Mahlke L, Oestern S, Drost J, et al. Prophylactic ventilation of severely injured patients with thoracic trauma – does it always make sense? Unfallchirurg. 2009;112:938–41.
116. Sutyak JP, Wohltmann CD, Larson J. Pulmonary contusions and critical care management in thoracic trauma. Thorac Surg Clin. 2007;17:11–23, v.
117. Bose D, Tejwani NC. Evolving trends in the care of polytrauma patients. Injury. 2006;37:20–8.
118. Harwood PJ, Giannoudis PV, Van Griensven M, et al. Alterations in the systemic inflammatory response after early total care and damage control procedures for femoral shaft fracture in severely injured patients. J Trauma. 2005;58:446; discussion 452-444.
119. O'brien PJ. Fracture fixation in patients having multiple injuries. Can J Surg. 2003;46:124–8.
120. Pape HC, Hildebrand F, Krettek C, et al. Experimental background – review of animal studies. Injury. 2006;37 Suppl 4:S25–38.
121. Pape HC, Rixen D, Morley J, et al. Impact of the method of initial stabilization for femoral shaft fractures in patients with multiple injuries at risk for complications (borderline patients). Ann Surg. 2007;246:491–9; discussion 499–501.
122. Weninger P, Figl M, Spitaler R, et al. Early unreamed intramedullary nailing of femoral fractures is safe in patients with severe thoracic trauma. J Trauma. 2007;62:692–6.
123. Gray AC, White TO, Clutton E, et al. The stress response to bilateral femoral fractures: a comparison of primary intramedullary nailing and external fixation. J Orthop Trauma. 2009;23:90–7; discussion 98–9.

124. Robinson CM. Current concepts of respiratory insufficiency syndromes after fracture. J Bone Joint Surg Br. 2001;83:781–91.
125. Taeger G, Ruchholtz S, Waydhas C, et al. Damage control orthopedics in patients with multiple injuries is effective, time saving, and safe. J Trauma. 2005;59:409–16; discussion 417.
126. Brundage SI, Mcghan R, Jurkovich GJ, et al. Timing of femur fracture fixation: effect on outcome in patients with thoracic and head injuries. J Trauma. 2002;52:299–307.
127. Dunham CM, Bosse MJ, Clancy TV, et al. Practice management guidelines for the optimal timing of long-bone fracture stabilization in polytrauma patients: the EAST Practice Management Guidelines Work Group. J Trauma. 2001;50:958–67.
128. Scalea TM, Boswell SA, Scott JD, et al. External fixation as a bridge to intramedullary nailing for patients with multiple injuries and with femur fractures: damage control orthopedics. J Trauma. 2000;48:613–21; discussion 621-613.
129. Rixen D, Grass G, Sauerland S, et al. Evaluation of criteria for temporary external fixation in risk-adapted damage control orthopedic surgery of femur shaft fractures in multiple trauma patients: "evidence-based medicine" versus "reality" in the trauma registry of the German Trauma Society. J Trauma. 2005;59:1375–94; discussion 1394-1375.
130. Pape HC, Hildebrand F, Pertschy S, et al. Changes in the management of femoral shaft fractures in polytrauma patients: from early total care to damage control orthopedic surgery. J Trauma. 2002;53:452–61; discussion 461-452.
131. Giannoudis PV. Surgical priorities in damage control in polytrauma. J Bone Joint Surg Br. 2003;85:478–83.
132. Pettiford BI, Luketich JD, Landreneau RJ. The management of flail chest. Thorac Surg Clin. 2007;17:25–33.
133. Voggenreiter G, Neudeck F, Aufmkolk M, et al. Operative chest wall stabilization in flail chest – outcomes of patients with or without pulmonary contusion. J Am Coll Surg. 1998;187:130–8.

9 Abdominal Injuries: Indications for Surgery

Clay Cothren Burlew and Ernest E. Moore

Contents

9.1	Initial Evaluation of the Injured Patient	89
9.1.1	Primary Survey	89
9.1.2	Secondary Survey	90
9.2	Imaging for Abdominal Injuries	92
9.3	Penetrating Injuries	92
9.4	Blunt Abdominal Trauma	96
9.4.1	Liver and Spleen	96
9.4.2	Pancreatic Injuries	97
9.4.3	Bowel Injuries	98
9.4.4	Genitourinary	98
9.5	Post-injury Complications Requiring Abdominal Exploration	99
9.6	Collaboration in the Multiply Injured Patient	100
References		100

C.C. Burlew (✉) and E.E. Moore
Department of Surgery, Denver Health Medical Center and the University of Colorado Denver School of Medicine, 777 Bannock Street, MC 0206, Denver, CO 80204, USA
e-mail: clay.cothren@dhha.org

This overview addresses the indications for laparotomy following trauma. The authors will suggest algorithms and tenants of care, but there is not a cookie-cutter approach that incorporates all trauma patients or their injuries. Laparotomy for trauma is an individualized decision based collectively upon clinical evaluation and diagnostic adjuncts. Multiple tools exist within the surgeon's armamentarium, including focused abdominal sonography for trauma (FAST) exam, diagnostic peritoneal aspirate (DPA)/diagnostic peritoneal lavage (DPL), imaging, and laparoscopy, to facilitate diagnosis and management of the trauma patient. Care for each injured patient requires experienced clinical evaluation, time-honed judgment, and individualized treatment. Junior trainees are often reminded of the value of experience in the trauma bay when a misstep in management occurs. Appropriate and timely intervention will limit the number of nontherapeutic laparotomies and their attendant morbidity.

9.1 Initial Evaluation of the Injured Patient

9.1.1 Primary Survey

The initial management of seriously injured patients consists of the primary survey, concurrent resuscitation, the secondary survey, diagnostic evaluation, and definitive care as promulgated by the Advanced Trauma Life Support (ATLS) course of the American College of Surgeons Committee on Trauma [1]. The first step in patient management in the emergency department (ED) is the "ABCs" (*A*irway with cervical spine protection, *B*reathing, and *C*irculation) of the primary survey, and evaluating the patient's response to resuscitation.

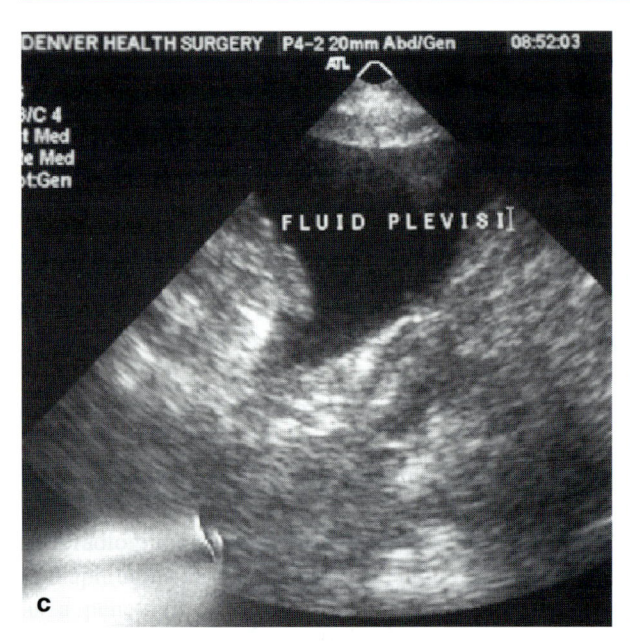

Fig. 9.2 (continued)

9.2 Imaging for Abdominal Injuries

Based upon mechanism, location of injuries identified on physical examination, screening radiographs, and the patient's overall condition, additional diagnostic studies are often indicated. Selective radiographs are done early in the patient's ED evaluation. For patients with severe blunt trauma, lateral cervical spine, chest, and pelvic radiographs should be obtained, often termed "The Big 3." Since its initial use in the early 1980s, CT scanning has become a routine part of trauma evaluation. With multi-slice helical scanning, the entire torso can be scanned in under 5 min. Patients with a positive FAST, who do not have immediate indications for laparotomy and are hemodynamically stable, undergo CT scan to quantify their injuries. Additionally, patients with persistent abdominal tenderness, significant abdominal wall trauma, distracting injuries, or altered mental status should undergo CT imaging. Although the majority of abdominal penetrating injuries that violate the peritoneum require laparotomy, the exception is penetrating trauma isolated to the right upper quadrant. In hemodynamically stable patients with the trajectory of penetrating trauma confined to the liver by CT scan, nonoperative observation is an option [7, 8].

CT scanning is excellent for identifying injuries of the solid organs (liver, spleen, kidney). If a diaphragmatic injury is not clearly identified on ED radiograph (Fig. 9.3), CT scan can also be used to delineate these injuries, particularly with sagittal or coronal reconstructions. Despite the increasing diagnostic accuracy of multi-slice CT scanners, CT still has limited sensitivity for identification of intestinal injuries. Bowel injury is suggested by findings of thickened bowel wall, "streaking" in the mesentery, free fluid without associated solid organ injury, or free intraperitoneal air [9].

The American Association for the Surgery Trauma (AAST) developed a grading scale to provide a uniform definition of solid organ injuries based upon the magnitude of anatomic disruption (Table 9.1) [10]. Solid organ injury grading permits effective transfer of information between treating physicians, and predicts failure rates and complication rates of nonoperative management (NOM). In addition to grading the injury, specific findings that should be noted on CT scan include contrast extravasation (i.e., a "blush"), the amount of intra-abdominal hemorrhage, and the presence of pseudoaneurysms (Fig. 9.4).

9.3 Penetrating Injuries

The diagnostic approach differs between penetrating and blunt abdominal trauma. As a rule, minimal evaluation is required prior to laparotomy for gunshot or shotgun wounds that violate the peritoneal cavity because over 90% of patients have significant internal injuries. Anterior truncal GSWs between the fourth intercostal space and the pubic symphysis, whose trajectory by x-ray or entrance/exit wound indicates peritoneal penetration, should undergo operative exploration (Fig. 9.5). GSWs to the back or flank are more difficult to evaluate because of the retroperitoneal location of the injured abdominal organs. Triple-contrast CT scan can delineate the trajectory of the bullet and identify peritoneal violation or retroperitoneal entry, but may miss specific injuries [11]. Similarly, in obese patients, if the GSW is thought to be tangential through the subcutaneous tissues, CT scan can delineate the tract and exclude peritoneal violation. Laparoscopy is another option to assess peritoneal penetration and is followed by laparotomy to repair injuries, if found. If in doubt, it is always safer to explore the abdomen than to equivocate, but a period

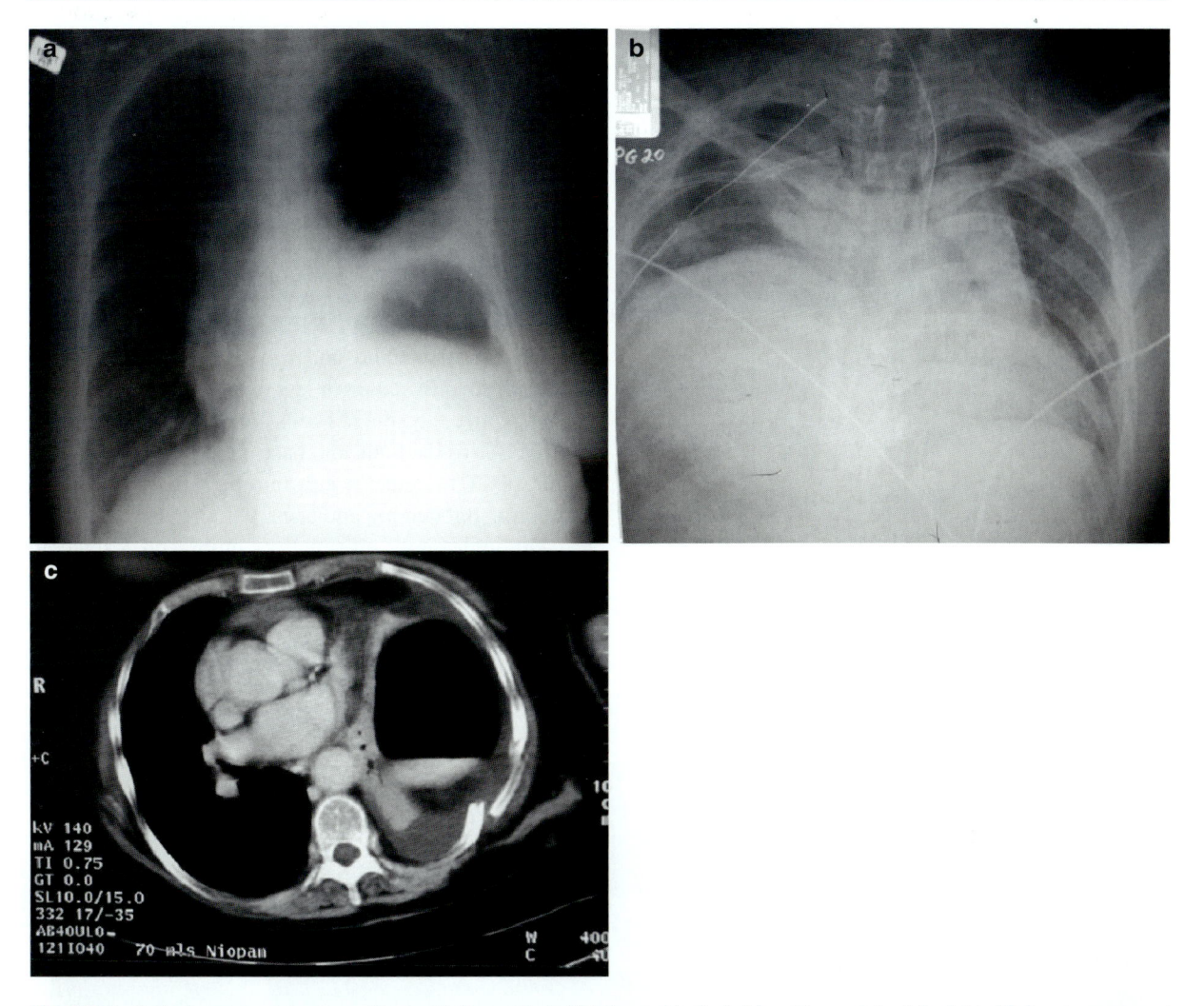

Fig. 9.3 Left diaphragm ruptures are evident with the gastric bubble located in the left hemithorax (**a**), while right-sided ruptures present with the appearance of an elevated hemidiaphragm (**b**). CT scanning may be used in questionable cases to better identify the injury (**c**)

of close observation of the patient, with a reliable examination and hemodynamic stability, may be considered.

In contrast to GSWs, SWs that penetrate the peritoneal cavity are less likely to injure intra-abdominal organs. Anterior abdominal SWs (from costal margin to inguinal ligament and bilateral mid-axillary lines) should be explored under local anesthesia in the ED to determine if the fascia has been violated. Injuries that do not penetrate the peritoneal cavity do not require further evaluation, and the patient is discharged from the ED. Patients with fascial penetration must be further evaluated for intra-abdominal injury, as there is up to a 50% chance of requiring laparotomy. The optimal diagnostic approach remains debated between serial examination, diagnostic peritoneal lavage (DPL), and CT scanning [12]. If DPL is pursued, an infraumbilical approach is used. Following placement of the catheter, a 10 cc syringe is connected and the abdominal contents aspirated (termed a diagnostic peritoneal aspirate or DPA). The aspirate is considered positive if more than 10 mL of blood is aspirated. If less than 10 mL is withdrawn, a liter of normal saline is instilled. The effluent is withdrawn via siphoning and sent to the laboratory for RBC count, WBC count, amylase, bilirubin, and alkaline phosphatase levels. Positive values are summarized in Table 9.2.

Table 9.1 AAST solid organ injury grading scales

	Subcapsular hematoma	Laceration
Liver injury grade		
I	<10% surface area	<1 cm in depth
II	10–50% surface area	1–3 cm
III	>50% or >10 cm	>3 cm
IV	25–75% of a hepatic lobe	
V	>75% of a hepatic lobe	
VI	Hepatic avulsion	
Spleen injury grade		
I	<10% surface area	<1 cm in depth
II	10–50% surface area	1–3 cm
III	>50% surface area	>3 cm
IV	>25% devascularization	Hilar injury
V	Shattered spleen	

Abdominal SWs of three body regions require a unique diagnostic approach: thoracoabdominal SWs, right upper quadrant SWs, and back/flank SWs. Occult injury to the diaphragm must be ruled out in patients with SWs to the lower chest. Patients undergoing DPL evaluation have different laboratory value cutoffs than those with standard anterior abdominal stab wounds (Table 9.2). An RBC count of more than 10,000/μL is considered positive, and an indication for laparotomy, while patients with a DPL RBC count between 1,000/μL and 10,000/μL should undergo laparoscopy or thoracoscopy. An RBC count of less than 1,000/μL is considered negative, i.e., the red cells are due to the procedure itself. SWs to the flank and back should undergo triple-contrast CT to detect occult retroperitoneal injuries of the colon, duodenum, and urinary tract [11].

Although not universally embraced, selected patients with penetrating injuries to the right upper quadrant may be candidates for nonoperative management [13–16]. Patients must have a CT scan that documents confinement of the injury to the liver

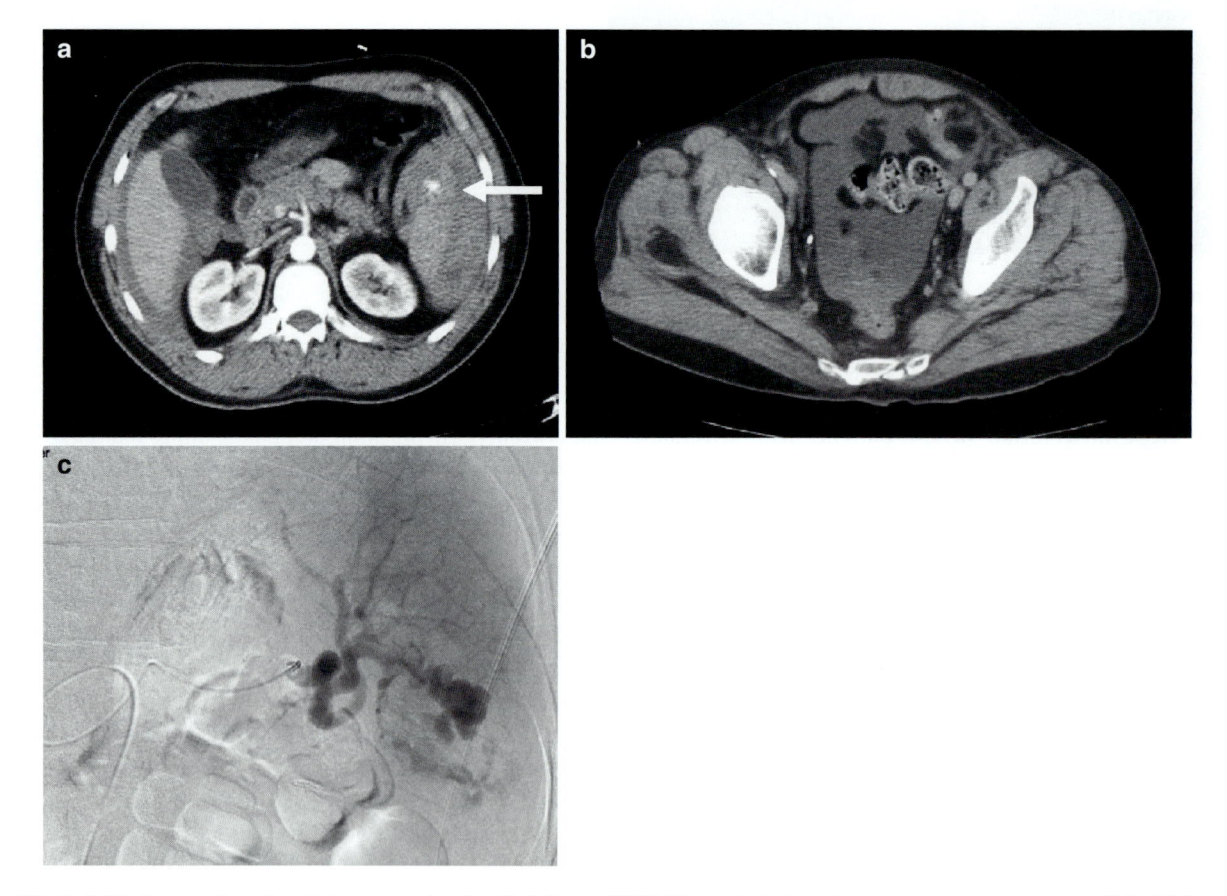

Fig. 9.4 Findings on imaging that are associated with failure of NOM for splenic injuries: contrast extravasation or "blush" (**a**), intra-abdominal hemorrhage extending into the pelvis (**b**), and pseudoaneurysms (**c**)

Fig. 9.5 Algorithm for the evaluation of penetrating abdominal injuries

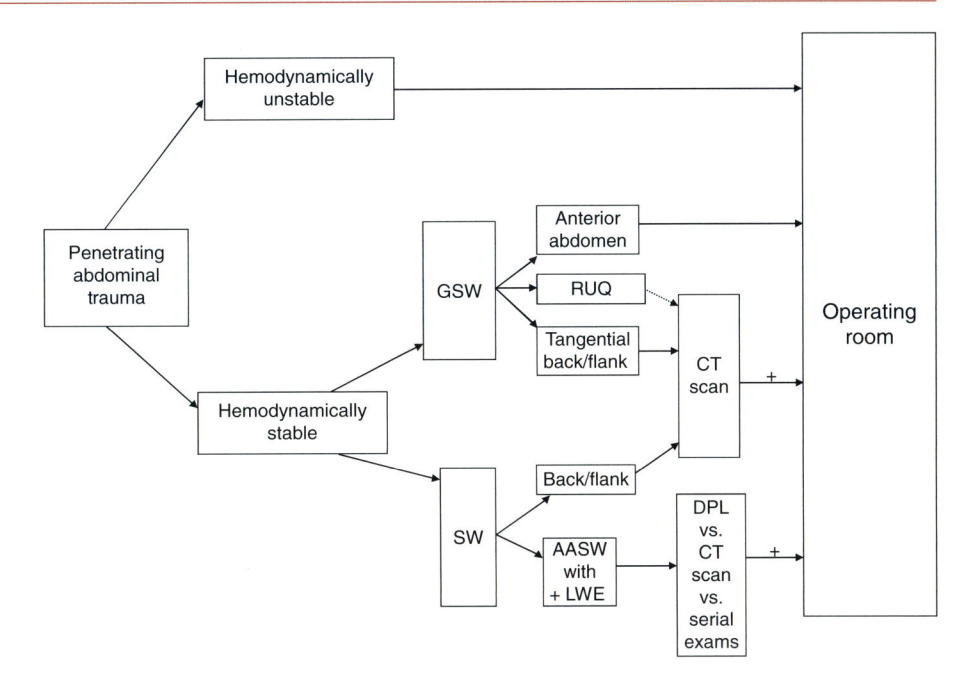

Table 9.2 A positive diagnostic peritoneal lavage following trauma is defined by specific laboratory values

Laboratory study	Positive value	
	AASW	TSW
White blood cell (WBC)	>500 cells/μL	>500 cells/μL
Red blood cell (RBC)	>100,000 cells/μL	>10,000 cells/μL
Amylase	>19 IU/L	>19 IU/L
Alkaline phosphatase	>2 IU/L	>2 IU/L
Bilirubin	>0.1 mg/dL	>0.1 mg/dL

AASW anterior abdominal stab wounds, *TSW* thoracoabdominal stab wounds

(Fig. 9.6). Additionally, the patient must be hemodynamically stable, have a reliable physical examination without evidence of peritonitis (i.e., cannot have depressed mental status), and not require blood products. Patients should be admitted for serial examination and hemoglobin monitoring; any alteration should prompt laparotomy. Violation of the diaphragm has the risk of a biliopleural fistula. An alternative approach is to perform laparoscopy to confirm trajectory of the missile or knife, and to repair the diaphragm. In addition to avoiding the morbidity of a laparotomy, the success of NOM for penetrating trauma has resulted in decreased hospital stays, lower transfusion requirements, and diminished abdominal infection rates.

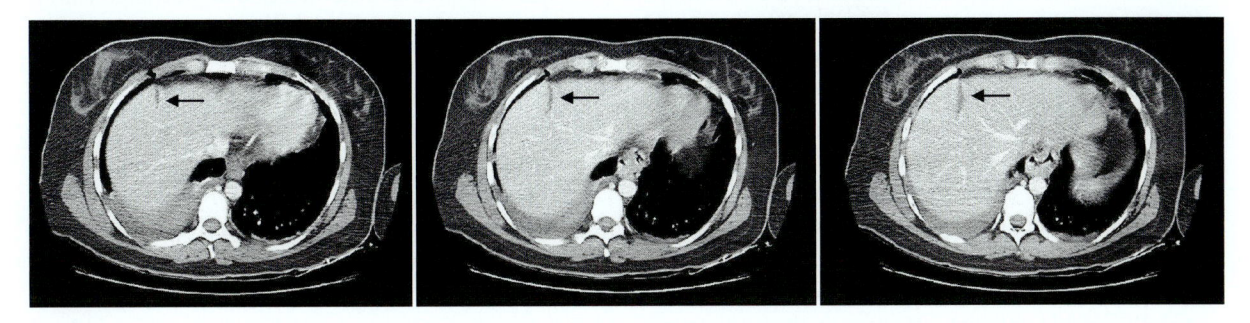

Fig. 9.6 Nonoperative management of penetrating abdominal trauma may be considered if the wound is isolated to the liver as documented by CT scan

9.4 Blunt Abdominal Trauma

9.4.1 Liver and Spleen

With the advent of CT scanning, nonoperative management of solid organ injuries has replaced routine operative exploration. Nonoperative management of blunt solid organ injuries is appropriate in hemodynamically stable patients that do not have overt peritonitis or other indications for laparotomy. High grade injuries, a large amount of hemoperitoneum, contrast extravasation, and pseudoaneurysms are not absolute contraindications for nonoperative management; however, these patients are at high risk for failure and are more likely to need angioembolization [17–21]. Likewise, there is not a patient age cutoff for the NOM of solid organ injuries. A multidisciplinary approach including angiography with selective angioembolization has improved NOM success rates as well as survival [19, 20, 22].

Over 80% of patients with liver injuries may be managed nonoperatively. Patients who require laparotomy for their liver injuries typically fail nonoperative management in the first 24–48 h [17, 22]. Patients with persistent hemodynamic instability despite red cell transfusions of 4 units in 6 h or 6 units in 24 h should undergo laparotomy. Patients that develop peritonitis following admission should also undergo laparotomy with concern of a missed bowel injury. Of the minority (8%) of patients that fail NOM, half require operation due to associated injuries (i.e., enteric or pancreatic injuries), while the other half undergo laparotomy for hepatic-related hemorrhage [17]. Prediction of which patients will ultimately require laparotomy has yet to be accomplished. Perhaps not surprisingly, those patients who fail NOM have increasing rates of failure associated with increasing grades of hepatic injury, with grade V injuries having a greater than 20% failure rate. Subsequent studies have reported failure rates of 14% in grade IV injuries and 23% in grade V injuries [18]. Similarly, the amount of hemoperitoneum appears to correlate with successful management; patients with a large amount of hemoperitoneum (i.e., blood extending into the pelvis) are more likely to fail NOM.

An indication for angioembolization to address ongoing hepatic bleeding is transfusion of 4 units of RBCs in 6 h or 6 units of RBCs in 24 h in the hemodynamically stable patient. Recurrent hemodynamic instability, however, often requires laparotomy with perihepatic packing for hemostasis. Patients with contrast extravasation identified on CT scanning, indicating arterial hemorrhage, should also be considered as a candidate for hepatic angiography. Originally, evidence of extravasation was an indication for laparotomy; however, the advent of endovascular techniques has resulted in effective hemostasis in selected cases. Angioembolization is particularly helpful in hemodynamically stable patients with contrast pooling within the hepatic parenchyma [19]. Patients with contrast extravasation into the peritoneal cavity are more likely to require laparotomy [20], but cases of successful embolization have been reported [21].

Until the 1970s, splenectomy was considered mandatory for all splenic injuries. Recognition of the immune function of the spleen refocused efforts on splenic salvage in the 1980s [23, 24]. Following success in pediatric patients, NOM of splenic injuries was adopted in the adult population and has become the prevailing strategy for blunt splenic trauma [25]. Nonoperative management of solid organ injuries is pursued in hemodynamically stable patients that do not have overt peritonitis or other indications for laparotomy [26–30]. As in the case of liver injuries, there is no cutoff age for patients for the NOM [31, 32], and high-grade injuries, a large amount of hemoperitoneum, contrast extravasation and pseudoaneurysms are not absolute contraindications for nonoperative management; however, these patients are at high risk for failure [33–36]. The identification of contrast extravasation as a risk factor for failure of NOM led to liberal use of angioembolization in an attempt to avoid laparotomy. The true value of angioembolization in splenic salvage has not been rigorously evaluated. Patients with intraparenchymal splenic blushes who are otherwise asymptomatic may be considered for a period of observation rather than empiric angioembolization [37]; it is thought that the contained hemorrhage within the splenic capsule may result in tamponade of the bleeding (Fig. 9.7).

It is clear, however, that 20–30% of patients with splenic trauma deserves early splenectomy, and that failure of NOM often represents poor patient selection [38, 39]. In adults, indications for prompt laparotomy include initiation of blood transfusion within the first 12 h, considered to be secondary to splenic injury, or hemodynamic instability. In the pediatric population, blood transfusions up to half the patient's blood

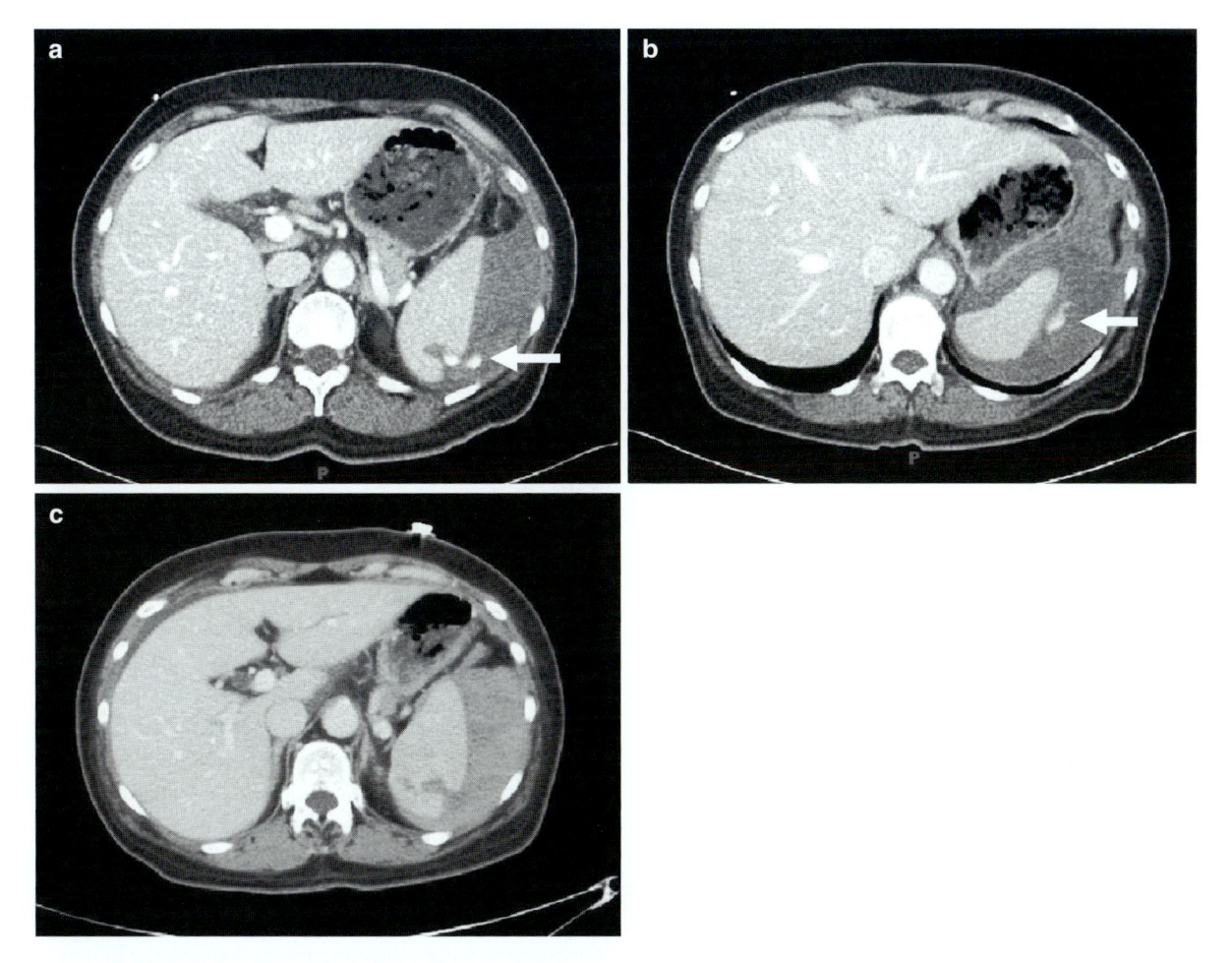

Fig. 9.7 Intraparenchymal splenic blush noted on initial CT scan (**a**, **b**) may resolve following a period of close observation (**c**)

volume are utilized prior to operative intervention. Following the first 12 post-injury hours, indications for laparotomy are not as black and white. Determination of the patient's age, comorbidities, current physiology, degree of anemia, and associated injuries will determine the use of transfusion alone versus intervention with either embolization or operation. Unlike hepatic injuries, which rebleed in 24–48 h, delayed hemorrhage or rupture of the spleen can occur up to weeks following injury. Overall, nonoperative treatment obviates laparotomy in more than 90% of cases.

9.4.2 Pancreatic Injuries

Pancreatic contusions, with or without associated ductal disruption, are difficult to diagnose in patients with blunt abdominal trauma [40]. Patients clearly at risk include those with significant mechanisms including high force, a seatbelt sign on physical examination, or a blow to the epigastrium [41]. The initial CT scan may show nonspecific stranding of pancreas. Associated fluid around the pancreas should prompt further invasive studies such as ERCP or MRCP to rule out a biliary or pancreatic duct injury. With a tentative diagnosis of a pancreatic contusion, one may consider following serial determinations of amylase/lipase; although these lab studies do not have a reliable sensitivity [42], increasing values over time combined with an alteration in clinical exam should prompt a repeat CT scan, duodenal C-loop study, DPL, or an ERCP depending upon the suspected lesion.

Historically, injuries to the pancreas were managed with operative intervention [43]. With the recent evolution of nonoperative management for solid organ injuries, a non-resectional management schema has developed for select pancreatic injuries [44, 45]. Observation of pancreatic contusions, particularly those in the head of the pancreas that may involve ductal disruption, includes serial exams and monitoring of serum amylase. Pancreatic injuries involving the major ducts, originally a strict indication for operative intervention, may be managed with ERCP and stenting in select patients; the durability of this approach is currently under investigation [46].

9.4.3 Bowel Injuries

Diagnosing a hollow viscus injury is notoriously difficult [47], and even short delays in diagnoses result in increased morbidity [48, 49]. Findings suggestive of a bowel injury include thickening of the bowel wall, "streaking" in the mesentery, or free intraperitoneal air [9]. If a patient's initial CT scan of the abdomen shows free fluid without evidence of a solid organ injury to explain such fluid, evaluation for a bowel injury should be performed [50–52]. DPL should also be considered in a patient if there is increasing intra-abdominal fluid on bedside ultrasound in patients with a solid organ injury but a stable hematocrit, and/or in patients with unexplained clinical deterioration. Particular attention should be paid to elevations in the DPL effluent of bilirubin, alkaline phosphatase, and amylase when pursuing a diagnosis of bowel injury, with specific laboratory values indicating the need for laparotomy (Table 9.2) [53, 54]. A rectal injury may be life-threatening in patients with pelvic fractures. While some patients have clear findings on physical examination, ranging from hematochezia to overt degloving of the perineum, others may have occult injuries that are missed on initial evaluation in the trauma bay. Flexible or rigid sigmoidoscopy should rule out blood within the canal, clear intestinal perforation, or ischemic mucosa [55].

Following blunt trauma, patients may develop hematomas in the duodenal wall which obstruct the lumen. Clinical exam findings include epigastric pain associated with either emesis or high nasogastric tube (NGT) output; CT scan imaging with oral contrast failing to pass into the proximal jejunum is diagnostic. Patients with suspected associated perforation, suggested by clinical deterioration or imaging with retroperitoneal free air or contrast extravasation, should be explored operatively. Nonoperative management includes continuous NGT decompression and nutritional support with total parenteral nutrition (TPN) [56, 57]. A marked drop in NGT output heralds resolution of the hematoma, which typically occurs within 2 weeks; repeat imaging to document these clinical findings is optional. If the patient does not improve clinically or radiographically within 4 weeks, operative evaluation is warranted.

9.4.4 Genitourinary

Over 90% of all blunt renal injuries are treated nonoperatively. Operative intervention following blunt trauma is limited to renovascular injuries and destructive parenchymal injuries that result in hypotension. The renal arteries and veins are uniquely susceptible to traction injury caused by blunt trauma. As the artery is stretched, the inelastic intima and media may rupture, causing thrombus formation and resultant stenosis or occlusion. The success of renal artery repair approaches 0%, but an attempt is reasonable if the injury is less than 5 h old, or if the patient has a solitary kidney or bilateral injuries [58]. Early CT with Interventional Radiology placement of a stent should improve outcomes. Reconstruction of blunt renal injuries, however, may be difficult because the injury is typically at the level of the aorta. If repair is not possible within this time frame, leaving the kidney in situ does not necessarily lead to hypertension or abscess formation. The renal vein may be torn or completely avulsed from the vena cava due to blunt trauma. Typically, the large hematoma causes hypotension, leading to operative intervention. The majority of penetrating wounds to kidneys are explored. Renal vascular injuries are common following penetrating trauma, and they may be deceptively tamponaded, resulting in delayed hemorrhage. For destructive parenchymal or irreparable renovascular injuries, nephrectomy may be the only option; palpation of a normal contralateral kidney must be performed as unilateral renal agenesis occurs in 0.1% of patients. Bladder injuries are subdivided based upon intraperitoneal versus extraperitoneal extravasation. Ruptures or lacerations of the intraperitoneal bladder are operatively closed with a running, single-layer, 3–0 absorbable monofilament suture. Laparoscopic repair is becoming common in patients not requiring laparotomy for other injuries. Extraperitoneal ruptures are treated nonoperatively with bladder decompression for 2 weeks.

9.5 Post-injury Complications Requiring Abdominal Exploration

Following hepatic injuries, the most common complication is a bile leak or biloma, occurring in up to 20% of patients (Fig. 9.8) [59, 60]. Clinical presentation includes abdominal distension, intolerance of enteral feeds, and elevated liver functions tests. CT scanning effectively diagnoses the underlying problem, and the vast majority is treated with percutaneous drainage and ERCP with sphincterotomy. Occasionally, laparoscopy or laparotomy with drainage of biliary ascites is indicated, particularly if the patient fails to resolve their ileus and fever [61]. Patients undergoing angioembolization for liver trauma must be carefully monitored for hepatic necrosis and may occasionally require delayed formal hepatic resection.

The most common problem in patients with splenic injuries is delayed bleeding, although as noted previously, the majority fails over an established timeframe. Patients undergoing splenic embolization can fail with rebleeding with 13% of patients requiring splenectomy [62].

Missed bowel injuries are the most commonly pursued injury, not due to their frequency (less than 5% of blunt trauma) but rather their associated morbidity. Observation for a missed small or large bowel injury is critical; clinical findings in such patients include a rising white blood cell count, fever, tachycardia, and increasing abdominal pain or frank peritonitis. After repair of bowel injuries, the most common intra-abdominal complications are anastomotic failure and abscess. Percutaneous versus operative therapy will be based on the location, timing, and extent of the collection.

The abdominal compartment syndrome (ACS) is defined as intra-abdominal hypertension plus end-organ sequelae (decreased urine output, increased pulmonary inspiratory pressures, decreased cardiac preload, and increased cardiac afterload). The ACS can be due to either intra-abdominal injury (primary) or massive resuscitation (secondary). A diagnosis of intra-abdominal hypertension cannot reliably be made by physical examination; therefore, it is obtained by measuring the intraperitoneal pressure. Organ failure can occur over a wide range of recorded bladder pressures, and except for >35 mmHg, there is no single measurement of bladder pressure that prompts therapeutic intervention. Rather, emergent decompression is warranted in the patient with intra-abdominal hypertension at the level it produces end-organ dysfunction. Decompression is performed operatively either in the ICU if the patient is hemodynamically unstable or in the operating room. ICU bedside laparotomy is easily accomplished, precludes transport in hemodynamically compromised patients, and requires minimal equipment (scalpel, suction, cautery, and abdominal temporary closure dressings). Patients with significant intra-abdominal fluid as the primary component of their ACS, rather than bowel or retroperitoneal edema, may be effectively decompressed via a percutaneous drain. This has been particularly applicable for nonoperative management of major liver injuries. These patients are identified by bedside ultrasound, and avoid the morbidity of a laparotomy. When operative decompression is required with egress of the abdominal contents, temporary coverage is obtained using a 1010 drape and ioban coverage (Fig. 9.9). It is to be noted that patients can develop recurrent abdominal compartment syndrome despite a widely open abdomen. Therefore, bladder pressures should be monitored every 4 h, with significant increases in pressures alerting the clinician to the possible need for repeat operative decompression.

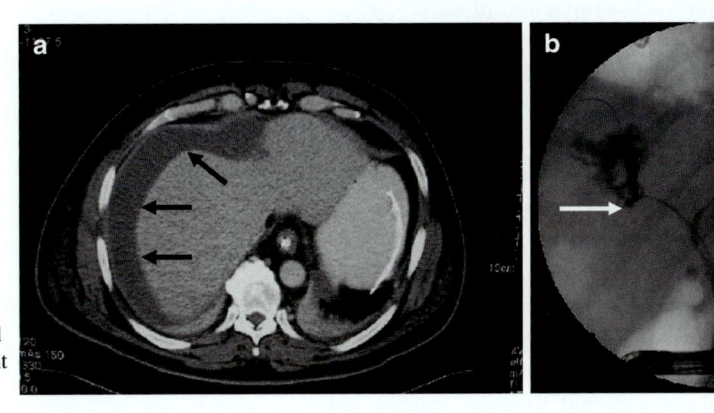

Fig. 9.8 A biloma, evident on CT scan (**a**), with an associated right hepatic duct injury evident on ERC (**b**)

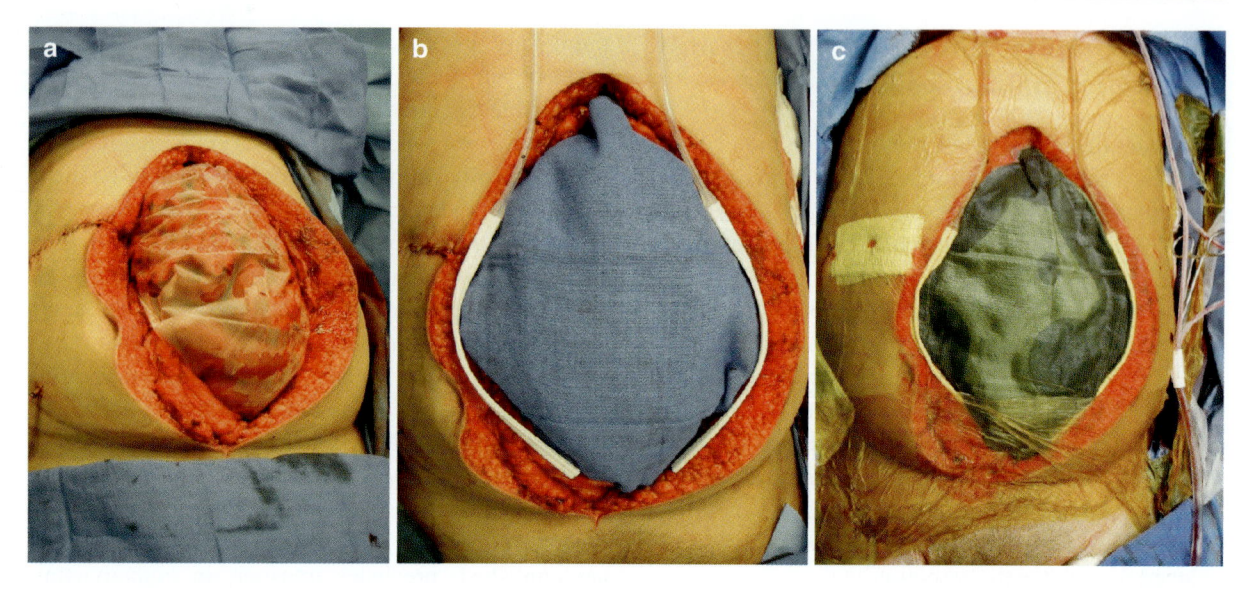

Fig. 9.9 Temporary closure of the abdomen entails covering the bowel with a fenestrated 1010 drape (**a**), placement of JP drains and a blue towel (**b**), followed by ioban occlusion (**c**)

9.6 Collaboration in the Multiply Injured Patient

Patients with abdominal trauma often have associated fractures of the pelvis and extremities due to the required energy transfer to produce an abdominal injury warranting operative care. Early dialog between the trauma and orthopedic teams is critical to coordinate patient care and optimize patient outcomes. One illustrative example of this collaboration is the patient with hemodynamic instability and an unstable pelvic fracture. Protocols for care, with the early involvement of both the trauma and orthopedic teams in the trauma bay and in the operating room, has been shown to reduce mortality [63]. In these multiply injured patients, the orthopedic team can stabilize fractures and place C-clamps in the ED, while the trauma team evaluates the patient for thoracoabdominal trauma and the need for operative management. In patients requiring emergent laparotomy who also require intervention for an unstable pelvic fracture, the two teams can operate simultaneously; the trauma team performs the laparotomy, while the orthopedic team places an external fixator and performs preperitoneal pelvic packing (PPP) [64, 65]. Alternatively, if the patient's hemodynamic instability is related to a pelvic fracture with concurrent extremity injuries, the trauma team can perform PPP, while the orthopedic team places external fixators, washes out open fractures, and performs necessary fasciotomies. Timely communication can ensure appropriate resuscitation and permit simultaneous operations [66, 67].

References

1. American College of Surgeons. Advanced trauma life support. 7th ed. Chicago: American College of Surgeons; 2004.
2. Dolich MO, McKenney MG, Varela JE, et al. 2, 576 ultrasounds for blunt abdominal trauma. J Trauma. 2001;50: 108–12.
3. Rozycki GS, Ochsner MG, Schmidt JA, et al. A prospective study of surgeon-performed ultrasound as the primary adjuvant modality for injured patient assessment. J Trauma. 1995;39:492–8.
4. Branney SW, Wolfe RE, Moore EE, et al. Quantitative sensitivity of ultrasound in detecting free intraperitoneal fluid. J Trauma. 1995;39:375–80.
5. Ochsner MG, Knudson MM, Pachter HL, et al. Significance of minimal or no intraperitoneal fluid visible on CT scan associated with blunt liver and splenic injuries: a multicenter analysis. J Trauma. 2000;49:505–10.
6. Rozycki GS, Ballard RB, Feliciano DV, Schmidt JA, Pennington SD. Surgeon-performed ultrasound for the assessment of truncal injuries: lessons learned from 1540 patients. Ann Surg. 1998;228:557–67.
7. Renz BM, Feliciano DV. Gunshot wounds to the liver. A prospective study of selective nonoperative management. J Med Assoc Ga. 1995;84:275–7.
8. Demetriades D, Gomez H, Chahwan S, et al. Gunshot injuries to the liver: the role of selective nonoperative management. J Am Coll Surg. 1998;188:343–8.

9. Malhotra AK, Fabian TC, Katsis SB, et al. Blunt bowel and mesenteric injuries: the role of screening computed tomography. J Trauma. 2000;48:991–8.
10. Moore EE, Cogbill TH, Jurkovich GJ, et al. Organ injury scaling: spleen and liver. J Trauma. 1995;38:323–4.
11. Boyle Jr EM, Maier RV, Salazar JD, et al. Diagnosis of injuries after stab wounds to the back and flank. J Trauma. 1997;42:260–5.
12. Biffl WL, Cothren CC, Brasel KJ, et al. A prospective observational multicenter study of the optimal management of patients with anterior abdominal stab wounds. J Trauma. 2008;64:250.
13. Renz BM, Feliciano DV. Gunshot wounds to the right thoracoabdomen: a prospective study of nonoperative management. J Trauma. 1994;37:737–44.
14. Demetriades D, Hadjizacharia P, Constantinou C, et al. Selective nonoperative management of penetrating abdominal solid organ injuries. Ann Surg. 2006;244:620–8.
15. Nance FC, Cohn I. Surgical judgment in the management of stab wounds of the abdomen: a retrospective and prospective analysis based on a study of 600 stabbed patients. Ann Surg. 1969;170:569–80.
16. Velmahos GC, Constantinou C, Tillou A, et al. Abdominal computed tomographic scan for patients with gunshot wounds to the abdomen selected for nonoperative management. J Trauma. 2005;59:1155–60.
17. Croce MA, Fabian TC, Menke PG, et al. Nonoperative management of blunt hepatic trauma is the treatment of choice for hemodynamically stable patients. Results of a prospective trial. Ann Surg. 1995;221:744–55.
18. Malhotra AK, Fabian TC, Croce MA, Gavin TJ, Kudsk KA, Minard G, et al. Blunt hepatic injury: a paradigm shift from operative to nonoperative management in the 1990 s. Ann Surg. 2000;231:804–13.
19. Pachter HL, Knudson MM, Esrig B, et al. Status of nonoperative management of blunt hepatic injuries in 1995: a multicenter experience with 404 patients. J Trauma. 1996;40:31–8.
20. Fang JF, Chen RJ, Wong YC, et al. Classification and treatment of pooling of contrast material on computed tomographic scan of blunt hepatic trauma. J Trauma. 2000;49:1083–8.
21. Ciraulo DL, Luk S, Palter M, et al. Selective hepatic arterial embolization of grade IV and V blunt hepatic injuries: an extension of resuscitation in the nonoperative management of traumatic hepatic injuries. J Trauma. 1998;45:353–8.
22. Richardson JD, Franklin GA, Lukan JK, et al. Evolution in the management of hepatic trauma: a 25-year perspective. Ann Surg. 2000;232:324–30.
23. Feliciano DV, Spjut-Patrinely V, Burch JM, et al. Splenorrhaphy: the alternative. Ann Surg. 1990;211:569–82.
24. Pickhardt B, Moore EE, Moore FA, et al. Operative splenic salvage in adults: a decade perspective. J Trauma. 1989;29:1386–91.
25. Richardson JD. Changes in the management of injuries to the liver and spleen. J Am Coll Surg. 2005;200:648–69.
26. Hurtuk M, Reed RL, Espositio TJ, Davis KA, Luchette FA. Trauma surgeons practice what they preach: the NTDB story on solid organ injury management. J Trauma. 2006;61:243–55.
27. Peitzman AB, Heil B, Rivera L, et al. Blunt splenic injury in adults: multi-institutional study of the Eastern association for the surgery of trauma. J Trauma. 2000;49:177–87.
28. Velmahos GC, Toutouzas KG, Radin R, Chan L, Demetriades D. Nonoperative treatment of blunt injury to solid abdominal organs: a prospective study. Arch Surg. 2003;138:844–51.
29. Pachter HL, Guth AA, Hofstett SR, Spencer FC. Changing patterns in the management of splenic trauma: the impact of nonoperative trauma. Ann Surg. 1998;227:708–17; discussion 717–9.
30. Rojani RR, Claridge JA, Yowler CJ, et al. Improved outcome of adult blunt splenic injury: a cohort analysis. Surgery. 2006;140:625–31; discussion 631–2.
31. Myers JG, Dent DL, Stewart RM, et al. Blunt splenic injuries: dedicated trauma surgeons can achieve a high rate of nonoperative success in patients of all ages. J Trauma. 2000;48:801–5; discussion 805–6.
32. Harbrecht BG, Peitzman AB, Rivera L, et al. Contribution of age and gender to outcome of blunt splenic injury in adults: multicenter study of the Eastern Association for the Surgery of Trauma. J Trauma. 2001;51:887–95.
33. Goan YG, Huang MS, Lin JM. Nonoperative management for extensive hepatic and splenic injuries with significant hemoperitoneum in adults. J Trauma. 1998;45:360–4; discussion 365.
34. Nwomeh BC, Nadler EP, Meza MP, Bron K, Gaines BA, Ford HR. Contrast extravasation predicts the for operative intervention in children with blunt splenic trauma. J Trauma. 2004;56:537–41.
35. Malhotra AK, Latifi R, Fabian TC, et al. Multiplicity of solid organ injury: influence on management and outcomes after blunt abdominal trauma. J Trauma. 2003;54:925–9.
36. Schurr MJ, Fabian TC, Gavant M, et al. Management of blunt splenic trauma: computed tomographic contrast blush predicts failure of nonoperative management. J Trauma. 1995;39:507–12; discussion 512-3.
37. Zumwinkle LE, Cothren CC, Moore EE, Kashuk JL, Johnson JL, Biffl WL. Blunt trauma induced splenic blushes are not created equal. Presented at the Western Trauma Association Annual Meeting, Crested Butte, CO. February 2009.
38. McIntyre LK, Schiff M, Jurkovich GJ. Failure of nonoperative management of splenic injuries: causes and consequences. Arch Surg. 2005;140:563–8.
39. Smith HE, Biffl WL, Majercik SD, et al. Splenic artery embolization: have we gone too far? J Trauma. 2006;61:541–4.
40. Leppaniemi AK, Haapiainen RK. Risk factors of delayed diagnosis of pancreatic trauma. Eur J Surg. 1999;165:1134–7.
41. Arkovitz MS, Johnson N, Garcia VF. Pancreatic trauma in children: mechanisms of injury. J Trauma. 1997;42:49–53.
42. Takishima T, Sugimoto K, Hirata M, Asari Y, Ohwada T, Kakita A. Serum amylase level on admission in the diagnosis of blunt injury to the pancreas: its significance and limitations. Ann Surg. 1997;226:70–6.
43. Patton Jr JH, Lyden SP, Croce MA, et al. Pancreatic trauma: a simplified management guideline. J Trauma. 1997;43:234–9; discussion 239–41.
44. Wales PW, Shuckett B, Kim PC. Long-term outcome after nonoperative management of complete traumatic pancreatic transection in children. J Pediatr Surg. 2001;36:823–7.
45. Jobst MA, Canty TG, Lynch FP. Management of pancreatic injury in pediatric blunt abdominal trauma. J Pediatr Surg. 1999;34:818–23.

46. Lin BC, Liu NJ, Fang JF, Kao YC. Long-term results of endoscopic stent in the management of blunt major pancreatic duct injury. Surg Endosc. 2006;20:1551–5.
47. Fakhry SM, Watts DD, Luchette FA. EAST Multi-Institutional Hollow Viscus Injury Research Group. Current diagnostic approaches lack sensitivity in the diagnosis of perforated blunt small bowel injury: analysis from 275,557 trauma admissions from the EAST multi-institutional HVI trial. J Trauma. 2003;54:295–306.
48. Fakhry SM, Brownstein M, Watts DD, Baker CC, Oller D. Relatively short diagnostic delays (<8 hours) produce morbidity and mortality in blunt small bowel injury: an analysis of time to operative intervention in 198 patients from a multicenter experience. J Trauma. 2000;48:408–14.
49. Niederee MJ, Byrnes MC, Helmer SD, Smith RS. Delay in diagnosis of hollow viscus injuries: effect on outcome. Am Surg. 2003;69:293–8.
50. Ng AK, Simons RK, Torreggiani WC, et al. Intra-abdominal free fluid without solid organ injury in blunt abdominal trauma: an indication for laparotomy. J Trauma. 2002;52:1134–40.
51. Miller PR, Croce MA, Bee TK, Malhortz AK, Fabian TC. Associated injuries in blunt solid organ trauma: implications for missed injury in nonoperative management. J Trauma. 2002;53:238–42.
52. Rodriguez C, Barone JE, Wilbanks TO, Rha CK, Miller K. Isolated free fluid on computed tomographic scan in blunt abdominal trauma: a systematic review of incidence and management. J Trauma. 2002;53:79–85.
53. McAnena OJ, Marx JA, Moore EE. Peritoneal lavage enzyme determinations following blunt and penetrating abdominal trauma. J Trauma. 1991;31:1161–4.
54. Heneman PL, Marx JA, Moore EE, Cantrill SV, Ammons LA. Diagnostic peritoneal lavage: accuracy in predicting necessary laparotomy following blunt and penetrating trauma. J Trauma. 1990;30:1345–55.
55. Velmahos GC, Gomez H, Falabella A, Demetriades D. Operative management of civilian rectal gunshot wounds: simpler is better. World J Surg. 2000;24:114–8.
56. Cogbill TH, Moore EE, Feliciano DV. Conservative management of duodenal trauma: a multicenter perspective. J Trauma. 1990;30:1469–75.
57. Huerta S, Bui T, Porral D, Lush S, Cinat M. Predictors of morbidity and mortality in patients with traumatic duodenal injuries. Am Surg. 2005;71:763–7.
58. Knudson MM, Harrison PB, Hoyt DB, et al. Outcome after major renovascular injuries: a Western trauma association multicenter report. J Trauma. 2000;49:1116–22.
59. Kozar RA, Moore FA, Cothren CC, et al. Risk factors for hepatic morbidity following nonoperative management: multicenter study. Arch Surg. 2006;141:451–9.
60. Giss SR, Dobrilovic N, Brown RL, Garcia VF. Complications of nonoperative management of pediatric blunt hepatic injury: diagnosis, management, and outcomes. J Trauma. 2006;61:334–9.
61. Goldman R, Zilkowski M, Mullins R, Mayberry J, Deveney C, Trunkey D. Delayed celiotomy for the treatment of bile leak, compartment syndrome, and other hazards of nonoperative management of blunt liver injury. Am J Surg. 2003;185:492–7.
62. Cocanour CS, Moore FA, Ware DN, Marvin RG, Clark JM, Duke JH. Delayed complications of nonoperative management of blunt adult splenic trauma. Arch Surg. 1998;133:619–24; discussion 624–5.
63. Biffl WL, Smith WR, Moore EE, et al. Evolution of a multidisciplinary clinical pathway for the management of unstable patients with pelvic fractures. Ann Surg. 2001;233(6):843–50.
64. Smith WR, Moore EE, Osborn P, Agudelo JF, Morgan SJ, Parekh AA, et al. Retroperitoneal packing as a resuscitative technique for hemodynamically unstable patients with pelvic fractures: report of two representative cases and a description of technique. J Trauma. 2005;59: 1510–4.
65. Cothren CC, Osborn PM, Moore EE, Morgan SJ, Johnson JL, Smith WR. Preperitoneal pelvic packing for hemodynamically unstable pelvic fractures: a paradigm shift. J Trauma. 2007;62(4):834–42.
66. Hak DJ, Smith WR, Suzuki T. Management of hemorrhage in life-threatening pelvic fracture. J Am Acad Orthop Surg. 2009;17(7):447–57.
67. Stahel PF, Smith WR, Moore EE. Current trends in resuscitation strategy for the multiply injured patient. Injury. 2009;40 Suppl 4:S27–35.

Management of Pelvic Ring Injuries

David J. Hak and Sean E. Nork

Contents

10.1	Introduction	103
10.2	Anatomy	103
10.3	Classification	105
10.4	Physical Examination	107
10.5	Emergent Treatment/Bony Stabilization	108
10.5.1	Pelvic Binders	108
10.5.2	Military Antishock Trousers (MAST)	108
10.5.3	Anterior External Fixation	108
10.5.4	C-Clamp	109
10.6	Hemorrhage Control	109
10.6.1	Angiography	109
10.6.2	Pelvic Packing	110
10.7	Treatment Algorithm	110
10.8	Definitive Treatment	112
10.8.1	Internal Fixation: Anterior Pelvic Ring	112
10.8.2	Internal Fixation: Posterior Pelvic Ring	113
	References	113

D.J. Hak (✉)
Denver Health/University of Colorado, 777 Bannock Street,
MC 0188, Denver, CO 80204, USA
e-mail: david.hak@dhha.org

S.E. Nork
Department of Orthopaedic Surgery, Harborview Medical
Center, 325 Ninth Avenue, P.O. Box 359798, Seattle,
WA 98104, USA
e-mail: nork@u.washington.edu

10.1 Introduction

High-energy pelvic fractures are life-threatening injuries. Approximately 20% of patients with high-energy pelvic injuries develop hemodynamic instability directly related to blood loss from the pelvic injury, and hemorrhage remains a leading cause of death in patients sustaining high-energy pelvic fractures. Evaluation and management of patients with pelvic fractures is a multidisciplinary responsibility, requiring efficient assessment and rapid intervention. Although the general surgery trauma specialist ultimately directs the management of multiply injured patients, it is important for the Orthopaedic surgeon to be involved in every phase of management of patients with pelvic fractures, including primary resuscitation. Early assessment by an Orthopaedic surgeon familiar with pelvic fracture patterns allows the treatment team to establish diagnostic and treatment priorities, and expedites the institution of life-saving maneuvers. A thorough understanding of potential sources of bleeding and awareness of treatment options is essential for all physicians involved in the care of patients with pelvic fractures.

10.2 Anatomy

The sacrum and two innominate bones (composed of the ilium, ischium, and pubis) are firmly connected by several strong ligaments to form the ring-like structure of the pelvis. Anteriorly, the innominate bones are joined at the pubic symphysis, which consists of a hyaline cartilage articulation with multiple supporting ligaments. Posteriorly, the innominate bones are joined

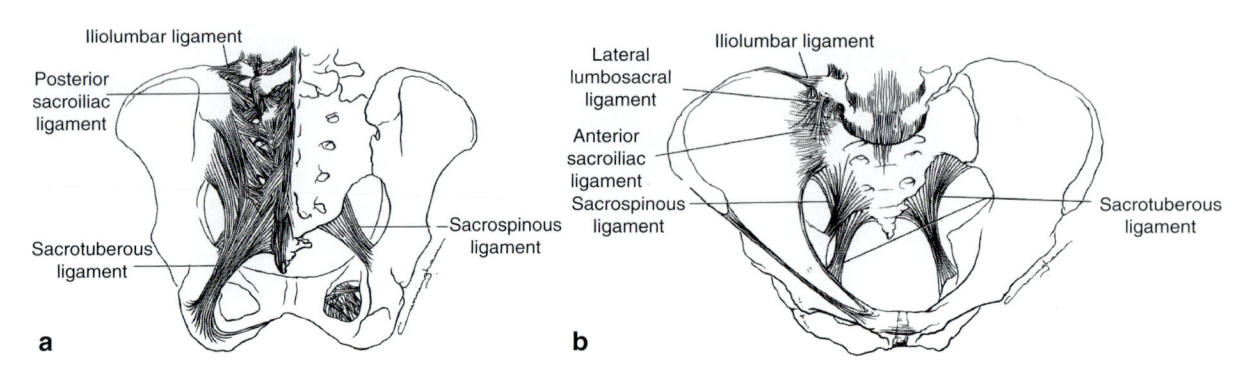

Fig. 10.1 (**a**) Posterior view of the pelvis showing the strong posterior ligaments which provide critical stability of the pelvic ring. (**b**) Anterior view of the pelvis showing the important ligamentous structures that stabilize the pelvic ring (From Tile [1])

to the sacrum at the sacroiliac joint. The sacroiliac joint consists of an articular portion anteriorly and the fibrous or ligamentous portion posteriorly.

The bones of the pelvis have no intrinsic stability and are stabilized by several strong ligamentous structures (Fig. 10.1a, b). The soft tissue connection at the pubic symphysis consists of fibrocartilage spanning the two pubic bones and the arcuate ligament inferiorly. The posterior pelvic ring ligaments are critical for pelvic stability. The strongest of these ligaments are the posterior sacroiliac ligaments. These ligaments are made up of short oblique fibers that run from the posterior ridge of the sacrum to the posterosuperior and posteroinferior iliac spines, and longer longitudinal fibers that run from the lateral sacrum to the posterosuperior iliac spine combining with the sacrotuberous ligament. The sacrotuberous ligament is a strong band of tissue that runs from the posterolateral sacrum and dorsal aspect of the posterior iliac spine to the ischial tuberosity. The sacrotuberous ligament, along with the posterior sacroiliac ligaments, provides vertical stability to the pelvis. The sacrospinous ligament runs from the lateral edge of the sacrum and coccyx to the sacrotuberous ligament and inserts onto the ischial spine. The iliolumbar ligaments run from the fourth and fifth lumbar transverse processes to the posterior iliac crest; the lumbosacral ligaments run from the fifth lumbar transverse process to the sacral ala. The anterior sacroiliac ligaments are relatively weak compared to the strong posterior sacroiliac ligaments.

Anatomically, the pelvis structures can be separated into the true pelvis, located below the iliopectineal line (pelvic brim), and the false pelvis, located above the iliopectineal line. Numerous anatomical structures, including vascular supply for the buttocks and lower extremities, pass between the false and true pelvis. The true pelvis contains the floor of the pelvis along with the urethra, rectum, prostate, and vagina. The false pelvis surrounds the lower intra-abdominal contents along with the iliacus muscle.

It is important to understand the location of the major blood vessels that lie on the inner wall of the pelvis, as injury to these vessels is commonly associated with severe hemorrhage (Fig. 10.2). An understanding of pelvic anatomy will help the orthopaedic surgeon recognize the fracture patterns that are more likely to cause direct damage to major vessels and result in significant bleeding. The common iliac artery divides into the external and internal branches. The external iliac artery exits the pelvis anteriorly over the pelvic brim to become the femoral artery. The internal iliac artery lies over the pelvic brim, and courses anterior and in close proximity to the sacroiliac joint. The posterior branches of the internal iliac artery include the iliolumbar, superior gluteal, and lateral sacral arteries. The superior gluteal artery, which is the largest branch of the internal iliac artery, courses across the sacroiliac joint in the true pelvis, and exits through the greater sciatic notch to supply the gluteus medius, gluteus minimus, and tensor fascia lata muscles. It is the most commonly injured vessel in pelvic fractures with posterior ring disruptions. Anterior branches of the internal iliac artery include the obturator, umbilical, vesical, pudendal, inferior gluteal, rectal, and hemorrhoidal arteries. The inferior gluteal artery exits the pelvis through greater sciatic notch inferior to the piriformis and supplies the gluteus maximus. The pudendal and obturator arteries are adjacent to the pubic rami. In addition to the arteries, there is an associated large venous plexus which drains into the internal iliac vein. Injury to this venous plexus is the major source of hemorrhage in most pelvic fractures.

Fig. 10.2 Internal aspect of the pelvis showing the major blood vessels that lie on the inner wall of the pelvis (From Kellam and Browner [2]; Chap. 31, Fig. 31-6)

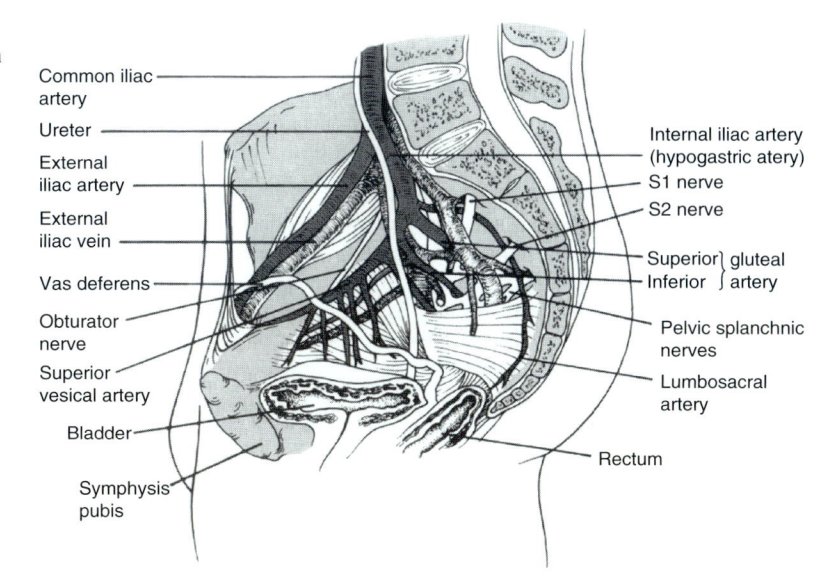

The neural structures that traverse the pelvis can also be injured in displaced pelvic fractures, leading to long-term morbidity. The sciatic nerve is formed by roots from the lumbosacral plexus (L4, L5, S1, S2, S3), and exits the pelvis deep to the piriformis muscle. The lumbosacral trunk is formed from the anterior rami of L4 and L5, and it crosses anterior to the sacral ala and SI joint. Fractures of sacral ala or dislocations of SI joint are most likely to injure the lumbosacral trunk. Typical displacement patterns in posterior pelvic fractures include cranial and posterior displacement of the hemipelvis. This may actually decrease the tension on the nerve roots exiting the pelvis posteriorly. More concerning are pelvic injuries with anterior (and caudal) displacement of the hemipelvis, as these displacement patterns potentially put the nerve roots on continued and significant stretch. The L5 nerve root exits below the L5 transverse process and crosses the sacral ala approximately 2 cm medial to the sacroiliac joint. It may be injured in SI joint disruptions and during anterior surgical approaches to the SI joint.

Significant anterior ring disruption can also damage the urethra and/or bladder. The female urethra is short and not rigidly fixed to the pubis or pelvic floor. Because it is more mobile, it is less susceptible to injury from shear forces associated with pelvic fractures. The male urethra is less mobile and is more susceptible to injury in pelvic fractures. Stricture is the most common long-term complication observed in male patients who have sustained a urethral injury, but impotence may also occur in 25–47% of patients with urethral rupture, likely due to associated injury of the parasympathetic nerves (S2–S4). In males, the bladder neck is attached to the pubis by puboprostatic ligaments and is contiguous with prostate, whereas in females, the bladder lies on the pubococcygeal portion of levator ani muscles. The superior and upper posterior portion of bladder are covered by peritoneum, while the remainder of the bladder is extraperitoneal and covered with loose areolar tissue. Bladder injuries may be caused by a variety of mechanisms including bony spicules from pubic rami fractures, blunt force injuries causing rupture, or shearing injuries. Intraperitoneal bladder ruptures require operative repair. Extraperitoneal bladder ruptures can usually be managed nonoperatively unless there is a bony spicule invading the bladder. Nonoperative management consists of catheter drainage and broad-spectrum antibiotics. Most bladder injuries heal by 3–6 weeks, and a cystogram is obtained prior to catheter removal to confirm bladder healing.

10.3 Classification

Classification systems are useful aids in decision making and treatment following high-energy pelvic fractures [3]. Several pelvic fracture classification systems have been developed, including the Pennal, Letournel, Bucholz, Tile, and Young and Burgess. The two classification systems commonly used are the Tile classification and the Young and Burgess classification.

Table 10.1 Tile classification of pelvic ring injuries

Type A:	Stable pelvic fractures
Type A1:	Avulsion fractures with no disruption of the pelvic ring
Type A2:	Nondisplaced or minimally displaced pelvic ring fracture (for example, a superior and inferior pubic ramus fracture)
Type A3:	Transverse fractures of the inferior sacrum or coccyx with no disruption of the pelvic ring
Type B:	Rotationally unstable, vertically stable
Type B1:	Anterior posterior compression injury (open book)
	Stage 1: Pubic symphysis diastasis less than 2.5 cm, no disruption of posterior pelvic ring ligaments
	Stage 2: Pubic symphysis diastasis greater than 2.5 cm, unilateral disruption of posterior pelvic ring ligaments
	Stage 3: Pubic symphysis diastasis greater than 2.5 cm, bilateral disruption of posterior pelvic ring ligaments
Type B2:	Lateral compression injury affecting only one side of the pelvic. Ipsilateral anterior and posterior ring involvement with instability in internal rotation
Type B3:	Lateral compression injury affecting both sides of the pelvis. Posterior pelvic ring injury with contralateral anterior ring involvement. Unstable in internal rotation. This type of injury has been called the "bucket-handle" fracture
Type C:	Rotational and vertically unstable
Type C1:	Ipsilateral anterior and posterior injury that results in rotational and vertical instability of the hemipelvis
Type C2:	Bilateral pelvic injury that results in rotational instability on one side and vertical instability on the other side
Type C3:	Bilateral pelvic injury in which both sides are both rotationally and vertically unstable

The Tile classification primarily describes pelvic instability based on the anterior and posterior injury pattern(s) [4, 5]. Injuries are divided into three broad categories using an ABC classification similar to the AO/OTA classification system. These three main categories are further divided into specific subtypes. Type A injuries are stable pelvic fractures. Type B injuries are rotationally unstable, but vertically stable fractures. Type C injuries are both rotationally and vertically unstable (Table 10.1).

The Young and Burgess classification is primarily a mechanistic system based on the perceived applied force necessary to produce the injury pattern observed. This classification system should alert the surgeon to common associated injuries, the resuscitation needs of the patient, and may direct clinical care. The pelvic fracture mechanism is categorized into anterior posterior compression (APC), lateral compression (LC), vertical shear (VS), and combined mechanism (CM). Within each category, subtypes indicate the severity of injury (Table 10.2 and Fig. 10.3).

The Young and Burgess pelvic fracture classification has been found to correlate with the pattern of organ injury, resuscitative requirements, and mortality [6, 7]. A rise in mortality has been shown as the APC grade increases, and the APC-III pattern of injuries has been correlated with the greatest 24-h fluid resuscitation requirements.

In a series of 210 consecutive patients with pelvic fractures, Burgess and colleagues reported that transfusion requirements for patients with APC injuries averaged 14.8 units, compared to a mean of 3.6 units for patients with LC injuries, and 5 units for patients with combined mechanism injuries [6]. The overall mortality rate in this series was 8.6%. A higher mortality rate was seen in the APC (20%) and CM patterns (18%), compared to the LC (7%) and VS (0%) patterns. Burgess and colleagues noted that exsanguination from pelvic injuries was rare in the lateral compression pattern in which mortality was typically due to other injuries, most commonly a severe closed head injury.

In a study of 343 trauma patients with pelvic fractures, investigators found that as the APC type increased from I to III, there was an increasing percentage of injury to the spleen, liver, and bowel [7]. In addition, there was an increasing incidence of pelvic vascular injury, retroperitoneal hematoma, shock, sepsis, and acute respiratory distress syndrome. Similarly, as the LC type increased from I to III, the authors found an increased incidence of pelvic vascular injury, retroperitoneal hematoma, shock, and 24-h volume needs. Organ injury patterns and mortality in patients with vertical shear injuries were similar to those with high-grade APC injuries. Patients with combined mechanisms of injury had an associated injury pattern similar to the lower grades of APC and LC injuries. The pattern of injury in the APC-III was correlated with the greatest 24-h fluid requirements. The investigators also reported major differences in the causes of

Table 10.2 Young and Burgess classification

Anterior posterior compression (APC)	
APC type I:	Slight widening of the symphysis pubis (<2.5 cm) but intact posterior pelvic ligaments
APC type II:	Widening of the symphysis pubis >2.5 cm with anterior opening of the sacroiliac joint. The posterior sacroiliac ligaments are intact, but the anterior sacroiliac, sacrotuberous, and sacrospinous ligaments have been torn
APC type III:	This is complete disruption of the ipsilateral ligaments including the posterior sacroiliac ligaments, resulting in both rotational and vertical instability of the hemipelvis
Lateral compression (LC)	
LC type I:	Crush of the sacrum and a ipsilateral horizontal pubic ramus fracture caused by a direct lateral force
LC type II:	Crush injury of the sacrum with either disruption of the posterior sacroiliac joint or a fracture of the iliac wing. The posterior fracture pattern is referred to as a "crescent" fracture. This is caused by a more anteriorly directed lateral force than the LC-I pattern
LC type III:	In addition to the LC-II fracture pattern, the force continues across the opposite hemipelvis resulting in an external rotation injury of the opposite hemipelvis
Vertical shear (VS)	
Caused by a vertically directed force which results in disruption of all the ligamentous structures of the hemipelvis. The posterior ring disruption may occur through the sacroiliac joint, or through a vertical fracture of the sacrum	
Combined mechanism (CM)	
High-energy pelvic fractures may also be caused by more than a single force directed in one plane. The combined mechanism of injury may have combined components of any of the above fracture patterns	

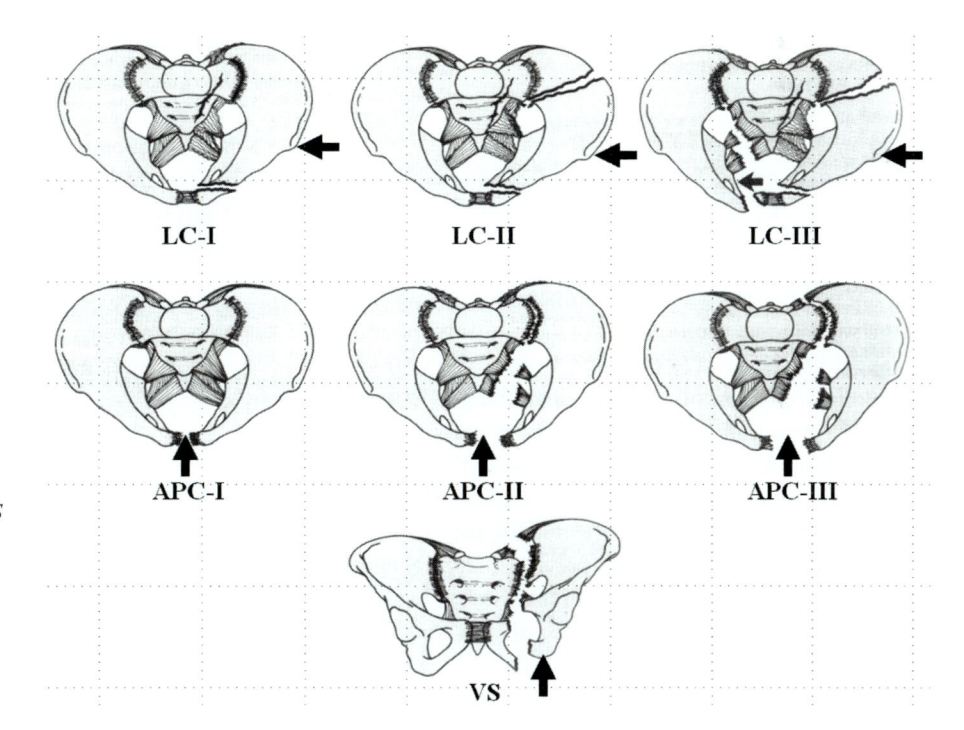

Fig. 10.3 The Young and Burgess classification of pelvic fracture. *LC* lateral compression type pattern, *APC* anteroposterior compression type pattern, *VS* vertical shear type pattern. The *arrow* in each panel indicates the direction of force producing the fracture pattern (From Kellam and Browner [2]; Chap. 31, Fig. 31-12)

death between patients with LC patterns compared to APC patterns. Brain injury was the major cause of death in LC injuries, while in APC patterns, the most common causes of mortality were shock, sepsis, and Acute Respiratory Distress Syndrome (ARDS) related to massive torso forces.

10.4 Physical Examination

The orthopaedic examination of the pelvis should be methodical and complete. An associated limb deformity (shortening or rotation) may be indicative of a pelvic injury with displacement. The skin about the entire pelvis should be examined to ensure that there are not any associated open wounds. This includes special attention to the perineum and gluteal folds where open fractures frequently occur. A digital rectal examination is required to detect rectal injury and open injuries in this location. In women, a vaginal examination should be performed to rule out an open injury. Manual palpation of the pelvis should be carefully performed, and repeated examinations should be avoided.

The potential of an associated urethral injury should be considered in all pelvic fractures with significant anterior ring disruption (APC-II and APC-III type patterns). Signs of potential urethral injury include: (1) inability to void despite a full bladder, (2) blood at urethral meatus, (3) high riding or abnormally mobile prostate, and (4) elevated bladder on IVP. However, the absence of meatal blood or a high riding prostate does not rule out urethral injury. A retrograde urethrogram should be obtained to rule out urethral injury prior to insertion of a urinary catheter, since passing a urinary catheter in the presence of a urethral injury can cause additional iatrogenic injury.

10.5 Emergent Treatment/Bony Stabilization

It is uncommon for bleeding from a pelvic fracture to be the sole source of blood loss in the multiply injured patient. In fact, massive bleeding from a pelvic fracture alone is uncommon. Nevertheless, the pelvic fracture must potentially be considered as a major source of bleeding in the hemodynamically unstable patient, particularly when initial attempts to control bleeding from other sources fail to stabilize the patient. Provisional stabilization of the pelvic fracture should occur immediately during the patient's initial evaluation and resuscitation using one of the methods described in the following section.

10.5.1 Pelvic Binders

Circumferential pelvic compression can be easily achieved in the prehospital setting with some form of commercially available pelvic binders, providing early and beneficial pelvic stabilization during transport and resuscitation. In lieu of a commercial binder, a folded sheet wrapped circumferentially around the pelvis can also be used [8] (Fig. 10.4). The use of pelvic binders has been shown to reduce transfusion requirements, length of hospital stay, and mortality in patients with APC injuries [9]. External rotation of the legs is commonly seen in displaced pelvic fractures, and forces acting through the hip joint may contribute to pelvic deformity. Correction of lower extremity external rotation can be easily achieved by taping the feet and knees together, which may improve the pelvic reduction provided through use of a pelvic binder.

10.5.2 Military Antishock Trousers (MAST)

In the 1970s and 1980s, Military antishock trousers (MAST) were commonly used to provide temporary compression and immobilization of the pelvic ring and lower extremity via pneumatic pressure. Although still useful for stabilization of patients with pelvic fractures, MAST has largely been replaced by the use of commercially available pelvic binders. In the past, the use of MAST has been associated with other complications including lower extremity compartment syndrome.

10.5.3 Anterior External Fixation

Several studies have reported the benefit of emergent pelvic external fixation in the resuscitation of the hemodynamically unstable patient with an unstable pelvic fracture [6, 10]. Several factors may contribute to the beneficial effects of external fixation in pelvic fractures. Immobilization helps limit pelvic displacement during patient movements and transfers, decreasing the possibility of clot disruption. In certain patterns (e.g., APC-II), reduction of pelvic volume is often achieved by application of the external fixator. Experimental studies have shown that reduction of an APC-II pelvic injury increases the retroperitoneal pressure, which may help tamponade venous bleeding [11]. Finally, the apposition of the displaced fracture surfaces can help facilitate the hemostatic pathway to control bony bleeding.

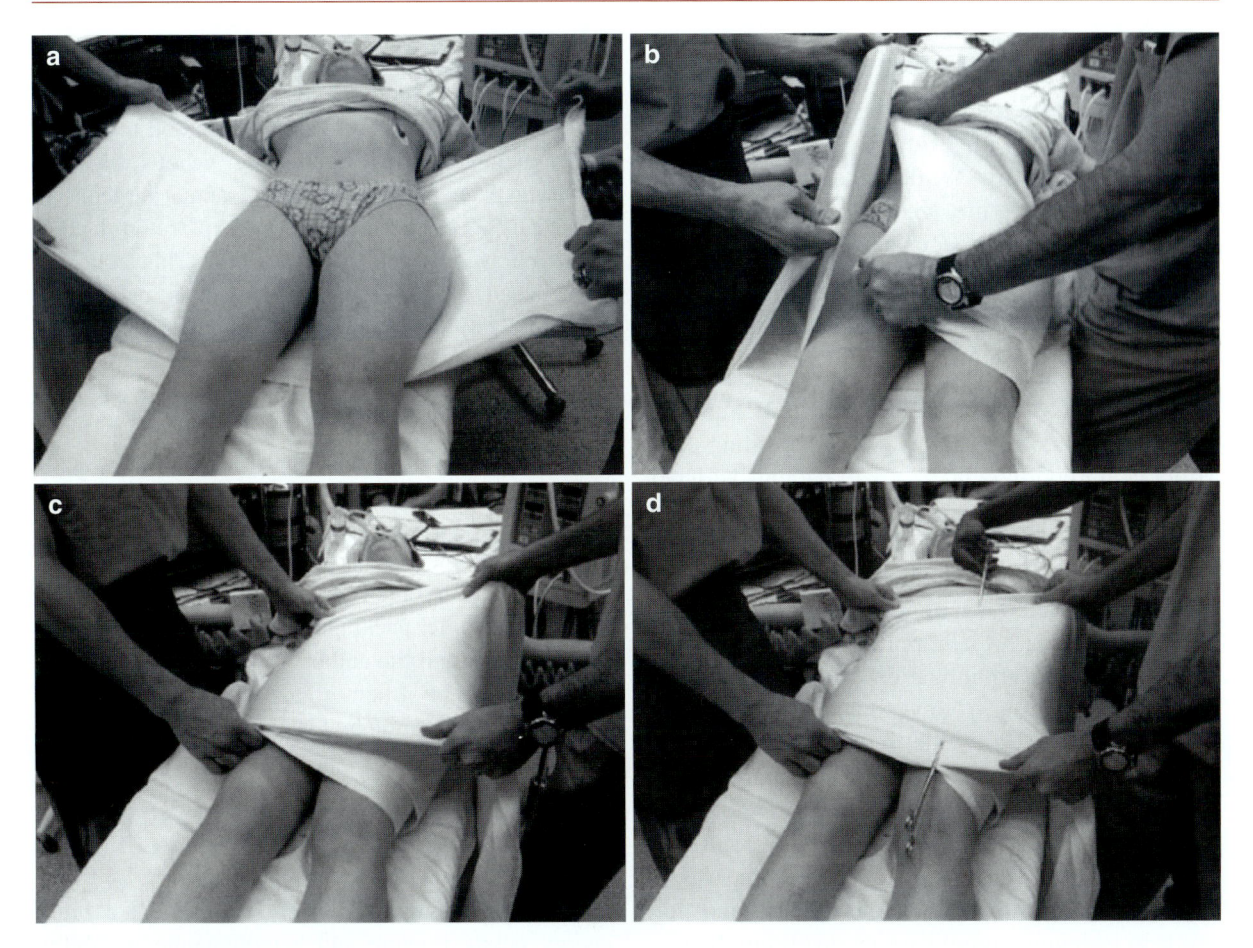

Fig. 10.4 Application of circumferential pelvic antishock sheeting. (**a**) A sheet is folded smoothly to a width of approximately 2 ft and placed beneath the patient's pelvis. (**b**) and (**c**) The ends of the sheet are crossed in an overlapping manner and pulled taut. (**d**) Clamps are placed proximally and distally to secure the sheet in position (From Routt et al. [8])

10.5.4 C-Clamp

Standard anterior external pelvic fixation does little to provide posterior pelvic stabilization. This limits the effectiveness of standard anterior external fixators in fracture patterns involving significant posterior disruption or in cases in which the iliac wing is fractured. The posteriorly applied pelvic C-clamp was developed to address these injury patterns. The C-clamp allows prompt application of a compressive force posteriorly across the sacroiliac joints; however, extreme care must be exercised to avoid iatrogenic injury during its application, and it should generally be done with fluoroscopic guidance [12]. Alternative applications of the C-clamp to the trochanteric region of the femur and to the gluteus medius pillars have also been described as alternative methods of reducing the pelvis in specific circumstances. These methods can be performed more safely without fluoroscopic guidance, but may not be feasible in patients with associated acetabular fractures [13].

10.6 Hemorrhage Control

While stabilization of the bony pelvis is the first stage in hemorrhage control, additional interventions may also be required in selected patients.

10.6.1 Angiography

The overall prevalence of patients with pelvic fractures who need embolization is reported to be <10%. In one review of 162 patients with high-energy pelvic fractures, only 8% underwent angiography. Embolization was more commonly performed in APC and VS patterns (performed in 20% of cases), but was infrequent in LC patterns (performed in only 1.7% of cases) [6]. While most pelvic fracture patients do not require angiography, angiographic exploration should be considered in patients with continued hypotension despite pelvic fracture stabilization and aggressive fluid resuscitation. Eastridge et al. reported that 58.7% of patients with persistent hypotension and a severely unstable pelvic fracture, including APC-II, APC-III, LC-II, LC-III, and VS injury patterns, had active arterial bleeding [14]. Miller et al. reported that 67.9% of patients with pelvic injuries and persistent hemodynamic instability had active arterial bleeding [15].

Early angiography and arterial embolization has been demonstrated to improve patient outcomes [16, 17]. However, it is important to remember that angiography and embolization are not effective in controlling bleeding from venous injuries and bony sites, which represents the predominant source of hemorrhage in high-energy pelvic fractures. Time spent in the angiography suite for hypotensive patients without arterial injury may not contribute to survival. In addition, the aggressive use of angiography is not without consequence and may result in ischemic complications involving the gluteal musculature and subsequent wound healing problems [18].

10.6.2 Pelvic Packing

Pelvic packing was developed as a method to achieve direct hemostasis by controlling venous bleeding resulting from pelvic fractures. Trauma surgeons in Europe have long been advocating exploratory laparotomy followed by pelvic packing [19]. This technique is believed to be especially useful in patients in extremis.

More recently, a modified method of pelvic packing, referred to as retroperitoneal packing, has been introduced in North America [20] (Fig. 10.5). In this approach, the intraperitoneal space is not entered, leaving the peritoneum intact to help provide a tamponade effect. Pelvic packing can be performed quickly with minimal blood loss. In one recent series, only 4 of 24 (16.7%) patients failed to stabilize hemodynamically following pelvic packing and required subsequent embolization, and the authors concluded that packing can quickly control hemorrhage and reduce the need for emergent angiography [21].

10.7 Treatment Algorithm

Patients presenting to Denver Health with a high-energy pelvic fracture and hemodynamic instability are initially given 2 L of crystalloid solution (Fig. 10.6). A portable chest radiograph, along with radiographic

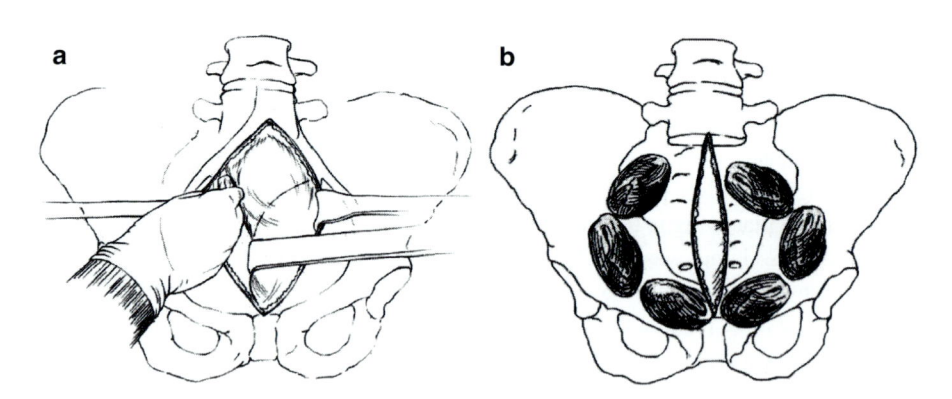

Fig. 10.5 Illustrations demonstrating the retroperitoneal packing technique. (**a**) An 8-cm midline vertical incision is made. The bladder is retracted to one side, and three unfolded lap sponges are packed into the true pelvis (below the pelvic brim) with a forceps. The first is placed posteriorly, adjacent to the sacroiliac joint. The second is placed anterior to the first sponge at a point corresponding to the middle of the pelvic brim. The third sponge is placed in the retropubic space just deep and lateral to the bladder. The bladder is then retracted to the other side, and the process is repeated. (**b**) General location of the six lap sponges following pelvic packing (Adapted from Smith et al. [20])

Fig. 10.6 Algorithm for the treatment of patients with pelvic fracture who present with hemodynamic instability. *Patients in whom a laparotomy was not done usually have an abdominal CT scan en route to the intensive care unit (*ICU*). In the ICU, the patient receives further fluid resuscitation and is warmed; attempts are made to normalize the coagulation status. Recombinant factor VIIa should be considered if the patient is recalcitrant to all other interventions. *FAST* focused abdominal sonography for trauma, *PRBCs* packed red blood cells

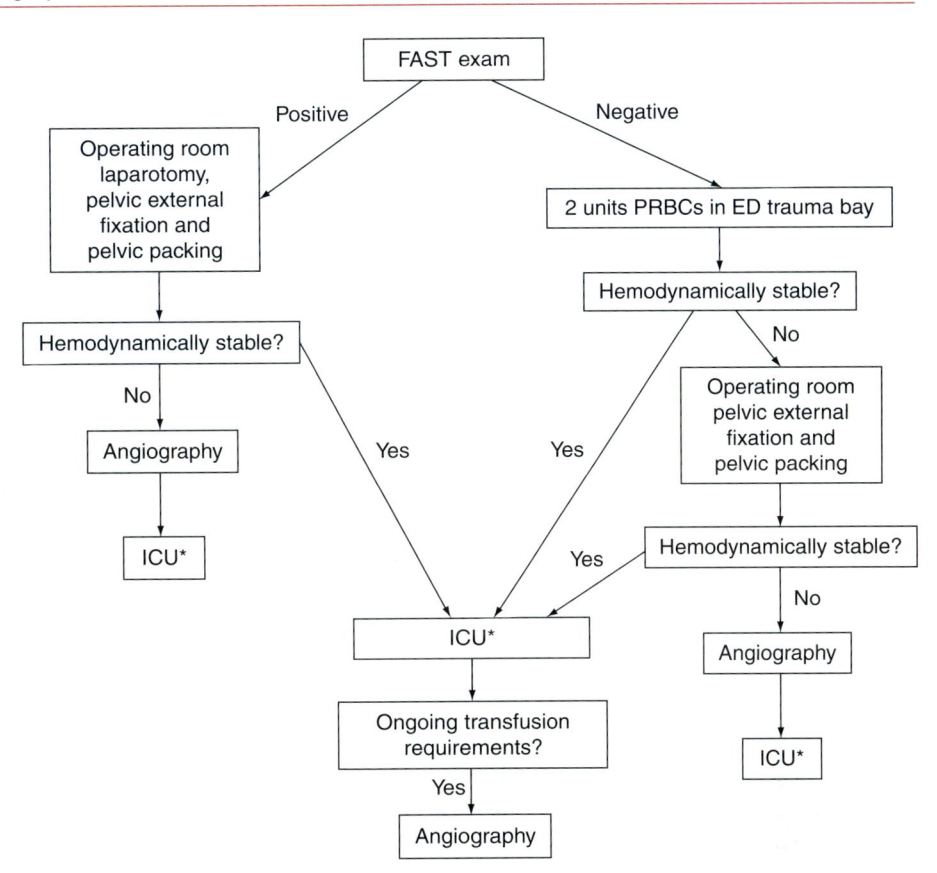

views of the pelvic and lateral cervical spine, is obtained to rule out a thoracic source of blood loss. A central venous pressure line is placed, and base deficit is measured.

A FAST examination is performed, and if positive, the patient is taken directly to the operating room for an exploratory laparotomy. A pelvic external fixator is placed, and pelvic packing is performed. If the patient remains hemodynamically unstable, he or she undergoes pelvic angiography prior to transfer to the intensive care unit (ICU). If hemodynamic stability is restored, the patient is transferred directly to the ICU. In the ICU, the patient receives further fluid resuscitation, is warmed, and attempts are made to normalize the coagulation status. If the patient requires ongoing transfusion while in the ICU, angiographic assessment, if not previously done, should be performed. Recombinant factor VIIa should be considered if the patient is recalcitrant to all other interventions.

If the FAST is negative, transfusion of PRBC is begun in the emergency department. If the patient remains hemodynamically unstable following the second unit of PRBC, he or she is taken to the operating room for pelvic external fixation and pelvic packing. If the patient remains hemodynamically unstable, he or she undergoes pelvic angiography prior to transfer to the intensive care unit (ICU). If hemodynamic stability is restored, the patient is transferred directly to the ICU. An abdominal computed tomography scan can be performed at this point in time. If the patient requires ongoing transfusion while in the ICU, angiographic assessment, if not previously done, should be performed.

The experience at Harborview Medical Center has evolved similarly in many respects, especially with regards to resuscitation and ICU management. Additionally, the overall concept of combining pelvic stability with hemorrhage control is adhered to. However, the use of pelvic packing and external fixation is much less commonly performed. Typically, pelvic stability is provided with a circumferentially wrapped sheet while the patient undergoes his or her initial abdominal and radiographic evaluations. These sheets are left in position for up to 24–48 h if necessary. However, frequent evaluation of the skin is necessary to avoid focal pressure and soft tissue necrosis. For patients with identified intra-abdominal pathology requiring exploratory laparotomy, pelvic stability is maintained either by retention of the circumferential pelvic sheet, by application of an external fixator, or by primary percutaneous pelvic stabilization of the posterior and/or anterior pelvic ring as indicated. Individualized care is directed by the fracture pattern. For patients who do not respond to a combination of pelvic stabilization and treatment of any identified intra-abdominal sources of bleeding, angiography is typically performed.

Clear and direct communication between the general trauma surgeon, orthopaedic trauma specialist, and other care providers is essential in the management of these severely injured patients. Such communication can help care providers understand each others concerns and the critical issues which each provider has identified. This communication can lead to improvements in the timing and order of the patient's subsequent diagnostic, interventional, and definitive management.

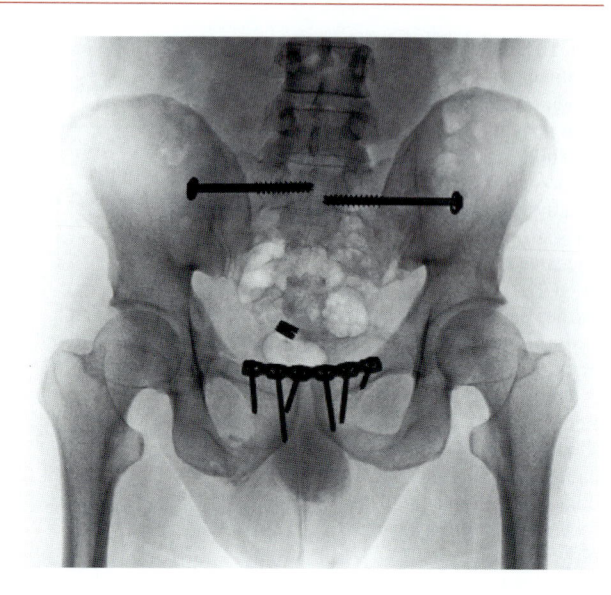

Fig. 10.7 Radiograph following plate fixation of anterior pelvic ring and bilateral percutaneous iliosacral screw fixation of an APC-III pelvic fracture

10.8 Definitive Treatment

10.8.1 Internal Fixation: Anterior Pelvic Ring

Reduction and fixation of a pubic symphysis diastasis may be performed using either a midline incision (extending any prior laparotomy incision) or a Pfannenstiel incision. A separate Pfannenstiel approach is preferred whenever possible to allow for extension laterally, if needed. The midline raphe is identified, and dissection occurs between the two bellies of rectus abdominis muscle. The insertion of the rectus is often traumatically avulsed from one of the rami. Surgical release of the rectus from its insertion should be avoided. A Hohmann type retractor can be placed beneath the rectus abdominus and over the anterior of the rami to assist with retraction of the rectus and reduction of the hemipelvis. Relaxation of retraction from one side often allows improved retraction and visualization on the opposite side. For "open book" type injuries, a Weber tenaculum is commonly placed anteriorly at the same level of the pubic body to achieve the reduction. Counterforce may need to be applied to correct any flexion or extension deformity of one hemipelvis with respect to the other. If one hemipelvis is posteriorly displaced, an anteriorly directed force may be obtained using a Jungbluth pelvic reduction clamp, which is applied with screws placed from anterior to posterior in the pubic body.

Several different plate and screw options may be used. Commonly, a six-hole 3.5-mm curved reconstruction plate is used (Fig. 10.7). Other options include the use of a two- or four-hole plate with large fragment cortical or cancellous screws. One advantage of a two-hole plate is that it permits some mobility, which may be useful in staged fixation when additional posterior reduction is required. However, in a clinical study comparing the use of a two-hole plate to a multi-hole plate fixation construct, investigators found a higher rate of implant failure and a significantly higher rate of pelvic malunion in patients treated with a two-hole symphyseal plate [22]. Locked plate fixation is now available; however, it has no clearly defined benefits over non-locked plating in the anterior pelvic ring. Double plating has also been described to improve stability if posterior internal fixation cannot be performed and the patient will be treated definitively with external fixation [23]. This is rarely used, requires a significant anterior soft tissue dissection, and has largely been replaced with a more aggressive approach to fixation of any associated posterior ring injuries.

If there is an associated fracture of the pubic ramus, a longer plate can be used to span across the fracture site. Given the multiple associated soft tissue attachments at the pubic ramis that provide some local stability, the associated rami fractures can sometimes be ignored and the anterior ring is treated with standard symphyseal fixation alone. Alternatively, a retrograde ramus screw can be used for internal fixation, but technically this is somewhat demanding as the available corridor for screw placement is quite narrow [24].

10.8.2 Internal Fixation: Posterior Pelvic Ring

Injury to the posterior pelvic ring can occur through a dislocation of the sacroiliac joint or through a fracture of the sacrum. These injuries can be addressed through either closed reduction or open reduction and subsequent internal fixation with cannulated or noncannulated screws.

It is important to obtain an anatomical reduction of the SI joint as long-term pain is associated with malreduction. The patient can be positioned either supine or prone, depending on the overall surgical plan and the comfort of the surgeon. A closed reduction can be attempted using a combination of limb traction, a fracture table, or direct manipulation using an external fixator. If an accurate reduction is obtained, percutaneous stabilization of the SI joint with large screws can be performed. When open reduction is required, either a posterior or anterior approach may be used. The posterior approach has been associated with a higher rate of wound healing complications, while the anterior approach has a higher risk of L5 nerve root injury as it runs less than 2 cm medial to the SI joint. However, with careful dissection and strategic posterior incision placement, the soft tissue complications associated with open approaches to the posterior pelvis have been significantly reduced. A combination of direct visualization, palpation of the SI joint, and radiographic evaluation is used to judge the reduction through either approach. Cannulated or noncannulated iliosacral screws can be used following either approach (Fig. 10.7). Alternatively, following the anterior approach, plate fixation can be used, but this is not as strong as iliosacral screws.

Crescent fractures involve a fracture in which a portion of the ilium remains attached to the sacrum. If the intact portion of the ilium is large, the fracture can be reduced through an open posterior approach and fixed with interfragmentary lag screws. Occasionally, if the fracture is quite anterior, an iliac approach may be used. In instances where the fragment is small or the posterior ligaments are injured, then stabilization with iliosacral screws is typically performed.

Posterior transiliac plate fixation may be selected for cases in which there is no available corridor for safe placement of SI screws. Usually, a 4.5-mm reconstruction plate is used and tunneled subcutaneously, securing fixation to both posterior iliac spines. Postoperative wound complications remain a concern, especially in the presence of a closed internal degloving injury [25].

Displaced or unstable fractures of the iliac wing may require fixation through the iliac portion of an ilioinguinal approach. Fixation of the iliac wing can be difficult as the available bone for screw fixations is limited. The iliac wing is very narrow except along the crest and as it widens near the acetabulum. Fixation can be accomplished either with plates (on the inner or outer aspect of the ilium), screws (placed between the inner and outer tables of the ilium), or combinations thereof.

References

1. Tile M, editor. Fractures of the pelvic and acetabulum. 2nd ed. Baltimore: Williams & Wilkins; 1995.
2. Kellam JF, Browner BD. Fractures of the pelvic ring. In: Browner BD, Jupiter JB, Levine AM, Trafton PG, editors. Skeletal trauma. Philadelphia: W.B. Saunders; 1992.
3. Olson SA, Burgess A. Classification and initial management of patients with unstable pelvic ring injuries. Instr Course Lect. 2005;54:383–93.
4. Tile M. Pelvic ring fractures: should they be fixed? J Bone Joint Surg Br. 1988;70(1):1–12.
5. Tile M. Acute pelvic fractures: I: Causation and classification. J Am Acad Orthop Surg. 1996;4(3):143–51.
6. Burgess AR, Eastridge BJ, Young JWR, et al. Pelvic ring disruptions: effective classification system and treatment protocols. J Trauma. 1990;30(7):848–56.
7. Dalal SA, Burgess AR, Siegel JH, et al. Pelvic fracture in multiple trauma: classification by mechanism is key to pattern of organ injury, resuscitative requirements and outcome. J Trauma. 1989;29(7):981–1000.
8. Routt Jr ML, Falicov A, Woodhouse E, Schildhauer TA. Circumferential pelvic antishock sheeting: a temporary resuscitation aid. J Orthop Trauma. 2002;16:45–8.

9. Croce MA, Magnotti LJ, Savage SA, Wood II GW, Fabian TC. Emergent pelvic fixation in patients with exsanguinating pelvic fractures. J Am Coll Surg. 2007;204:935–42.
10. Riemer BL, Butterfield SL, Diamond DL, et al. Acute mortality associated with injuries to the pelvic ring: the role of early patient mobilization and external fixation. J Trauma. 1993;35:671–7.
11. Grimm MR, Vrahas MS, Thomas KA. Pressure-volume characteristics of the intact and disrupted pelvic retroperitoneum. J Trauma. 1998;44:454–9.
12. Ganz R, Krushell RJ, Jakob RP, Küffer J. The antishock pelvic clamp. Clin Orthop Relat Res. 1991;267:71–8.
13. Archdeacon MT, Hiratzka J. The trochanteric C-clamp for provisional pelvic stability. J Orthop Trauma. 2006;20:47–51.
14. Eastridge BJ, Starr A, Minei JP, O'Keefe GE, Scalea TM. The importance of fracture pattern in guiding therapeutic decision-making in patients with hemorrhagic shock and pelvic ring disruptions. J Trauma. 2002;53:446–51.
15. Miller PR, Moore PS, Mansell E, Meredith JW, Chang MC. External fixation or arteriogram in bleeding pelvic fracture: initial therapy guided by markers of arterial hemorrhage. J Trauma. 2003;54:437–43.
16. Agolini SF, Shah K, Jaffe J, Newcomb J, Rhodes M, Reed III JF. Arterial embolization is a rapid and effective technique for controlling pelvic fracture hemorrhage. J Trauma. 1997;43:395–9.
17. Balogh Z, Caldwell E, Heetveld M, et al. Institutional practice guidelines on management of pelvic fracture-related hemodynamic instability: do they make a difference? J Trauma. 2005;58:778–82.
18. Yasumura K, Ikegami K, Kamohara T, Nohara Y. High incidence of ischemic necrosis of the gluteal muscle after transcatheter angiographic embolization for severe pelvic fracture. J Trauma. 2005;58:985–90.
19. Pohlemann T, Bosch U, Gänsslen A, Tscherne H. The Hannover experience in management of pelvic fractures. Clin Orthop Relat Res. 1994;305:69–80.
20. Smith WR, Moore EE, Osborn P, et al. Retroperitoneal packing as a resuscitation technique for hemodynamically unstable patients with pelvic fractures: report of two representative cases and a description of technique. J Trauma. 2005;59:1510–4.
21. Cothren CC, Osborn PM, Moore EE, Morgan SJ, Johnson JL, Smith WR. Preperitonal pelvic packing for hemodynamically unstable pelvic fractures: a paradigm shift. J Trauma. 2007;62:834–42.
22. Sagi HC, Papp S. Comparative radiographic and clinical outcome of two-hole and multi-hole symphyseal plating. J Orthop Trauma. 2008;22:373–8.
23. Ponson KJ, Hoek van Dijke GA, Joosse P, Snijders CJ, Agnew SG. Improvement of external fixator performance in type C pelvic ring injuries by plating of the pubic symphysis: an experimental study on 12 external fixators. J Trauma. 2002;53:907–12.
24. Routt Jr ML, Simonian PT, Grujic L. The retrograde medullary superior pubic ramus screw for the treatment of anterior pelvic ring disruptions: a new technique. J Orthop Trauma. 1995;9:35–44.
25. Suzuki T, Hak DJ, Zran BH, et al. Outcome and complications of posterior transiliac plating for vertically unstable sacral fractures. Injury: Int J Care Injured. 2009;40:405–9.

Urological Injuries in Polytrauma

David Pfister and Axel Heidenreich

Contents

11.1	Introduction	115
11.2	Renal Trauma	115
11.2.1	Clinical Symptoms	115
11.2.2	Imaging Studies	116
11.2.3	Treatment	117
11.3	Ureteral Trauma	117
11.3.1	Clinical Symptoms	117
11.3.2	Imaging	118
11.3.3	Management	118
11.4	Bladder Trauma	119
11.4.1	Clinical Symptoms	119
11.4.2	Imaging	119
11.4.3	Treatment	121
11.5	Urethral Trauma	121
11.5.1	Clinical Symptoms	123
11.5.2	Radiographic Examination	123
11.5.3	Treatment	123
References		125

11.1 Introduction

In approximately 10% of all patients with multiple traumas, urological components are regularly involved [1]. Genitourinary injuries may result in significant morbidity and mortality [1–3]. In general, one must distinguish between blunt and penetrating injuries to the urogenital organs necessitating urgent intervention. The incidence of injuries to the various organs varies with the kidney being the most commonly injured organ in 1–5% of trauma cases. Most urethral injuries are iatrogenic, while about 18% result in blunt and 7% in penetrating traumas.

11.2 Renal Trauma

Renal trauma occurs in about 1–5% of all cases with blunt trauma accounting for the most common mechanism of renal injury about 90% of the time [1–7]. While penetrating injuries are much less frequent, they tend to be more severe and result in a higher rate of nephrectomies [8]. Possible indicators for renal trauma are falls, blunt trauma to the flank region, and high-speed motor-vehicle accidents [1, 5, 6]. The Committee on the Organ Injury Scaling of the American Association for Surgery of Trauma (AAST) has classified renal injuries as shown in Table 11.1.

11.2.1 Clinical Symptoms

Gross hematuria might be present, but it does not correlate with the degree of injury since major injuries such as renal pedicle lacerations or disruption of the ureteropelvic junction may occur without hematuria. Blood transfusion requirements are an indirect indication of the rate of blood loss.

D. Pfister and A. Heidenreich (✉)
Department of Urology, RWTH University Aachen,
Pauwelsstr. 30, 52074 Aachen, Germany
e-mail: aheidenreich@ukaachen.de

Table 11.1 AAST organ injury severity scale for the kidney

1	Contusion or non-expanding subcapsular hematoma. No laceration
2	Non-expanding perirenal hematoma, cortical laceration < 1 cm deep w/o extravasation
3	Cortical laceration > 1 cm w/o urinary extravasation
4	Laceration: through corticomedullary junction into collecting system or Vascular: segmental renal artery or vein injury with contained hematoma
5	Laceration: shuttered kidney or Vascular: renal pedicle injury or avulsion

11.2.2 Imaging Studies

Patients with blunt renal trauma, a microscopic hematuria, and stable vital signs in the absence of deceleration trauma need not undergo any type of imaging studies [1, 4, 9].

Patients with gross hematuria, penetrating injuries with suspected renal involvement and instable vital signs must undergo immediate imaging studies (Fig. 11.1) [1, 5]. CT represents the gold standard for radiographic assessment in suspected renal injury because it (1) defines the location and the extent of

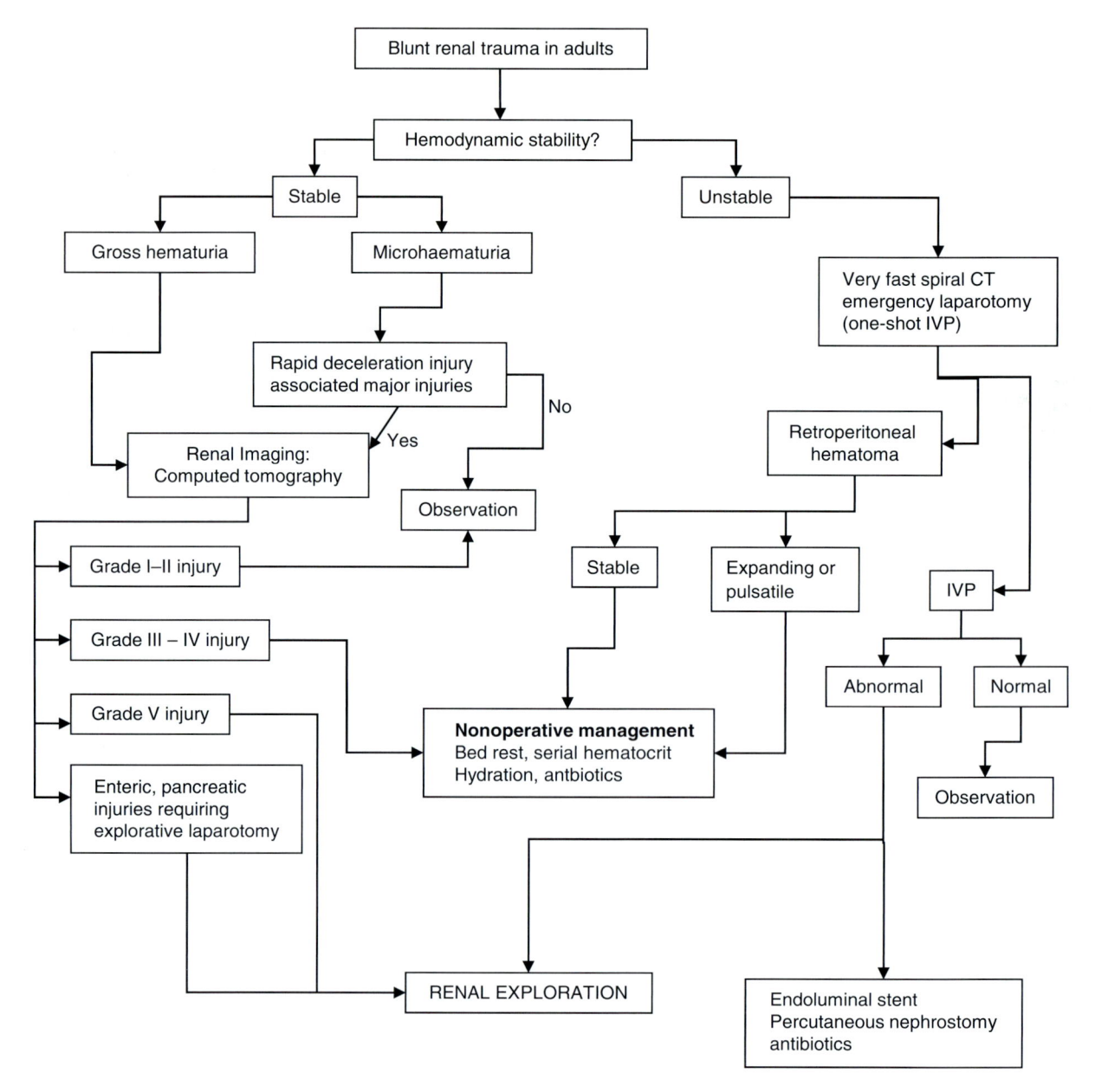

Fig. 11.1 Diagnostic and therapeutic algorithm for suspected blunt renal trauma in adults

injuries, (2) detects contusions and devitalized segments, (3) allows visualization of the entire retroperitoneum, (4) allows assessment of the renal pedicle, and (5) detects urinary extravasations [1, 5, 9, 10]. Spiral CT scans are advantageous due to shorter scanning times, but do not allow the identification of injuries to the renal collecting system, thereby necessitating the use of delayed scans. Angiography is important only for superselective embolization in the management of persisting or delayed hemorrhage.

11.2.3 Treatment

A summary of the various therapeutic approaches is presented in Fig. 11.1. Life-threatening hemodynamic instability or expanding or pulsatile retroperitoneal hematoma during explorative laparotomy usually represents an AAST grade 5 injury and requires immediate surgery [1, 3]. A transperitoneal approach with early occlusion of the renal pedicle prior to opening of Gerota's fascia is strongly recommended. In patients with avulsion of the renal pedicle close to the aorta or the inferior vena cava, it may be necessary to clamp the major vessels just above and below the renal pedicle to control bleeding and explore the retroperitoneum. In patients with significant injuries to the vascular pedicle, nephrectomy is the treatment of choice unless the kidney can be preserved in cases of solitary organ or bilateral injuries. In patients demonstrating significant bleeding from the renal parenchyma due to penetrating injuries or induced arteriovenous fistula, a superselective embolization is the treatment of choice [4, 6, 11].

Persistent bleeding, injuries to the renal collecting system, the renal pelvis, or the ureter with urinary extravasation, all present relative indications for surgery [1]. Although urinary extravasations may be treated by endoluminal stenting and/or placement of a percutaneous nephrostomy only, surgical reconstruction may be advisable in the presence of devitalized fragments and associated enteric and pancreatic injuries [12]. Expectant management for renal lacerations resulted in only a 23% urological morbidity rate, whereas watchful waiting for combined renal and enteric or pancreatic lacerations resulted in an 85% urological morbidity rate. However, if patients undergo surgical repair of the renal collecting system, watertight closure and the intraoperative placement of an endoluminal stent are mandatory.

Hemodynamically stable patients with AAST grade 1 and 2 injuries can be managed nonoperatively with supportive care, bed-rest, hydration, and prophylactic antibiotics [4–6].

Stable patients with renal gunshot injuries or stab wounds must be explored if the renal hilum and the collecting system are involved, or if persistent bleeding exists.

In patients with significant renal injuries, postoperative observation is especially and extremely important because a variety of delayed complications may occur within the first 30 days of injury, including, but not limited to, bleeding, perinephric abscess, urinary fistula, arteriovenous fistula, and pseudoaneurysms [2, 13]. Patients must undergo imaging studies if they develop clinical symptoms such as fever, increasing flank pain, persistent bleeding, and arterial hypertension. As for the primary diagnosis, CT scan of the abdomen is the preferred imaging modality.

11.3 Ureteral Trauma

Trauma to the ureter is rare and accounts for only about 1% of all genitourinary injuries. Most commonly, ureteral lesions result from iatrogenic injuries (75%), and only 18% and 7% result from blunt and penetrating trauma, respectively. The majority of iatrogenic injuries occur after gynaecologic interventions (70–75%), while about 15–20% occur after general surgery and about 10–15% occur due to urologists.

As with all other genitourinary organs, the AAST has classified ureteral injuries according to their severity as indicated in Table 11.2.

11.3.1 Clinical Symptoms

There are no specific clinical symptoms; unspecific symptoms include meteorism, abdominal distension, and flank pain caused by retroperitoneal urinoma. Ureteral injury should always be suspected in patients

Table 11.2 Classification of ureteral injury

Grade	Description of injury
I	Hematoma only
II	Laceration < 50% of circumference
III	Laceration > 50% of circumference
IV	Complete tear < 2 cm of devascularization
V	Complete tear > 2 cm of devascularization

with penetrating abdominal or retroperitoneal injuries and in patients with blunt deceleration traumas.

11.3.2 Imaging

The most common imaging modality is intravenous pyelography, which is performed in two-thirds of the patients with suspected ureteral injuries. Typically, IVP demonstrates retroperitoneal extravasation of contrast material. In about 30–50% of cases, additional retrograde ureteropyelography is performed to verify the location and the extent of the ureteral injury. Small lesions may be managed by placement of an endoluminal DJ-catheter. In very rare cases, the suspicion of a ureteral injury is based on ultrasound findings of a retroperitoneal fluid collection (urinoma) or a hydronephrosis (Fig. 11.2).

11.3.3 Management

In patients with partial tears of the ureter, the most common, simple, and effective measurement is to place a ureteral stent and/or a percutaneous nephrostomy tube.

If iatrogenic ureteral injuries are detected intraoperatively, an endoluminal DJ stent should be placed and the ureteral laceration closed by interrupted sutures with a monofil suture. Postoperatively, no drain or suction should be placed in order to prevent the development of a urinary fistula.

Reconstruction of grade III–V injuries depends on the anatomic localization of the injury. Usually, grade III and IV injuries may be treated by an end-to-end anastomosis once debridement and spatulation of the ureteral ends have been performed. The anastomosis is reconstructed with absorbable sutures after placement of a ureteral

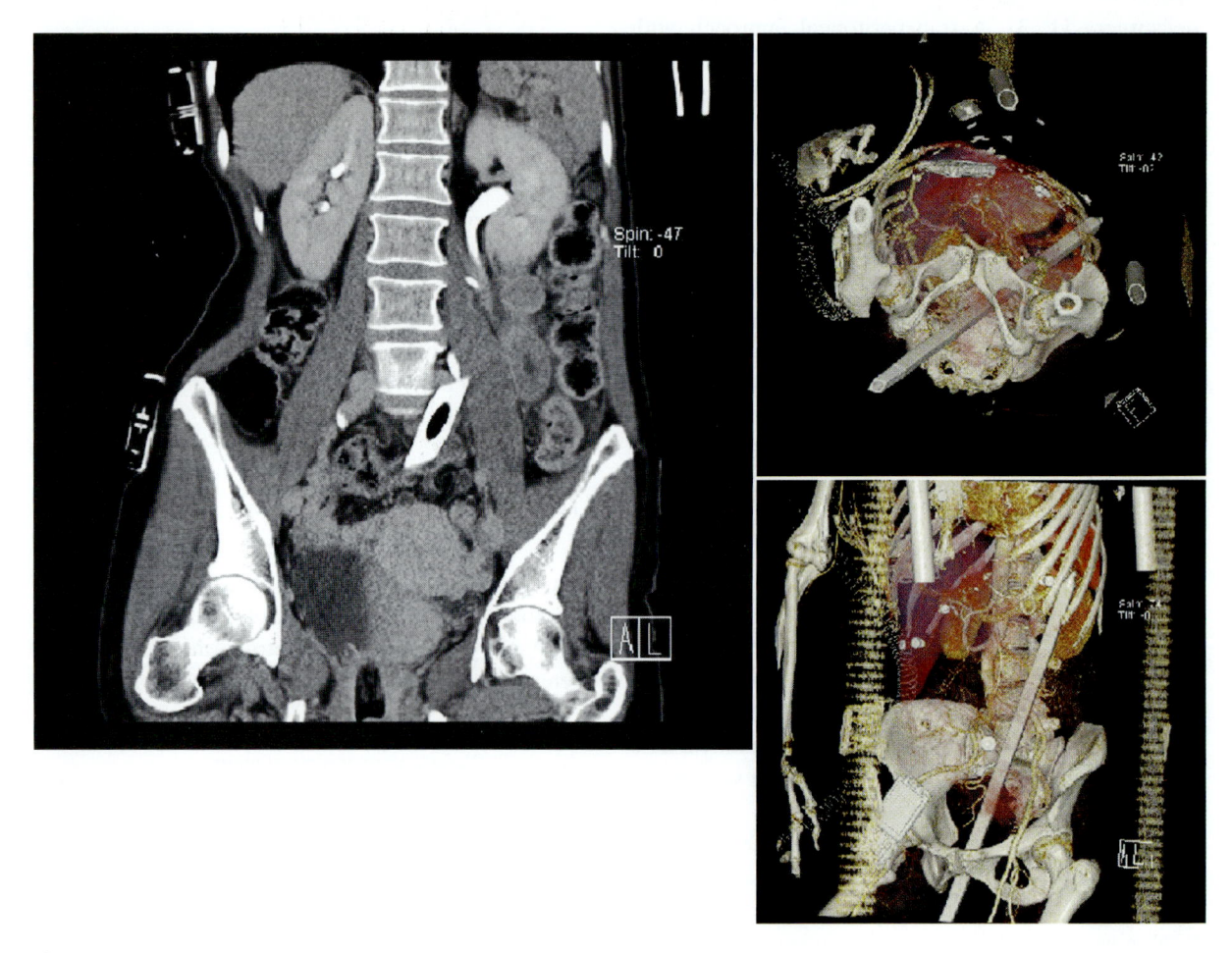

Fig. 11.2 Left ureteral injury with urinoma and hematoma in the small pelvis

Table 11.3 Surgical options to reconstruct ureteral injuries depending on the anatomic level of injury

Level of urethral injury	Options of reconstruction
Upper third	Transuretero-ureterostomy
	Ureterocalycostomy
	Ileal replacement of the ureter
	Percutaneous pyelovesical bypass prosthesis
	Renal autotransplantation
Middle third	Transuretero-ureterostomy
	Boari flap and intravesical reimplantation
	Ileal replacement of the ureter
Lower third	Direct intravesical reimplantation
	Psoas hitch reimplantation
Complete ureteral loss	Ileal replacement (delayed)[a]
	Renal autotransplantation (delayed)[a]
	Percutaneous pyelovesical bypass (delayed)[a]

[a]For urinary drainage, a percutaneous nephrostomy tube should be placed together with occlusion of the ureter by sutures, clips, or occluding catheters

Table 11.4 AAST organ injury severity scale for the bladder

I	Hematoma	Contusion, intramural hematoma
I	Laceration	Partial thickness
II	Laceration	Extraperitoneal bladder wall laceration < 2 cm
III	Laceration	Extraperitoneal (>2 cm) or intraperitoneal (<2 cm) bladder wall laceration
IV	Laceration	Intraperitoneal bladder wall laceration > 2 cm
V	Laceration	Intraperitoneal or extraperitoneal bladder wall laceration extending into the bladder neck or ureteral orifices

catheter, which can stay in place for about 3–4 weeks. Other surgical options are listed in Table 11.3.

11.4 Bladder Trauma

Bladder injuries are among the most frequent urological injuries in trauma patients. Among abdominal injuries needing surgical repair, about 2% involve the bladder [1, 14, 15]. Blunt trauma accounts for about 65–85% of bladder ruptures, whereas penetrating trauma accounts for only about 25% (14–33%) of all bladder injuries. Bladder ruptures in the setting of blunt traumas are classified as extra- or intraperitoneal, triggering the choice between a conservative approach and a surgical correction. Most commonly, extraperitoneal bladder ruptures occur in about 55% of cases, followed by intraperitoneal bladder ruptures in 38%. Combined injuries are rare, occurring in only 5–8% of cases. Motor vehicle accidents contribute significantly to bladder rupture by blunt trauma. Seventy to ninety-seven percent of patients with bladder trauma have accompanied pelvic fractures, whereas only 5–30% of the pelvic fractures are associated with bladder injuries [14–19].

The Committee on the Organ Injury Scaling of the American Association for Surgery of Trauma (AAST) has classified bladder injuries as shown in Table 11.4.

11.4.1 Clinical Symptoms

The two most common signs and symptoms for bladder injuries are gross hematuria (80–100%) and abdominal tenderness (60–70%) [14]. Other findings may include the inability to void (rule out: intrapelvic urethral rupture!), bruises over the suprapubic region, and abdominal distension. Depending on the type and extent of associated injuries to the pelvic floor, extravasation of urine may result in swelling of the perineum, scrotum, thighs, and the anterior abdominal wall.

11.4.2 Imaging

The classic combination of pelvic fracture and gross hematuria requires immediate cystourethrography to rule out urethral and/or bladder ruptures (Fig. 11.3) [14, 16, 20, 21]. All patients with pelvic ring fractures and gross hematuria should undergo immediate cystography (Figs. 11.4 and 11.5). Since microscopic hematuria is a relative indicator for significant injury, recommendations for the most appropriate imaging studies are sparse in existing guidelines. Imaging of the bladder may be reserved for those with anterior rami fractures (straddle fractures) or Malgaigne type severe ring disruption (Tile III).

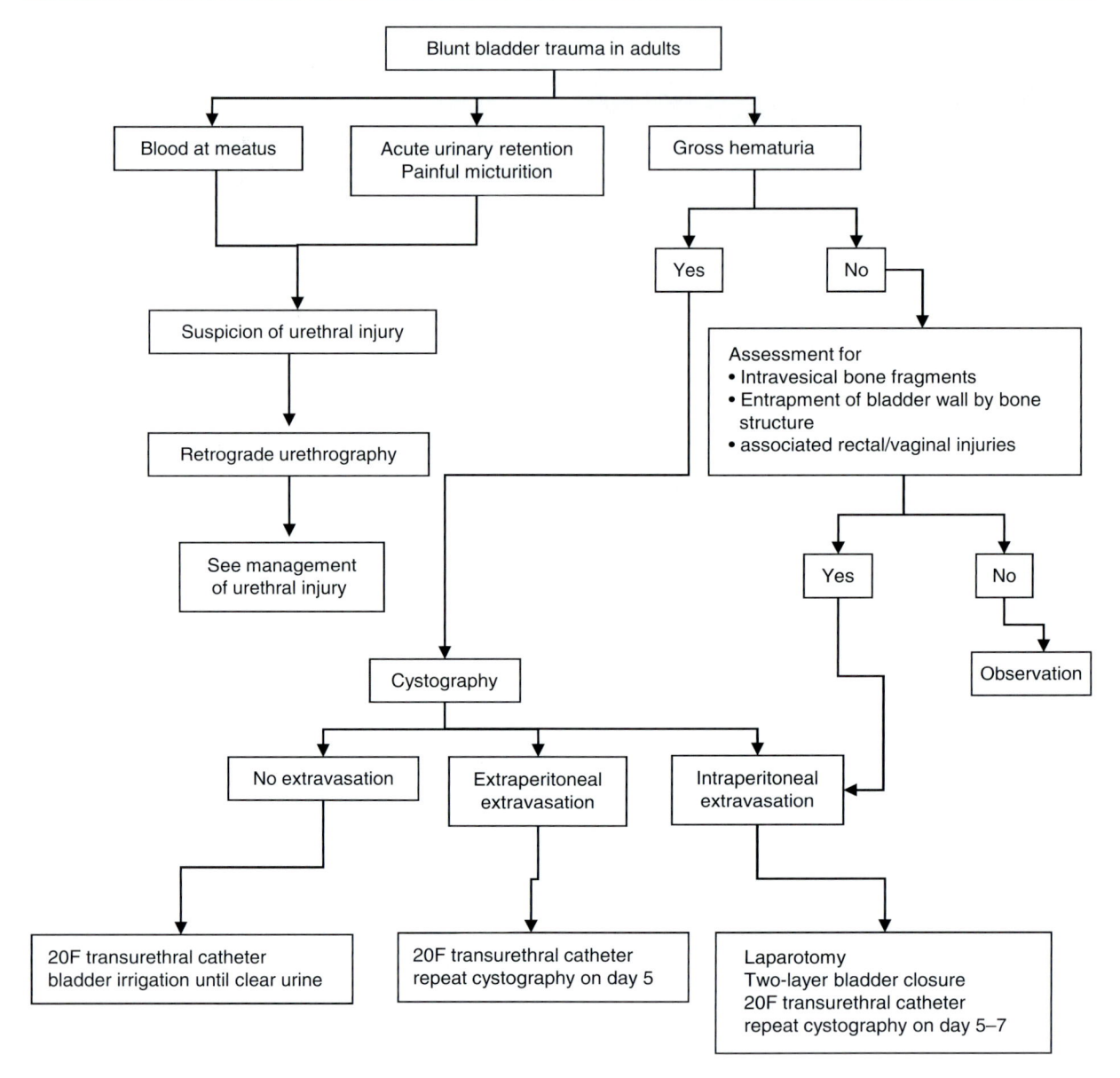

Fig. 11.3 Diagnostic and therapeutic algorithm for suspected blunt bladder trauma in adults

Retrograde cystography in the evaluation of bladder trauma represents the imaging procedure of choice [14, 16, 18–20]. With adequate filling and post-void images taken, cystography has an accuracy of 85–100% in the identification of bladder ruptures. For the highest degree of diagnostic accuracy, the bladder should be filled with at least 350 cc of contrast agent. Bladder rupture may be identified on the post-drainage film in only about 10% of patients. Thus, images must always include x-rays upon maximal distension and a completely emptied bladder.

Blood at the urethral meatus may be a sign of significant urethral injury. Retrograde urethrography should be performed prior to catheterization of the bladder to exclude associated urethral lesions, which can occur in 10–30% of cases [1, 16].

Other imaging studies such as ultrasonography, intravenous pyelography, standard CT scans, or magnetic resonance imaging are inadequate for the evaluation of the bladder and the urethra after trauma [1, 14, 16]. As CT scan is performed in most patients who present with

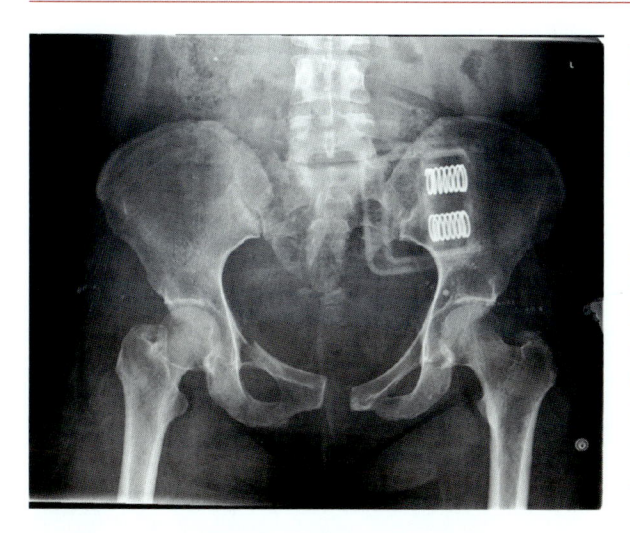

Fig. 11.4 Decelaeration trauma after a jump from the third floor

multiple trauma, CT cystography is an excellent substitute for standard cystography. The bladder should be filled with at least 350 cc of dilute (2%) contrast dye [21].

ureteral orifices requires immediate surgical repair. Bladder neck reconstruction, transurethral placement of an endoluminal catheter, or even ureteral reimplantation (Psoas-Hitch technique) may be required in cases of severe ureteral orifice damage.

In contrast to extraperitoneal bladder ruptures, all penetrating and intraperitoneal injuries should undergo immediate surgical repair [1, 14, 15]. In most cases, intraperitoneal bladder perforations are accompanied by other intra-abdominal injuries. Peritonitis might develop because of the urinary leakage. In this scenario, an overlooked bladder perforation may be mimicked by a significant rise in serum creatinine levels due to peritoneal reabsorbtion. Antibiotic prophylaxis is administered for 3 days. Standard cystography is feasible on postoperative days 7–10 [16]. A suprapubic catheter is superior to a transurethral catheter for urinary drainage. In case of concomitant rectal or vaginal injuries, the ruptured organs are closed separately with a two-layer technique, and a peritoneal flap of a vascularized omentum flap is interposed between bladder, vagina, and rectum.

11.4.3 Treatment

The therapeutic approach to treat any bladder rupture depends on the type of injury, the coexisting injuries, and the condition of the patient (Fig. 11.3).

Most patients with extraperitoneal bladder ruptures may be treated nonoperatively by catheter drainage even in the presence of large extravasations [1, 18, 19, 22]. More than two-thirds of the ruptures resolve within 2 days and almost all within 3 weeks. From the day of catheterization until 3 days after removal of the catheter, antibiotic prophylaxis is recommended.

If a laparotomy is performed for other reasons, the extraperitoneal bladder ruptures should be closed with a single layer running suture of 2–0 or 3–0. The bladder is usually drained using a 20 F transurethral catheter before a cystography is performed post operatively on day 5. Following internal fixation of the pelvic fracture, a direct repair of the extraperitoneal rupture is advised. Concomitant rectal and/or vaginal injuries, open pelvic fractures, the presence of bone fragments in the bladder wall, and entrapment of the bladder wall between bone fragments necessitate immediate surgical repair even in extraperitoneal bladder rupture [1, 14, 15]. Involvement of the bladder neck or the

11.5 Urethral Trauma

Urethral injuries occur most commonly in about 6–10% of pelvic fractures [1, 23, 24]. Unstable diametric pelvic fractures and bilateral ischiopubic rami fractures carry the highest risk of injury to the posterior urethra. In particular, the combination of straddle injuries with diastasis of the sacroiliac joint poses a risk about seven times higher for urethral injuries. The bulbomembranous junction is more vulnerable, as the posterior urethra is fixed at the urogenital diaphragm as well as the puboprostatic ligaments. In children, these are more frequently localized proximally and interfere with the bladder neck, as the prostate is still rudimentary. In rare cases, a urethral disrupture may be diagnosed by the existence of the triad: blood at the external urethral meatus, inability to void, and palpable full bladder. It is usually detected by false catheterization or by the inability to place a transurethral catheter by the emergency department. Additional symptoms may include perineal hematoma and inability to palpate the prostate. In cases of a large pelvic hematoma, the symptom of an impalpable prostate may be misdiagnosed, as the contour of the prostate is smudged. In females with urethral injuries, vulvar edema and blood at the vaginal introitus may be signs of urethral disorders.

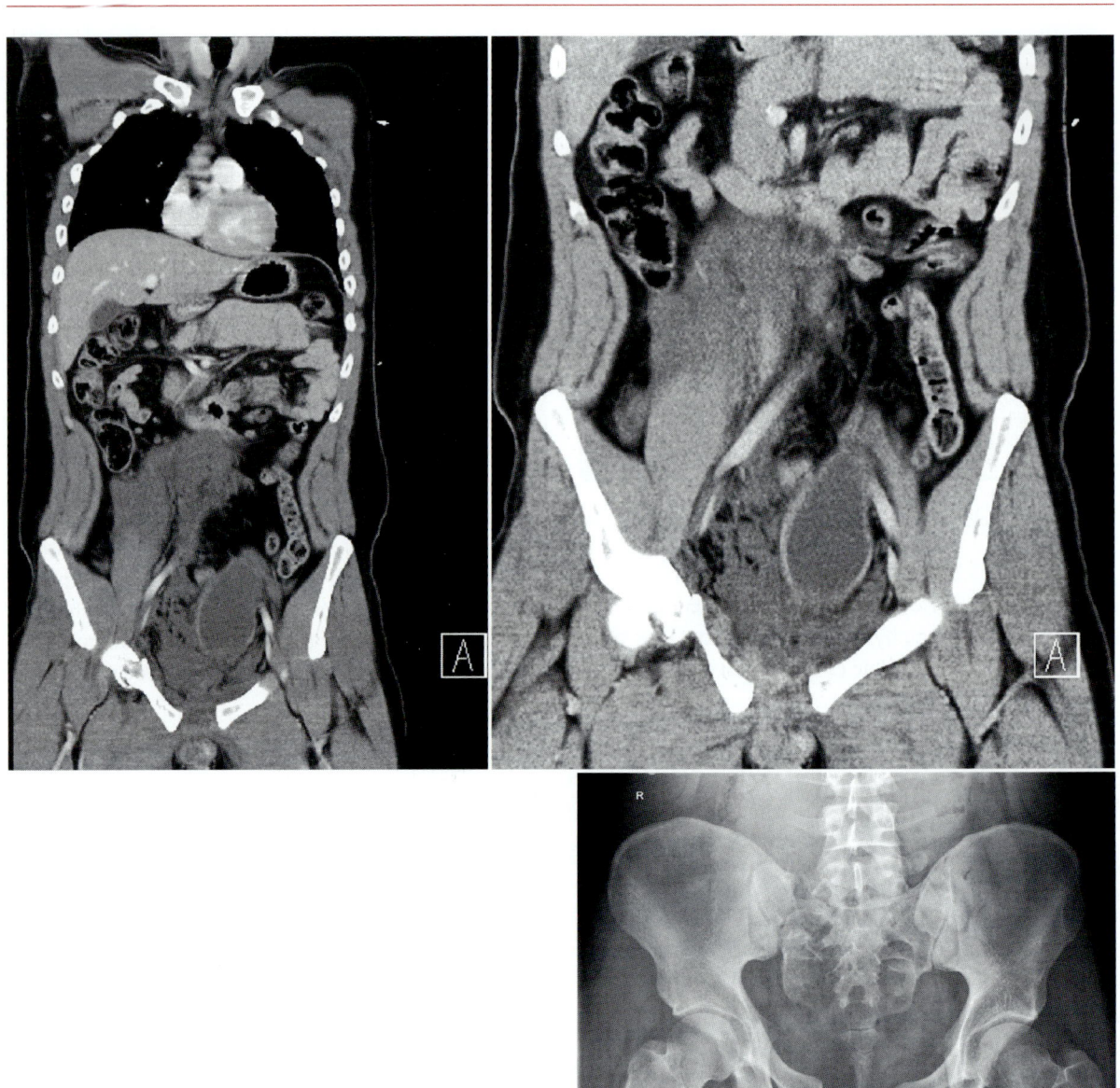

Fig. 11.5 Rupture of the symphysis following a motor bicycle accident: hematoma of the small pelvis, cranial dislocation of the bladder due to intrapelvic rupture of the urethra

The Committee on Organ Injury Scaling of the American Association for the Surgery of Trauma (AAST) has developed a reliable urethral-injury scaling system (Table 11.5).

No treatment is required for type I and II injuries [1, 23–31]. Usually, types II and III can be managed nonoperatively. A transurethral and a suprapubic catheter are placed. Types IV and V will require either endoscopic realignment or delayed urethroplasty.

Penetrating injuries to the anterior urethra most commonly derive from gunshots and involve the pendulous and bulbar urethral segments.

Table 11.5 AAST organ injury severity scale for the urethra

I	Contusion	Blood at the urethral meatus, normal urethrogram
II	Stretch injury	Elongation of the urethra w/o extravasation on urethrography
III	Partial disruption	Extravasation of contrast at injury site with contrast visualized in the bladder
IV	Complete disruption	Extravasation of contrast at injury site without visualization in the bladder; <2 cm urethral separation
V	Complete disruption	Complete transsection with >2 cm urethral separation, or extension into the prostate or vagina

11.5.1 Clinical Symptoms

Blood at the meatus is present in about 40–95% of patients with posterior urethral injuries and in about 75% of patients with anterior urethral trauma. Its presence should preclude any attempts of urethral manipulation until the entire urethra is adequately imaged. Partial urethral disruption can be very easily transformed into complete urethral disruption due to several attempts of forced transurethral catheterization. In unstable patients, one attempt of transurethral catheterization is justified; if there is any difficulty, a suprapubic tube should be inserted instead. If a urethral injury is suspected, a retrograde urethrogram should be performed.

Gross or microscopic hematuria is a nonspecific clinical sign and the amount of bleeding does not correlate with the extent of injury [1, 24]. Pain on urination or acute urinary retention suggests urethral intrapelvic disrupture with temporary spasm of the internal bladder sphincter. Any of the above-mentioned symptoms necessitates immediate radiographic evaluation [30], precludes transurethral manipulation, and prompts placement of a suprapubic catheter for urinary drainage.

Blood at the external urethral meatus is present in more than 80% of female patients with pelvic fractures and urethral injuries.

11.5.2 Radiographic Examination

When a urethral injury is suspected, immediate retrograde urethrography should be performed (Fig. 11.6) [1, 24, 30]. In females direct urethroscopy can be performed. In cases of subsequent urethral strictures a combined urethrogram and cystogram is appropriate to delineate the pelvic anatomy. Also, magnetic resonance tomography or antegrade cystourethroscopy via the suprapubic tract can be performed to visualize the anatomy of the urethra.

11.5.3 Treatment

Treatment differs with regard to involvement of the anterior vs. posterior urethra and differs between males and females.

11.5.3.1 Treatment for Urethral Injuries in Males

Type I and II injuries of the anterior urethra can be easily managed by the placement of a transurethral catheter [1]. Type III injuries of the anterior urethra can be managed by the placement of a suprapubic catheter or a transurethral catheter, with the advantage that the suprapubic tube avoids urethral manipulation and diverts urine from the place of injury [23, 24]. In more than 50% of the cases, spontaneous recanalization occurs; in all other cases, strictures can be managed by internal urethrotomy. Alternatively, delayed urethral reconstructive surgery may be performed with anastomotic urethroplasty or buccal mucosa grafts in strictures <1 cm or longer than 1 cm.

Type IV injuries can be repaired by an end-to-end anastomosis, whereas type V injuries should be reconstructed by flap urethroplasty or by buccal mucosa grafts.

In females, most anterior urethral injuries can be sutured primarily from a transvaginal approach [23, 24]. Proximal urethral injuries are best approached transvesically, with an optimal view of the bladder neck, the ureteral orifices, and the proximal urethra.

A treatment algorithm for the management of anterior and posterior male urethral injuries is presented in Fig. 11.6.

Partial tears or short disruptions of the posterior urethra can be by a suprapubic or transurethral catheter for about 2 weeks. The majority of injuries heal and the risk of urethral strictures is low.

The management for complete disruption of the posterior urethra is variable [25–31]:

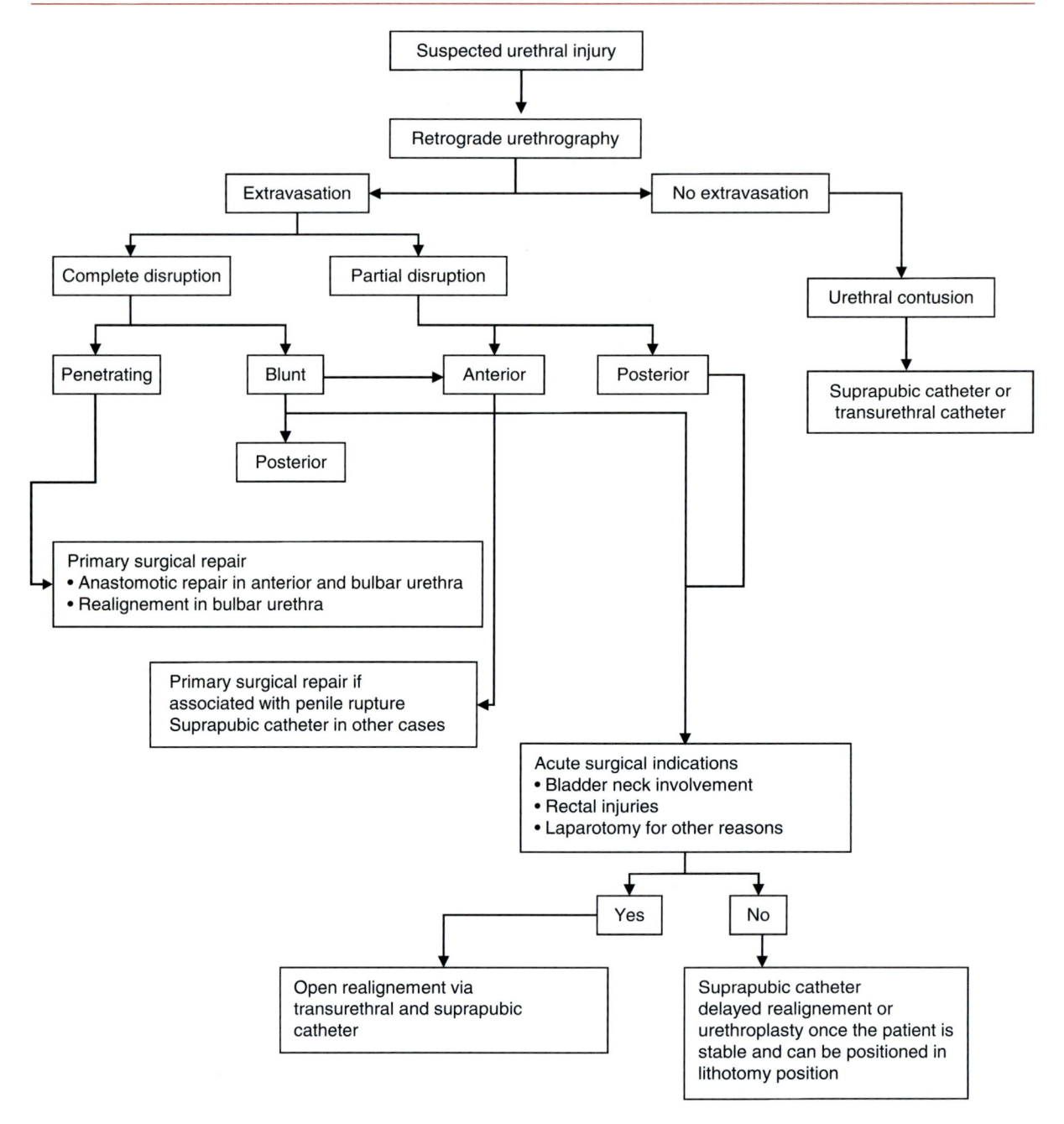

Fig. 11.6 Diagnostic and therapeutic algorithm for suspected blunt urethral injury in male adults

1. Immediate open repair in case of any associated injury to the rectum double-layer closure of urethral and rectal lesion and interposition of a flap from the greater omentum
2. Primary endoscopic realignment by antegrade (using the canal of the suprapubic catheter) or retrograde approach
3. Primary open realignment with evacuation of the pelvic hematoma is not recommended; it is associated with frequent postoperative incontinence and impotence

The most common result of posterior urethral disruption is the development of a short prostatobulbar urethral gap filled with dense fibrotic tissue. Delayed surgical repair of a posterior urethral disrupture should be performed after 3 months. Surgery requires proper positioning of the patient in the lithotomy position.

Preoperatively, a retrograde urethrogram and a simultaneous cystogram should be performed to determine the length of the stricture or fibrotic discontinuation of the urethra. If involvement of the bladder neck is suspected, a flexible or rigid urethroscopy is helpful for examining anatomy. In patients who did not undergo primary realignment, the urethral dislocation as well as the length of the defect can be visualized by MRI. In selected patients with short urethral strictures, an endoscopic strategy may follow. In case of complete urethral obstructions, some have favored endoscopic interventions. However, there is a high risk of undermining the urethra and bladder neck and the restructure rate is 80%. Furthermore, the endoscopic procedure often requires several interventions and long-term repetitive dilatations with recurrent strictures and obliterations.

Usually, long posterior urethral strictures are best managed by an open surgical repair via a perineal approach. The urethra is accessed by a midline or lambda incision. The urethra is then mobilized from the beginning of the fibrotic defect to the midscrotum, allowing a tension-free anastomosis. The scar tissue as well as the fibrotic tissue of the proximal urethra must be excised completely to prevent restrictures. For long strictures, a flap urethroplasty of buccal mucisa grafts is used. Adjunctive maneuvers are infrequently needed. In rare cases, pubectomy can be helpful for cases with extended fibrosis, failed former urethroplasty, or accompanied bladder neck involvement.

Erectile dysfunction is a complication of urethral distraction injuries described in 30–60% of the patients with pelvic fracture [31]. It is questionable as to whether posttraumatic impotence is a result of the injury itself or due to the surgical management. The frequency of posttreatment erectile dysfunction remains the same, independent of initial therapy (early realignment, open surgery, or no treatment). The overall rate of incontinence, anejaculation and areflexic bladder is low (2–4%). Another problem is recurrent urethral strictures, which arise in 15–23% of patients. Minimally invasive treatment by endoscopic incision of the stricture is often sufficient.

11.5.3.2 Treatment of Urethral Injuries in Females

Vaginal inspection should be performed in every female patient to assess the extent and localization of the urethral injury and the presence, localization, and extent of potentially associated vaginal injuries. Vaginal injuries are further evaluated with an abdominal CT scan to screen for associated intrapelvic or intra-abdominal injuries.

In complete urethral ruptures, immediate surgical repair is recommended to avoid urethrovaginal fistulas and complete urethral obliteration. A complete obliteration with an embedded urethra in scar tissue results in a significantly more complicated surgery with an increased frequency of severe complications. Injuries of the distal urethra can be easily repaired via a transvaginal approach. Injuries of the proximal or the bladder neck are best reconstructed via a retropubic approach. Only in unstable patients should a suprapubic catheter be used and is delayed primary reconstruction justified.

References

1. Lynch TH, Martinez-Pineiro L, Plas E, Serafetinides E, Türkeri L, Santucci RA, et al. EAU guidelines on urological trauma. Eur Urol. 2005;47:1–15.
2. Starnes M, Demetriades D, Hadjizacharia P, Inaba K, Best C, Chan L. Complications following renal trauma. Arch Surg. 2010;145:377–81.
3. Chow SJ, Thompson KJ, Hartman JF, Wright ML. A 10-year review of blunt renal artery injuries at an urban level I trauma centre. Injury. 2009;40:844–50.
4. Broghammer JA, Fisher MB, Santucci RA. Conservative management of renal trauma: a review. Urology. 2007;70: 623–9.
5. Alsikafi NF, Rosenstein DI. Staging, evaluation, and nonoperative management of renal injuries. Urol Clin North Am. 2006;33:13–9.
6. Baverstock R, Simons R, McLoughlin M. Severe blunt renal trauma: a 7-year retrospective review from a provincial trauma centre. Can J Urol. 2001;8:1372–76.
7. Santucci RA, McAninch JM. Grade IV renal injuries: evaluation, treatment, and outcome. World J Surg. 2001;25: 1565–72.
8. Velmahos GC, Demetriades D, Cornwell III EE, Belzberg H, Murray J, Asensio J, et al. Selective management of renal gunshot wounds. Br J Surg. 1998;85:1121–4.
9. Eastham JA, Wilson TG, Ahlering TE. Radiographic evaluation of adult patients with blunt renal trauma. J Urol. 1992;148(2 Pt 1):266–7.
10. Mee SL, McAninch JW, Robinson AL, Auerbach PS, Carroll PR. Radiographic assessment of renal trauma: a 10-year prospective study of patient selection. J Urol. 1989;141: 1095–8.
11. Umbreit EC, Routh JC, Husmann DA. Nonoperative management of nonvascular grade IV blunt renal trauma in children: meta-analysis and systematic review. Urology. 2009; 74:579–82.
12. Husmann DA, Gilling PJ, Perry MO, Morris JS, Boone TB. Major renal lacerations with a devitalized fragment following blunt abdominal trauma: a comparison between nonoperative (expectant) versus surgical management. J Urol. 1993;150:1774–7.

13. Malcolm JB, Derweesh IH, Mehrazin R, DiBlasio CJ, Vance DD, Joshi S, et al. Nonoperative management of blunt renal trauma: is routine early follow-up imaging necessary? BMC Urol. 2008;8:11.
14. Gomez RG, Ceballos L, Coburn M, Corriere Jr JN, Dixon CM, Lobel B, et al. Consensus statement on bladder injuries. BJU Int. 2004;94:27–32.
15. Dreitlein DA, Suner S, Basler J. Genitourinary trauma. Emerg Med Clin North Am. 2001;19:569–90.
16. Morey AF, Iverson AJ, Swan A, Harmon WJ, Spore SS, Bhayani S, et al. Bladder rupture after blunt trauma: guidelines for diagnostic imaging. J Trauma. 2001;51:683–6.
17. Paparel P, Badet L, Tayot O, Fessy MH, Bejui J, Martin X. Mechanisms and frequency of urologic complications in 73 cases of unstable pelvic fractures. Prog Urol. 2003;13: 54–9.
18. Hsieh CH, Chen RJ, Fang JF, Lin BC, Hsu YP, Kao JL, et al. Diagnosis and management of bladder injury by trauma surgeons. Am J Surg. 2002;184:143–7.
19. Corriere Jr JN, Sandler CM. Mechanisms of injury, patterns of extravasation and management of extraperitoneal bladder rupture due to blunt trauma. J Urol. 1988;139:43–4.
20. Carlin BI, Resnick MI. Indications and techniques for urologic evaluation of the trauma patient with suspected urologic injury. Semin Urol. 1995;13:9–24.
21. Deck AJ, Shaves S, Talner L, Porter JR. Computerized tomography cystography for the diagnosis of traumatic bladder rupture. J Urol. 2000;164:43–6.
22. Corriere Jr JN, Sandler CM. Management of the ruptured bladder: seven years of experience with 111 cases. J Trauma. 1986;26:830–3.
23. Kulkarni SB, Barbagli G, Kulkarni JS, Romano G, Lazzeri M. Posterior urethral stricture after pelvic fracture urethral distraction defects in developing and developed countries, and choice of surgical technique. J Urol. 2010;183: 1049–54.
24. Bjurlin MA, Fantus RJ, Mellett MM, Goble SM. Genitourinary injuries in pelvic fracture morbidity and mortality using the National Trauma Data Bank. J Trauma. 2009; 67:1033–9.
25. Mundy AR, Andrich DE. Pelvic fracture-related injuries of the bladder neck and prostate: their nature, cause and management. BJU Int. 2010 May, 105(9):1302-8.
26. Koraitim MM. Predictors of surgical approach to repair pelvic fracture urethral distraction defects. J Urol. 2009;182: 1435–9.
27. Andrich DE, Day AC, Mundy AR. Proposed mechanisms of lower urinary tract injury in fractures of the pelvic ring. BJU Int. 2007;100:567–73.
28. Ball CG, Jafri SM, Kirkpatrick AW, Rajani RR, Rozycki GS, Feliciano DV, et al. Traumatic urethral injuries: does the digital rectal examination really help us? Injury. 2009;40: 984–6.
29. Myers JB, McAninch JW. Management of posterior urethral disruption injuries. Nat Clin Pract Urol. 2009;6:154–63.
30. Ingram MD, Watson SG, Skippage PL, Patel U. Urethral injuries after pelvic trauma: evaluation with urethrography. Radiographics. 2008;28:1631–43.
31. Anger JT, Sherman ND, Dielubanza E, Webster GD, Hegarty PK. Erectile function after posterior urethroplasty for pelvic fracture-urethral distraction defect injuries. BJU Int. 2009; 104:1126–9.

Fracture Management

Bernhard Schmidt-Rohlfing, Roman Pfeifer, and Hans-Christoph Pape

Contents

12.1	Introduction	127
12.2	Assessment of the Fracture and the Degree of Soft Tissue Injury	127
12.2.1	Soft Tissue Injury in Closed Fractures	127
12.2.2	Open Fractures	128
12.2.3	Upper Versus Lower Extremity Injuries	129
12.2.4	Fracture Care in Serial Extremity Fractures	129
12.3	Staged Approach to Severely Injured Patients	130
12.3.1	Acute Phase (1–3 h After Admission)	130
12.3.2	Primary Phase: Stabilization of Fractures	130
12.3.3	Secondary Period: Regeneration	130
12.3.4	Assessment of the Patient	130
12.3.5	Borderline Conditions	131
12.3.6	Unstable	131
12.3.7	In Extremis Condition	131
12.3.8	Patient Assessment for Initial Definitive Surgery Versus Temporizing Orthopaedic Surgery	131
12.3.9	Surgical Priorities in the Presence of Additional Head Injuries	131
12.3.10	Surgical Priorities in the Presence of Additional Chest Injuries	132
12.3.11	Surgical Priorities in the Presence of Additional Pelvic Ring Injuries	133
12.3.12	Surgical Priorities Depending on Trauma System	133
References		134

B. Schmidt-Rohlfing, R. Pfeifer and H.-C. Pape (✉)
University of Aachen Medical Center,
Pauwelsstr. 30, 52074 Aachen, Germany
e-mail: papehc@aol.com, hpape@ukaachen.de

12.1 Introduction

There is a general consensus that in isolated fractures, early fixation is essential to avoid complications such as pneumonia, fat embolism, or thromboembolism. Fracture fixation should allow for early mobilization of the patient. However, in the multiply injured patient with fractures, there are life-threatening conditions and priorities that may postpone external or internal fixation.

12.2 Assessment of the Fracture and the Degree of Soft Tissue Injury

12.2.1 Soft Tissue Injury in Closed Fractures

Proper diagnosis and assessment of the true degree of soft tissue damage in closed fractures is crucial. Contusions may raise more therapeutic questions than simple inside-out puncture wounds. Weakening of the skin barrier may be followed by necrosis and infection. Assessment of the severity of a closed fracture helps guide the timing and type of osteosynthesis (Table 12.1). Early detection and evaluation of neural, vascular, and muscular injuries also affects the overall outcome.

Specific attention has to be dedicated to the occurrence of compartment syndromes. These should be anticipated when the capillary perfusion pressure is less than intracompartmental pressure. Pain out of proportion in responsive patients is the hallmark indicator. In sedated patients, measurement of intracompartmental pressure is mandatory. If in doubt, early fasciotomy has to be performed as a surgical emergency.

Table 12.1 Classification of soft tissue injuries in closed fractures [1]

Closed fracture G0: No injury or very minor soft tissue injury. The G0 classification covers simple fractures, i.e., fractures caused by indirect injury mechanisms
Closed fracture G1: Inside-out contusions caused by fracture fragments
Closed fracture G2: Deep, contaminated abrasions or local dermal and muscular contusions. Impending compartment syndrome is usually associated with a G2 lesion. These injuries usually are caused by direct forces that shear off soft tissue and are often associated with moderate-to-severe fracture types
Closed fracture G3: Extensive skin contusions, muscular disruption, decollement, and obvious compartment syndrome combined with any closed fracture are graded as G3. In this subgroup, severe fracture types and comminuted fractures are usually seen

12.2.2 Open Fractures

The standard classification system for open fractures was described by Gustillo [2]. It ranges from bone piercing from inside to outside with 1 cm or less in length (Type I), to open fractures with major vascular injuries that require repair to salvage the limb (classified as Type IIIc)(see the Chap. 18).

Initial care of open fractures consists of thorough irrigation, debridement, and assessment of the soft tissues damage, followed by fracture fixation. Exposed bone requires soft tissue coverage which should be performed as soon as possible.

The extent of vascular and nerve damage and the general condition of the patient are important. In severe soft tissue trauma, planned re-evaluation is often required, especially in highly contaminated wounds.

Amputation versus reconstruction of upper and lower extremity fractures associated with severe open injuries remains a question [3]. Time-consuming reconstructive surgery in severely injured patients may increase morbidity and mortality. In cases of pending amputation, the MESS score (Mangled Extremity Severity Score) can be of some help as it provides an objective evaluation [4].

Open fractures caused by low-energy trauma may be treated like closed injuries if associated with little soft tissue damage. After the initial debridement, the fracture is stabilized with the most suitable implant and method of fixation.

Open fractures caused by high-energy trauma are usually associated with severe soft tissue damage and commonly combined with extensive bone loss or destruction. This injury requires a graded concept of care. Usually, a temporal fixation strategy is used, if soft tissue coverage of the hardware cannot be achieved. Placement of the external fixator should be considered the definitive stabilization until closure of the wound. The personality of each fracture requires individual treatment. In multiply injured patients, the overall injury severity has to be considered as well as the extent of shock and any initial blood loss.

During initial debridement, all soft tissues should be assessed. If necrotic tissue is left in place, further contamination, bacterial growth, and infection are likely to occur. Sufficient surgical exposure of the injury is essential for adequate assessment.

Special situations include the following:

1. Local Soft Tissue Injury vs. Degloving
   A degloving injury has to be ruled out or diagnosed properly. The assessment includes the degree of soft tissue laceration and periosteal stripping. Thereby, assessment of osseous vascularity is helpful to decide whether fragments should be maintained or removed.

2. Treatment of Morel-Lavallée lesions (subcutaneous degloving)
   Morel-Lavallé lesions are defined as large subcutaneous tissue degloving injuries induced by shearing forces. This mechanism causes a large underlying hematoma. In contrast to other soft tissue injuries, Morel-Lavallé lesions should *not* be debrided aggressively. Small incisions allow complete evacuation of the hematoma. The cutaneous skin flap is decompressed and has a better chance to survive.

3. Consultation of the Plastic Surgeon
   Exposed bone and tendons in an area with limited soft tissue coverage often require early treatment with soft tissue flaps. If severe muscle injury or nerve damage is present, muscle or tendon transfer procedures can be performed in a timely fashion to avoid severe disabilities secondary to loss of motion.

In multiply injured patients, there is a higher risk of increasing soft tissue necrosis due to impaired soft tissue perfusion (in posttraumatic edema and increased capillary permeability caused by massive volume resuscitation). Therefore, multiple planned operative revisions have to be scheduled. These "second look" surgeries allow for recurrent assessment of the soft tissues and any additional muscle or skin necrosis. This strategy enables the surgeon to do a timely repeat debridement if required (e.g., with high-pressure irrigation). These operative revisions of soft tissue injures should be scheduled every 48 h as long as there is an impairment of local perfusion. The traumatic wound should be left open and covered with a synthetic saline-soaked dressing or by vacuum therapy. Local vacuum therapy may save the patient some of the planned "second look" surgeries. It has been shown to be successful in treatment of a variety of wounds including extensive degloving injuries [5, 6]. Subatmospheric pressure on the wound site enhances wound healing, reduces the amount of fluid, and increases local blood flow [7, 8]. These effects have been shown to minimize the risk for wound infection [9].

When definitive internal fixation is possible from the soft tissue point of view, the insertion of stable devices is preferred. In case of shaft fractures of the femur or tibia, the use of intramedullary nails is recommended whenever possible.

For intra-articular open fractures, most surgeons prefer a two-step strategy. Some authors recommend limited internal fixation and gross reduction of severely displaced fragments for soft tissue decompression. The minimally invasive fixation comprises the reconstruction of the joint itself and temporary stabilization with K-wires followed by stabilization with lag screws and adjusting/set screws. Definitive fixation is carried out secondarily following consolidation of the soft tissues.

12.2.3 Upper Versus Lower Extremity Injuries

In severe open fractures of the upper extremity, certain principles are different from those of the lower extremities. It is widely accepted that surgical management of lower extremities precedes the treatment of upper limb injuries. Moreover, the maintenance of correct length is less important in the treatment of upper extremity fractures. Severe upper extremity injuries, such as open fractures, compartment syndrome, and concomitant vascular injuries, require immediate surgical management. In general, splinting or definitive fixation is more frequently performed in the upper extremity because soft tissue coverage is usually easier.

12.2.4 Fracture Care in Serial Extremity Fractures

The sequence of fracture care in patients with serial extremity injuries is important. Simultaneous treatment of extremity injuries can be achieved if the logistic conditions allow the surgeon to do so. The recommendations for the timing of fixation are summarized as follows:

In serial injuries of the upper extremity, immobilization of humeral shaft fractures is an adequate option unless the injuries are open or if neurovascular injuries require surgical intervention. In forearm fractures, early fixation is advised due to limited soft tissue coverage.

In periarticular fractures, early fixation should be performed if the patient condition is adequate. If no definitive fixation can be performed and if the patient goes to the OR for other causes, transarticular external fixation (TEF) is preferred over casting. External fixation allows for better stability and assessment of soft tissues. This is of utmost importance due to the risk of compartment syndrome in these injuries.

In serial injuries of the lower extremities, definitive fixation should be achieved whenever possible. In floating knee injuries, retrograde femoral nails and an antegrade tibial nails can be placed using the same incision. In unstable patients, closed reduction and transarticular external fixation is performed for temporary fracture stabilization.

In metadiaphyseal and periarticular fractures, the priorities of care are dictated by the degree of soft tissue damage. The orthopaedic emergencies that require operative care are:

- Compartment Syndrome
- Vascular Injuries
- Irreducible hip dislocation
- Open fractures

Among the higher priorities are femoral head fractures (Pipkin I–III) and fractures of the talus. Any other periarticular fracture is of lower priority, if no further

Table 12.2 Classification system of complex extremity injuries [10]

Fracture-associated injury	Points	
Severe soft tissue damage	2	
+ Hemorrhagic shock	3	
ISS 16–25	1	
ISS > 25	2	
Neurovascular injury	1	
Articular involvement	1	
Type of complex extremity fracture	Points	Fracture care
Low risk	1–2	Definitive internal
Moderate risk	3–4	External
High risk	>4	Consider amputation

complication is evident (compartment syndrome, pulseless extremity, or open fracture).

In the care of upper extremity fractures, similar principles are applied. In bilateral fractures, simultaneous treatment should be considered. Both extremities can be draped at the same time. Some parts of the procedure may require operative treatment of only one extremity at the time because of fluoroscopy, or handling issues. If the vital signs of the patient deteriorate during the operation, the second extremity may just be temporarily stabilized using external fixation.

The classification system of complex extremity fractures is shown in Table 12.2.

12.3 Staged Approach to Severely Injured Patients

Initial fracture care of severely injured patients requires anticipation of potential problems and decision making about the timing of interventions using a systematic approach [11]. Four different phases of the posttraumatic course are separated:

1. Acute phase (1–3 h): resuscitation
2. Primary phase (1–48 h): stabilization
3. Secondary period (2–10 days): regeneration
4. Tertiary period (weeks to months after trauma): reconstruction & rehabilitation

12.3.1 Acute Phase (1–3 h After Admission)

Initially, the focus of treatment is on the control of acute life-threatening conditions. Complete patient assessment is required to identify all life-threatening conditions. This involves airway control, thoracocentesis, rapid control of external bleeding, and fluid and/or blood replacement therapy. Prioritization of the orthopaedic injuries is crucial as well. The orthopaedic fractures that require immediate surgery are listed above. Spinal and pelvic fractures are covered in different chapters.

12.3.2 Primary Phase: Stabilization of Fractures

The primary phase is the usual time where major extremity injuries are managed. These include acute stabilization of major extremity fractures associated with arterial injuries and compartment syndrome. Fractures can be temporally stabilized by external fixation and the compartments released where appropriate.

12.3.3 Secondary Period: Regeneration

During the secondary phase, the general condition of the patient is stabilized and monitored. In most cases, this implies days 2–4 after trauma. Surgical interventions should be limited to those that are absolutely necessary ("second look," debridement), and lengthy procedures should be avoided. Physiological and intensive care scoring systems help monitor the clinical progress.

12.3.4 Assessment of the Patient

Once the initial assessment is completed, patients can be categorized into one of four categories. Overall injury severity, the presence of specific injuries, and the hemodynamic status are among the most critical. Then, volume requirements, inflammation, and coagulation can be addressed. These include stable hemodynamics, stable oxygen saturation, lactate level <2 mmol/l, no coagulopathy, normal body temperature, urinary output >1 ml/kg/h, and no requirement for inotropic support.

12.3.5 Borderline Conditions

Borderline conditions are defined as indicated in Table 12.3.

In this group of patients, a cautious operative strategy should be used. Additional invasive monitoring should be instituted preoperatively. A low threshold should be used for conversion to a "damage control" approach to the patient management, as detailed below, at the first sign of deterioration.

12.3.6 Unstable

Patients who are hemodynamically unstable despite initial intervention are at risk of rapid deterioration, subsequent multiple organ failure, and death. In these patients, a "damage control" approach is required. This entails rapid life-saving surgery only when absolutely necessary and timely transfer to the intensive care unit for further stabilization and monitoring. Temporary stabilization of fractures using external fixation, hemorrhage control, and exteriorization of gastrointestinal injuries is advocated. Complex reconstructive extremity procedures should be delayed until stable conditions are achieved and the acute immunoinflammatory response to injury has subsided.

Table 12.3 Clinical parameters used to identify patients in uncertain condition, named "borderline." Usually, at least three of these have to be present to allow for classification as borderline [12]

Factors to identify the borderline patient
• Injury Severity Score >40
• Multiple injuries (ISS >20) in association with thoracic trauma (AIS >2)
• Multiple injuries in association with severe abdominal or pelvic injury and hemorrhagic shock at presentation (systolic BP <90 mmHg)
• Patients with bilateral femoral fractures
• Radiographic evidence of pulmonary contusion
• Hypothermia below 35 °C

12.3.7 In Extremis Condition

These patients have ongoing uncontrolled blood loss. They remain severely unstable despite ongoing resuscitative efforts and are usually suffering from the "deadly triad" (hypothermia, acidosis, and coagulopathy). The patients should then be transferred directly to the intensive care unit for invasive monitoring and advanced hematologic, pulmonary, and cardiovascular support. Orthopaedic injuries can be stabilized rapidly in the emergency department or intensive care unit using external fixation.

12.3.8 Patient Assessment for Initial Definitive Surgery Versus Temporizing Orthopaedic Surgery

The initial patient assessment usually is performed using scoring systems such as the ISS or NISS. For life-threatening conditions, which are frequently due to penetrating trauma, the "triad of death" (blood loss, coagulopathy, and loss of temperature) approach has been used. In patients with blunt orthopaedic injuries, it is important to account for soft tissue injuries as well and parameters of oxygenation to assess the clinical status of the patient [11].

Table 12.4 documents the parameters and scoring systems that can be used to categorize a patient's condition. Three out of the four criteria should be present to qualify a patient for a specific category [12]. It is important to note that the combination of these parameters is a suggestion only and has a low level of evidence. Nevertheless, most of the components are scores that have been routinely used in the past and are widely accepted. For screening purposes, the following threshold levels have been used: pulmonary dysfunction (PaO$_2$/FiO$_2$ <250), platelet count (<95.000), hypotension unresponsive to therapy >10 blood units per 6 h, and vasopressor requirement. Inflammatory parameters have also been described to have predictive power for the development of complications, but they are currently not available for routine use in most trauma centers [13].

12.3.9 Surgical Priorities in the Presence of Additional Head Injuries

According to the pathophysiology of head injury, the brain loses the autoregulation of blood flow in zones of

Table 12.4 Classification system for clinical patient assessment. Three out of the four categories must be met to classify for a certain category. It is to be noted that patients who respond to resuscitation qualify for early definitive fracture care, as long as prolonged surgeries are avoided [12]

	Parameter	Stable (GRADE I)	Borderline (Grade II)	Unstable (Grade III)	In extremis (Grade IV)
Shock	Blood pressure (mmHg)	100 or more	80–100	60–90	<50–60
	Blood units (2 h)	0–2	2–8	5–15	>15
	Lactate levels	Normal range	Around 2.5	>2.5	Severe acidosis
	Base deficit mmol/l	Normal range	No data	No data	>6–8
	ATLS classification	I	II–III	III–IV	IV
Coagulation	Platelet count (µg/ml)	>110,000	90,000–110,000	<70,000–90,000	<70,000
	Factor II and V (%)	90–100	70–80	50–70	<50
	Fibrinogen (g/dl)	>1	Around 1	<1	DIC
	D-Dimer	Normal range	Abnormal	Abnormal	DIC
Temperature		<33°C	33–35°C	30–32°C	30°C or less
Soft tissue injuries	Lung function; PaO_2/FiO_2	350–400	300–350	200–300	<200
	Chest trauma scores; AIS	AIS I or II (e.g., abrasion)	AIS 2 or more (e.g., 2–3 rib fractures)	AIS 3 or more (e.g., serial rib fx. >3)	AIS 3 or more (e.g., unstable chest)
	Chest trauma score; TTS	0	I–II	II–III	IV
	Abdominal trauma (Moore)	< or = II	< or = III	III	III or >III
	Pelvic trauma (AO class.)	A type (AO)	B or C	C	C (crush, rollover abd.)
	External (AIS)	AIS I–II (e.g., abrasion)	AIS II–III (e.g., mult. >20 cm tears)	AIS III–IV (e.g., <30% burn)	(Crush injury, >30% burn)

contusion. Also, an increase in the utilization of glucose occurs, adding to the susceptibility to ischemic injury [14]. Head trauma patients are at greatest risk for decreased cerebral blood flow during the first 12–24 h following injury [15]. Intraoperative hypotension is an important risk factor for secondary brain injury ("second hit" to the brain) [16]. The primary goal in the management of traumatic brain injury is the avoidance of secondary insults (hypoperfusion) [17].

The management needs to be performed in close cooperation with the neurosurgical team, and sudden changes in the strategy can occur according to the degree of cerebral swelling, imminent herniation, or increase in bleeding.

The orthopaedic surgeon and the neurosurgeon need to reveal how much operative time, blood loss, and temperature loss can be accepted for each individual case. General rules are currently not available. If in doubt, monitoring of the intracranial pressure (ICP) is safer and should be performed. During fracture fixation, secondary insults should be avoided by maintaining adequate cerebral perfusion.

12.3.10 Surgical Priorities in the Presence of Additional Chest Injuries

The pathophysiology in chest trauma is well described. A lung contusion is a separate entity from rib fractures and has a higher association with Acute Respiratory Distress Syndrome (ARDS) than rib fractures [18]. In isolated rib fractures, a decrease in biomechanical (lack of rib cage motion) and pain-related hypoxemia is reversed by artificial ventilation. With lung contusion despite ventilation, intrapulmonary edema can develop.

This is mediated by inflammatory cells and causes a local immunologic reaction [19]. The progressive nature of a pulmonary contusion can cause problems and is frequently underestimated. Early after injury, the blood gas parameters can still be within normal limits, and the chest X-ray may also present as a false negative. The immunologic mechanisms initiated by pulmonary contusions are comparable to those seen after severe injury [20, 21]. Thus, the host response to pulmonary contusion is similar to non-pulmonary injury, resulting in an increased risk of ARDS.

Patient evaluation focuses on the following clinical criteria: presence of a lung contusion on the initial chest X-ray or CT scan, worsening oxygenation (requirement of increased $FiO_2 > 40\%$ or $PaO_2/FiO_2 < 250$), and increased airway pressures (e.g., >25–30 cm H_2O). The pulmonary function can change within hours after the injury, and repeated blood gases should be obtained.

12.3.11 Surgical Priorities in the Presence of Additional Pelvic Ring Injuries

The pathophysiology of systemic effects in severe pelvic injuries is dictated by the degree of local blood loss from the pelvic floor, the presacral venous plexus, and any arterial damage. Unlike other injuries, autotamponade does not occur and retroperitoneal bleeding may mimic intra-abdominal injury. Soft tissue disruption can have more severe side effects than in the extremities since a higher degree of kinetic energy is required to cause substantial displacement. In open injuries with intestinal damage, a substantial increase in the risk of infection and late sepsis occurs [21, 22].

Timing of pelvic fixation is based on the hemodynamic status and the presence of associated abdominal injuries. The decision to attempt definitive fixation within 24–48 h appears to be dependent upon the pelvic ring fracture pattern [23] and can be attempted in stable and borderline patients. In unstable patients, the use of sheets wrapped about the pelvis or a pelvic binder allows for rapid circumferential splinting of the pelvic ring most effectively at the level of the greater trochanter [24].

The paucity of studies in the literature seems to support early surgical management of such injuries. Favorable patterns may be treated by percutaneous fixation when several factors coincide: Closed reduction can be achieved, the injury pattern is amenable to screw fixation alone, and the surgeon and operating team are available and experienced [25]. In cases of exsanguinations from a pelvic ring injury, direct packing of the true pelvic space has been described [26]. This technique is dependent upon achieving provisional stability of the pelvic ring with a binder, external fixation or internal fixation.

Current recommendations are to identify the source of pelvic hemorrhage and to stop the bleeding, followed by stabilization of the pelvic ring. The use of a binder is often successful for achieving a physiologic state that allows surgery unless a single artery is damaged. This may be treated by coiling.

12.3.12 Surgical Priorities Depending on Trauma System

Some authors have argued that the trauma system dictates patient care. The early total care of all fractures was advocated by certain clinicians in the 1980s. However, a recent survey on the management of major fractures in multiply injured patients demonstrates that the timing of fracture fixation is similar in two groups

Table 12.5 Mean duration until definitive treatment of major fractures in patients with multiple injuries, specified according to body regions [27]

Duration until definitive treatment	USA $n=77$	GER $n=93$	P-value
All fractures	5.5 days ± 4.2	6.6 days ± 8.7	n.s
Humerus fractures	5 days ± 3.7	6.6 days ± 6.1	n.s
Radius fractures	6 days ± 4.7	6.1 days ± 8.7	n.s
Femur fractures	7.9 days ± 8.3	5.5 days ± 7.9	n.s
Tibia fractures	6.2 days ± 5.6	6.2 days ± 9.1	n.s
Pelvis fractures	5 days ± 2.8	7.1 days ± 9.6	n.s

of trauma centers in both the United States and Germany. Thereby, a staged approach toward fracture management appears to be the rule in both systems [27] (Table 12.5).

References

1. Oestern HJ, Tscherne H. Pathophysiology and classification of soft tissue injuries associated with fractures. In: In fractures with soft tissue injuries. 1st ed. Berlin: Spinger; 1984.
2. Gustilo RB, Mendoza RM, Williams DN. Problems in the management of type III (severe) open fractures: a new classification of Type III open fractures. J Trauma. 1984;24(742):746.
3. Pape HC, Probst C, Lohse R, et al. Predictors of late clinical outcome following orthopedic injuries after multiple trauma. J Trauma. 2010;69(5):1243–51.
4. Johansen K, Daines M, Howey T, Helfet D, Hansen Jr ST. Objective criteria accurately predict amputation following lower extremity trauma. J Trauma. 1990;30(5):568–72.
5. Meara JG, Guo L, Smith JD, Pribaz JJ, Breuing KH, Orgill DP. Vacuum-assisted closure in the treatment of degloving injuries. Ann Plast Surg. 1999;42(6):589–94.
6. DeFranzo AJ, Marks MW, Argenta LC, Genecov DG. Vacuum-assisted closure for the treatment of degloving injuries. Plast Reconstr Surg. 1999;104(7):2145–8.
7. Mullner T, Mrkonjic L, Kwasny O, Vecsei V. The use of negative pressure to promote the healing of tissue defects: a clinical trial using the vacuum sealing technique. Br J Plast Surg. 1997;50(3):194–9.
8. Banwell P, Withey S, Holten I. The use of negative pressure to promote healing. Br J Plast Surg. 1998;51(1):79.
9. Fleischmann W, Lang E, Russ M. Treatment of infection by vacuum sealing. Unfallchirurg. 1997;100(4):301–4.
10. Kobbe P, Lichte P, Pape HC. Complex extremity fractures following high energy injuries: the limited value of existing classifications and a proposal for a treatment-guide. Injury. 2009;40 Suppl 4:S69–74.
11. Pape HC, Tornetta III P, Tarkin I, Tzioupis C, Sabeson V, Olson SA. Timing of fracture fixation in multitrauma patients: the role of early total care and damage control surgery. J Am Acad Orthop Surg. 2009;17(9):541–9.
12. Pape HC, Giannoudis PV, Krettek C, Trentz O. Timing of fixation of major fractures in blunt polytrauma: role of conventional indicators in clinical decision making. J Orthop Trauma. 2005;19(8):551–62.
13. Pape HC, Remmers D, Grotz M, et al. Reticuloendothelial system activity and organ failure in patients with multiple injuries. Arch Surg. 1999;134(4):421–7.
14. Reinert M, Hoelper B, Doppenberg E, Zauner A, Bullock R. Substrate delivery and ionic balance disturbance after severe human head injury. Acta Neurochir Suppl. 2000;76:439–44.
15. Miller JD. Head injury and brain ischaemia – implications for therapy. Br J Anaesth. 1985;57(1):120–30.
16. Chesnut RM, Marshall LF, Klauber MR, et al. The role of secondary brain injury in determining outcome from severe head injury. J Trauma. 1993;34(2):216–22.
17. Siegel JH, Gens DR, Mamantov T, Geisler FH, Goodarzi S, MacKenzie EJ. Effect of associated injuries and blood volume replacement on death, rehabilitation needs, and disability in blunt traumatic brain injury. Crit Care Med. 1991;19(10):1252–65.
18. Stellin G. Survival in trauma victims with pulmonary contusion. Am Surg. 1991;57(12):780–4.
19. Regel G, Dwenger A, Seidel J, Nerlich ML, Sturm JA, Tscherne H. Significance of neutrophilic granulocytes in the development of post-traumatic lung failure. Unfallchirurg. 1987;90(3):99–106.
20. Tate RM, Repine JE. Neutrophils and the adult respiratory distress syndrome. Am Rev Respir Dis. 1983;128(3): 552–9.
21. Weiland JE, Davis WB, Holter JF, Mohammed JR, Dorinsky PM, Gadek JE. Lung neutrophils in the adult respiratory distress syndrome. Clinical and pathophysiologic significance. Am Rev Respir Dis. 1986;133(2):218–25.
22. Keel M, Trentz O. Pathophysiology of polytrauma. Injury. 2005;36:691–709.
23. Olson SA, Burgess A. Classification and initial management of patients with unstable pelvic ring injuries. Instr Course Lect. 2005;54:383–93.
24. Bottlang M, Simpson T, Sigg J, Krieg JC, Madey SM, Long WB. Noninvasive reduction of open-book pelvic fractures by circumferential compression. J Orthop Trauma. 2002;16(6):367–73.
25. Routt Jr ML, Falicov A, Woodhouse E, Schildhauer TA. Circumferential pelvic antishock sheeting: a temporary resuscitation aid. J Orthop Trauma. 2006;20(1 Suppl):S3–6.
26. Cothren CC, Osborn PM, Moore EE, Morgan SJ, Johnson JL, Smith WR. Preperitonal pelvic packing for hemodynamically unstable pelvic fractures: a paradigm shift. J Trauma. 2007;62(4):834–9.
27. Schreiber V, Tarkin HI, Hildebrand F, et al. The timing of definitive fixation for major fractures in polytrauma – a matched pair comparison between a US and European level I centers. Injury. 2010 Aug 10. [Epub ahead of print] doi:10.1016/j.injury.2010.07.248.

Mangled Extremity: Management in Isolated Extremity Injuries and in Polytrauma

Mark L. Prasarn, Peter Kloen, and David L. Helfet

Contents

13.1	Introduction	135
13.2	Mechanism of Injury	136
13.3	Common Injury Patterns	136
13.4	Scoring Systems	136
13.5	Management	138
13.6	Complications	145
13.7	Predictive Ability of Scoring Systems to Predict Final Outcome	145
13.8	Outcomes Following Limb Salvage Versus Amputation	146
13.9	Cost of Care	147
13.10	The Mangled Upper Extremity	147
13.11	The Mangled Extremity and Polytrauma	147
13.12	Conclusions	148
References		148

M.L. Prasarn (✉)
Department of Orthopaedics and Rehabilitation,
University of Rochester/Strong Memorial Hospital,
601 Elmwood Avenue, Box 665, Rochester, NY 14642, USA
e-mail: markprasarn@yahoo.com,
mark_prasarn@urmc.rochester.edu

P. Kloen
Academic Medical Center, Meibergdreef 9, Amsterdam,
The Netherlands
e-mail: p.kloen@amc.uva.nl

D.L. Helfet
Orthopedic Trauma Service, Hospital for Special Surgery,
535 E. 70th Street, New York, NY 10021, USA
e-mail: helfetd@hss.edu

13.1 Introduction

Clinical decision making for trauma patients with extremity injuries is typically straightforward, resulting in maintenance of viability and function of the involved limb. Damage control orthopaedics (DCO) has produced similar outcomes in the severely injured, unstable trauma victim with a relatively simple extremity injury. Numerous reports have described the beneficial effects of such temporizing measures that then allow the patient to be stabilized [1–5]. The decision process becomes much more clouded when dealing with trauma victims with severe extremity injuries, i.e., mangled extremities. There has been much debate as to whether limb salvage or amputation results in the best clinical outcomes in such a patient.

The emergent management of severe extremity trauma poses a difficult clinical decision for the entire treating surgical team. Resuscitation and management of all life-threatening injuries always must take precedence over any extremity injury. In a small subset of patients with complete traumatic disruption and clearly irreparable injuries, an immediate completion amputation should be performed. Likewise, in the setting of prolonged limb ischemia, severe soft-tissue loss that cannot be reconstructed, or concurrent life-threatening injuries elsewhere in an unstable polytrauma patient, a primary amputation is likely indicated. Also, patients with severe ipsilateral foot and ankle crush injuries may be better served with immediate amputation.

There exists a significant population of trauma patients in whom such clear indications for amputation are absent. It has been questioned whether or not attempted preservation of the limb in such patients is appropriate, or whether the patient would be better served with primary amputation. In many circumstances,

13.5 Management

Initial management of the patient with a limb-threatening injury begins with ATLS protocol emphasizing a primary survey with immediate assessment of ABC's (Table 13.2). Following this, the field dressing should be removed and any significant bleeding immediately controlled. This should be done with direct pressure, tourniquet, a compressive dressing, or proximal clamping (in that order of preference). Once the resuscitative effort is underway, further assessment of other injuries should be undertaken as well as a thorough neurovascular examination. If there is disruption to the arterial flow to the extremity, and salvage is being considered, an intraluminal shunt may be used. Wound dressing, gross alignment, and splinting should be performed. Following this, any radiographic studies may be obtained (including vascular studies if necessary), and intravenous antibiotic and tetanus prophylaxis administered. We always calculate a MESS for each patient at the onset of treatment.

If an early amputation is deemed necessary, it is often advantageous to take medical record photographs to document the severity of the injury. We also recommend keeping a photographic record throughout the course of treatment if reconstruction is performed, to document both progress and decline. Our indications for early amputation include: unreconstructable osseous or soft-tissue injuries, irreparable vascular injuries, and severe loss of the plantar soft tissue. Previous authors have recommended amputation if plantar sensation is absent. Recent evidence has suggested that initially absent plantar sensation does not predict a poor functional outcome, and that it may return in more than half of patients followed out to 24 months [31]. We therefore do not use absent plantar sensation as criteria for a primary amputation alone.

The amputation should be performed at the most distal level possible, but should not include clearly nonviable tissues. Examining color, consistency, contractility, and bleeding determine tissue viability. It has been shown that transtibial amputations have significantly better functional outcomes and lower energy expenditure than more proximal levels of amputation [11, 32]. A thorough irrigation and debridement should be performed without any attempt to close the wound at this time. A sterile dressing or wound vacuum assisted closure VAC can be

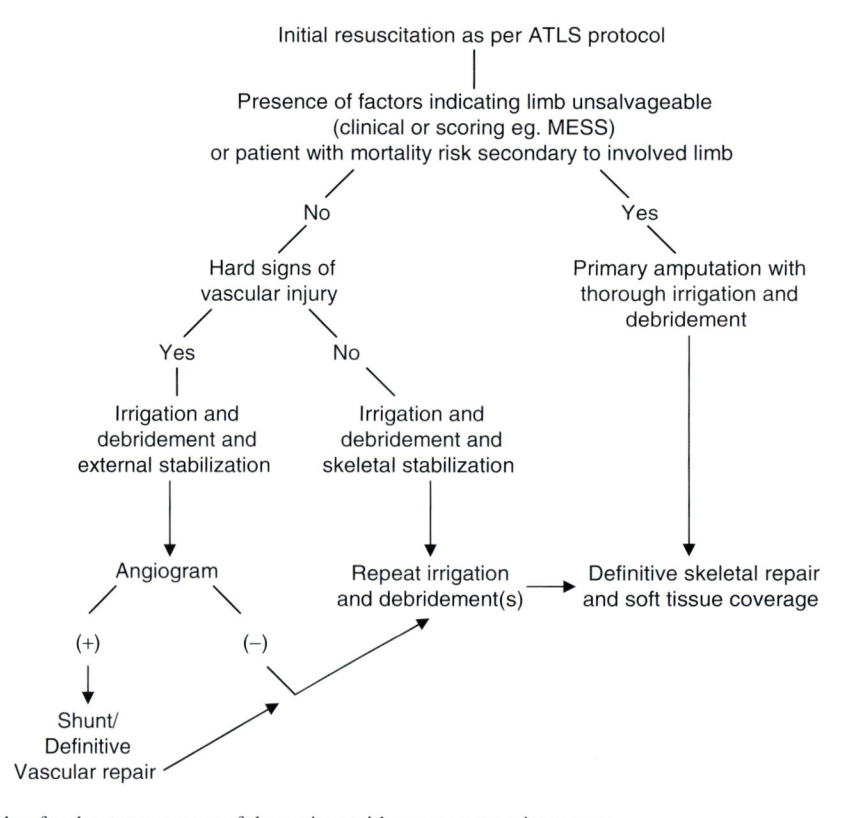

Table 13.2 Algorithm for the management of the patient with severe extremity trauma

applied, and a splint placed if the amputation is below the level of the knee or elbow (Fig. 13.1). Repeat surgical debridements as deemed necessary should be performed on return to the operating room. In most instances, several irrigation and debridements are undertaken prior to closure of the stump site.

If the need for amputation is not clear upon initial examination, then limb salvage should be attempted. Once again a thorough irrigation and debridement with removal of any contaminants and nonviable tissue performed emergently. External fixation to gain stability of fractures and to aid in wound care is typically performed at this time. If necessary, a definitive vascular repair should be performed following skeletal stabilization. Ex-fix pins should be placed strategically away from the zone of injury and based on future incisions for definitive open reduction and internal fixation (ORIF). Compromise of formal ORIF after DCO using external fixation is generally not an issue [5]. Fasciotomies should be performed as necessary. Antibiotic bead pouches and negative pressure wound therapy can be used to help decrease infection and assist with wound care [33–38]. The extremity is closely monitored over the next 24–72 h for soft-tissue viability and sensorimotor function. Wounds should be regularly inspected, and repeat irrigation and debridements performed based on wound appearance (tissue viability, presence of contaminants, infection, etc.). VAC dressings are changed every 48–72 h.

If at any point the limb is deemed unsalvageable, or the patient's life is in jeopardy secondary to the extremity injury, amputation should be performed. If the extremity remains viable for reconstruction and the patient's condition permits, then definitive skeletal stabilization and early soft-tissue coverage should be performed [39, 40]. The use of BMP-2 has been approved in complex open tibia fractures. It was shown to accelerate fracture healing, reduce infection rate, and decrease the need for secondary procedures to obtain union in a randomized, prospective study

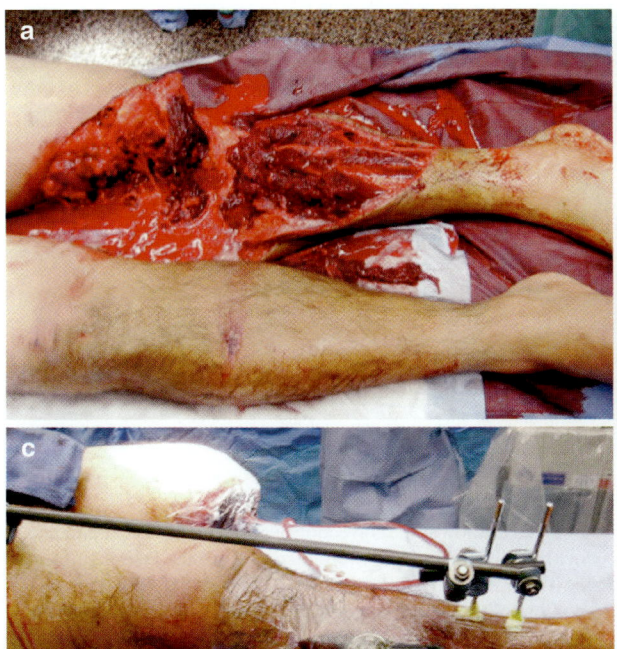

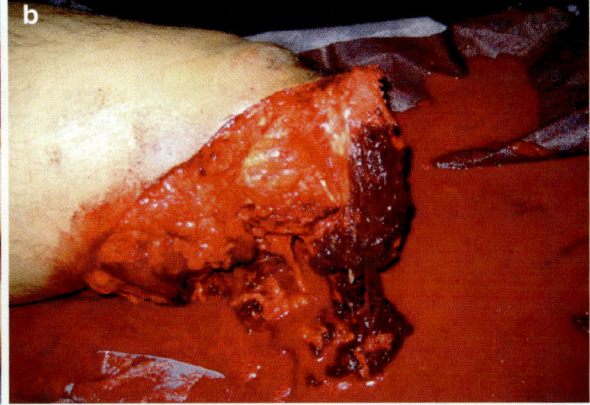

Fig. 13.1 A 21-year-old male presented to the emergency department following a motorcycle collision with bilateral lower extremity injuries. (**a**) Left-sided pulse-less (Grade IIIC) "mangled" knee/lower extremity injuries and a right-sided bicondylar closed tibial plateau fracture with compartment syndrome (*top image*). (**b**) Left-sided completion of the above knee amputation retaining as much viable soft tissue as possible (*middle image*). (**c**) Application of negative pressure wound therapy dressing to left-sided amputation site, as well as external fixation of right bicondylar tibial plateau fracture and leg fasciotomies for compartment syndrome (*bottom image*)

involving 450 open tibia fractures [41]. Further research involving a larger cohort of patients with longer follow-up is necessary to confirm these results, and analyze the long-term complications and outcomes. Until more data is available, the utility and safety of BMP in the setting of open fractures is still uncertain. Various modalities are available for surgical fixation including: uniplanar external fixators, hybrid external fixators, thin-wire ring external fixators, plate and screw constructs, and intramedullary nails. There are pros and cons of each modality. It is beyond the scope of this chapter to recommend the type of fixation to use in the setting of complex extremity trauma. Many patients may require additional surgery in order to achieve osseous union and this should be thoroughly discussed with the patient along with potential complications [8, 19, 42] (Figs. 13.2 and 13.3).

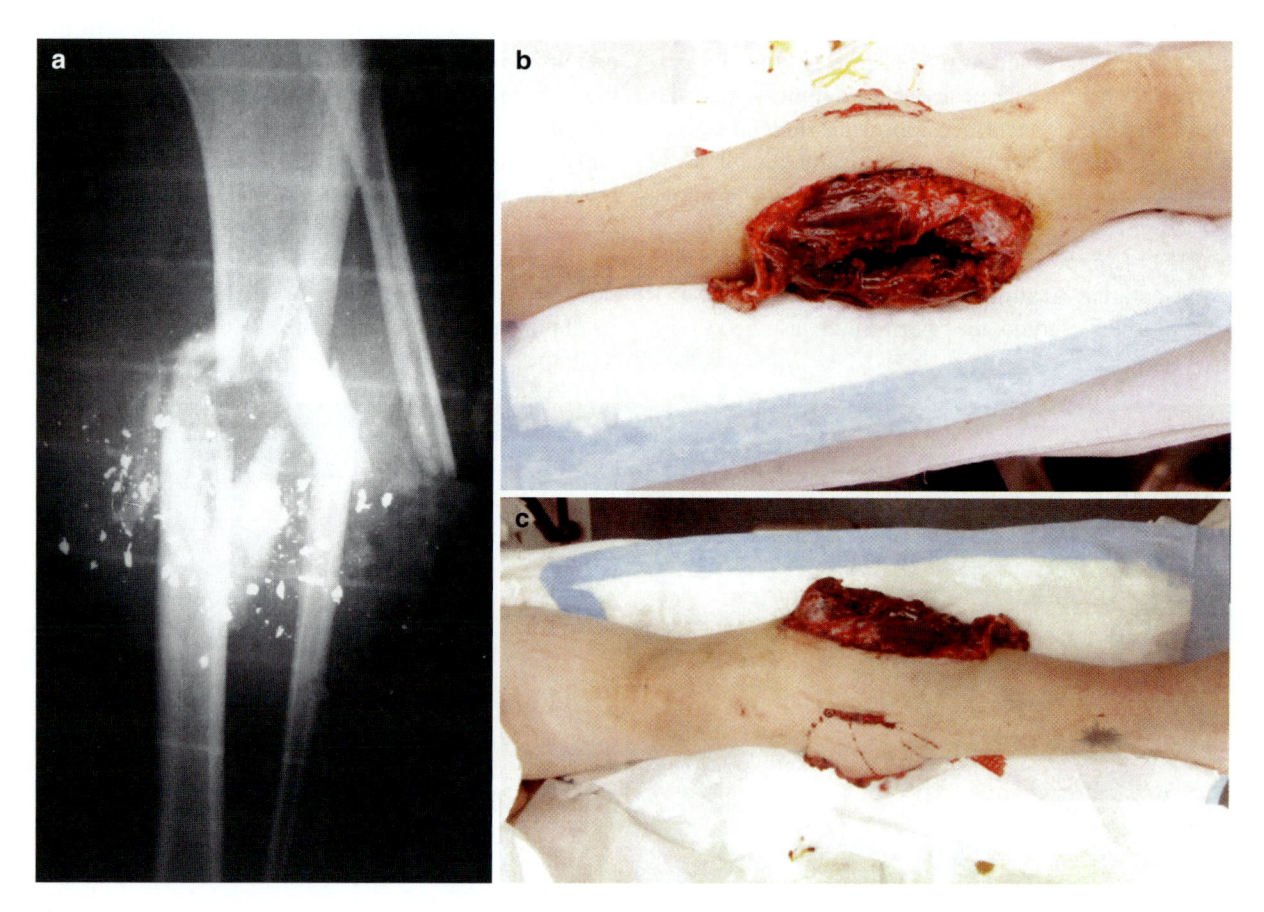

Fig. 13.2 A 36-year-old male was accidentally shot in the leg with a shotgun during a hunting trip. (**a–c**) He suffered an open, left-sided grade IIIC tibial shaft fracture with marked comminution. He also presented with complete functional deficit to his anterior compartment. He was taken to a local trauma center for irrigation and debridement (*I and D*), stabilization with and external fixation and a saphenous vein revascularization of the popliteal artery. Subsequent multiple I and D procedures were performed (including compromised bone). A negative pressure wound therapy dressing was placed over the wound sites. An Inferior Vena Cava (*IVC*) filter was also inserted. (**d**) On day 3, a reamed, locked tibial intramedullary nail was inserted. (**e**) At 2 weeks following the injury, the patient was transferred to our institution for definitive management of his injuries. Repeat I and D was performed, the proximal interlocking screw was then removed to allow some correction of alignment and a percutaneous locking plate and screws were placed along the lateral surface of the tibia and a VAC dressing was applied. (**f**) Radiographs 7 months following revision surgery illustrate progressive healing. (**g**) Radiographs at 19 months illustrate some callus formation and a broken proximal interlocking screw. (**h, i**) Exchange IM nailing was planned and performed with placement of Demineralized Bone Matrix (*DBM*) and a Bone Morphogenic Protein-2 (BMP-2) supplement. (**j**) At the latest follow-up visit at 29 months following revision surgery, he presented with good radiographic and clinical findings including increased callus formation and consolidation of the fracture, well-healed soft tissues, resolution of most pain symptoms, a return to activities of daily living, and some recreational activities including weight training and skiing. A slight dorsiflexion lag was still present

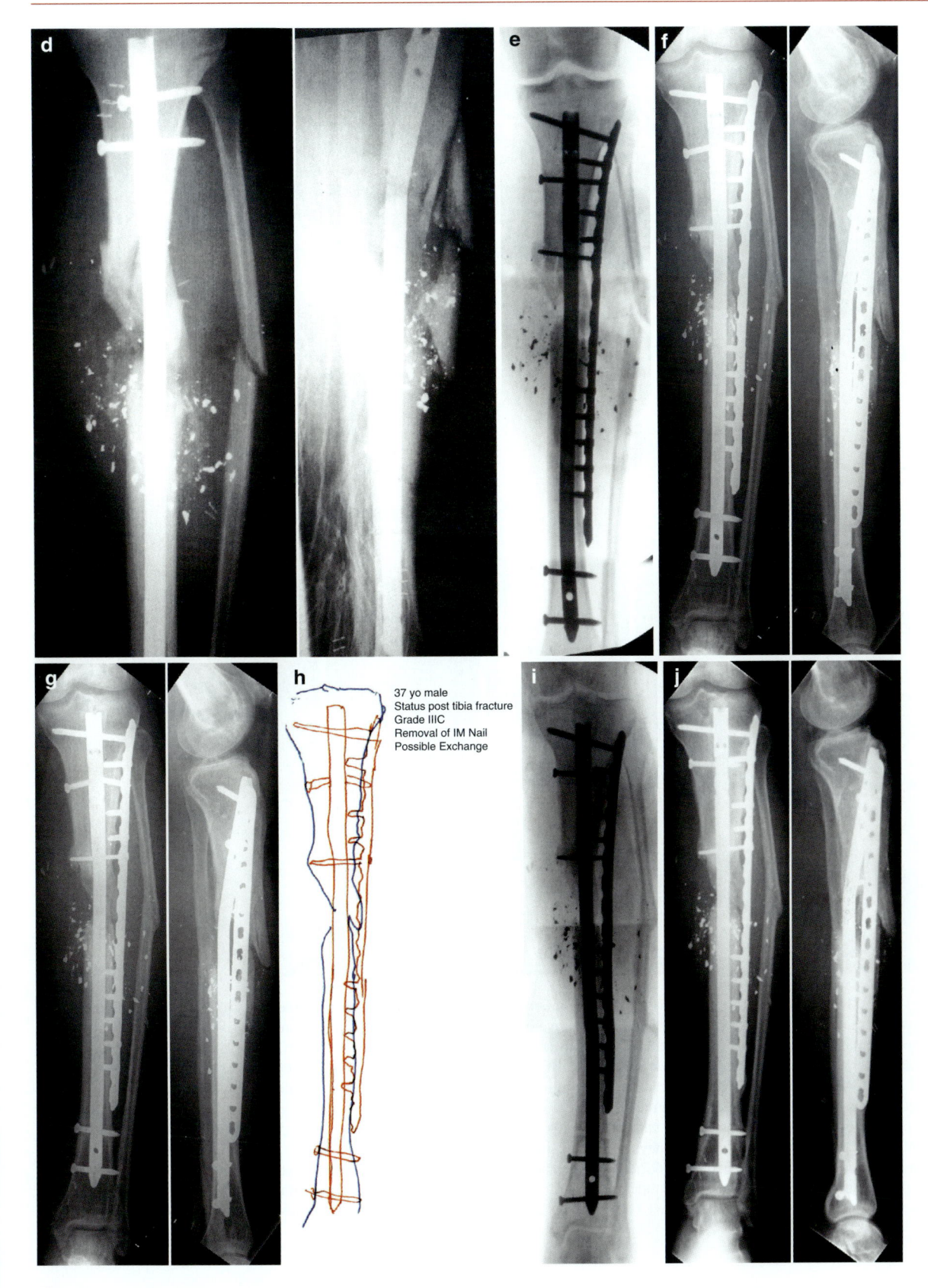

13 Mangled Extremity: Management in Isolated Extremity Injuries and in Polytrauma   141

37 yo male
Status post tibia fracture
Grade IIIC
Removal of IM Nail
Possible Exchange

Fig. 13.2 (continued)

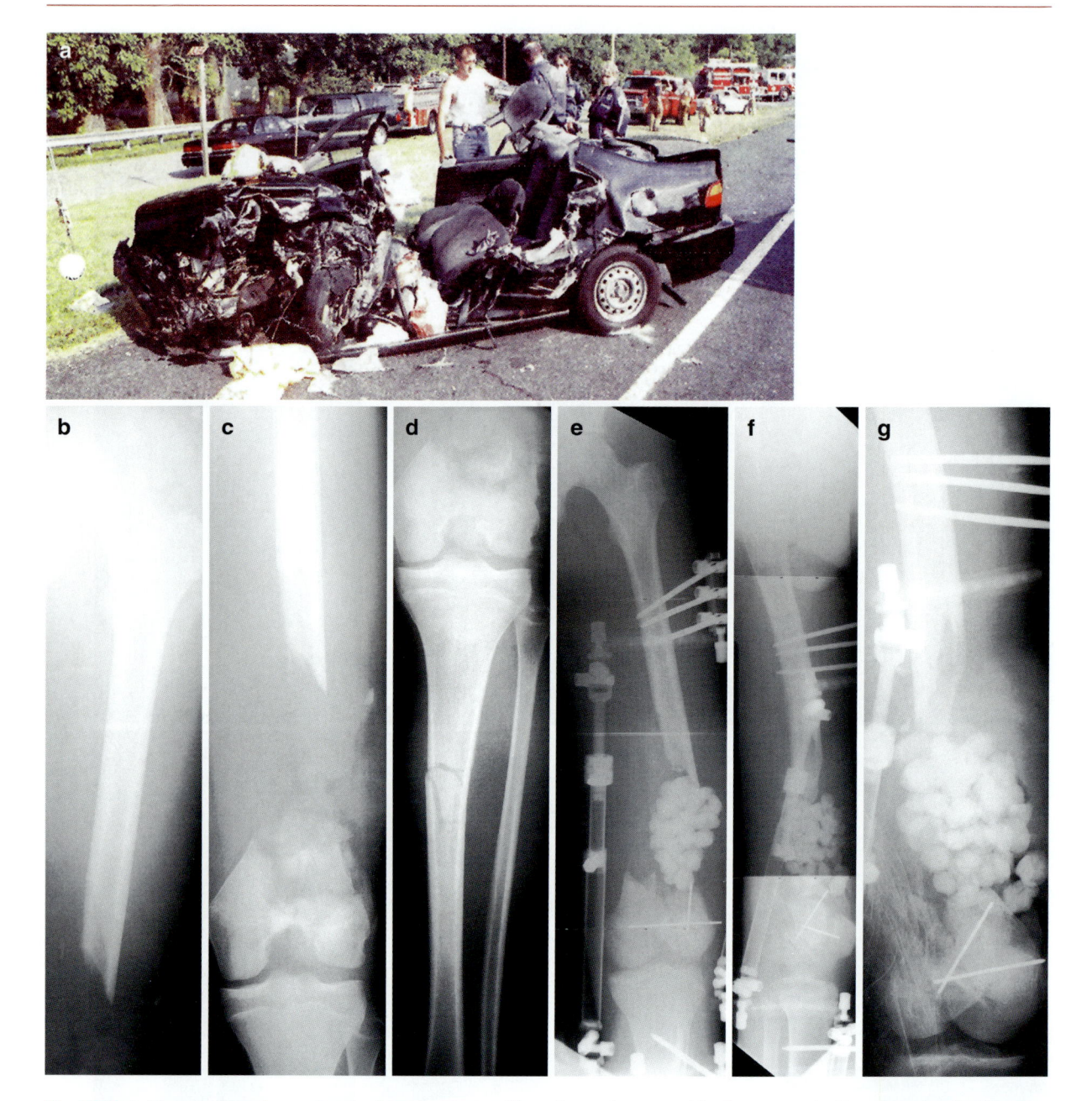

Fig. 13.3 A 17-year-old male was involved in a head-on collision with a tractor trailer. After being trapped inside the vehicle for approximately 1 h, he was extricated and flown to a local trauma center. He was diagnosed with an open, Grade IIIC left-sided AO/OTA Type C3.3 distal femur fracture with segmental defect and an ipsilateral tibial shaft fracture. External fixation was placed for initial stabilization and antibiotic beads were subsequently placed in the defect at 3 days following injury. Open Reduction and Internal Fixation (*ORIF*) was performed with placement of an intramedullary (*IM*) locked nail for treatment of the tibial shaft fracture and then ORIF of the distal femur fracture with placement of a Less Invasive Stabilization System (*LISS*) locking plate and screws. One week later, the antibiotic beads were removed and the defect was prepared for bone graft placement. A second incision was made along the lateral border of the ipsilateral fibula and a free vascularized fibula bone graft was harvested for transplant to the femoral defect. It was docked in a double barrel fashion and stabilized using screw fixation. Following surgery, he returned for regular follow-up visits. Three months after surgery, all of the fractures were healing with incorporation of bone graft. The LISS plate was removed 4.5 years following the initial surgery. The clinical

and radiographic follow-up illustrated excellent results with bony union, full range of motion, and complete resolution of pain and return to pre-injury activities. (**a**) Photograph of the vehicle and the scene following the accident. (**b–d**) Anteroposterior (*AP*) X-rays illustrating an AO/OTA Type C3.3 distal femur fracture with segmental bone defect and an ipsilateral tibial shaft fracture. (**e–g**) AP and lateral radiographs following placement of external fixation and antibiotic beads at the site of the segmental bone defect. (**h**) Counterclockwise from top-left; preoperative plan, fluoroscopic images showing placement of intramedullary nail for the tibial shaft fracture and locking screws and open reduction and internal fixation (*ORIF*) of the distal femur fracture with placement of a LISS locking plate and screws. (**i–k**) Immediate postoperative radiographs demonstrating adequate fixation and alignment. (**l**) AP radiographs illustrating preparation of distal femoral bone defect for placement of vascular bone graft. (**m**) AP X-radiograph following free vascularized fibular bone and placement of screw fixation. (**n–q**) AP and lateral X-rays 3.5 years following ORIF showing a healed distal femur fracture with incorporation of the fibular bone graft and a healed tibial shaft fracture. (**r**, **s**) AP and lateral X-rays 8 months following removal of LISS plate and screws and 4.5 years following fracture surgery

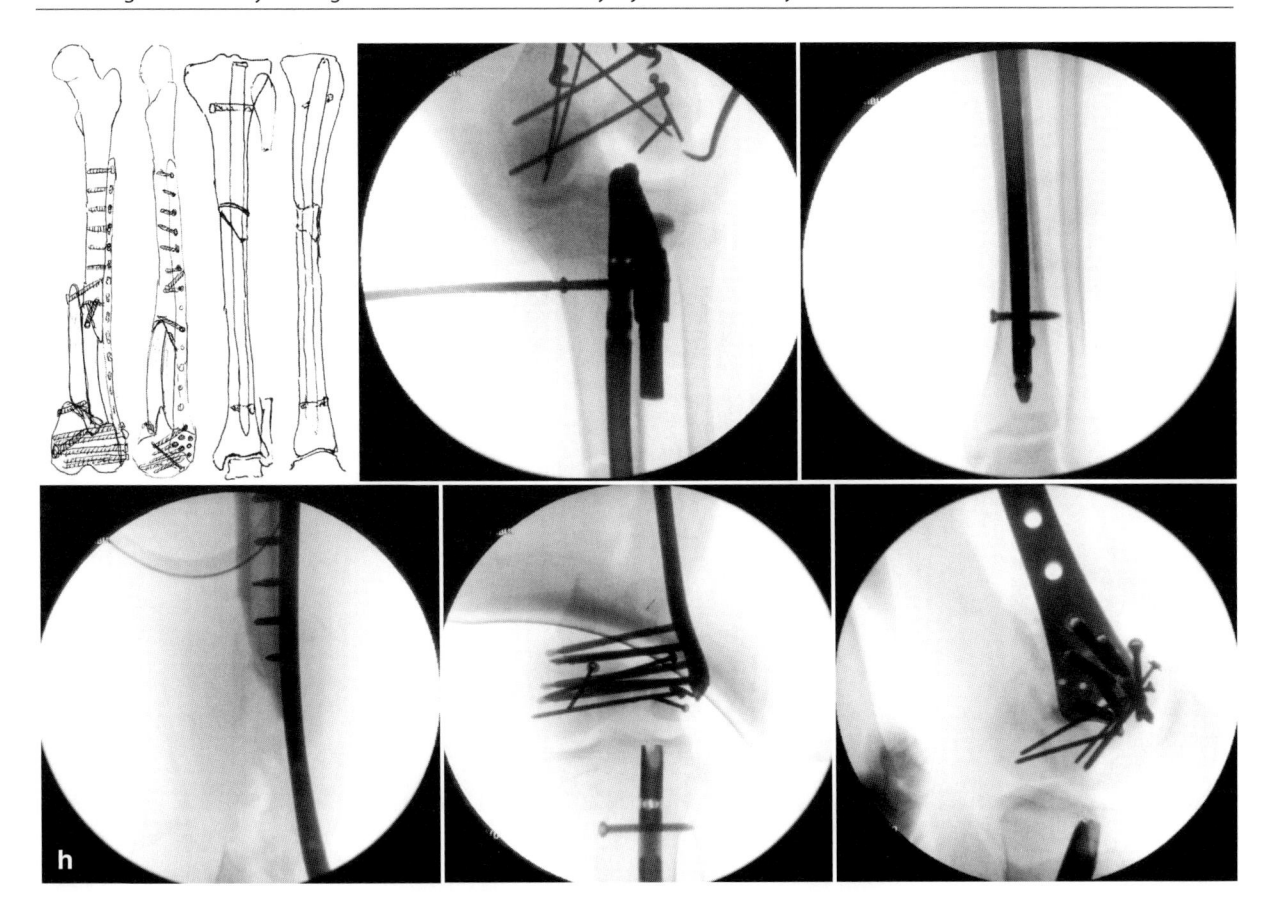

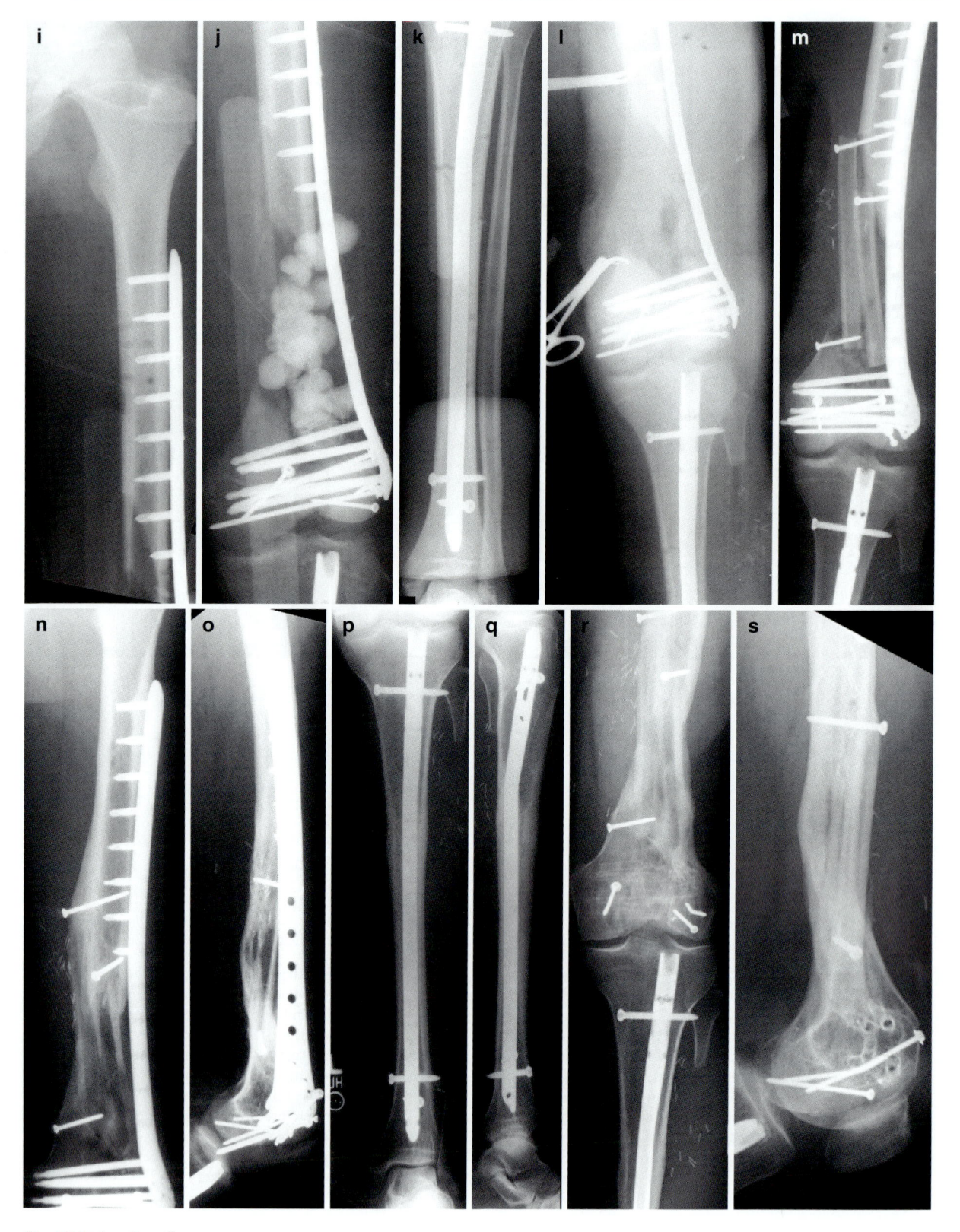

Fig. 13.3 (continued)

13.6 Complications

A major factor in the decision making in the treatment of the mangled extremity is the possible major complications associated with each treatment arm. Harris et al. reported the nature and incidence of major complications for patients enrolled in the LEAP study group. Their cohort consisted of 545 patients with severe lower extremity injuries followed prospectively for 24 months. A physician examined each patient at 3-, 6-, 12-, 24-month intervals and major complications recorded. The two most common complications were wound infection (28.3%) and nonunion (23.7%), and the majority of each of these required operative intervention and inpatient care. Approximately, a quarter of each of these complications were considered severe enough to compromise long-term function. The overall incidence of wound dehiscence was 8.6% and that of osteomyelitis 7.7%. There was also a 5.3% incidence of symptomatic hardware [19].

The complication data from the cohort was further examined based on treatment arm in the study. A total of 149 patients underwent amputations, and the revision amputation rate was 5.4%. The most common complications in this group were wound infection (34.2%), followed by stump revision (14.5%), phantom limb pain and wound breakdown (13.4% each), and stump complications (10.7%). In the limb reconstruction group, the most common complication was nonunion (31.5%), followed by wound infection (23.2%). Of these infections, 8.6% developed into osteomyelitis. There was an incidence of posttraumatic arthrosis of 9.4% and wound necrosis or breakdown of 6.5%. The late amputation group (patients amputated after initial discharge) experienced the highest rate of major complications (85%) [19].

This fact clearly highlights the need for appropriate decision making in the patient with a mangled extremity at the onset of treatment. Although there were no late mortalities reported, an incidence of up to 21% has been reported in the literature. Bondurant et al. undertook an investigation looking at the effects of delayed versus primary amputation. There was a significant increase in length of hospital stay (22 versus 53 days) and number of surgical interventions (1.6 versus 6.9). The cost was almost double ($28,964 versus $53,462), and there was a 21% mortality rate in the delayed amputation group [43]. It is quite evident that every effort should be made to avoid a late amputation given such high costs for all involved.

In a prospective cohort study (using LEAP study patients), Castillo et al. examined the specific effect of smoking on complication rate in severe open tibia fractures. A total of 268 patients with unilateral injuries were followed prospectively. Nonunion rates were significantly higher in both the current and previous smoking groups (37% and 32%, respectively). The authors were able to demonstrate that current smokers were more than twice as likely to develop an infection, and 3.7 times more likely to have osteomyelitis. Previous smoking history was detrimental as well, and this group was 2.8 times as likely to develop osteomyelitis than nonsmokers. Their recommendation was that orthopaedic surgeons should encourage patients to enter smoking cessation programs [44].

13.7 Predictive Ability of Scoring Systems to Predict Final Outcome

Some authors have examined the ability of the previously discussed scoring systems to predict functional outcome following treatment. Durham et al. performed a retrospective analysis of upper and lower severe extremity injuries to determine the validity and ability to predict outcome of the above discussed predictive indices. For each of the four systems analyzed, there were no significant differences between patients with good or poor functional outcomes [45]. Ly et al. reported on the ability of the five most commonly used predictive indices (above plus Hannover Fracture Scale-98) to determine functional recovery following limb salvage in a cohort of 507 patients (LEAP study group). The authors showed that none of the scoring systems analyzed were able to determine outcome based on the Sickness Impact Profile (SIP) out to 24 months following injury [46]. One can conclude, based on these two studies, that the commonly applied predictive indices may be useful in early decision making, but are unable to predict functional recovery.

(=injury), and its effectiveness in the context of major orthopaedic fractures has been shown [5, 54, 55].

The question whether amputation of a mangled limb is advisable for a severely injured patient cannot be answered [56]. There are no clear guidelines with respect to the *isolated* mangled extremities, let alone the polytrauma patient. As an exception, utilizing DCO guidelines, salvage of the *stable* polytrauma patient's mangled limb is possibly the most relevant. For these, techniques involving early free tissue transfer and internal fixation as proposed by the "fix-and-flap" technique might be successful, but require a highly specialized trauma center [40]. Still, for these patients, the decision whether to salvage or amputate faces the same dilemmas as for the patient with the isolated mangled limb as described elsewhere in this chapter.

Borderline patients that stabilize after resuscitation can undergo early total care (ETC), but reconstructive efforts need to anticipate potential deterioration. Long procedures (e.g., "fix-and-flap") are not justified in these patients. Wound debridement, revascularization, and external fixation are all that can be done while a rapid turn for the worse should be anticipated. In the *unstable* or *in extremis* polytrauma patient, there might be a role for primary amputation as prolonged revascularization and stabilization procedures add to the patient's catabolic state and will increase the second hit enormously. Any other reconstructive efforts for the extremities are not justified.

Next steps in limb salvage should not be undertaken until the patient has stabilized and is beyond the systemic inflammatory response syndrome (SIRS) stage. As a rule, timing of second and subsequent major procedures (longer than 3 h) should be at least after 4 days [3]. If the limb develops evidence of sepsis, early amputation should still be considered. The use of fresh warm blood, plasma, and recombinant factor VII defined as Damage Control Resuscitation before surgery helps to optimize the physiologic parameters and theoretically allows for more prolonged surgical procedures such as revascularization [57].

13.12 Conclusions

The combination of osseous, vascular, soft-tissue, and nerve injury present following severe trauma to an extremity makes such injuries a challenge to treat. Unfortunately, the data regarding the management of the mangled extremity are conflicting, and the literature is without Class I studies. It is therefore imperative that an experienced surgical team at a trauma center that cares for such patients with some regularity care for the patient with a complex extremity injury [58]. The treating team must always keep in mind the high prevalence of associated multisystem trauma and systemic problems related to these injuries. Even though the treatment goal is limb salvage, it must be kept in mind that in many instances, a primary amputation might provide the best outcome. New insights, therapies, and techniques will improve outcomes in even the most severely injured patients with complex extremity injuries. As for the mangled limb in these patients, it is unlikely a scoring system will allow a clear cutoff point for amputation versus salvage. What has become clear is that primary amputation should not be considered a treatment failure but rather a means of meeting goals of treatment [59]. As Hansen pointed out long ago, we should not let heroism triumph over reason [47].

Disclaimer None of the authors claim any conflicts of interest or received any funding for this manuscript.

References

1. Giannoudis PV, Dinopoulos H, Chalidis B, et al. Surgical stress response. Injury. 2006;37 Suppl 5:S3–9.
2. Giannoudis PV, Giannoudi M, Stavlas P. Damage control orthopaedics: lessons learned. Injury. 2009;40 Suppl 4:S47–52.
3. Hildebrand F, Giannoudis P, Kretteck C, et al. Damage control: extremities. Injury. 2004;35:678–89.
4. Pape HC. Effects of changing strategies of fracture fixation on immunologic changes and systemic complications after multiple trauma: damage control orthopedic surgery. J Orthop Res. 2008;26:1478–84.
5. Taeger G, Ruchholtz S, Waydhas C, et al. Damage control orthopedics in patients with multiple injuries is effective, time saving, and safe. J Trauma. 2005;59:409–16; discussion 17.
6. Ball CG, Rozycki GS, Feliciano DV. Upper extremity amputations after motor vehicle rollovers. J Trauma. 2009;67:410–12.
7. Beatty ME, Zook EG, Russell RC, et al. Grain auger injuries: the replacement of the corn picker injury? Plast Reconstr Surg. 1982;69:96–102.
8. Bosse MJ, MacKenzie EJ, Kellam JF, et al. An analysis of outcomes of reconstruction or amputation after leg-threatening injuries. N Engl J Med. 2002;347:1924–31.
9. Campbell II DC, Bryan RS, Cooney III WP, et al. Mechanical cornpicker hand injuries. J Trauma. 1979;19:678–81.

10. Dente CJ, Feliciano DV, Rozycki GS, et al. A review of upper extremity fasciotomies in a level I trauma center. Am Surg. 2004;70:1088–93.
11. Dirschl DR, Dahners LE. The mangled extremity: when should it be amputated? J Am Acad Orthop Surg. 1996;4:182–90.
12. Gorsche TS, Wood MB. Mutilating corn-picker injuries of the hand. J Hand Surg Am. 1988;13:423–7.
13. Gupta A, Wolff TW. Management of the mangled hand and forearm. J Am Acad Orthop Surg. 1995;3:226–36.
14. Korompilias AV, Beris AE, Lykissas MG, et al. The mangled extremity and attempt for limb salvage. J Orthop Surg Res. 2009;4:4.
15. Roberts CS, Pape HC, Jones AL, et al. Damage control orthopaedics: evolving concepts in the treatment of patients who have sustained orthopaedic trauma. Instr Course Lect. 2005;54:447–62.
16. Togawa S, Yamami N, Nakayama H, et al. The validity of the mangled extremity severity score in the assessment of upper limb injuries. J Bone Joint Surg Br. 2005;87:1516–19.
17. Bartlett CS, Helfet DL, Hausman MR, et al. Ballistics and gunshot wounds: effects on musculoskeletal tissues. J Am Acad Orthop Surg. 2000;8:21–36.
18. Brown KV, Ramasamy A, McLeod J, et al. Predicting the need for early amputation in ballistic mangled extremity injuries. J Trauma. 2009;66:S93–7; discussion S7–8.
19. Harris AM, Althausen PL, Kellam J, et al. Complications following limb-threatening lower extremity trauma. J Orthop Trauma. 2009;23:1–6.
20. Hoogendoorn JM, van der Werken C. Grade III open tibial fractures: functional outcome and quality of life in amputees versus patients with successful reconstruction. Injury. 2001;32:329–34.
21. Helfet DL, Howey T, Sanders R, et al. Limb salvage versus amputation. Preliminary results of the Mangled Extremity Severity Score. Clin Orthop Relat Res. 1990;256:80–6.
22. Howe Jr HR, Poole Jr GV, Hansen KJ, et al. Salvage of lower extremities following combined orthopedic and vascular trauma. A predictive salvage index. Am Surg. 1987;53:205–8.
23. Johansen K, Daines M, Howey T, et al. Objective criteria accurately predict amputation following lower extremity trauma. J Trauma. 1990;30:568–72; discussion 72–3.
24. Lange RH, Bach AW, Hansen Jr ST, et al. Open tibial fractures with associated vascular injuries: prognosis for limb salvage. J Trauma. 1985;25:203–8.
25. Russell WL, Sailors DM, Whittle TB, et al. Limb salvage versus traumatic amputation. A decision based on a seven-part predictive index. Ann Surg. 1991;213:473–80; discussion 80–1.
26. Bonanni F, Rhodes M, Lucke JF. The futility of predictive scoring of mangled lower extremities. J Trauma. 1993;34:99–104.
27. Roessler MS, Wisner DH, Holcroft JW. The mangled extremity. When to amputate? Arch Surg. 1991;126:1243–8; discussion 8–9.
28. O'Sullivan ST, O'Sullivan M, Pasha N, et al. Is it possible to predict limb viability in complex Gustilo IIIB and IIIC tibial fractures? A comparison of two predictive indices. Injury. 1997;28:639–42.
29. Robertson PA. Prediction of amputation after severe lower limb trauma. J Bone Joint Surg Br. 1991;73:816–18.
30. McNamara MG, Heckman JD, Corley FG. Severe open fractures of the lower extremity: a retrospective evaluation of the Mangled Extremity Severity Score (MESS). J Orthop Trauma. 1994;8:81–7.
31. Bosse MJ, McCarthy ML, Jones AL, et al. The insensate foot following severe lower extremity trauma: an indication for amputation? J Bone Joint Surg Am. 2005;87:2601–8.
32. MacKenzie EJ, Bosse MJ, Pollak AN, et al. Long-term persistence of disability following severe lower-limb trauma. Results of a seven-year follow-up. J Bone Joint Surg Am. 2005;87:1801–9.
33. Dedmond BT, Kortesis B, Punger K, et al. The use of negative-pressure wound therapy (NPWT) in the temporary treatment of soft-tissue injuries associated with high-energy open tibial shaft fractures. J Orthop Trauma. 2007;21:11–7.
34. Henry SL, Ostermann PA, Seligson D. The antibiotic bead pouch technique. The management of severe compound fractures. Clin Orthop Relat Res. 1993;295:54–62.
35. Herscovici Jr D, Sanders RW, Scaduto JM, et al. Vacuum-assisted wound closure (VAC therapy) for the management of patients with high-energy soft tissue injuries. J Orthop Trauma. 2003;17:683–8.
36. Ostermann PA, Henry SL, Seligson D. The role of local antibiotic therapy in the management of compound fractures. Clin Orthop Relat Res. 1993;295:102–11.
37. Ostermann PA, Seligson D, Henry SL. Local antibiotic therapy for severe open fractures. A review of 1085 consecutive cases. J Bone Joint Surg Br. 1995;77:93–7.
38. Prasarn ML, Zych G, Ostermann PA. Wound management for severe open fractures: use of antibiotic bead pouches and vacuum-assisted closure. Am J Orthop (Belle Mead NJ). 2009;38(11):559–63.
39. Godina M. Early microsurgical reconstruction of complex trauma of the extremities. Plast Reconstr Surg. 1986;78:285–92.
40. Gopal S, Majumder S, Batchelor AG, et al. Fix and flap: the radical orthopaedic and plastic treatment of severe open fractures of the tibia. J Bone Joint Surg Br. 2000;82:959–66.
41. Govender S, Csimma C, Genant HK, et al. Recombinant human bone morphogenetic protein-2 for treatment of open tibial fractures: a prospective, controlled, randomized study of four hundred and fifty patients. J Bone Joint Surg Am. 2002;84-A:2123–34.
42. Gopal S, Giannoudis PV, Murray A, et al. The functional outcome of severe, open tibial fractures managed with early fixation and flap coverage. J Bone Joint Surg Br. 2004;86:861–7.
43. Bondurant FJ, Cotler HB, Buckle R, et al. The medical and economic impact of severely injured lower extremities. J Trauma. 1988;28:1270–3.
44. Castillo RC, Bosse MJ, MacKenzie EJ, et al. Impact of smoking on fracture healing and risk of complications in limb-threatening open tibia fractures. J Orthop Trauma. 2005;19:151–7.
45. Durham RM, Mistry BM, Mazuski JE, et al. Outcome and utility of scoring systems in the management of the mangled extremity. Am J Surg. 1996;172:569–73; discussion 73–4.
46. Ly TV, Travison TG, Castillo RC, et al. Ability of lower-extremity injury severity scores to predict functional outcome after limb salvage. J Bone Joint Surg Am. 2008;90:1738–43.

47. Hansen Jr ST. Overview of the severely traumatized lower limb. Reconstruction versus amputation. Clin Orthop Relat Res. 1989;243:17–9.
48. Georgiadis GM, Behrens FF, Joyce MJ, et al. Open tibial fractures with severe soft-tissue loss. Limb salvage compared with below-the-knee amputation. J Bone Joint Surg Am. 1993;75:1431–41.
49. MacKenzie EJ, Bosse MJ, Kellam JF, et al. Characterization of patients with high-energy lower extremity trauma. J Orthop Trauma. 2000;14:455–66.
50. Smith JJ, Agel J, Swiontkowski MF, et al. Functional outcome of bilateral limb threatening: lower extremity injuries at two years postinjury. J Orthop Trauma. 2005;19:249–53.
51. Hertel R, Strebel N, Ganz R. Amputation versus reconstruction in traumatic defects of the leg: outcome and costs. J Orthop Trauma. 1996;10:223–9.
52. MacKenzie EJ, Jones AS, Bosse MJ, et al. Health-care costs associated with amputation or reconstruction of a limb-threatening injury. J Bone Joint Surg Am. 2007;89:1685–92.
53. Slauterbeck JR, Britton C, Moneim MS, et al. Mangled extremity severity score: an accurate guide to treatment of the severely injured upper extremity. J Orthop Trauma. 1994;8:282–5.
54. Nowotarski PJ, Turen CH, Brumback RJ, et al. Conversion of external fixation to intramedullary nailing for fractures of the shaft of the femur in multiply injured patients. J Bone Joint Surg Am. 2000;82:781–8.
55. Scalea TM, Boswell SA, Scott JD, et al. External fixation as a bridge to intramedullary nailing for patients with multiple injuries and with femur fractures: damage control orthopedics. J Trauma. 2000;48:613–21; discussion 21–3.
56. Kobbe P, Lichte P, Pape HC. Complex extremity fractures following high energy injuries: the limited value of existing classifications and a proposal for a treatment-guide. Injury. 2009;40 Suppl 4:S69–74.
57. Fox CJ, Gillespie DL, Cox ED, et al. Damage control resuscitation for vascular surgery in a combat support hospital. J Trauma. 2008;65:1–9.
58. Mackenzie EJ, Rivara FP, Jurkovich GJ, et al. The impact of trauma-center care on functional outcomes following major lower-limb trauma. J Bone Joint Surg Am. 2008;90:101–9.
59. Cannada LK, Cooper C. The mangled extremity: limb salvage versus amputation. Curr Surg. 2005;62:563–76.

Management of Spine Fractures

Karl-Åke Jansson and Kevin Gill

Contents

14.1	Incidence	151
14.1.1	Associated Injuries and Premorbid Factors	151
14.2	Mortality	152
14.3	Definition of Spinal Instability	152
14.4	Prehospital Management	152
14.4.1	Initial Management	152
14.4.2	Clinical History and Examination	154
14.4.3	Immobilization	154
14.4.4	Management During Transport	154
14.5	In-Hospital Management	154
14.5.1	History	154
14.5.2	Physical Examination and Initial Treatment	154
14.5.3	Spinal Imaging	157
14.5.4	Hospital Resuscitation: Workup	158
14.5.5	Cervical Traction	158
14.6	Treatment	159
14.6.1	Nonsurgical Treatment	159
14.6.2	Surgical Treatment	160
14.6.3	Special Situations	162
14.7	Clinical Outcome	163
References		164

Karl-Åke Jansson (✉)
Department of Orthopedic Surgery, Karolinska Institutet at Karolinska University Hospital, SE-171 76 Stockholm, Sweden
e-mail: karl-ake.jansson@karolinska.se

Kevin Gill
Department of Orthopaedic Surgery
Southwestern University
Dallas, TX, USA

14.1 Incidence

Injuries of the spine include a broad spectrum of injuries, ranging from pure soft tissue lesions to fracture dislocations with associated spinal cord injury.

Spine fractures represent 1% of all skeletal fractures [1], and up to 30% in multiply injured patients [2]. The annual vertebral fracture incidence varies from 7.5 to 90 per 100,000 inhabitants [3, 8]. Spine fractures are often associated with other severe injuries and should be managed according to the general principles for severely injured patients. In every high-energy injury patient, clinicians should have a high suspicion for spinal trauma. Motor vehicle accidents account for most of the fractures in younger patients, while falling is the most common cause of injuries in elderly patients.

14.1.1 Associated Injuries and Premorbid Factors

Spine fractures tend to have other severe musculoskeletal injuries (40%) [1], and only 20% of patients with spinal cord pathology have an isolated injury to the spine [9]. A large proportion of spine fractures have associated brain and chest injuries. The combination of abdominal injuries and spine fractures is even more rare. Special care has to be taken not to miss a spinal injury in intubated patients with closed head injuries. Also, despite the options of CT scanning, certain local factors such as ankylosing spondylitis can interfere with the diagnostics of a spinal fracture [10].

H.-C. Pape et al. (eds.), *The Poly-Traumatized Patient with Fractures*,
DOI: 10.1007/978-3-642-17986-0_14, © Springer-Verlag Berlin Heidelberg 2011

14.2 Mortality

In patients who die on scene, the spine injuries are rarely the major cause of death [11]. Among those with an identifiable injury, only 4% are due to spine injuries [12]. The in-hospital deaths related to spinal cord injury are as low as 3%, and the reported 90-day mortality rate after thoracolumbar spine fracture surgery is 1.4% [6]. Although the mortality rate has decreased over the last years, this may be due to multiple causes, such as improved trauma management and resuscitation and multidisciplinary rehabilitation programs help prevent late deaths.

14.3 Definition of Spinal Instability

Spinal instability is defined as failure to withstand normal physiological loads and/or inability to support the spinal cord. This in turn leads to deformity, neurologic deficit, and pain. Instability of the spine injury is defined by the mechanism of injury and various anatomical and pathological classification systems. Evaluation of the degree of spinal injury and its inherent instability relies upon clinical examination, radiologic evaluation, and appropriate classification of the injury. See Table 14.1 guidelines for interpreting instability of the spine.

The most important sign of instability is deformity, followed by neurological deficit.

> Close cooperation between spine surgeon, the trauma leader, and radiologist is a key factor. Unstable injuries of the spine should be rendered for emergency surgery according to a protocol following the damage control approach, while stable patients with unstable spine fracture should undergo surgery as soon as possible.

14.4 Prehospital Management

14.4.1 Initial Management

Up to 25% of patients with spinal cord injuries develop neurological deterioration prior to hospitalization. As a rule, patients with suspected spine injury can be managed as if they had an unstable fracture. An algorithm to the spine-injured trauma victim is shown in Fig. 14.1.

Table 14.1 Guidelines for interpreting instability of the spine

General considerations

This checklist is not validated in an applied clinical setting

It was designed to determine which patient subpopulations have to undergo immediate surgery or whether immobilization of their spinal injury is required

Neurologic considerations

Patients with initial neurological deficit usually have an unstable spine injury

Nerve root involvement is a weaker indicator for instability

Anatomic and biochemical considerations

A narrow spinal canal lowers the threshold for neurological complications in patients with spinal trauma

When all anterior or all posterior elements are damaged, the injury should be considered potentially unstable

An anterior injury is usually more unstable in flexion
A posterior injury is usually more unstable in extension

Radiological considerations

A displacement of more than 3.5 mm in the cervical sagittal CT as well as segmental kyphosis of more than 11° may account for instability

A widened intervertebral space and facet joint distraction of more than 50% resemble unstable discoligamentous injury

Bony avulsion injuries of the anterior or posterior upper and lower vertebral endplates may indicate rupture of the anterior or posterior longitudinal ligaments

In the thoracolumbar region, loss of more than 50% of vertebral height, sagittal angulation of more than 25°, spinal canal encroachment more than 50%, and increased interspinous process distances are associated with unstable spine injuries

Patient-related considerations

Age, osteoporosis, ankylosing spondylitis, DISH (Diffuse Idiopathic Skeletal Hyperostosis), pulmonary diseases, noncompliance to treatment (i.e., psychiatric disease, drug dependence)

Physiological considerations

Intractable pain may be a useful indicator for instability

Associated injuries

Multiple rib fractures and/or injuries to sternum affect the stability of the thoracic spine. These injuries may cause a higher need for operative treatment of spine injury

Multiple fractures of the transverse processes may indicate rotational instability

The oxygen supply should be secured to the patients according to ATLS (advance trauma life support) principles [13]. The neurological examination follows immediately after examination of mental status, motor deficit, radiculopathy, and sensory loss. If the patient is

14 Management of Spine Fractures

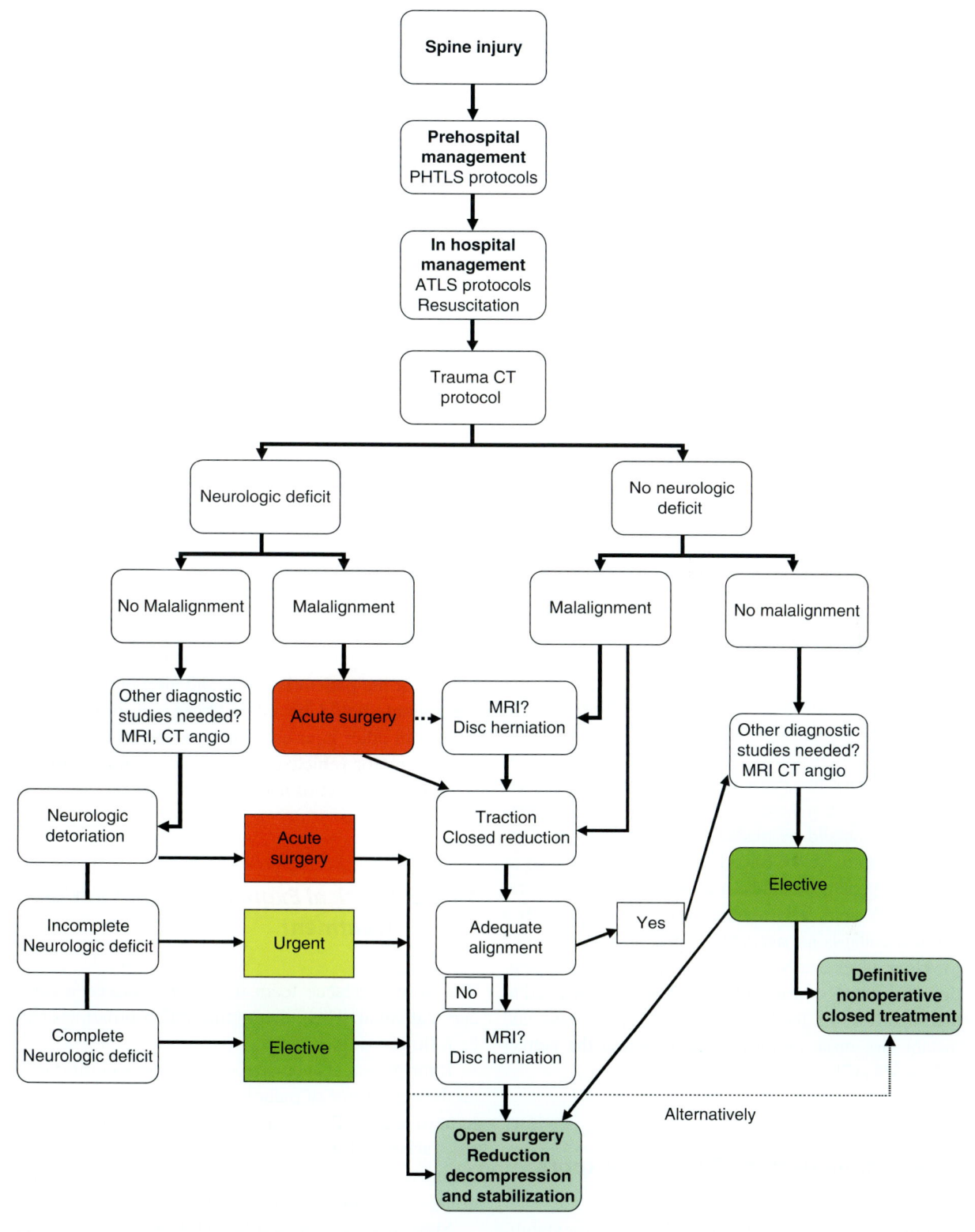

Fig. 14.1 An algorithmic approach to the spine injury patient. PHTLS, prehospital trauma life support, ATLS, advance trauma life support, CT computed tomography, MRI magnetic resonance imaging

hypotensive, hypertensive neurogenic shock should be considered and one should be aware of signs of hypotension, bradycardia, and warm and dry skin along with normal mental status.

14.4.2 Clinical History and Examination

The trauma mechanism can be a hint toward a spinal cord injury [14]. A history of a high-energy injury, high-speed motor vehicle accident (MVA), fall from heights (>4 m), and physical signs of a head injury with or without unconsciousness, pain from the spine, and or neurological signs (weakness, radiculopathy, sensory loss) can define the degree of injury [14]. However, if the patient has a low risk of spine injuries, the Canadian C-spine rule can be used to decide if further investigation is required [15, 16]. The Canadian C-spine rule uses age, mechanism of injury, and physical examination to determine the need for CT scan.

14.4.3 Immobilization

Immediate immobilization should be achieved at the scene of the accident.

Patients with suspected spine injury should be treated as if the injury has caused spinal instability. A spine board or a vacuum mattress should be applied. The cervical spine should be placed in neutral position. This maneuver must not be forced, and if neurological signs occur the patient should be immobilized in non-neutral position. A rigid cervical collar should be applied. If a cervical collar is not available or does not fit, blankets/towels or tapes can be used to secure the neutral position. In patients wearing a helmet it is recommended to take it off. Some football helmets allow for easy and instant face mask removal while retaining the helmet (PHTLS®) [17].

14.4.4 Management During Transport

A spine board fixation with special devices for stabilization of the neck is preferable during transport. There is a risk for pressure ulcers especially if the patient is unconscious or has neurological deficit; therefore a 2-h limit is required. If a longer transport is necessary, the patient has to be turned regularly. A patient on a spine board is unable to secure his or her own airway and should be under supervision during transportation.

14.5 In-Hospital Management

The management in the hospital continues according to the principles of ATLS (Fig. 14.2).

14.5.1 History

The patient, eyewitnesses, paramedics, and emergency physicians should be questioned regarding the circumstances of the accident in order to determine the direction of force and mechanism of injury. Extrication from motor vehicle and traumatic brain injuries are associated with high risk of spinal injury [18].

In the ER setting, it is important to request information on the injury to continue the workup of spinal trauma. If the patient is stable and alert on admission, the patient should be asked about age, drug intake, pain from other injuries masking spine injury, as well as if the motor vehicle collision was a simple rear-end type, and the onset of neck pain.

14.5.2 Physical Examination and Initial Treatment

The primary rescue team usually has placed a rigid cervical collar. Then, the regular ATLS principles can be followed (Fig. 14.2).

If the patient is unconscious, the examiner must rely on the occurrence of pathological reflexes and changes in muscle tone. Priapism and low rectal sphincter tone may account for impairment. Patients with delayed diagnosis are often more hypotensive, critically injured, or have low Glasgow Coma Scale scores [19].

Since hypotension is a known factor for exacerbation of unfavorable secondary immunologic events, the restoration of a sufficient cardiopulmonary function

14 Management of Spine Fractures

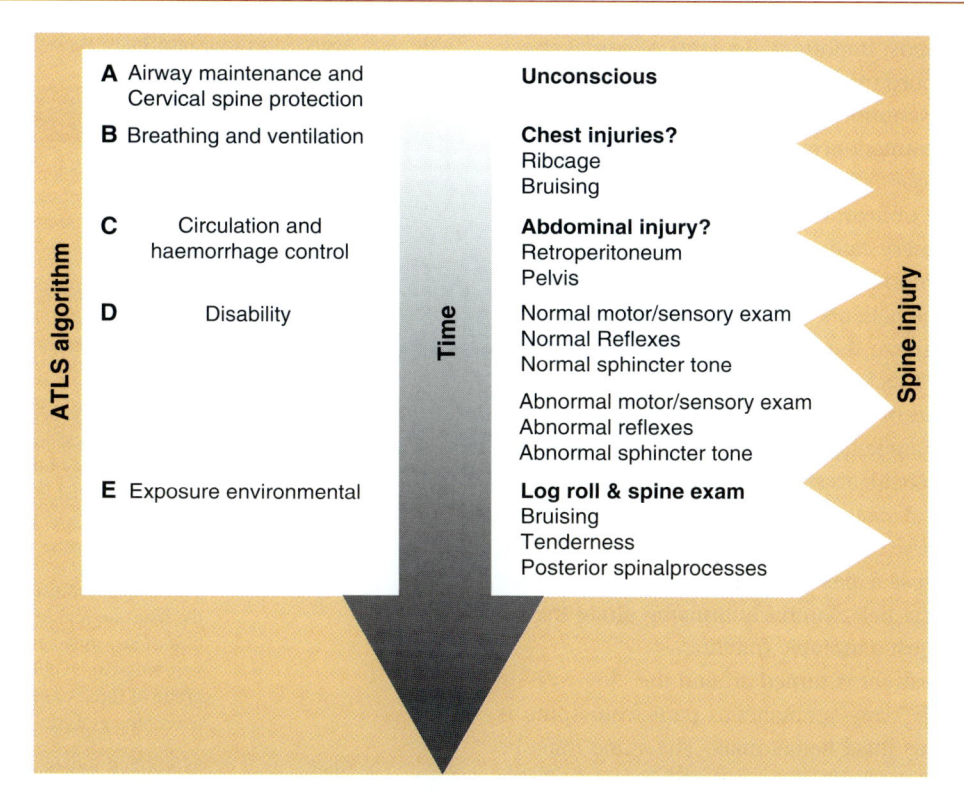

Fig. 14.2 ATLS® algorithm and spine trauma assessment. In step A, cervical spine (C-Spine) protection is essential. Every unconscious patient is stabilized by a stiff-neck orthosis. Patients with signs of chest injury in step B and abdominal injury in step C, especially retroperitoneal, are highly suspicious for thoracic and/or lumbar spine injury. Normal motor examination and reflexes do not rule out significant spine injury in the comatose patient. Abnormal neurologic examination is a sign for substantial spinal column injury including spinal cord injury. Log roll in step E is important to assess the posterior elements of the cervical to the sacral spine and looking for any signs of bruising, open wounds, tender points, and palpation of paravertebral tissue and posterior spinous processes in search for distraction injury. Spine precautions should only be discontinued when patients regain consciousness and are able to communicate sufficiently on spinal discomfort or neurologic sensations before the spine is cleared

and constant arterial mean pressure is essential to maintain sufficient organ perfusion with special regard toward injuries of the central nervous system including brain and spinal cord [20]. It has also been shown that secondary immunologic events with systemic immune reactions follow mechanical injuries to the spinal cord [21]. In steps B and C, early oxygenation and volume replacement is very important.

14.5.2.1 Ventilation

Maintenance of an adequate airway and breathing remains an important priority in the trauma patient. Spinal cord injured patients may suffer from inadequate respiratory function due to paralysis of the intercostal muscles or diaphragm. The diaphragm is innervated from C3–C5 level. With diaphragmatic injury the patients lose about two thirds of the vital capacity that is compensated by an increased breading frequency. Concomitant injuries may also compromise respiratory function. Maintenance of spinal alignment is critical during intubation. If endotracheal intubation is needed, it is best performed in conjunction with inline cervical traction, or by nasotracheal tube or by fiber-optic procedures.

14.5.2.2 Circulation

A spinal cord injury may cause vasospasm due to dysfunction of blood flow autoregulation. An injury above Th6 involves the sympathetic nerve system and increases the risk for neurogenic shock. Hypotension, due to loss of sympathetic vascular tone, and bradycardia, due to loss of sympathetic innervations of the heart, are the most important elements of spinal shock due to spinal cord injury. If neurogenic shock is present, fluid resuscitation is a vital first intervention and follows the treatment principles used for brain injury.

Central venous catheter and arterial lines are required for assessment of heart rate, blood pressure, and perfusion, while urinary catheter monitors urine output. The early use of blood products is recommended in the multiple injured patients with an associated spinal cord injury to maximize the oxygen-carrying capacity and to minimize the secondary ischemic injury to the spinal cord. Early use of vasopressors such as dopamine or atropine is recommended to maintain the systolic blood pressure. The goal is to attain a pressure >90 mmHg.

The physical examination continues with inspection. A transverse band of ecchymosis across the abdomen can suggest a flexion-distraction type of injury caused by a seat belt. Similarly bruising along the rib cage may suggest a thoracic fracture.

When the patient is turned around the "log roll" in ATLS® step "E," any spontaneous pain from spine is noted as well as local hematomas. The spine must be palpated systematically for tenderness, step-off, or interspinous process gapping. If the patient is kept in the rigid collar and posture changes are performed in axial alignment, additional injury to the spinal column is prevented and life-saving intervention can safely be performed.

A detailed neurological examination, including motor and sensory function, should then be performed. A quick and easy way to do this early on is to ask the patient to move all four extremities. The neurological examination could be difficult to perform due to many factors. Unconscious patients can be evaluated with pain stimulation and noted reactions. Spinal shock could mask improvement of neurological recovery. Peripheral nerve injuries or fractures also influence the interpretation of the examination.

14.5.2.3 Classification of Neurological Injury

The initial responsibility of the physician evaluating a patient with spinal cord injury is to determine the extent of neurological deficit. The neurological status should be assessed according to standardized scores, i.e., the ASIA (American Spinal Injury Association) [22], a modification of Frankel grading system, see Table 14.2.

Table 14.2 ASIA (American Spinal Injury Association) impairment scale

Scale	Type of spinal cord injury (SCI)	Description of SCI
A	Complete	No motor or sensory function below the level of injury including the sacral segments S4–S5
B	Incomplete	Sensory but no motor function is preserved below the neurological level and includes the sacral segments S4–S5
C	Incomplete	Motor function is preserved below the neurological level, and more than half of key muscles below the neurological level have a muscle grade less than three (cannot overcome gravity)
D	Incomplete	Motor function is preserved below the neurological level, and at least half of key muscles below the neurological level have a muscle grade of three or more (can at least overcome gravity)
E	Normal	Motor and sensory functions are normal

Sacral Sparing

Sacral sparing represents at least partial structural continuity of the white matter long tracts. Clinically, it is demonstrated by perianal sensation, rectal motor function, and great toe flexor activity.

A rectal examination is mandatory in every evaluation of spinal injury.

Spinal Shock

In complete transections of the spinal cord, spinal areflexia occurs. This state is named spinal shock. It is clinically graded by testing the bulbocavernosus reflex, a spinal reflex mediated by the S3–S4 region of the medullary cone. This reflex is often absent for the first 4 h after injury and usually returns within 24 h. If no evidence of spinal cord function is noted below the level of injury, and the bulbocavernosus reflex has not returned, no determination can be made regarding the lesion. After 24 h, 99% of the patients emerge from spinal shock, as observed by the return of sacral reflexes. If no sacral function exists at this point, the injury is considered. Ninety-nine percent of patients with complete injuries have no functional recovery. One exception is a direct injury to the conus medullaris where some functional recovery occurs.

Incomplete Spinal Cord Injury Syndrome

Incomplete spinal cord injury can present as one of the following syndromes.

Anterior cord syndrome implies complete motor and sensory loss except retained trunk and lower extremity deep pressure sensation and proprioception. Only one out of ten patients has a chance of recovery.

Central cord syndrome represents central gray matter destruction with preservation of just the peripheral spinal cord structures. The patient usually is tetraplegic with preserved perianal sensation. Often, there is early return of bowel and bladder control. The neural axons nourishing the upper extremity pass more medial than the axons to the lower extremity. Therefore, the leg is stronger than the arm. The most common cause is cervical hyperextension injury in patients with narrow spinal canals. This injury can be mechanically stable. The syndrome has a good prognosis with recovery up to 75%.

Brown-Séquard syndrome (lateral cord syndrome) is a unilateral cord injury, often caused by missiles. It is characterized by loss of motor deficit ipsilateral to the spinal cord injury and contralateral pain and temperature hypoesthesia. This syndrome usually has a good prognosis. Most patients regain bowel and bladder function and ability to walk.

14.5.3 Spinal Imaging

Clearing the injured spine is a challenge for any trauma unit. What modalities to use? Timing of investigations? Multiply injured patients or unconscious patients and/or presence of neurological deficits determine the radiographic protocol.

14.5.3.1 Plain Film Radiography: Primary Assessment

Conventional plain films have been used as a screening tool in the primary assessment of spinal injury. However, the examination takes time and has a low specificity; therefore, in modern trauma care, it has been replaced by computer tomography (CT). It is difficult to perform adequate conventional X-rays in the severely injured patient. The first cervical vertebrae and the cervicothoracic junction are difficult to visualize. Only 52% of cervical spine fractures are identified by plain films, while 98% can be visualized by CT [23]. Primary survey emergency room cervical plain radiographs are often of poor quality. If conventional lateral cervical spine view is performed and there is doubt, computed tomography should be performed.

14.5.3.2 Computed Tomography: Secondary Assessment

The development and accessibility of CT has discarded the use of plain radiography. The sensitivity and specificity are higher with CT. Thus, most trauma centers no longer include the plain cervical radiographs into the primary trauma assessment [24, 25]. Whole-body scans from head to pelvis can quickly be obtained in a spiral-imaging pattern. This is recommended for severely injured patients in case of suspicion of spinal trauma [26].

Modern CT-scanners with 64 scales (MDDT multislice-DT) are capable of obtaining a full body scan (190 cm) in seconds – slice thickness is as low as of 0.6–0.8 mm [27]. This allows for high-quality imaging and various planes. This delivers more information on the condition of the spine than any conventional plain film [28, 66]. The risk of cervical discoligamentous injuries when using a conventional scanner is approximately 1% and does not require emergency MRI [29]. CT is also helpful for the surgeon in the preoperative planning. The coronal and sagittal plane reconstructions can assist the surgeon in appreciating the degree of deformity and severity of injury. Additional 3D CT reconstruction can be used for complex spinal anatomic areas such as the upper cervical spine. Numerous sets of radiographic criteria have been developed in an attempt to predict which patients are or will become unstable after a spinal injury.

In a cervical sagittal CT scan, a displacement of more than 3.5 mm as well as segmental kyphosis of more than 11° may account for instability [30]. A widened intervertebral space and facet joint distraction of more than 50% resemble unstable discoligamentous injury [31]. Bony avulsion injuries of the anterior or posterior upper and lower vertebral endplate might indicate to rupture of the anterior or posterior longitudinal ligaments. At C1, this accounts for bony avulsion injuries of the transverse ligament. The frontal and axial CT-reconstructions should rule out rotational offset of the vertebral segment, which indicates rotational instability with special attention to the C1-2 area. In the thoracolumbar region, a loss of more than 50% of vertebral height, sagittal angulations of more than 25°, spinal canal encroachment more than 50%, and increased interspinous distances are associated with unstable spine injuries [32, 33].

In addition to the radiological findings on spinal CT scans, additional injuries may reveal unstable spine trauma. Fractures of the transverse processes and ribs account for rotational injury. Sternal fracture following hyperflexion might be an upper thoracic posterior column injury. Retroperitoneal bleeding shown in CT scan is often associated with hyperextension to the thoracolumbar region.

14.5.3.3 Computed Tomography Contrast Angiography

Blunt cerebral vascular injuries (BCVI), primarily arterial dissection, may occur in association with cervical spine trauma [34]. Early diagnosis and treatment reduces morbidity (stroke) and mortality in patients with vertebral artery injuries [20, 61]. Catheter-angiography has been gold standard, but it is invasive. Routine screening with MR-angiography and 16-slice CT angiography can be performed in the initial radiologic workup [64].

Trauma victims with any of the following signs or symptoms should be considered to have BCVI until proven otherwise [36, 37]: coma unexplained by CT, neurologic deficit, including hemiparesis, transient ischemic attack, Horner's syndrome, oculosympathetic paresis or vertebrobasilar insufficiency, evidence of cerebral infarction on CT; arterial hemorrhage from neck, mouth, nose, ears, large or expanding cervical hematoma, cervical bruit in a patient younger than 50 years; fracture subluxation in cervical spine at any level, fractures from C1 to C3, and fractures into the transverse foramen at any level; displaced mid-face fracture (LeFort II or III), basilar skull fracture with carotid canal involvement, closed head injury with consistent diffuse axonal injury with Glasgow Coma Scale <6, neck belt sign or significant swelling, near hanging with anoxia. To be "stroke fighters" in managing trauma patients, we must continue to screen patients with defined risk factors with multislice CT angiography.

14.5.3.4 Magnetic Imaging

MRI is superior to CT in visualizing the spinal cord, intervertebral disk, and spinal ligaments. In the absence of visible bone lesions, a patient with a neurological deficit should undergo MRI examination as early as possible to detect a possible spinal cord compression amiable to surgical treatment, such as disk herniation or extradural spinal hematoma. In a patient with neurological deficit unrelated to the spine fracture level, a MRI is also indicated.

Spinal cord contusions are frequent in patients with a congenitally narrow spinal canal (spinal stenosis) or with a severely spondylitic spine. An additional application for MRI is the ability to visualize vascular structures. MR arteriogram can therefore be used to assess the patency of the vertebral arteries. Multiple spinal injuries are sometimes evident on screening MRI images of the whole spine, but often these lesions do not have a relation with the mechanism of the main injury, and careful consideration of any further action must be considered [17, 38]. The major drawbacks of MRI are the logistic problems with the magnetic field, and the need for special monitoring equipment for the severely injured patient. It is also time consuming and there is a risk associated with delayed investigations while keeping patients in cervical collars [37, 39, 40]. The role of prereduction MRI for facet dislocation remains controversial.

14.5.4 Hospital Resuscitation: Workup

Individually adapted care for the patient is preferable. However, the spinal cord injury patients need intensive care at least during the first 24 h to maintain adequate assessment of critical parameters and treatment options.

14.5.5 Cervical Traction

Cervical spine injuries can often be treated with traction initially. It can improve cervical spine deformity, decompress nerves, and provide stability. Acute stabilization of the cervical spine with a halo ring has been advocated [41]. Once the emergent surgical care has been completed, the definitive treatment of the cervical injury can be determined with the use of the halo vest as an alternative [42]. Hearly et al. reported that six out of ten patients had undergone surgical procedures performed after halo ring application, and none of the patients had any neurological deterioration. This result exemplifies the importance of effective communication among the many disciplines involved in the treatment of the severely injured patient. The spinal surgeon provides safety in treatment of the spinal injury, while trauma surgeons can address the life-threatening injuries. The principles for halo ring/cervical tong application have been well described [7, 43, 62, 63]. Adherence to established application guidelines is critical to minimize morbidity.

14.5.5.1 Spinal Cord Injury Units

Neuroprotective Drugs

The objective of pharmacological treatment is reduction of symptom, prophylaxis, and treatment of complications. Patient with spinal cord injury should be treated at intensive care units and be transferred as soon as possible to spinal cord units. The secondary injury mechanism has been studied, and different neuroprotective substances have been tried in order to decrease the negative consequences of the tissue trauma. In clinical practice, corticosteroids have been used. The role of steroids remains controversial and should not be recommended as standard treatment unless incomplete spinal cord injury is suspected [44].

Stroke Prevention

Blunt cerebral vascular injuries (BCVI), primarily arterial dissection, may occur in association with cervical spine trauma [34]. Early diagnosis and treatment reduces morbidity and mortality in patients with vertebral artery injuries [45].

Antithrombotic therapy in form of antiplatelet (aspirin) and or anticoagulation (heparin) should be started if there are no contraindications, and in some cases endovascular stent therapy is an option.

Thrombosis Prophylaxis

Patients with instable spine injuries will often be immobilized for the first days in the hospital. It is therefore important to prevent deep venous thrombosis (DVT). Spinal cord injury causes low smooth muscle tone in the vessels and blood pooling in the extremities. This increases the risk of DVT. Early mobilization and exercise is important. Stockings, intermittent pneumatic compression devices, and pharmacological anti-thrombosis prophylaxis are used, if not contraindicated.

14.6 Treatment

The goal of treatment is to restore mechanical and neurological functions, initiate rehabilitation, reduce pain, and prevent spinal deformity and complications. No universal guideline is available today, so we rely primarily on common sense protocols to answer the following critical questions: Can I securely remove the neck brace? Can the patient be mobilized safely? Is urgent surgery required?

14.6.1 Nonsurgical Treatment

14.6.1.1 External Orthosis

The major objective of nonoperative treatment is the same as for surgical treatment: Avoid neurological deterioration, and if it arises take action to reverse it, while maintaining an acceptable spine anatomy during the treatment to allow healing of the injury in reasonable time under physiologic loads. Optimal management must also consider early patient mobilization. To achieve these important goals, good patient selection, resource utilization, and competence to complete the nonsurgical treatment are needed.

Spinal orthosis are frequently used in nonsurgical treatment. They can restrict motion of the spine by acting indirectly to reinforce the intervening soft tissue. Despite the heterogeneity of designs, the functions of all braces are analogous and include restriction of spinal movements, maintenance of spinal alignment, reduction of pain, and support of the trunk musculature.

14.6.1.2 Cervical Braces Rigid: Cervical Collars

Rigid cervical collars can be used as definitive therapy for some spinal injuries, as a temporary immobilizer for postinjury transport or during the early hospital management. Rigid cervical collars do not adequately immobilize by their use alone and must be properly sized for each patient. The Stifneck® Select™ Collars ease of application favors its use in the prehospital setting, and its effectiveness of cervical stabilization is comparable to other high cervicothoracic orthoses. The limitation of Stifneck is that it is uncomfortable for the patient and could cause skin ulcer. Therefore should the Stifneck be replaced by other rigid collars (Philadelphia, Newport/Aspen, Miami J.) during the first 24 h. Cervical bracing with the addition of a thoracic vest (SOMI and Minerva braces) and halo-vest immobilization increases the stability.

14.6.1.3 Thoracolumbar Orthosis

In the thoracic spine, the rib cage provides some natural support for thoracic spine fractures. The upper thoracic region (TH5) and above is a very difficult region to immobilize with an external orthosis, often requiring immobilization with a halo orthosis and a long thoracic vest. Spinal fractures from T6 to L2 are typically braced with a three-point fixation system (Jewett brace) that maintains extension of the thoracolumbar area or with a custom molded, hard shell orthosis (Body Jacket). Below L3, a lumbosacral orthosis is used for support. In order to increase the immobilization at the lumbosacral junction, a leg extension can be fitted to the orthosis to assist in limiting motion across the pelvis. Casting is another option for lumbar and thoracolumbar fractures and can provide better support and eliminate concerns of noncompliance.

14.6.2 Surgical Treatment

Most spine fractures can be treated nonsurgically. Only a small select group of unstable spine injuries with or without neurologic association merit surgical treatment. Two primary goals for the surgical treatment are: decompression of compromised/threatened neuronal elements and maintenance of spinal stability. A clearcut treatment recommendation does not exist which is partially a result of inconsistent injury description in the literature that makes extrapolation of data difficult. The spinal fracture, patient, and associated injury/factors have to be interpreted before surgery is chosen as treatment option. Controversy persists in the surgical community regarding the optimal treatment of many traumatic spinal injuries, especially regarding timing of surgical intervention and type of surgical approach (Fig. 14.3a, b).

14.6.2.1 Damage Control Spine Surgery

Frequently, the question arises as to which patient needs definitive surgery according to the principles of early total spine care and which patient is in need of a staged procedure after initial stabilization. Since no data exists for the multiple injured patients with spine trauma, one has to adopt information from general trauma [46, 47, 65]. Hemodynamically unstable patients with signs of shock, suffering from the lethal triad of hypothermia, coagulopathy, and acidosis, have high mortality rates and should be submitted to staged definitive fixation [48]. Since no cutoff parameters are defined to separate each treatment principle, the decision making has to be done on an individual basis.

14.6.2.2 Secondary Surgery After Resuscitation and Restoration of Immunologic Homoeostasis

Following life-saving management of thoracic or abdominal injuries including also damage control stabilization of pelvis and femoral fractures, definitive surgery can be performed. In spine trauma, the initial stabilization of the cervical spine with halo/traction tongs could be converted to halo vest or open surgery [41]. In the thoracolumbar spine primary stabilized with posterior internal fixations, additional anterior surgery could be performed safely at day 7–10 post trauma assuming an uneventful recovery period [49, 50].

Patients suffering from prolonged inflammatory reactions (SIRS) are scheduled for secondary surgery as recovery dictates.

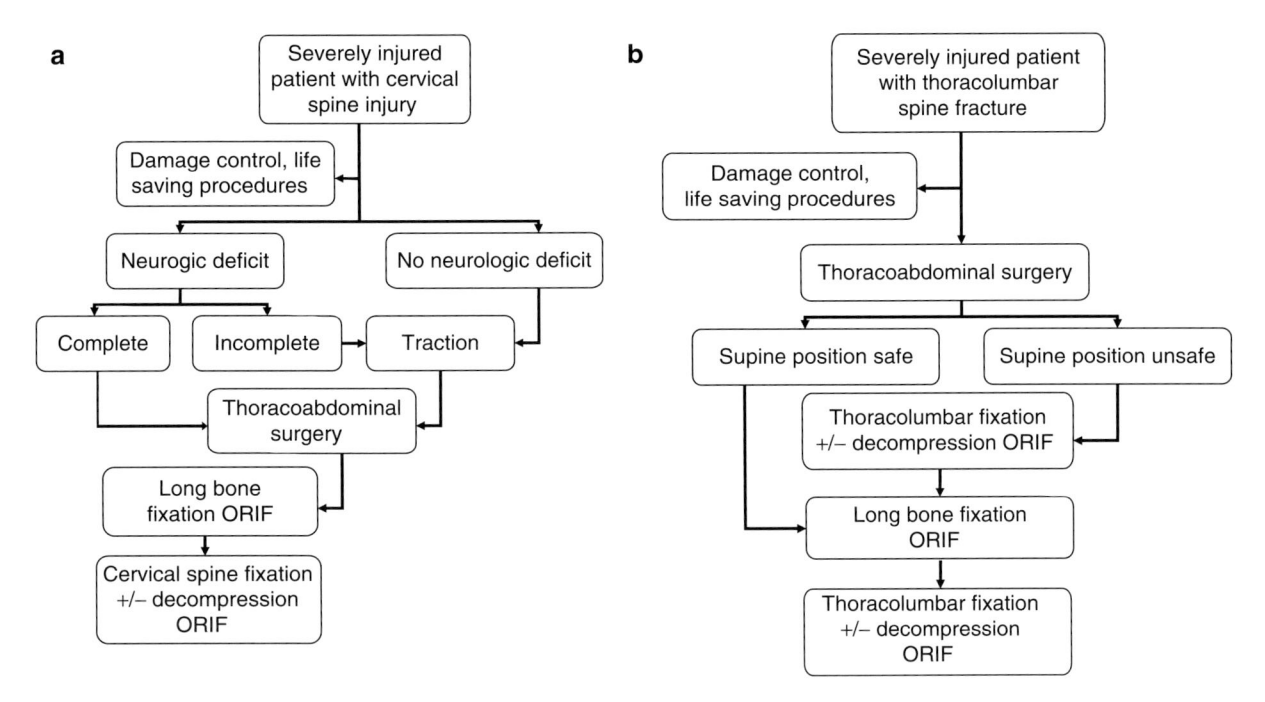

Fig. 14.3 Algorithm for the surgical management of a severely injured patient with (**a**) cervical fractures and (**b**) thoracolumbar fractures. *ORIF* open reduction and internal fixation

14.6.2.3 Surgical Timing

Surgical timing is an important but difficult consideration, especially in multiply injured patients. The optimal timing of surgery after spinal injury remains controversial. Animal studies have suggested a significant benefit from early decompression after acute spinal cord injury. Little human clinical evidence is available to support the belief that early surgical decompression and stabilization improves neurological recovery rates. Management of the severely injured patient depends on other injuries and the subsequent consequences of different treatments, which makes the timing of surgical strategies a matter for a professional cooperation. The only randomized, controlled trial states that surgery performed for cervical spinal cord injuries less than 72 h versus more than 5 days after the injury demonstrated no significant difference in motor scores at final follow-up [51]. Early spinal stabilization can be performed safely in the multiple-trauma patient in medical centers, where the medical and ancillary staff are available on a 24-h basis and are familiar with these procedures [52]. A meta-analysis provided the following guidelines: urgent decompression of bilateral locked facets in patients with incomplete tetraplegia or in patients with spinal cord injury, and neurological deterioration [53]. Urgent decompression in any acute cervical spinal cord injury remains a reasonable practice option and can be performed safely. Indications for urgent (within 24 h) spinal stabilization have been advocated in the presence of extensive polytrauma that predisposes to severe pulmonary and/or metabolic derangement if not mobilized and if associated injuries dictate acute surgical treatment and chest trauma and pulmonary contusions predict pulmonary deterioration [32]. They concluded that urgent spinal stabilization is safe and appropriate in polytrauma patients when progressive neurologic deficit, thoracoabdominal trauma, or fracture instability increases the risks of delayed treatment. However, there was small sample in their study and it did not reach statistical significances in outcome measures. Another study of severely injured patients with spinal trauma [54] reported contrasting outcome of early stabilization (within 72 h); however, this study's findings were also not significant. Their findings were discussed and could be due to the fact that the stabilization procedure represented the critical "second hit" popularized by Pape et al. [48].

In most institutions, stabilization of the other spinal fractures is performed in a semi-urgent fashion once medical optimization of the patient has been accomplished, preferably within 3 days of the injury. Late surgical intervention may require more extensive surgery to achieve spinal alignment, decompression, and stability.

Surgical Options

Anterior, posterior, and combined anterior and posterior approaches can be used to treat traumatic spinal instability. The surgical approach selected may depend on the fracture type, neurological status, and the individual preference of the surgeon. Anterior approaches may be favored in situations where a herniated disk or bone fragment is causing ventral compression on the spinal cord. If in addition, fracture patterns are significantly compromised, they may be best addressed by an anterior approach to restore the structural stability of the anterior spinal column. The surgical approach includes in most cases spinal instrumentation as a method of straightening and stabilizing the spine. Hooks, rods, and wires to the spine rearrange the stresses on the bone and keep them in proper alignment. Posterior surgical approaches and instrumentation allow for better reduction when deformities are present and may be beneficial in restoring the posterior tension band in distraction injuries. With posterior instrumentation, there is restitution of the biomechanical forces needed to hold the spine in normal alignment. In fracture dislocations, when there is severe disruption of the spinal column, combined anterior-posterior instrumentation procedures may be used to maximize stability of the spinal column and increase fusion rates. There is no single preferred approach to many types of spinal fractures; often the preferences of the individual surgeon take precedence. Despite the maturation of surgical techniques and development of sophisticated instrumentation devices, there is a lack of good guidelines for the treatment of many fractures. In general, posterior approaches are favored for the thoracic and lumbar spine because of the ease and familiarity of approach. Today, pedicle screw fixation allows better fixation with fewer contact points than prior treatment, which required longer fusion constructs due to poor spinal element capture. Anterior approaches to the thoracic and lumbar spine tend to be more technically challenging since they involve mobilization of the lung, viscera, and great vessels.

14.6.3 Special Situations

14.6.3.1 Gunshot/Open Injury

Decompression does not improve recovery if the bullet traverses the canal without any residual mass effect on neural elements [55]. Evidence of acute lead intoxication, an intracanal copper bullet, or new onset of neurologic deficit can justify operative decompression and/or bullet removal. Overzealous laminectomy can destabilize the spine and lead to late postoperative deformity. For complete and incomplete neural deficits at the cervical and thoracic levels, operative decompression is of little benefit and can lead to higher complication rates than nonoperative management. With gunshots to the T12 to L5 levels, better motor recovery has been reported after intracanal bullet removal versus nonoperative treatment [56]. Surgery may also be necessary for dural repair in patients with a persistent cerebrospinal fluid leak. Debridement and removal of the bullet is an option during laparotomy for abdominal injury. If the projectile traverses the oropharynx or intestine, intravenous broad-spectrum antibiotics should be administered for 3 days as prophylaxis.

14.6.3.2 Ankylosing Spondylitis (AS), Diffuse Idiopathic Skeletal Hyperostosis (DISH)

Fractures in patients with AS or DISH are deemed unstable until proven otherwise and should be treated as such. Patients should be immobilized as soon as the diagnosis is made. These patients usually have a preinjury deformity, which should be kept in place during the workup. Strict logroll precautions are used until definitive management has been decided.

The spine is commonly fused to a solid piece of bone and the level arm strongly influences the fracture, causing a potentially severely unstable spine.

14.6.3.3 Spinal Cord Injury Without Instability in the Spondylotic Spine

In patients with complete or incomplete spinal cord injury without radiographic signs of an injury, fracture or ligament instability, a cervical spinal stenosis frequently occurs. The role and timing of surgery is controversial.

14.6.3.4 Pediatric Patients

In children, ligamentous injuries are more frequent than bony injury. These pediatric injury patterns transition to adult types at 11 years of age. Most pediatric injuries occur in the upper cervical spine between the occiput and C3 because the ratio of mass between the head and the body is disproportionate at this location. Spinal cord injury without radiographic abnormality (SWICORA) commonly occurs in children younger than 11 years. The mechanism of these injuries is not fully understood but is likely to be a fracture of the cartilaginous vertebral endplate, which in turn leads to distraction of the cord and ischemic injury. Children with spinal tenderness or questionable radiographic findings should be treated by immobilization until their symptoms resolve or until reliable radiographic review has been made.

14.6.3.5 Geriatric Patients

Spondylosis is more frequent in elderly patients and results in a higher prevalence of associated spinal cord injury. What would otherwise be a minor, low-energy injury mechanism can result in markedly unstable injuries in an older patient. Treatment is often demanding, older patients poorly tolerate external bracing, and surgical interventions often carry an additional risk of complications due to age-related medical conditions. Halo therapy is almost impossible in these elderly patients. Commonly osteoporosis compromises stabilization procedures. All in all the elderly spine management often leads to a combined nonoperative and operative treatment in order to complete the treatment course.

14.7 Clinical Outcome

The clinical outcome of patients with spinal injuries is difficult to assess. Most of the available literature focuses on isolated spinal injuries. It is common sense that patients with spine injuries and other severe multiple injuries have a higher rate of disability, occupational handicap, and risk for ongoing incapacitating pain [57].

A 5-year follow-up study by Mclain et al. assessed functional outcome in patients with thoracic, thoracolumbar, or lumbar fractures as a result of all high-energy trauma [35]. Thirty-eight percent of these patients were polytrauma patients (ISS = 26 used for threshold definition of polytrauma). Patients limited by pain were more often impaired by residual radicular and neuropathic symptoms than by back pain. Mclain noted that patients with persistent back pain generally had an identifiable and correctable mechanical problem, such as sagittal imbalance, pseudarthrosis, or persistent instability. Forty-four percent of patients had functional limitations at follow-up, and it was found that neurologic injury, more than any other factor, determined functional outcome.

A long-term follow-up in 52 spine fracture patients is in concordance with the previous literature, in that higher ISS and severe initial neurologic injury are associated with worse outcome [58]. Thereby, a longer time interval for follow-up does not appear to be associated with a better outcome. This seems to suggest that no further improvement occurs in the long run. The authors found no difference in outcome between patients who had minimal neurologic deficit after cervical, thoracic, or lumbar spine fractures, when the injury occurred in isolation. This may be a surprising finding since one might expect differences in outcome following different injury levels. However, these patients all had minimal neurological deficits and statistically comparable ISS scores. Studies in the literature which have categorized spine patients according to fracture level have noted dissimilar initial injury severities and found dissimilar outcomes among the groups. A study by Saboe et al. found a significant difference in the presence or absence of associated injuries and spine fracture level and concluded that the presence of associated injuries meant patients were less likely to have neurological deficits [59]. Spine trauma patients were also assessed according to fracture level by Schinkel et al. and a difference in accompanied trauma injuries was found, that was then also related to in-hospital stay and short-term outcome [60]. A 10-year follow-up has demonstrated that patients who suffered multiple level spinal fractures had worse general outcomes in comparison with those in the isolated single region injury category, and significantly better than the paraplegic group (Table 14.3). Patients with spinal fractures continue to be a medical challenge.

Table 14.3 General outcome variables in patients with spinal fractures at the 10-year time point

Outcomes	Groups						p-value
	Cervical	Thoracic	Lumbar	Single	Multiple	Paraplegia	(<0.05)*
Limp	2/9	3/7	5/19	10/35	3/6	N/A	n.s.
Use of sp. aids	2/9	2/7	4/19	8/35	4/6	10/11	0.001
Polytrauma outcome score (overall)	76.8 (15.3–190.5)	65.3 (38.2–85.1)	60.3 (13.6–153.0)	67.0	106.6 (59.2–148.9)	137.1 (80.5–181.3)	0.001
Polytrauma outcome score (patient assessed)	57.8 (11.1–133.5)	44.5 (20.362.4)	43.7 (8.6–95.2)	48.3	69.0 (45.0–88.9)	72.5 (34.1–106.2)	0.02
Polytrauma outcome score (physician assessed)	19 (4.2–57.0)	20.8 (8.9–34.1)	16.7 (0.7–67.0)	18.6	37.6 (14.2–67.1)	64.6 (28.8–119.3)	0.001
SF-12 (PCS)	42.0 (25.4–56.3)	46.4 (37.2–57.6)	43.9 (25.1–56.9)	43.6	40.5 (28.3–50.5)	34.6 (19.8–45.1)	0.02
SF-12 (MCS)	50.7 (30.9–67.3)	49.7 (32.3–58.1)	49.2 (24.6–59.9)	49.4	47.5 (39.9–57.4)	56.7 (39.0–69.8)	n.s.
Use of meds before accident	0/9	0/7	1/19	1/35	1/6	1/11	n.s.
Use of meds after accident	1/9	1/7	8/19	10/35	4/6	7/11	0.05

n.s. Not significant

*p-value comparing all five unshaded groups (excluding group "Single")

References

1. Court-Brown CM, Caesar B. Epidemiology of adult fractures: a review. Injury. 2006;37:691–7.
2. Laurer H, Maier B, El Saman A, et al. Distribution of spinal and associated injuries in multiple trauma patients. Eur J Trauma Emerg Surg. 2007;33:476–81.
3. Chen HY, Chiu WT, Chen SS, et al. A Nationwide epidemiological study of spinal cord injuries in Taiwan from July 1992 to June 1996. Neurol Res. 1997;19:617–22.
4. Cooper C, Atkinson EJ, O'Fallon WM, et al. Incidence of clinically diagnosed vertebral fractures: a population-based study in Rochester, Minnesota, 1985–1989. J Bone Miner Res. 1992;7:221–7.
5. Hu R, Mustard CA, Burns C. Epidemiology of incident spinal fracture in a complete population. Spine. 1996;21: 492–9.
6. Jansson KÅ, Blomqvist P, Svedmark P, et al. Thoracolumbar vertebral fractures in Sweden: an analysis of 13,496 patients admitted to hospital. Eur J Epidemiol. 2010;6:431–7.
7. Kang M, Vives MJ, Vaccaro AR. The Halo vest: principles of application and management of complications. J Trauma. 2003;33:445–51.
8. Kanis JA, Johnell O, Oden A, et al. Long term risk of osteoporotic fracture in Malmo. Osteoporos Int. 2000;11: 669–74.
9. National Spinal Cord Injury Data Base, Spinal Cord Injury Information Network. http://www.spinalcord.uab.edu/show.asp?durki=24480 (2009).
10. Levi AD, Hurlbert RJ, Anderson P, et al. Neurologic deterioration secondary to unrecognized spinal instability following trauma–a multicenter study. Spine. 2006;15:451–8.
11. De Knegt C, Meylaerts SAG, Leenen LPH. Applicability of the trimodal distribution of trauma deaths in a Level I trauma centre in the Netherlands with a population of mainly blunt trauma. Injury. 2008;9:993–1000.
12. Gomes E, Araújo R, Carneiro A, et al. Mortality distribution in a trauma system: from data to health policy recommendations. Eur J Trauma Emerg Surg. 2008;34:561–9.
13. American College of Surgeons Committee on Trauma. Advanced trauma life support for doctors, student course manual, 8th ed. Chicago: American College of Surgeons; 2007.
14. Eastern Association for the Surgery of trauma (EAST). Determination of cervical spine stability in trauma patients. http://www.east.org/tpg/chap3u.pdf (2009).
15. Stiell IG, Clement CM, Grimshaw J. Implementation of the Canadian C-Spine Rule: prospective 12 centre cluster randomised trial. BMJ. 2009;339:b4146.
16. Stiell IG, Clement CM, McKnight RD, et al. The Canadian C-spine rule versus the Nexus low risk criteria in patients with trauma. N Engl J Med. 2003;25:2510–18.
17. PHTLS basic and advanced prehospital trauma life support, 6th ed. St. Louis: Mosby Jems; 2007.
18. Holly LT, Kelly DF, Counelis GJ, et al. Cervical spine trauma associated with moderate and severe head injury: incidence, risk factors, and injury characteristics. J Neurosurg. 2002;96: 285–91.

19. Anderson S, Biros MH, Reardon RF. Delayed diagnosis of thoracolumbar fractures in multiple-trauma patients. Acad Emerg Med. 1996;3:832–9.
20. Schmidt OI, Heyde CE, Ertel W, et al. Closed head injury-an inflammatory disease? Brain Res Brain Res Rev. 2005;48: 388–99.
21. Baptiste DC, Fehlings MG. Update on the treatment of spinal cord injury. Prog Brain Res. 2007;161:217–33.
22. American Spinal Injury Association (ASIA). http://www.asia-spinalinjury.org/publications/2006_Classif_worksheet.pdf (2006).
23. Holmes JF, Akkinepalli R. Computed tomography versus plain radiography to screen for cervical spine injury: a meta-analysis. J Trauma. 2005;5:902–5.
24. Antevil JL, Sise MJ, Sack DI, et al. Spiral computed tomography for the initial evaluation of spine trauma: a new standard of care? J Trauma. 2006;61:382–7.
25. Hauser CJ, Visvikis G, Hinrichs C, et al. Prospective validation of computed tomographic screening of the thoracolumbar spine in trauma. J Trauma. 2003;55:228–35.
26. Hessmann MH, Hofmann A, Kreitner KF, et al. The benefit of multislice CT in the emergency room management of polytraumatized patients. Acta Chir Belg. 2006;106:500–7.
27. Lennquist S, editor. Traumatologi. Stockholm: Liber AB; 2007. p. 113–6. ISBN 978-91-47-05216-5.
28. Brown CV, Antevil JL, Sise MJ, et al. Spiral computed tomography for the diagnosis of cervical, thoracic, and lumbar spine fractures: its time has come. J Trauma. 2005; 58:890–5.
29. Qaiyum M, Tyrrell PN, McCall IW, et al. MRI detection of unsuspected vertebral injury in acute spinal trauma: incidence and significance. Skeletal Radiol. 2001;30: 299–304.
30. White III AA, Panjabi MM. The problem of clinical instability in the human spine: a systematic approach. In: White III AA, Panjabi MM, editors. Clinical biomechanics of the spine. Philadelphia: JB Lippincott; 1990. p. 277–378.
31. Blauth M, Knop C, Bastian L, et al. Complex injuries of the spine. Orthopade. 1998;27:17–31.
32. McLain RF, Benson DR. Urgent surgical stabilization of spinal fractures in polytrauma patients. Spine. 1999;24: 1263–654.
33. Rihn JA, Anderson DT, Harris E, et al. A review of the TLICS system: a novel, user-friendly thoracolumbar trauma classification system. Acta Orthop. 2008;79:461–6.
34. Fassett DR, Dailey AT, Vaccaro AR. Vertebral artery injuries associated with cervical spine injuries: a review of the literature. J Spinal Disord Tech. 2008;21:252–8.
35. Mclain RF, Burkus JK, Benson DR. Segmental instrumentation for thoracic and thoracolumbar fractures: prospective analysis of construct survival and five-year follow-up. Spine J. 2001;1(5):310–23.
36. Cothren CC, Moore EE, Ray Jr CE, et al. Cervical spine fracture patterns mandating screening to rule out blunt cerebrovascular injury. Surgery. 2007;141:76–82.
37. Dunham CM, Brocker BP, Collier BD, et al. Risks associated with magnetic resonance imaging and cervical collar in comatose, blunt trauma patients with negative comprehensive cervical spine computed tomography and no apparent spinal deficit. Crit Care. 2008;12:R89.
38. Green RA, Saifuddin A. Whole spine MRI in the assessment of acute vertebral body trauma. Skeletal Radiol. 2004;33: 129–35.
39. Como JJ, Thompson MA, Anderson JS, et al. Is magnetic resonance imaging essential in clearing the cervical spine in obtunded patients with blunt trauma? J Trauma. 2007;63: 544–9.
40. Hogan GJ, Mirvis SE, Shanmuganathan K, et al. Exclusion of unstable cervical spine injury in obtunded patients with blunt trauma: is MR imaging needed when multi-detector row CT findings are normal? Radiology. 2005;237: 106–13.
41. Heary RF, Hunt CD, Krieger AJ, et al. Acute stabilization of the cervical spine by halo/vest application facilitates evaluation and treatment of multiple trauma patients. J Trauma. 1992;33:445–51.
42. Perry J, Nickel VL. Total cervical-spine fusion for neck paralysis. J Bone Joint Surg Am. 1959;41:37–60.
43. Barnett GH, Hardy RW. Gardner tongs and cervical traction. Med Instrum. 1982;16:291–2.
44. Sayer FT, Kronvall E, Nilsson OG. Methylprednisolone treatment in acute spinal cord injury: the myth challenged through a structured analysis of published literature. Spine J. 2006;6:335–43.
45. Schneidereit NP, Simons R, Nicolaou S, et al. Utility of screening for blunt vascular neck injuries with computed tomographic angiography. J Trauma. 2006;60:209–15.
46. Pape HC, Grimme K, Van Greinsven M, et al. Impact of intramedullary instrumentation versus damage control for femoral fractures on immunoinflammatory parameters: prospective randomized analysis by the EPOFF Study Group. J Trauma. 2003;55:7–13.
47. Scalea TM, Boswell SA, Scott JD, et al. External fixation as a bridge to intramedullary nailing for patients with multiple injuries and with femur fractures: damage control orthopedics. J Trauma. 2000;48:613–21.
48. Pape HC, Giannoudis P, Krettec C. The timing of fracture treatment in polytrauma patients: relevance of damage control orthopedic surgery. Am J Surg. 2002;183:622–9.
49. Keel M, Labler L, Trentz O. Damage control in severely injured patients: why, when and how? Eur J Trauma. 2005; 31:212–21.
50. Kossman T, Trease L, Freedman I, et al. Damage control surgery for spine trauma. Injury. 2004;35:661–70.
51. Vaccaro AR, Daugherty RJ, Sheehan TP, et al. Neurologic outcome of early versus late surgery for cervical spinal cord injury. Spine. 1997;22:2609–13.
52. Harris MB, Sethi RK. The initial assessment and management of the multiple-trauma patient with an associated spine injury. Spine. 2006;31(11 Suppl):S9–15.
53. Fehlings MG, Perrin RG. The role and timing of early decompression for cervical spinal cord injury: update with a review of recent clinical evidence. Injury. 2005;36(2): B13–26.
54. Kerwin AJ, Frykberg ER, Schinco MA, et al. The effect of early spine fixation on non-neurologic outcome. J Trauma. 2005;58:15–21.
55. Stauffer ES, Kelly EG. Gunshot wounds of the spine. The effects of laminectomy. J Bone Joint Surg Am. 1976;61: 389–92.

56. Bono CM, Heary RF. Gunshot wounds to the spine. Spine J. 2004;4:230–40.
57. Hebert JS, Burnham RS. The effect of polytrauma in persons with traumatic spine injury. A prospective database of spine fractures. Spine. 2000;25(1):55–60.
58. Darwiche SS, Probst C, Steel JL, et al. Spinal fractures in multiple trauma patients – what is the long term outcome? (Abstract AAST 2009).
59. Saboe LA, Reid DC, Davis LA, Warren SA, Grace MG. Spine trauma and associated injuries. J Trauma. 1991;31(1):43–8.
60. Schinkel C, Frangen TM, Kmetic A, Andress HJ, Muhr G, der DGU AG Polytrauma. Spinal fractures in multiply injured patients: an analysis of the German Trauma Society's Trauma Register. Unfallchirurg. 2007;110(11):946–52.
61. Biffl WL, Cothren CC, Moore EE, et al. Western Trauma Association critical decisions in trauma: screening for and treatment of blunt cerebrovascular injuries. J Trauma. 2009;67:1150–3.
62. Gardner WJ. The principle of spring-loaded points for cervical traction. Technical note. J Neurosurg. 1973;39:543–4.
63. Manthey DE. Halo traction device. Emerg Med Clin North Am. 1994;12:771–8.
64. NORDTER, Nordic trauma forum for trauma and emergency radiology. Handling Blunt Cerebro-Vascular Injuries (BCVI) carotid and vertebral – An evidence based recommendation. www.nordictraumarad.com/concensus/FINAL%20BCVI%20consensus%20Aronsborg%2020071023.pdf (2007).
65. Rupp RE, Ebraheim NA, Chrissos MG, et al. Thoracic and lumbar fractures associated with femoral shaft fractures in the multiple trauma patient. Occult presentations and implications for femoral fracture stabilization. Spine. 1994;19: 556–60.
66. Wintermark M, Mouhsine E, Theumann N, et al. Thoracolumbar spine fractures in patients who have sustained severe trauma: depiction with multi-detector row CT. Radiology. 2003;227:681–9.

The Management of the Multiply Injured Elderly Patient

Charles M. Court-Brown and N. Clement

Contents

15.1	Introduction	167
15.2	**Multiple Injuries**	168
15.2.1	Epidemiology	168
15.2.2	Motor Vehicle Accidents	169
15.2.3	Falls from a Height	170
15.2.4	Falls	171
15.3	**Treatment**	171
15.4	**Predictors of Mortality**	171
15.5	**Outcome**	172
15.5.1	Polytrauma	172
15.5.2	Falls	173
15.6	**Types of Injury**	173
15.6.1	Head Injury	174
15.6.2	Multiple Fractures	174
15.6.3	Fall-Related Multiple Fractures	175
References		177

C.M. Court-Brown (✉) and N. Clement
Department of Orthopaedic Surgery, Royal Infirmary
of Edinburgh, Old Dalkeith Road, Edinburgh, EH16 4SU, UK
e-mail: courtbrown@aol.co.uk

15.1 Introduction

The management of the multiply injured patient improved significantly in the 1960s and 1970s in a number of countries. Specialist trauma centres were established, and the importance of early resuscitation and surgical treatment was appreciated. However, very little interest was taken in the management of the severely injured elderly patient until the 1980s, when a number of papers on this topic were published. In 1984, Oreskovich et al. [1] published the results of the treatment of 100 consecutive patients who were older than 70 years of age. They documented a 15% mortality but noted that while 85% of their patients survived, 88% of them did not return to their previous level of independence. They also observed that the Injury Severity Score (ISS) [2] was not predictive of survival in this elderly group.

DeMaria and his colleagues [3] took a somewhat more optimistic view of the benefits of aggressive trauma care in the multiply injured elderly. In 1987, they published the results of 63 survivors of blunt trauma who were over 65 years of age. They pointed out that the overall level of injury was moderate, with a mean ISS of 15.8; they noted that only 62% of their patients had injuries in two or more body regions and that 71% of the patients had pre-existing cardiovascular disease. Prior to injury, 97% of the patients were independent; but after treatment and rehabilitation, 89% of patients returned to an independent existence although they pointed out that these patients tended to be younger, and to have had a shorter hospital stay and fewer complications. Of the 12 patients in their study who were aged 80 years or more, only 8 (66.6%) returned home. Their conclusion was that aggressive support of the elderly was justified as few required permanent nursing home care and the majority returned to independent living.

This study also examined the factors related to failure to survive trauma in older patients. The authors showed that non-survivors were older and had more severe overall injury. They also had more serious head and neck trauma, but there was no difference in the severity of non-head and neck trauma, the mechanism of injury, or the requirement for surgery. Non-survivors had more frequent complications including a higher prevalence of cardiovascular complications and a greater requirement for ventilation for 5 or more days. They took the view that a number of complications were potentially avoidable and therefore aggressive treatment of geriatric trauma was indicated.

In 1989, Champion et al. [4] analysed data from 3,833 patients aged 65 years or more in the Major Trauma Outcome Study (MTOS) and showed that 20.7% of older patients injured in motor vehicle accidents died. In this analysis, they pointed out that 28.2% of the elderly patient group had been injured in motor vehicle accidents compared with 40.6% who had been injured in falls and that 11.7% of the latter group had died. They concluded that the perception of injury as a disease of the young resulted in people failing to recognise the importance of trauma in the elderly. They suggested that trauma systems and trauma centres might be put in place to treat elderly patients. Champion and his colleagues [5] also analysed a group of 180 elderly trauma patients aged 65 years or more and compared their results with a similarly injured group of younger patients. They also used a nationally collected database to analyse mortality at different ages. They showed that mortality increased with age and that this increase occurred at all ISS scores, in all mechanisms of injury and in all body regions. Older patients had higher complication rates, and this was particularly true for pulmonary and infectious complications. They theorised that triaging elderly trauma patients to trauma centres at a lower threshold of injury to similarly injured younger patients would be beneficial.

Since these papers were published, there has been an increasing awareness of the importance of trauma in the elderly population, this group usually being defined as patients aged at least 65 years. However, there are difficulties in defining what constitutes severe trauma in the elderly population. Superficially, the concept of severe injury is straightforward and one can specify that the ISS should be at least 16 or that there should be injuries in multiple body systems. However, Champion et al. [4] pointed out that there was a significant mortality following simple falls and that in the elderly population, an ISS of 0–8 was associated with a mortality of 2.9% and a complication rate of 16.2%. An ISS of 9–15 was associated with a mortality of 6.9% and a complication rate of 31.1%. It is now generally accepted that in the elderly population, the mortality of low-energy injury is relatively high and the common fragility fractures, particularly those of the proximal femur, are associated with significant mortality. It is also accepted that minor head injuries in the elderly may prove fatal.

One of the consequences of the high mortality associated with low-energy injuries in the elderly is that, understandably, many of these patients are admitted to trauma centres where they can receive specialist trauma management. This has resulted in some confusion in papers discussing the problem of trauma in the elderly population. Some studies have specifically looked at polytraumatised older patients with injuries in more than one body system or an ISS of at least 16 whereas other studies have examined all patients admitted to certain types of hospital. Obviously, the results from these two types of study will be different. In this chapter, we have accepted that it is difficult to define what constitutes multiple trauma or severe injury in the elderly population and we have examined both patients with multiple body system injures and those with multiple fractures.

15.2 Multiple Injuries

15.2.1 Epidemiology

It is generally assumed that the incidence of polytrauma in the elderly is increasing and, indeed, this does seem to be the case. There is no doubt that the incidence of the elderly in the population is increasing rapidly. In 2000, 12% of the population of the United States was at least 65 years of age, with 5.9% being 75 years or older and 1.5% being 85 years or older. It has been postulated that by 2030, 20% of the population will be aged 65 years or more and 2.5% will be aged 85 years or more [6]. In the United Kingdom, it has become clear that the fastest growing group in the population are the nonagenarians (≥90 years), who made up 0.58% of the population in 2001 but will probably comprise 1.2% of the population in 2025 [7].

United Kingdom statistics have also shown that the increase in the population of the elderly is not being matched by improved health. In 2008, the National Office of Statistics stated that while the population of the United Kingdom had been living longer over the previous 23 years, the time that both sexes could be expected to be in poor health or have a limiting illness or disability had risen between 1988 and 2004 [8]. There were some minor improvements after 2004, but it is clear that increased longevity will be matched by poorer health and an increasing incidence of medical comorbidities. This is particularly important in severe or multiple trauma as medical comorbidities help to dictate the prognosis in the elderly. The fact is that the problem is already occurring in orthopaedic trauma. Figures from Edinburgh, Scotland in 2000 show that while nonagenarians make up 0.58% of the population, they account for 3.02% of the fractures in the community, 8.7% of the in-patient admissions and 7.6% of the acute orthopaedic trauma surgery [9].

However, the increase in the elderly population has to be balanced against a presumed decrease in motor vehicle accidents in many countries. In the United Kingdom in 2001, 9.7% of motor vehicle accident casualties were 60 years or more, but this represents a decline of 2.1% since 1994–1998 [10]. As there is no formalised trauma system in the United Kingdom, this improvement shows the value of accident prevention. It seems reasonable to assume that accident prevention will improve in other countries and the incidence of motor vehicle accident casualties will decline. However, a contrary view has been put forward by the World Health Organisation, which listed motor vehicle trauma as the 11th most common cause of death in 2002 but forecast that it would become the 3rd most common cause of death by 2020 [11].

It is difficult to be precise about the future epidemiology of multiple trauma in the elderly, but there is no doubt that low-energy multiple fractures will be an increasing problem because of the increasing number of falls in a progressively older, less fit population. It has been estimated that about 10% of falls cause severe injury [12], and a recent Swedish study has shown that 7% of falls in the elderly result in fracture [13]. It is likely that fall-related fractures will increase in frequency in the future and the Center of Disease Control and Prevention in the United States has suggested that in 2020, the cost of falls may reach $54.9 billion [14].

As has already been pointed out, it is difficult to estimate the prevalence of severe injury in the elderly population as the published data comes from hospitals that admit different categories of patients and different severities of injury. However, a review of the Trauma Audit and Research Network (TARN) database in the United Kingdom, which reviews all injured patients who arrive alive at hospitals and who are admitted for more than 72 h or who die within the 72 h period, shows that only 1.8% of patients have an ISS ≥16 and are 65 or more years of age [15]. Forty-two percent of the injuries followed motor vehicle accidents.

If one simply examines fractures in the 65+ year group data from the Royal Infirmary of Edinburgh in 2007/2008 [16] show that 36.9% of fractures occur in patients who are aged at least 65 years. However, 85.6% of these fractures follow a simple fall, only 1.3% of fractures occurring as a result of a motor vehicle accident and 0.6% occurring as a result of a fall from a height, these being the two common causes of high-energy injury. It is therefore apparent that severe injury in the elderly population is relatively rare whether this be polytrauma or high-energy fracture.

15.2.2 Motor Vehicle Accidents

Motor vehicle accidents are the cause of most high-energy injuries in the elderly although as has previously been discussed their overall prevalence is relatively low. If one excludes the studies that have included fall-related accidents, it becomes clear that the other causes of high-energy injury are relatively rare. Tornetta et al. [17] showed that 73.9% of high-energy polytrauma in the elderly was caused by motor vehicle accidents compared with 18.1% which were caused by falls from a height and 8% by crush injury and other causes. In this study, only 31.1% of the motor vehicle accident polytrauma cases were in elderly pedestrians. These figures are similar to European figures but, generally speaking, there are more pedestrian injuries in Europe. Broos et al. [18] studied 126 multiply injured elderly patients in Belgium. If the 30 fall-related injuries are excluded, 75% of the injuries followed motor vehicle accidents, with 44% being pedestrians. A further 28% were car occupants, 21% were bicyclists, and 7% were motorcyclists. In a large study from Germany, Kuhne et al. [19] showed that 53.2% of patients aged 56–75 years and 44.9% aged 76–95 years sustained multiple injuries as a result of motor vehicle accidents.

In view of the relatively high numbers of pedestrian injuries and fatalities in the elderly population, it is worth examining these injuries in more detail. A study from Los Angeles of 5,000 pedestrian versus motor vehicle accidents between 1994 and 1996 [20] showed that only 8% of the victims were aged 65 years or more. The average ISS of the elderly group was 12.3 which was higher than the paediatric and adult groups. The highest prevalence of injuries was musculoskeletal (40%) followed by head and neck injuries (31%) and external injuries (13.9%). There were very few spinal (5.4%) or chest injuries (3.4%). An analysis of the musculoskeletal injuries showed that in the elderly group, there were twice as many upper limb as lower limb fractures. The overall mortality for the 5,000 patients was 7.7%, but it varied greatly with age, with 3.1% mortality in the paediatric group, 8.1% in the adult group, and 27.8% in the elderly group.

Another analysis of a trauma registry in Los Angeles between 1993 and 2003 [21] involving 5,838 patients showed that 9.3% of pedestrians injured in motor vehicle accidents were older than 65 years. The authors analysed two groups of patients, those with an ISS >15 and those with an ISS >30. In both groups, patients over 65 years of age had the highest prevalence of injury. The elderly showed a high prevalence of severe head injury with an AIS >3 (23.7%), but lower prevalences of severe chest injury (8.8%), spinal injury (8.5%), abdominal injury (8.3%), and extremity injury (1.3%). The main head injuries were subarachnoid haematomas and brain contusions. The main extremity injuries were fractures of the pelvis and tibia. There was a similar distribution of fractures of the cervical, thoracic and lumbar spines. The overall mortality for all age groups was 7.7%, but in the 65+ year group, the mortality was 25.1%.

Similar figures were seen in an Australian study [22], where pedestrians aged 17–39 years had an average ISS of 14.1 and a mortality of 3.7%. The 40–64 year group had an average ISS of 13.4 and a mortality of 5.5%, but the ≥65 year group had an average ISS of 14.9 and a mortality of 22.7%. The authors highlighted intoxication in young males and injuries in the elderly population as being the two most important causes of pedestrian injuries.

In a recent study from Ireland [23], the authors analysed 3,232 accidents involving adult pedestrians. They documented that older adults represent 36% of adult pedestrian fatalities and 23% of serious injuries although they only accounted for 19% of adult pedestrian motor vehicle accidents. In this study, they attempted to analyse which conditions were associated with a higher rate of elderly pedestrian injuries and deaths. They showed that most accidents involving elderly pedestrians occurred in daylight with good visibility (56%) and in good weather conditions (77%). Older adults were less likely to be injured at night than younger adults, but they were more likely to be struck by trucks or heavy goods vehicles than younger patients. Accidents involving older pedestrians occurred at every type of road crossing, but the elderly were less likely to be injured at traffic lights or roundabouts. The authors emphasised the need for specialised accident prevention schemes for the elderly.

Another potential problem is increasing cognitive dysfunction in the elderly population. There is evidence that elderly patients may have an impaired ability to judge automobile speed [24] and may show poorer attention at road crossings [25]. A recent study has provided evidence that more elderly patients killed in pedestrian accidents had symptoms of dementia than age-matched controls [26]. This may well prove to be a significant problem in an increasingly aging population.

15.2.3 Falls from a Height

The other cause of high-energy injury is falls from a height. The extent of injury depends on the height of the fall and the elderly patients tend to fall from lower heights than younger patients. However, it is likely that injuries caused by falls from a height are more common than they previously were. An analysis of the distribution of fractures between the 1950s and 2007/2008 in the United Kingdom [16] shows that a number of fractures that used to be seen in the young now often occur in older fractures. A good example of this is the calcaneal fracture which is often caused by a fall from a height. This fracture is now relatively common in older patients.

An analysis of 1,613 patients who had fallen more than 15 ft [27] showed that in the 65+ year group, severe head and spinal injuries were most common, with a prevalence of 18.9% and 16.2%, respectively. The frequency of pelvic, femoral and tibial fractures increased with age such that the prevalence of these fractures in the 65+ year group was 18.7%, 18.9% and 8.1%, respectively.

15.2.4 Falls

In recent years, there has been an increase in the incidence of falls in the elderly. As has already been pointed out, there is good evidence that in older people, falls from a standing height may cause considerable injury and may be responsible for significant mortality. In an analysis of the changing epidemiology of injuries and mortality following falls in patients aged 50 years and above in Finland, Kannus et al. [28] showed significant changes between 1970 and 1995. They demonstrated that there had been a 284% increase in the number of older persons with a fall-induced injury during this period, and they showed that the annual increase in fall-induced injury was 9.9% for males and 12.1% for females. They did note that there had been a slight decline between 1970 and 1977 but found that there was a rapid and sharp increase in the incidence of fall-induced injury after 1977. They recorded that the mean age of older persons with a fall-induced injury had risen from 67.3 years in 1970 to 73.0 years in 1995. The figures for males were 63.6 and 68.0 years, respectively, and for females, they were 69.2 and 75.3 years, respectively. Analysis of the injuries caused by falls showed that the prevalence of long bone fractures had stayed constant in the study period but that soft tissue injuries and dislocations had increased although head injury, other than fracture, had apparently decreased. They thought that the incidence of fall-induced injury would continue to rise.

15.3 Treatment

The treatment of polytrauma in the elderly is essentially the same as that in young patients although there are two important caveats. Firstly, as Champion et al. [4] pointed out, elderly patients may well require more aggressive resuscitation and treatment than younger patients with equivalent injuries. This applies in particular to apparently less severe injuries. Secondly, the frequency of medical comorbidities is usually higher than may be seen in younger patients and a good history of associated medical conditions must be obtained. However, the principles of assessment, resuscitation, and treatment are similar to those for younger patients and are discussed elsewhere in this book. A good analysis of the principles of management of the multiply injured patient is contained in the chapter dealing with the 'Management of the multiply injured patient' by Giannoudis and Pape in the 7th edition of Rockwood and Green [29].

15.4 Predictors of Mortality

An analysis of medical comorbidities in the New York State Registry between 1994 and 1998 shows that, not unexpectedly, the frequency of medical comorbidities increases with age. In an analysis of 76,466 patients, Hannan et al. [30] showed that in their 13–39-year age group, only 3.5% of patients had associated comorbidities compared with 29.4% in the 65–74-year group, 34.7% in the 75–84-year group, and 37.3% in the 85+ year group. Their possible comorbidities included chronic obstructive pulmonary disease, congestive heart failure, acute myocardial infarction, other ischaemic heart disease, cerebrovascular disease and peripheral vascular disease. When combined with factors such as intubation status, low systolic blood pressure, low motor response, male gender and lower ICISS, the presence of comorbidities was associated with increased mortality. The adjusted odds ratios for mortality relative to the 13–39 year group were 2.67 for 40–64-year-old patients, 8.41 for 65–74-year-old patients, 17.4 for 75–84-year-old patients and 34.98 for the 85+ year group.

McGwin et al. [31] analysed the relationship between mortality and chronic medical comorbidities together with the severity of the injury in both younger and older patients. They showed that in older less severely injured patients, the presence of medical comorbidities increased mortality whereas the same effect was not noted in more severely injured patients with an ISS >26. They concluded that older patients with medical comorbidities should be considered to have an increased risk of death compared with their non-chronically ill counterparts. Older patients with minor injuries (ISS 1–15) had a significantly increased risk of death if they had coexisting haematological disease, diabetes, cardiac disease, renal disease, hepatic disease, neurological disease, respiratory disease or spinal injury. In moderately injured elderly patients (ISS 16–25), respiratory and cardiac diseases influenced mortality, but hypertension was protective. In severely injured patients (ISS ≥26), hypertension and spinal injury appeared to be protective. However, the authors pointed out that there may well have been underreporting of associated medical comorbidities, but they suggested that their results showed that elderly patients with minor injuries and associated medical comorbidities should be treated aggressively.

Similar results were reported by Broos et al. [18], who found that early survivors of multiple injuries had a significantly lower prevalence of diabetes and cardiopulmonary, neuropsychiatric and renal disease. Tornetta et al. [17] looked at other predictors of outcome in the multiply injured elderly. They showed that the requirement for transfusion and fluid replacement predicted outcome as did the type of surgery that the patient required. They found that patients who underwent only a general surgical procedure were 2.5 times more likely to die and patients who required both general surgery and orthopaedic surgery were 1.5 times more likely to die. Those who underwent an orthopaedic procedure were less likely to die than those who had no surgery. They could not demonstrate a positive correlation between mortality and early or late surgery.

The Injury Severity (ISS) [2] is the most widely used determinant of injury. Early studies suggested that it was less predictive of outcome in the elderly than in younger patients. However, Tornetta et al. [17] theorised that this was because minor fall-related injuries were included in these studies and that when they were excluded, elderly patients who died had a higher ISS than those who survived (33.1 and 16.4). They found that the Glasgow Coma Scale (GCS) [32] was also predictive of survival in the elderly. Giannoudis et al. [15] also showed that the ISS, GCS and blood pressure (BP) on admission were predictive of survival in elderly patients. They showed that a pulse rate of >90 on admission and severe (Abbreviated injury scale (AIS)[33] ≥3) head, chest, abdominal and spinal injury were associated with higher mortality in elderly patients. In the elderly group, cardiac arrest on admission was associated with 100% mortality. A list of predictors of mortality in elderly patients is given in Table 15.1.

Table 15.1 Factors that increase mortality in elderly patients

Injury severity score <25
GCS <9
Systolic blood pressure <90 mmHg
Pulse >90/min
Increased transfusion requirement
Increased volume replacement
Associated injuries (AIS >3)
Head
Chest
Abdomen
Spine
Comorbidities
Haematological disease
Diabetes
Cardiovascular disease
Renal disease
Hepatic disease
Neurological disease
Respiratory disease

Source: Data from Giannoudis et al. [15], Tornetta et al. [17] and McGwin et al. [31]

15.5 Outcome

15.5.1 Polytrauma

There is very little information about outcome, other than mortality, in the elderly admitted with severe injury. There is some evidence that older patients have fewer long-term psychological problems than younger patients [34], but these results were from patients who were not polytraumatised patients but those admitted with severe fractures. Studies on the outcome of elderly polytrauma survivors are required.

Mortality following polytrauma clearly varies with the degree of injury, and in the large multi-centre studies where a wide spectrum of injury has been included, the mortality is less than in studies that concentrate on polytrauma victims. There is also considerable variation between mortality in different countries. In countries such as the United States and Germany, where there are formal trauma systems, the results are better than in the United Kingdom where such a system is lacking. The literature suggests that the average mortality for elderly polytraumatised patients in countries with a formal trauma system is 15–25% [6, 17, 18], but of course, it depends on the age of the patients and the severity of injury. Kuhne et al. [19] analysed mortality in 5,375 patients in Germany who had an ISS ≥16 and were aged between 15 and 95 years. The overall mortality was 23%, but it was 8.1% if the ISS was 16–24, 27.2% if the ISS was 25–50 and 66.1% if the ISS was 51–75. Their results are shown in Fig. 15.1. The authors stated that mortality rose from 56 years onwards. These overall mortality figures are not dissimilar to those reported from other trauma centres, but higher figures have been reported. Aldrian et al. [35] reported a mortality of 53.3% in the elderly, with 31.1% dying within 24 h. Their average ISS was 32.1.

The statement by Kuhne et al. [19] that mortality in polytraumatised patients rose after the age of 56 once again highlights the polarisation of much of the literature dealing with severely injured patients. Their assessment of a group of polytraumatised patients admitted to trauma centres in Germany should be compared with the study of Caterino et al. [36] in the United States, who examined the Ohio State Registry that records a wider range of admissions from both trauma and non-trauma centres. They found that 70 years was the equivalent age at which mortality increased and recommended that in trauma studies, 70 years should be taken as the cut-off age for considering a patient to be elderly; but it is vital that the type of injury be accurately recorded, given the differences between these two papers.

In the United Kingdom, which lacks a formal trauma system, Giannoudis et al. [15] reported 42% mortality in elderly polytraumatised patients. As with other studies, the mortality was age dependent and it reached almost 50% in patients aged over 75 years. In their earlier study, DeMaria et al. [3] had reported 80% mortality in patients with an ISS ≥25 who were at least 80 years of age. More recently, it has been shown that elderly patients with an ISS >30 require less ICU facilities than younger patients because of their higher mortality [37]. It is also interesting to note that in the United States, mortality following injury in the very elderly (>80 years) is less in trauma centres than in acute care hospitals [38]. Mortality obviously increases with age and degree of injury, but it is also influenced significantly by the type of hospital and the trauma system within the country.

15.5.2 Falls

The mortality from falls has increased in the last few decades. As with the incidence of fall-induced injury, Kannus and his co-workers used the Finnish Cause-of-Death register to assess the incidence of fall-induced mortality between 1971 and 2002 [39]. They pointed out that in 2002, falls were responsible for 285% more deaths than motor vehicle accidents and that there had been an overall 136% increase in fall-induced deaths in the study period. The relevant figures for males and females were 201% and 97%, respectively. They also showed that while the incidence of fall-induced deaths had been relatively steady in females between 1975 and 2002, it had continued to increase in males. They theorised that there would be a 108% increase in mortality by 2030.

15.6 Types of Injury

In the elderly, there are two main types of serious injury that frequently occur with both low-energy and high-energy injuries and may be associated with significant mortality. These are head injuries and fractures.

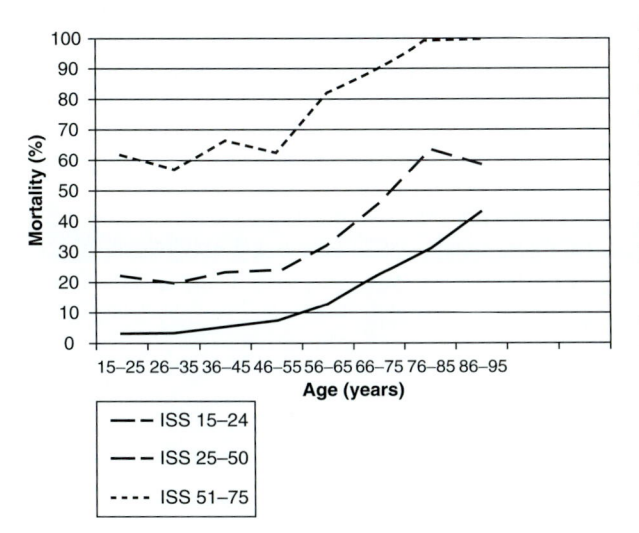

Fig. 15.1 Mortality following multiple injury for different ages and different injury severity. Note the increase in mortality in the sixth decade (Data taken from Kuhne et al. [19]. With permission)

Obviously, injuries may occur in other body systems, but they are usually caused by high-energy trauma and their characterisation and management is discussed elsewhere in the book.

15.6.1 Head Injury

In a recent study of head injury in the elderly, Mitra et al. [40] analysed 96 patients and showed that 31.2% of head injuries followed a low fall, 30.2% occurred because the patient was struck by a motor vehicle and 17.7% were caused by a high fall. All patients presented with an initial GCS <8, which had not been caused by sedation or paralysis. They reported that 62.2% of patients aged 65–74 years died compared with 68.2% aged 75–84 years and 100% of patients aged at least 85 years. Increasing age and brainstem injury were identified as predictors of mortality. Frankel et al. [41] analysed the outcome of traumatic brain injury in the elderly and showed that elderly patients were significantly less likely to be discharged home. However, they felt that the results of treatment were encouraging and stated that older patients exhibited the potential to achieve functional goals.

15.6.2 Multiple Fractures

Multiple fractures in the elderly may occur as a result of high-energy or low-energy injuries. The assumption is often made that they are mainly caused by motor vehicle accidents or falls from a height but this is simply not the case. In a review of 6,872 in-patient and out-patient fractures in the Royal Infirmary of Edinburgh in 2007/2008 [16], there were 2,335 patients aged at least 65 years. Of these 119 (5.1%) presented with multiple fractures. One hundred and nine (91.5%) had two fractures, 9 (7.6%) had three fractures and 1 (0.8%) 75-year-old pedestrian presented with four fractures after a motor vehicle accident. Table 15.2 shows the causes of multiple fractures in the elderly population. It can be seen that the highest prevalence is indeed related to motor vehicle accidents, with 36.4% of patients presenting with multiple fractures. Predictably, the next most common cause of multiple fractures in the elderly was falls from a height followed by falls down stairs. However, although the prevalence of multiple fractures following simple falls was only 4.4%, the frequency of fall-related fractures in the elderly population means that 92 patients presented with multiple fractures following a fall during the year, this constituting 78.6% of all the multiple fractures. Table 15.2 shows that the average of the multiple fracture group was 71.3 years and about 80% were female.

A review of the 32 fractures that resulted from motor vehicle accidents shows that they occurred in 22 patients, with 7 patients presenting with 2 fractures and 1 patient with 4 fractures. The average age was 80.2 years and 75% of the patients were male. Five (22.7%) of the 22 patients were bicyclists, all of whom presented with a single fracture. Another four (18.2%)

Table 15.2 The epidemiology of multiple fractures in patients aged at least 65 years presenting to the Royal Infirmary of Edinburgh over a 1-year period in 2007/2008

	Patients (n)	Multiple fractures	%	Average age (year)	Gender ratio
Simple fall	2,111	96	4.5	79.0	16/84
Fall from height	11	3	27.3	72.0	67/33
Fall down stairs	80	10	12.5	77.0	30/70
Motor vehicle accident	22	8	36.4	80.2	75/25
Direct blow/assault	45	2	4.4	77.5	0/100
Sport	17	0	–	–	–
Spontaneous	24	0	–	–	–
Others	25	0	–	–	–
	2,335	119	5.1	77.1	21/79

were vehicle occupants, and one vehicle passenger presented with two fractures. The remaining 13 (59.1%) elderly patients were pedestrians struck by a vehicle, of whom 7 (53.8%) presented with multiple fractures. The average age of this group was 78.9 years, and 14 (63.6%) of the fractures were in the lower limb or pelvis and 8 (36.4%) were in the upper limb. Three (13.6%) of the fractures were open.

Table 15.2 shows that the prevalence of multiple fractures following a fall from a height approaches that of motor vehicle accidents, but all the fractures were closed, suggesting either that falls from a height in the elderly are not as severe as in younger patients or possibly that many falls are fatal. Table 15.2 also shows that falls down stairs are associated with a high prevalence of multiple fractures. The results indicate that the highest frequency of multiple fractures in the 65+ year group follows motor vehicle accidents where the elderly patient is a pedestrian struck by a vehicle. However, the greatest number of multiple fractures in the elderly that present to orthopaedic surgeons follow a simple fall and these will be examined in more detail elsewhere in the book.

15.6.3 Fall-Related Multiple Fractures

A review of all patients aged at least 16 years who presented to the Orthopaedic Trauma Unit of the Edinburgh Royal Infirmary over a 1-year period between 2007/2008 shows that 3,843 fractures were caused by simple falls, this being 55.9% of all the fractures. Analysis of the patients of at least 65 years of age shows that 2,213 fractures were caused by simple falls.

These fractures occurred in 2,111 patients, with 2,015 patients presenting with a single fracture, 90 presenting with two fractures and six patients presenting with three fractures. Table 15.2 shows that the average age of patients presenting with multiple fractures after a fall was 79 years. The average age of males was 76.6 years, with 79.5 years being recorded for females. This compares with 79.2 years and 80.0 years for males and females who presented with single fractures. The gender ratio for single fractures was 20/80, indicating that multiple fractures are more common in elderly females, but the average ages of males and females are not dissimilar.

An analysis of multiple fractures of all ages in 2007/8 shows that they are much more common in older patients. Figure 15.2 shows the age-related incidence of multiple fall-related fractures in the whole population. There were none in the 15–19 years group, but Fig. 15.2 shows that the incidence starts to rise in the 6th decade of life and continues to rise until the tenth decade; it is presumed that this is mainly because of increased osteopenia and other medical comorbidities that predispose the patients to falls.

Only six (6.25%) of the elderly patients who presented with fall-related multiple fractures had three fractures. It was not possible to define any relationship between different fracture combinations. Two involved the upper limb only, and four involved both upper and lower limbs. Five (83.3%) of these fractures occurred in females with an average age of 78.6 years, with only one 71-year-old male presenting with three fractures after a fall.

A review of the 90 patients who presented with double fracture combinations showed there were three groups. Group 1 consisted of 29 (32.2%) patients who presented with two upper limb fractures. Group 2

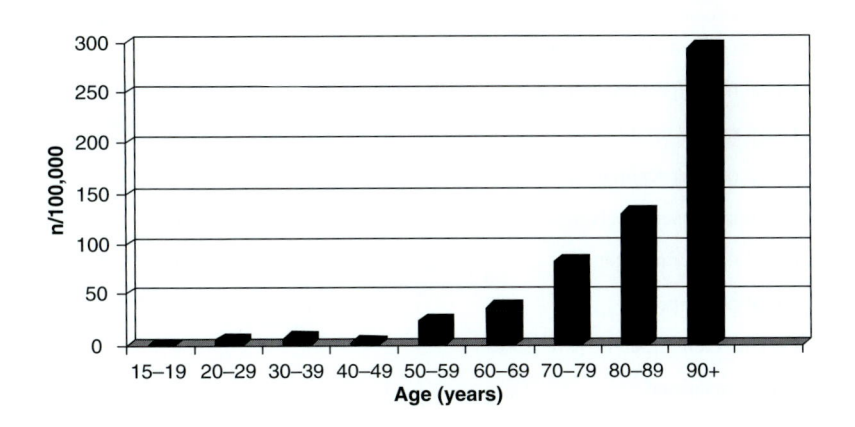

Fig. 15.2 The incidence of multiple fall-related fractures in different age groups (Data from the Royal Infirmary of Edinburgh, Scotland)

comprised 11 (12.2%) patients who presented with two lower limb fractures, and Group 3 consisted of the remaining 50 (55.6%) patients who presented with fracture combinations involving both upper and lower limbs. Pelvic fractures were included with the lower limb fractures. Group 1 had an average age of 75 years and a male/female gender ratio of 17/83. Group 2 had an average age of 83.4 years and a gender ratio of 18/82, and Group 3 had an average age of 80.6 years and a gender ratio of 14/86.

Analysis of the Group I patients showed that combinations of fractures involving the distal radius and proximal humerus were most commonly seen. Of the 29 upper limb double fracture combinations, 19 (65.5%) involved the distal radius and 11 (37.9%) the proximal humerus, with 4 (13.8%) patients presenting with fractures of the distal radius and proximal humerus. There were, in fact, only three double upper limb fracture combinations that did not involve the distal radius or proximal humerus. The commonest Group 1 combinations were bilateral distal radial fractures (27.5%), the distal radius/proximal humerus combination (13.8%) and the combination of distal radius and finger phalanx (10.3%).

Of the 11 Group 2 patients, 5 (45.4%) involved the proximal femur, 4 (36.4%) the pelvis and 4 (36.4%) involved the ankle. In fact, there was only one combination of midfoot and metatarsal fractures that did not involve the proximal femur, pelvis or ankle. The commonest lower limb combinations were fractures of the proximal femur and pelvis and fractures of the ankle and metatarsal which both occurred in 27.3% of Group 2 fractures.

Group 3 fractures were most commonly seen. Of the 50 Group 3 fractures, 34 (68%) involved the proximal femur and 17 (34%) presented with a combination of proximal femoral and proximal humeral fractures, this being the commonest double fracture combination. A further 11 (22%) patients presented with proximal femoral and distal radial fractures. Of the fracture combinations that did not involve the proximal femur, the common combination was that of the proximal humerus and pelvis, which presented in 8% of Group 3 cases followed by that of the distal radius and pelvis, which occurred in 6% of the patients.

The results show that the four commonest fractures in double fracture combinations involve fractures of the proximal femur, distal radius, proximal humerus and pelvis. Proximal femoral fractures occurred in 39 (43.3%) of the double fracture combinations with distal radius fractures being involved in 38 (42.2%). The average ages of these fracture groups were 81.4 and 77.6 years, respectively, and the gender ratios were 20/80 and 13/87. Proximal humeral fractures occurred in 34 (37.8%) of the double fracture combinations. These patients had an average age of 79.7 years and a gender ratio of 15/85. Pelvic fractures occurred in 11 (12.2%) patients with an average age of 87.7 years and a gender ratio of 8/92.

Table 15.3 shows the basic epidemiological data of the nine most common double fracture combinations, these being the fracture combinations that presented at least three times during the year. It is evident that fractures of the proximal femur, proximal humerus and distal radius are involved in all the common combinations except for the ankle metatarsal combination. It is also worth noting the extreme age of patients who

Table 15.3 Epidemiological criteria of the nine double fracture configurations that occurred at least three times in a 1-year period

Fracture combination	n	%	Age (year)	Gender ratio (%)
Proximal humerus/proximal femur	17	18.9	80.9	18/82
Distal radius/proximal femur	11	12.2	80.2	18/82
Distal radius/distal radius	8	8.9	74.2	20/80
Distal radius/proximal humerus	4	4.4	79.5	0/100
Proximal humerus/pelvis	4	4.4	87.2	25/75
Distal radius/finger phalanx	3	3.3	74.7	0/100
Distal radius/pelvis	3	3.3	85.0	0/100
Proximal femur/pelvis	3	3.3	92.3	0/100
Ankle/metatarsal	3	3.3	75.3	0/100

present with a combination of a fall-related pelvic fracture and a fracture of the proximal femur, distal radius and proximal humerus.

With increased longevity, it seems likely that multiple fall-related fractures will become more common and that they will present in patients who have multiple medical comorbidities and who require aggressive medical management to increase the chance of survival from these apparently straightforward injuries.

References

1. Oreskovich MR, Howard JD, Copass MK, et al. Geriatric trauma: injury patterns and outcomes. J Trauma. 1984;24:565–72.
2. Baker SP, O'Neill B, Haddon W, et al. The injury severity score: a method for describing patients with multiple injuries and evaluating emergency care. J Trauma. 1974;14:187–96.
3. DeMaria EJ, Kenney PR, Merriam MA, et al. Survival after trauma in geriatric patients. Ann Surg. 1987;206:738–43.
4. Champion HR, Copes WS, Buyer D, et al. Major trauma in geriatric patients. Am J Public Health. 1989;79:1278–82.
5. Finelli FC, Jonsson J, Champion HR, et al. A case control study for major trauma in geriatric patients. J Trauma. 1989;29:541–8.
6. US Census Bureau: International data base (IDB). Available at http://www.census.gov/ipc/www/idb.
7. National Statistics. http://www.statistics.gov.uk/cci/nugget_print.asp?ID=1875.
8. National Statistics. http://www.statistics.gov.uk/cci/nugget_print.asp?ID=934.
9. Court-Brown CM, Clement N. Four score years and ten. An analysis of the epidemiology of fractures in the very elderly. Injury. 2009;40:1111–4.
10. National Statistics. http://www.dft.gov.uk/pgr/statistics.
11. Safety on roads. What's the vision? OECD Publishing; 2002.
12. Tinetti ME, Speechley M, Ginter SF. Risk factors for falls among elderly persons living in the community. N Engl J Med. 1988;319:1701–7.
13. Von Heideken WP, Gustafson Y, Kallin K, et al. Falls in very old people: the population based Umeå study in Sweden. Arch Gerontol Geriatr. 2009;49:390–6.
14. Center of Disease Control and Prevention: Cost of falls among older adults. http://www.cdc.gov/homeandrecreationalsafety/falls/fallscost.html.
15. Giannoudis PV, Harwood PJ, Court-Brown C, et al. Severe and multiple trauma in older patients: incidence and mortality. Injury. 2009;40:362–7.
16. Court-Brown CM, Aitken SA, Forward D, RV O'Toole. The epidemiology of fractures. In: Bucholz RW, Heckman JD, Court-Brown CM, Tornetta P, editors. Rockwood and green's fractures in adults. 7th ed. Philadelphia: Lippincott, Williams & Wilkins; 2010.
17. Tornetta P, Mostavi H, Riina J, et al. Morbidity and mortality in elderly trauma patients. J Trauma. 1999;46:702–6.
18. Broos PLO, D'Hoore A, Vanderschot P, et al. Multiple trauma in elderly patients. Factors influencing outcome: importance of aggressive care. Injury. 1993;24:365–8.
19. Kuhne CA, Ruchholtz S, Kaise GN, et al. Mortality in severely injured elderly trauma patients-when does age become a risk factor. World J Surg. 2005;29:1476–82.
20. Peng RY, Bongard FS. Pedestrian versus motor vehicle accidents: an analysis of 5000 patients. J Am Coll Surg. 1999;189:343–8.
21. Demetriades D, Murray J, Martin M, et al. Pedestrians injured by automobiles: relationship of age to injury type and severity. J Am Coll Surg. 2004;199:382–7.
22. Small TJ, Sheedy JM, Grabs AJ. Cost, demographics and injury profile of adult pedestrian trauma in inner Sydney. ANZ J Surg. 2006;76:43–7.
23. Martin AJ, Hand EB, Trace F, et al. Pedestrian fatalities and injuries involving Irish older people. Gerontology. 2010;56(3):266–71.
24. Oxley J, Fildes B, Ihsen E, et al. Differences in traffic judgements between young and old adult pedestrians. Accid Anal Prev. 1997;29:839–47.
25. Sparrow WA, Bradshaw EJ, Lamoureux E, et al. Ageing effects on the attention demands of walking. Hum Mov Sci. 2002;21:961–72.
26. Gorrie CA, Rodriguez M, Sachdev P, et al. Increased neurofibrillary tangles in the brains of older pedestrians killed in traffic accidents. Dement Geriatr Cogn Disord. 2006;22:20–6.
27. Demetriades D, Murray J, Brown C, et al. High-level falls: type and severity of injuries and survival outcome according to age. J Trauma. 2005;58:342–5.
28. Kannus P, Parkkari J, Koskinen S, et al. Fall-induced injuries and deaths among older adults. JAMA. 1999;281:1895–9.
29. Giannoudis PV, Pape HC. Management of the multiply injured patient. In: Bucholz RW, Heckman JD, Court-Brown CM, Tornetta P, editors. Rockwood and green's fractures in adults. 7th ed. Philadelphia: Lippincott, Williams & Wilkins; 2010.
30. Hannan EL, Hicks Waller C, Szypulski Farrell L, et al. Elderly trauma inpatients in New York State: 1994–1998. J Trauma. 2004;56:1297–304.
31. McGwin G, MacLennan PA, Bailey Fife J, et al. Preexisting conditions and mortality in older trauma patients. J Trauma. 2004;56:1291–6.
32. Teasdale G, Jennett B. Assessment of coma and impaired consciousness. A practical scale. Lancet. 1974;2(7872):81–4.
33. Copes WS, Lawnick M, Champion HR, et al. A comparison of abbreviated injury scale 1980 and 1985 versions. J Trauma. 1988;28:78–86.
34. Ponsford J, Hill B, Karamitsios M, Bahar-Fuchs A. Factors influencing outcome after orthopaedic trauma. J Trauma. 2008;64:1001–9.
35. Aldrian S, Nau T, Koenig F, et al. Geriatric polytrauma. Wien Klin Wochenschr. 2005;117:145–9.
36. Caterino JM, Valasek T, Werman HA. Identification of an age cutoff for increased mortality in patients with elderly trauma. Am J Emerg Med. 2010;28:151–8.
37. Taylor MD, Tracy JK, Meyer W, et al. Trauma in the elderly: intensive care unit resource use and outcome. J Trauma. 2002;53:407–14.

38. Meldon SW, Reilly M, Drew BL, et al. Trauma in the very elderly: a community-based study of outcomes at trauma and nontrauma centers. J Trauma. 2002;52: 79–84.
39. Kannus P, Parkkari J, Niemi S, et al. Fall-induced deaths among elderly people. Am J Public Health. 2005;95: 422–4.
40. Mitra B, Cameron PA, Gabbe BJ, et al. Management and hospital outcome of the severely head injured elderly patient. ANZ J Surg. 2008;78:588–92.
41. Frankel JE, Marwitz JH, Cifu DX, et al. A follow-up study of older adults with traumatic brain injury: taking into account decreasing length of stay. Arch Phys Med Rehabil. 2006;87:57–62.

Polytrauma in Young Children

Hans Georg Dietz, Roman Pfeifer, and Hans-Christoph Pape

Contents

16.1	Definition and Epidemiology	179
16.2	Anatomic and Physiologic Specifics in Children and Adolescents	179
16.3	Patterns of Injury	180
16.4	Scoring	181
16.5	Prehospital Care	181
16.6	Emergency Room Management	182
16.7	Specific Injuries	182
16.7.1	Head Injury	182
16.7.2	Thoracic Trauma	183
16.7.3	Abdominal	183
16.7.4	Spine Trauma	184
16.7.5	Orthopaedic Injuries	184
References		186

Traumatic injuries are the main causes of morbidity and mortality in children up to the age of 14 years. Most of these deaths occur as a result of a combination of severe head, thoracic, abdominal, and/or skeletal trauma. Severe head injury is associated with the highest morbidity and mortality rates. Significant trauma in children up to the age of 5 years is most often caused by a fall from height at home. In older children, traffic accidents account for the majority of trauma. This can be broken down into three groups, with equal involvement of bicycle, pedestrian, and motor vehicle accidents. Importantly, nearly 30% of the deaths in children involved in an accident sustaining polytrauma could be avoided by correct medical and surgical management [1–3].

16.1 Definition and Epidemiology

Similar to adults, polytrauma in children is defined as a combination of injuries involving two or more organ systems as a result of a single incident that account for a life-threatening condition [3].

The incidence of polytraumatized children is estimated to be 360 per 100,000, which accounts for 6% of all polytrauma patients. Age breakdown is as follows: less than 5 years – 25%; 6–10 years – 25%; and 11–15 years – 50%. The overall mortality rate is about 12% [4].

16.2 Anatomic and Physiologic Specifics in Children and Adolescents

Children differ physiologically and anatomically from adults. A child's head is proportionally larger than an adult's, and accounts for a larger percentage of the

H.G. Dietz (✉)
Kindertraumatologie, Kinderchirurgie der LMU München,
Lindwurmstr. 4, D-80337 München, Germany
e-mail: hgdietz@med.uni-müenchen.de

R. Pfeifer and H.-C. Pape
Department of Trauma Surgery, University of Aachen
Medical Center, Pauwelsstr. 30, 52074 Aachen, Germany

H.-C. Pape et al. (eds.), *The Poly-Traumatized Patient with Fractures*,
DOI: 10.1007/978-3-642-17986-0_16, © Springer-Verlag Berlin Heidelberg 2011

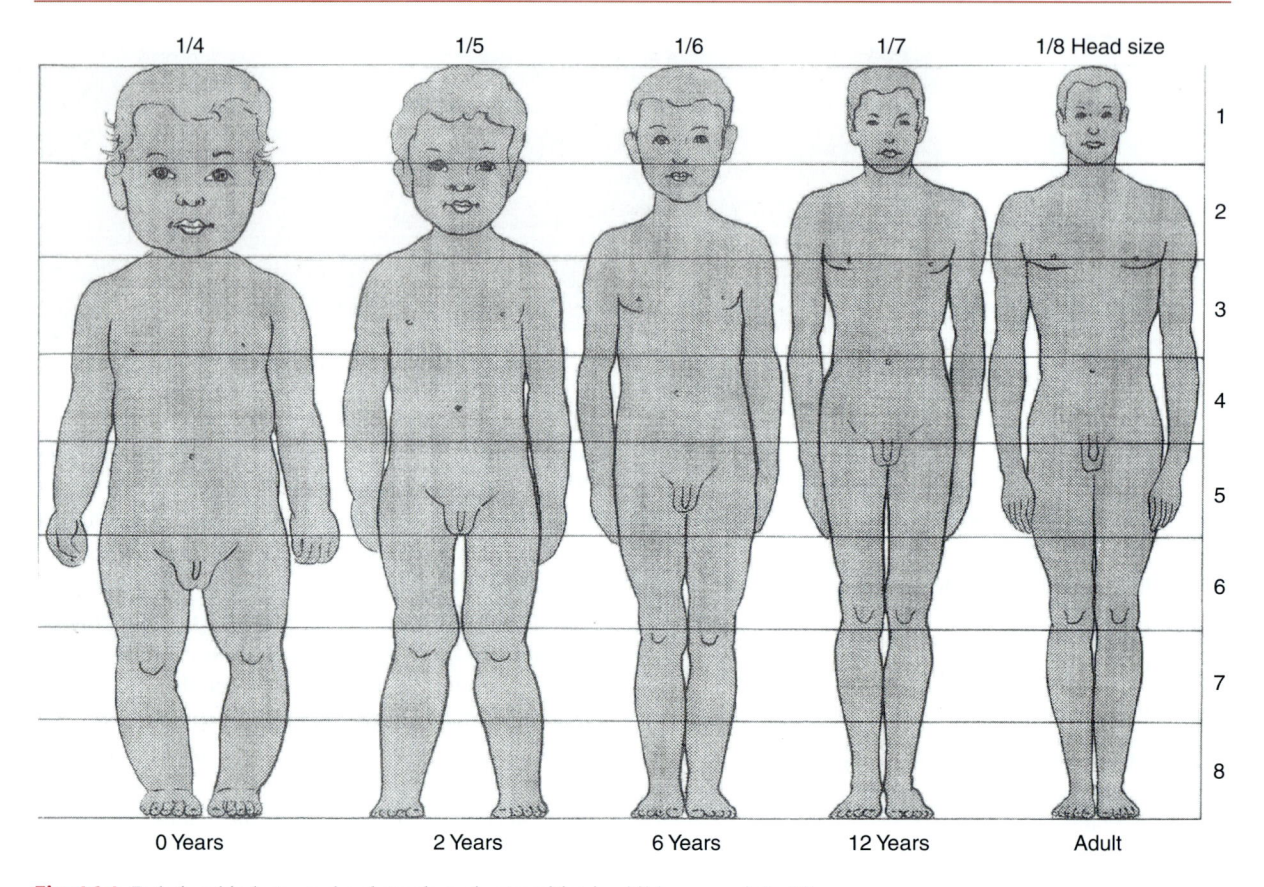

| 1/4 | 1/5 | 1/6 | 1/7 | 1/8 Head size |
| 0 Years | 2 Years | 6 Years | 12 Years | Adult |

Fig. 16.1 Relationship between head, trunk, and extremities in children vs. adults [5]

total body surface area (Fig. 16.1). This leads to a disproportionately higher risk of injuries to the skull and to the cervical spine. The airway is anatomically different from that of an adult, and there is less respiratory reserve capacity.

Since children have less body mass and less total blood volume, their cardiovascular response to injury may be less sustained than in adults. This difference is even greater in younger children and toddlers. In breast-fed infants, even small amounts of blood loss can lead to hypovolemic shock. Table 16.1 describes estimates of blood loss in children and adults.

Table 16.1 Relationship between age, blood loss, and % of the total blood volume

Age (years)	Blood loss (ml)	% total blood volume
4	500	40
8	500	25
Adult	500	10

Therefore, major bleeds may be easily missed, and the consequences can be severe [3, 6].

16.3 Patterns of Injury

Younger children sustain different injury patterns from adults. In the pediatric polytrauma population, head trauma combined with fractures is the most frequent pattern of injuries, followed by a combination of head and chest or abdominal trauma. In general, approximately 80% of all pediatric polytrauma patients suffer from head injuries, 60% have fractures, 40% have thoracic trauma, and 35% have abdominal trauma. The common combination of head trauma, thoracic injury, and femur fractures is termed "Waddell's triad."

In the very young child, head injuries and fractures of the lower limb are more frequent than thoracic, abdominal, or pelvic injuries. An insufficient safety belt can cause a lumbar spine shear fracture (Chance fracture). This injury is typically associated with abdominal trauma, including small bowel ruptures [4].

16.4 Scoring

Anatomic, physiologic, and prognostic trauma scores exist for adults, each of which can be adapted for children. However, scores seem to be more helpful in the retrospective evaluation of treatment, with no primary influence upon initial management [7]. Although the Injury Severity Score (ISS) is used for children, the Pediatric Trauma Score (PTS) has been developed and should be used preferentially for polytraumatized children. The PTS is a combination of anatomical and physiological values scoring weight, airway status, systolic blood pressure, level of consciousness, and the presence of open wounds and fractures. Each value is scored between −1 and +2, and added to yield a total score between −6 and +12. [8] (Table 16.2). Additionally, the Glasgow Coma Scale and the Pediatric Glasgow Coma Scale is available to assess neurologic status (Table 16.3).

16.5 Prehospital Care

Administration of first aid and basic life support directly at the injury site is crucial, and starts with airway support and oxygen administration with early intubation if needed. In general, the primary survey and resuscitation following the A-B-C-D-E's of the Advanced Trauma Life Support (ATLS) rules apply.

A-Airway: To secure adequate oxygenation, the airway should be assessed and a primary oxygenation mask should be started (12 L/minO$_2$). Complicating matters, in infants, the larynx is in a cephalad and anterior position, and the tongue is larger in relation to the mouth. Cervical spine precautions with a rigid collar should be utilized at all times.

B-Breathing: Hypoventilation is the most common cause of cardiac arrest in children. The pediatric chest is more compliant and compressible when compared with that of adults. Asymmetric thoracic movement and skin emphysema are signs of insufficient breathing (i.e., Pneumothorax). Insufficient respirations prompt immediate intervention such as CPR or artificial respirations.

Table 16.2 Pediatric trauma score

I. Scoring
  A. Weight
    1. Weight >20 kg: score +2
    2. Weight 10–20 kg: score +1
    3. Weight <10 kg: score −1
  B. Airway
    1. Normal airway: score +2
    2. Maintained airway: score +1
    3. Invasive airway (e.g., intubated): score −1
  C. Systolic blood pressure
    1. SBP >90 mmHg: score +2
    2. SBP 50–90 mmHg: score +1
    3. SBP <50 mmHg: score −1
  D. Central nervous system
    1. Awake: score +2
    2. Obtunded: score +1
    3. Coma: score −1
  E. Open wound
    1. No open wound: score +2
    2. Minor open wound: score +1
    3. Major open wound: score −1
  F. Skeletal trauma
    1. No skeletal trauma: score +2
    2. Closed fracture: score +1
    3. Open fracture or multiple fractures: score −1

II. Interpretation
  A. Score range: +12 to −6
  B. Trauma score <= 8 indicates significant mortality risk

III. References
  A. Tepas (1987) J Pediatr Surg 22:14

C-Circulation: Tachycardia, low systolic blood pressure, and pale skin are signs of insufficient perfusion. Large-bore intravenous access through two or more peripheral veins should be used; a central line should not be employed at this stage. In cases of insufficient peripheral venous access, intraosseous access through the tibia may be used.

Table 16.3 Modified Glasgow Coma Scale for infants and children

Area	Infants	Children	Score assessed[a]
Eye opening	Open spontaneously	Open spontaneously	4
	Open in response to verbal stimuli	Open in response to verbal stimuli	3
	Open in response to pain only	Open in response to pain only	2
	No response	No response	1
Verbal response	Coos and babbles	Oriented, appropriate	5
	Irritable cries	Confused	4
	Cries in response to pain	Inappropriate words	3
	Moans in response to pain	Incomprehensible words or nonspecific sounds	2
	No response	No response	1
Motor response[b]	Moves spontaneously and purposefully	Obeys commands	6
	Withdraws to touch	Localizes painful stimulus	5
	Withdraws in response to pain	Withdraws in response to pain	4
	Responds to pain with decorticate posturing (abnormal flexion)	Responds to pain with flexion	3
	Responds to pain with decerebrate posturing (abnormal extension)	Responds to pain with extension	2
	No response	No response	1

[a]Score: 12 suggests a severe head injury, 8 suggests need for intubation and ventilation, 6 suggests need for intracranial pressure monitoring

[b]If the patient is intubated, unconscious, or preverbal, the most important part of this scale is motor response. This section should be carefully evaluated

D-Disability: In general, the most important difference when assessing neurological function relates to the preverbal age group. The neurological investigation should include the pediatric Glasgow Coma Scale. It is important to consider the age-related modifications and the specifics of the pupil's reaction to light in children.

E-Exposure: In children, it is very important to maintain or regain normothermia. The high ratio of the infant's body surface area with respect to body volume makes them especially prone to hypothermia.

16.6 Emergency Room Management

The emergency room team in the hospital should follow strict ATLS protocols. The Trauma Team consists of a pediatric trauma surgeon, a pediatric surgeon, a pediatric anesthesiologist, as well as specialized nurses and technicians. Following initial resuscitation including airway control, pneumothorax treatment, bleeding control, and volume therapy, emergency diagnostic testing is initiated. Blood draws, nasogastric tube insertion, and bladder catheterization are performed. Abdominal ultrasonography for detection of free fluid and visceral injuries is the standard of care. Similar to adults, a whole body CT scan can be performed to allow for simultaneous evaluation of the spine and the pelvis [8–10].

16.7 Specific Injuries

16.7.1 Head Injury

Intracranial bleeding as well as brain swelling and edema can increase intracranial pressure and reduce cerebral perfusion. Cerebral blood flow (CBF) is related to the intracranial pressure (ICP) and the

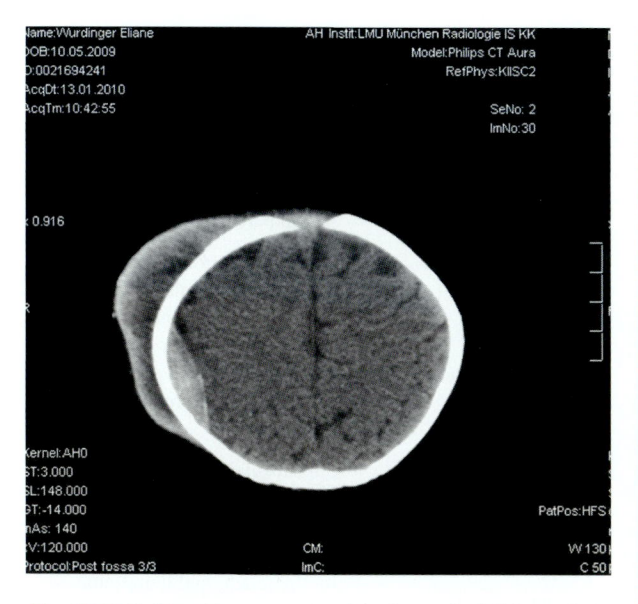

Fig. 16.2 Epidural hematoma, patient 8 month, fall from chair

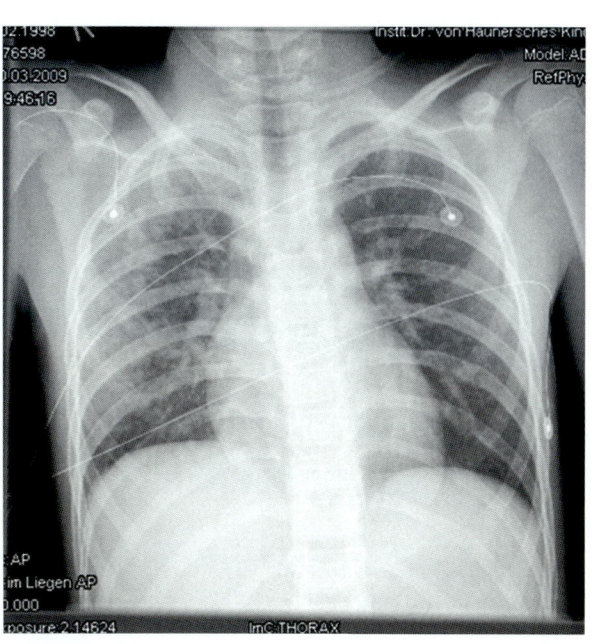

Fig. 16.3 Lung contusion in X-ray plain (**a**) and in CT scan (**b**), patient 5 years, car accident

cerebral perfusion pressure (CPP). The ICP value in children should be between 3 and 17 mmHg. It is mandatory to keep the ICP less than 20 mmHg. The CPP should be >50 mmHg up to 4 years of age, >60 mmHg between 5 and 8 years of age, and >70 mmHg for children over the age of 8. The current standard of care prompts a head computed tomography if the GCS value is less than 12 points. The indications for surgery are similar to adults, which include midline shifts (Fig. 16.2). For patients with a GCS of less than 8 points, monitoring with an intracranial ventricular or intraparenchymal device is recommended. In general, prognosis for recovery of the pediatric brain following head trauma is better than that of adults. If an intracranial hematoma is detected, emergent surgical evacuation is required. Initially, the head should be elevated up to 30. Respirator settings should aim at achieving O_2 saturations of 100%.

In children, increased chest wall compliance can cause severe pulmonary contusions in the absence of fractures, and life-threatening hemorrhage can occur. Therefore, a chest CT should be performed, followed by blood gas analysis to monitor the oxygenation index (P_aO_2/FIO_2 ratio, normal value 300–400) [11–13] (Fig. 16.3). Surgical intervention is rarely necessary, but a thoracotomy is performed when control of bleeding is necessary. If lung fistulas develop, they may be treated electively. Although diaphragmatic lesions are rare, care must be taken to rule them out as bowel herniations may occur with these injuries. The risk of Acute Respiratory Distress Syndrome (ARDS) is similar to that of adults and Extracorporeal Membrane Oxygenation (ECMO) may be required.

16.7.2 Thoracic Trauma

Approximately 50% of pediatric polytrauma patients sustain thoracic injuries, and 25% of these are associated with skeletal injuries. Mortality rises up to 39% if thoracic trauma is compounded with brain and abdominal injuries. The diagnosis of subcutaneous emphysema and/or paradoxical breathing requires rapid intubation and ventilation.

16.7.3 Abdominal

Approximately 45% of polytraumatized children have abdominal trauma. Abdominal wall ecchymosis is a sign of serious visceral injury. Because the spleen and liver of children are proportionally larger and the diaphragm is lower than in adults, intra-abdominal organs are more vulnerable to blunt trauma (Fig. 16.4). Diagnostic tests to evaluate these organs include ultrasound, commonly followed by a CT scan. Diagnostic

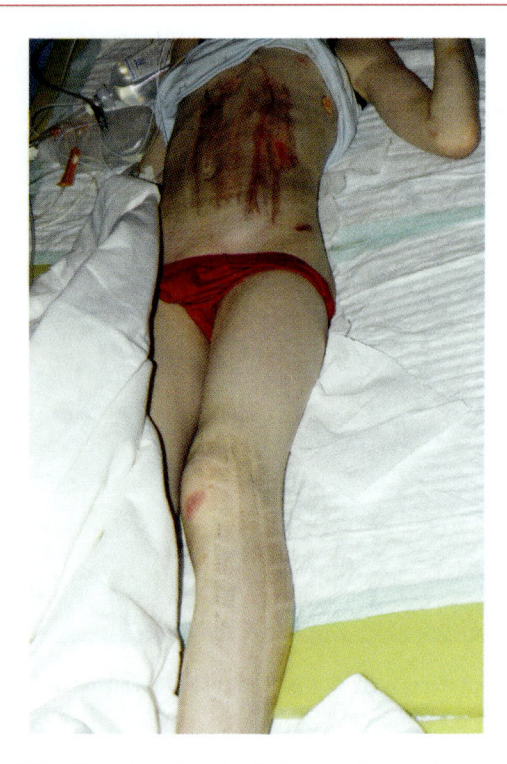

Fig. 16.4 Thoracic and abdominal marks in a patient ran over by a tractor

Table 16.4 Injury description liver

Grade	Injury description liver	
I	Hematoma	Subcapsular, nonexpanding, <10 cm surface area
	Laceration	Capsular tear, nonbleeding, <1 cm parenchymal bleeding
II	Hematoma	Subcapsular, nonexpanding, 10–50% surface area
		Intraparenchymal nonexpanding <10 cm in diameter
	Laceration	Capsular tear, active bleeding; 1–3 cm parenchymal dept <10 cm in length
III	Hematoma	Subcapsular, >50% surface area or expanding;
		Ruptured subcapsular hematoma with active bleeding;
		Intraparenchymal hematoma >10 cm or expanding
	Laceration	>3 cm parenchymal depth
IV	Hematoma	Ruptured intraparenchymal hematoma with active bleeding
	Laceration	Parenchymal disruption involving 25–75% of hepatic lobe
V	Laceration	Parenchymal disruption involving >75% of hepatic lobe
	Vascular	Just a hepatic venous injury (i.e., retrohepatic vena cava)
VI	Vascular	Vascular avulsion

peritoneal lavage and diagnostic laparoscopy are rarely performed if a CT scan is available. Once diagnosed, blunt liver trauma can be graded according to the classification of the American Association for the Surgery of Trauma (AAST) [6, 11, 14, 15] (Table 16.4).

Recent studies show that with most cases of solid organ injury, conservative treatment can be employed. In cases with vascular injuries and minor bleeding, interventional radiology may be useful. When laparotomy for hemorrhagic control of the liver is required, direct suture and ligation of the bleeding vessels is employed to control blood loss. In grade V liver injuries, abdominal packing can allow time for resuscitation with a planned second look at a later time. Although bowel lacerations and ruptures require surgery, intramural hematomas are usually well treated by conservative means. Pancreatic injuries such as contusions and ruptures usually heal, but may lead to the development of pseudocysts. Complete ruptures of the kidney or avulsed renal vessels require surgery and reconstruction. Hematomas and urinomas can easily be diagnosed by ultrasound, and ureteral or renal lesions can be managed by percutaneous drainage or endoscopically applied stents.

16.7.4 Spine Trauma

The relation between the head and the weak neck muscles in children is responsible for injuries to the cervical spine. Injuries from C1 to C3 are more frequent in young children compared to adults. The majority of pediatric thoracic and lumbar spine injuries are type A injuries according to the OTA/AO classification and are treated with a removable molded body jacket, or fiberglass body cast. Distraction and rotation lesions are rare and require internal fixation [16].

16.7.5 Orthopaedic Injuries

Extremity injuries in the growing skeleton have to be treated cautiously. Some fractures do not require anatomic reduction, depending on age and classification.

16.7.5.2 Articular Fractures

Articular fractures require meticulous reduction in order to avoid secondary deformities or early growth plate closure. These injuries should be treated by an expert in pediatric orthopaedic trauma.

16.7.5.3 Pelvic Fractures

Injuries to the pelvis are rare, but are frequently associated with injuries to the bladder, urethra, and the rectum. The greater plasticity and elasticity of the pediatric pelvic ring explains why these injuries are often overlooked initially. Hemorrhage in the retroperitoneal or intraperitoneal space originates from the fractured bone or from disrupted vessels (veins) and can lead to life-threatening bleeding. Techniques for surgical stabilization are different than in the adult, and external fixation is frequently the technique of choice [19].

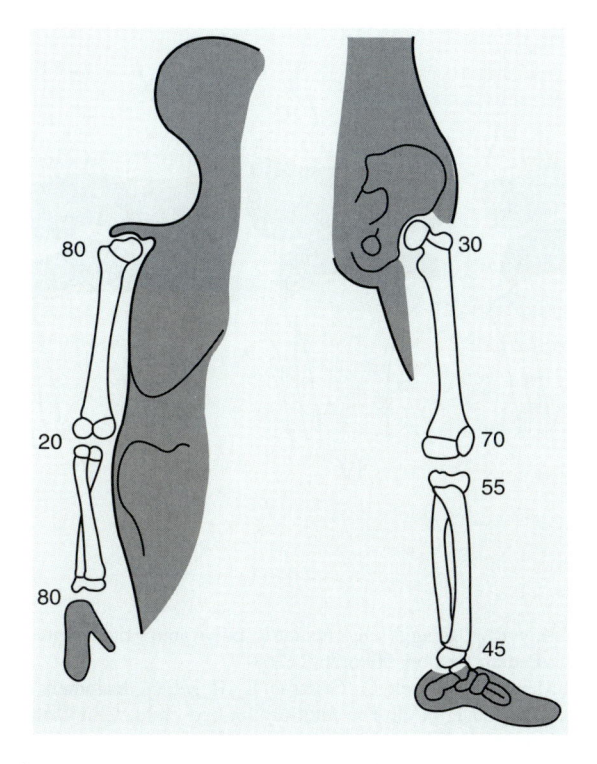

Fig. 16.5 Corrective potential (in %) of extremity injuries [17]

16.7.5.4 Physeal Injuries

Traumatic injuries to the growth plate (physis) may lead to growth arrest with length discrepancies or angular deformities. Numerous descriptive and prognostic classification schemes have been devised. The anatomical classification of Salter and Harris described in 1963 [20] is widely accepted and utilized routinely (Table 16.5 and Fig. 16.6).

The ability to correct varus deformities may be as high as 60°. However, rotational deformities do not have the potential to remodel, and this may pose challenges in the lower extremity. Moreover, transitional fractures during skeletal maturation should not be overlooked and may require surgical intervention to avoid inadequate growth plate recovery (Fig. 16.5).

Table 16.5 Salter Harris classification [20]

Type I
A complete physeal fracture with or without displacement
Type II
A physeal fracture that extends through the metaphysis, producing a chip fracture of the metaphysis, which may be very small
Type III
A physeal fracture that extends through the epiphysis
Type IV
A physeal fracture plus epiphyseal and metaphyseal fractures
Type V
A compression fracture of the growth plate

16.7.5.1 Diaphyseal Fractures

In closed diaphyseal fractures, the indications for elastic stable intramedullary nailing (ESIN) are more frequent than in adults. Given the short healing time of the growing skeleton, this technique is ideal to avoid injuries to the physis. Most surgeons prefer the ESIN technique because of higher patient comfort when compared with external fixation and plate osteosynthesis. The elastic properties of the nails support the biology of pediatric fracture healing by stimulating both periosteal and endosteal callus formation [18].

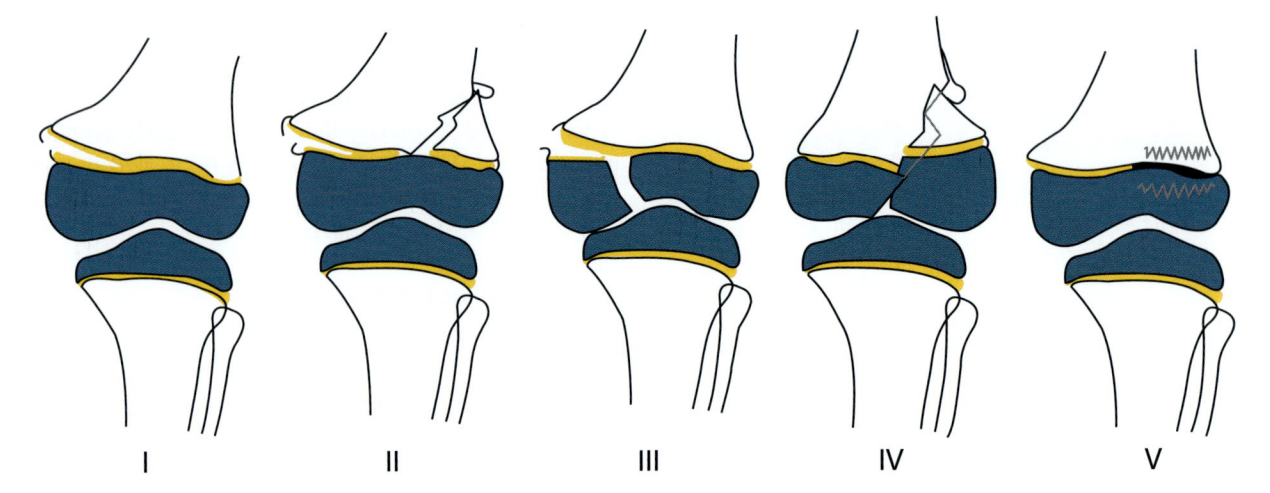

Fig. 16.6 Anatomical classification of Salter and Harris [20]

16.7.5.5 Corrective Potential

In the growing child, there is the potential of correcting angular deformities in all three planes. The corrective potential is dependent on the fracture type, location, age, degree of angulation, and the level of activity of the physis. Younger patients have greater metabolically active physes, with greater potential for correcting malunited fractures spontaneously. Sagittal plane angular deformities correct better than coronal plane deformities, and varus deformities correct better than valgus deformities. Bones remodel in response to body weight, muscle action, and by intrinsic control mechanisms of the periosteum. In meta-diaphyseal angular deformities, bone degradation will occur on the convex side and appositional bone formation occurs on the concave side. These biological mechanisms are described in the law of Roux and the thesis of Wolff. Although spontaneous correction is possible, accurate anatomic alignment should be attempted whenever reasonably achieved by conservative or operative means, especially in the lower limbs.

References

1. Wetzel RC, Bums RC. Multiple trauma in children: critical care overview. Crit Care Med. 2002;30(11 Suppl):S468–77.
2. Jakob H, Brand J, Marzi I. Multiple trauma in pediatric patients. Unfallchirurg. 2009;112(11):951–8.
3. Kay RM, Skaggs DL. Pediatric polytrauma management. J Pediatr Orthop. 2006;26(2):268–77.
4. Meier R, Krettek C, Grimme K, Regel G, Remmers D, Harwood P, et al. The multiply injured child. Clin Orthop Relat Res. 2005;432:127–31.
5. Bernbeck R, Dahmen G. Kinder-Orthopädie. 3rd ed. Stuttgart, New York: Thieme; 1983. p. 8.
6. Stylianos S, Nathens AB. Comparing processes of pediatric trauma care at children's hospitals versus adult hospitals. J Trauma. 2007;63(6 Suppl):S96–100.
7. Ott R, Kramer R, Martus P, Bussenius-Kammerer M, Carbon R, Rupprecht H. Prognostic value of trauma scores in pediatric patients with multiple injuries. J Trauma. 2000;49: 729–36.
8. Biarent D, Bingham R, Richmond S, Maconochie I, Wyllie J, Simpson S, et al. European resuscitation council guidelines for resuscitation (2005) Section 6 Pediatric life support. Resuscitation. 2005;67(1):97–133.
9. Degenhardt P, Kleber C, Bail HJ. Emergencies in pediatric traumatology – fractures in the growing age and pediatric polytrauma. Anasthesiol Intensivmed Notfallmed Schmerzther. 2009;44(6):445–9.
10. Sturm JA, Lackner CK, Bouillon B, Seekamp A, Mutschler WE. Advanced Trauma Life Support (ATLS). Unfallchirurg. 2002;105(11):1027–32.
11. Hörmann M, Scharitzer M, Philipp M, Metz VM, Lomoschitz F. First experiences with multidetector CT in traumatized children. Eur J Radiol. 2003;48(1):125–32.
12. Balci AE, Kazez A, Eren S, Ayan E, Ozalp K, Eren MN. Blunt thoracic trauma in children: review of 137 cases. Eur J Cardiothorac Surg. 2004;26(2):387–92.
13. Munk RD, Strohm PC, Saueressig U, Zwingmann J, Uhl M, Südkamp NP, et al. Effective dose estimation in whole-body multislice CT in paediatric trauma patients. Pediatr Radiol. 2009;39(3):245–52.
14. Stylianos S. Compliance with evidence-based guidelines in children with isolated spleen or liver injury: a prospective study. J Pediatr Surg. 2002;37(3):453–6.

15. Lutz N, Mahboubi S, Nance ML, Stafford PW. The significance of contrast blush on computed tomography in children with splenic injuries. J Pediatr Surg. 2004;39(3):491–4.
16. Carreon LY, Glassman SD, Campbell MJ. Pediatric spine fractures: a review of 137 hospital admissions. J Spinal Disord Tech. 2004;17(6):477–82.
17. von Laer Lutz. Frakturen und Luxationen im Wachstumsalter. 4th ed. Stuttgart, New York: Thieme Verlag; 2001. p. 12.
18. Dietz HG, Schmittenbecher P, Slongo T, Wilkins K. AO manual of fracture management elastic stable intramedullary nailing(ESIN) in children. Stuttgart: Thieme; 2005.
19. Vitale MG, Kessler MW, Choe JC, Hwang MW, Tolo VT, Skaggs DL. Pelvic fractures in children an exploration of practice and patient outcome. J Pediatr Orthop. 2005;25:581–7.
20. Salter RB, Harris WR. Injuries involving the epiphyseal plate. J Bone Joint Surg Am. 1963;45:587–622.

Fracture Management in the Pregnant Patient

Erich Sorantin, Nima Heidari, Karin Pichler, and Annelie-Martina Weinberg

Contents

17.1	Epidemiology	189
17.2	Anatomic and Physiologic Changes in Pregnancy	190
17.3	Assessment of the Injured Pregnant Patient	192
17.3.1	General Assessment	192
17.3.2	Radiological Assessment	193
17.4	Surgical Intervention	197
17.4.1	Anaesthesia	197
17.4.2	Intraoperative Radiology	198
17.4.3	Orthopaedic Surgical Management	199
17.5	Outcomes	201
References		201

E. Sorantin
Department of Radiology, Medical University of Graz,
Auenbruggerplatz 34, 8036 Graz, Austria
e-mail: erich.sorantin@medunigraz.at

N. Heidari
Paediatric Trauma Fellow, Department of Paediatric and Adolescent Surgery, Medical University of Graz,
Auenbruggerplatz 34, 8036 Graz, Austria
e-mail: n.heidari@gmail.com

K. Pichler
Medical University of Graz, Harrachgasse 21/7,
A-8010 Graz, Austria
e-mail: karin_pichler@hotmail.com

A.-M. Weinberg (✉)
Department of Paediatric and Adolescent Surgery, Medical University of Graz, Auenbruggerplatz 34, 8036 Graz, Austria
e-mail: annelie.weinberg@t-online.de

17.1 Epidemiology

Trauma in pregnancy is a relatively uncommon problem, but it is complicated due to the alterations of the maternal anatomy and physiology as well as the presence of the foetus in the gravid uterus. Between 4% and 8% of all pregnant women have an accident resulting in an injury [1–4], but only 0.3–0.4% require admission to a hospital [5]. Trauma is the leading non-obstetric cause of maternal mortality, accounting for 46% of maternal deaths [6]. This translates to approximately one million deaths/year worldwide. Pregnancy itself is not a risk factor for mortality following trauma; this has been shown to be a function of the severity of the injury [7, 8]. The risk of trauma to both the foetus and the mother increases as the pregnancy progresses with approximately 15% of injuries occurring in the first trimester and up to 55% in the third trimester. The pregnant patient seems to be more vulnerable to abdominal trauma and less prone to head or thoracic injury. It is not clear, however, whether the severity of the head injury is less or the potential for recovery greater [8]. The increase in the relative incidence of abdominal trauma with increasing gestation is most likely due to change in the shape of the patient as well as inappropriate positioning of seatbelts in motor vehicles. The leading cause for trauma is road traffic accidents, followed by falls [6]. Other important causes such as domestic violence should not be overlooked, and some studies suggest this to be the leading cause for maternal mortality [9]. These injury patterns are described in reports from western countries.

The leading cause in foetal death is road traffic accidents with the main aetiologies being maternal death and placental abruption. A combination of a non-viable pregnancy (less than 23 weeks gestation) and an injury severity score of greater than 8 has been shown to increase foetal mortality fivefold [10].

Several risk factors have been identified for the occurrence of injuries and trauma in the pregnant patient including young age, history of domestic violence and drug abuse [11]. It is interesting that some racial risk factors have been identified in the occurrence of trauma in pregnancy in the USA. It has been shown that African-American and Hispanic pregnant women are at higher risk for trauma in pregnancy [12]. This is more likely to be a function of the patient's socio-economic status. In addition to the high-energy injuries described above, pregnant women sustain low-energy fractures associated with falls. Osteoporosis of pregnancy has been implicated in these injuries [13, 14].

17.2 Anatomic and Physiologic Changes in Pregnancy

The most obvious and dramatic change during pregnancy is the enlargement of the uterus, brought about by the growth of the foetus (Table 17.1). The uterus becomes an intra-abdominal organ at approximately 12 weeks of gestation. At 20 weeks, the vertex of the uterus can be palpated at the level of the umbilicus, and by the 36th week, the uterus reaches the costal margin. In the last few weeks of pregnancy, fundal height decreases as the foetal head engages into the pelvis in preparation for the birth.

Anatomical changes during pregnancy should be borne in mind when interpreting initial radiological assessment of the patient. The elevation of the diaphragm by approximately 4 cm and its widening by 2 cm during late pregnancy should be appreciated on the chest radiograph. This may give the appearance of widened mediastinum and an enlarged heart. Increased levels of circulating progesterone lead to the softening of the sacroiliac ligaments, hence widening the joint space. The symphysis pubis may also be widened by 4–8 mm [16].

The changes in the cardiovascular system are numerous and begin from the eighth week of gestation. Progesterone induces relaxation of the smooth-muscle in walls of the peripheral vasculature. There is a gradual decline in blood pressure from week 10, reaching its lowest point by week 28 of gestation. In the third trimester, the blood pressure gradually returns to pre-pregnancy levels. The heart rate also shows an increase of 10–15 beats/min, driving an increase in the cardiac output of 30–50%. This gradually returns to normal over the first two post-partum weeks. There is a 50% increase in the blood volume which is mostly due to an expansion of the plasma volume with only 30% increase in the volume of red cells. This brings about a dilutional anaemia referred to as physiological anaemia of pregnancy. The hypervolaemic and hyperdynamic circulation allows the mother to tolerate blood loss of 500–1,000 ml with little change in blood pressure and pulse rate. This however is achieved to the detriment of the foetus following trauma. Vasoconstriction of uterine and splanchnic blood vessels and diversion of circulatory volume masks maternal blood loss although signs of foetal distress will be apparent prior to the mother showing the expected signs of shock [17].

Almost all the coagulation factors increase in pregnancy. These along with the expansion of blood volume and cardiac output are important adaptations for the expected blood loss at the time of delivery [11]. This hypercoagulable state predisposes the mother to thromboembolic disease.

The respiratory system also undergoes some changes. There is engorgement of the respiratory mucosa, which leads to difficulties in intubation and mucosal bleeding [18, 19]. This may result in severe airway compromise. There are also adaptations related to the increased metabolic demands. The presence of the foetus necessitates an increase of 15–20% in oxygen consumption. Progesterone stimulates the respiratory centre leading to hyperventilation, which brings about a compensated respiratory alkalosis with a concomitant drop in the PCO_2. There is a 4-cm elevation of the diaphragm, with a 2-cm increase in the thoracic anteroposterior diameter. This results in a 20–25% decrease in the functional residual capacity [15]. The pregnant patient is therefore much less tolerant of hypoxia and the associated acidosis. Foetal oxygenation remains constant if maternal PaO_2 is kept above 60 mmHg as below this level there is a profound drop in foetal oxygenation [11].

Progesterone reduces gastrointestinal motility and the gravid uterus displaces the stomach cephalad. This results in the incompetence of the gastroesophageal pinchcock mechanism, placing the pregnant patient at greater risk of regurgitation and aspiration [20]. Therefore, all pregnant patients should be assumed to have a full stomach and the threshold for insertion of a gastric tube lowered.

17 Fracture Management in the Pregnant Patient

Table 17.1 Changes in maternal anatomy and physiology in pregnancy [11, 15]

Conditions	Change during pregnancy	Normal pregnancy values
Cardiovascular		
Heart rate	Increases 15–20 bpm	75–95 bpm
Cardiac output	Increases 30–50%	6–8 l/min
Mean arterial blood pressure	Decreases 10 mmHg in midtrimester	80 mmHg
Systemic vascular resistance	Decreases 10–15%	1,200–1,500 dyn/s/cm^{-5}
ECG	Flat or inverted T waves in leads III, V1 and V2	
	Q waves in leads III and aVF	
Hematologic		
Blood volume	Increases 30–50%	4,500 ml
Erythrocyte volume	Increases 10–15%	
Haematocrit	Decreased	
White blood cell count	Increased	5,000–15,000/mm³
Factors I, II, V, VII, VIII, IX, X and XII	Increased	
Fibrinogen	Increased	>400 mg/dl
Prothrombin time	Decreased by 20%	
Partial thromboplastin time	Decreased by 20%	
Respiratory		
Tidal volume	Increased 40%	700 ml
Minute ventilation	Increased 40%	10.5 ml
Expiratory reserve volume	Decreased 15–20%	550 ml
Functional residual capacity	Decreased 20–25%	1,350 ml
Upper airway	Increased oedema; capillary engorgement	
Diaphragm	Displaced 4 cm cephalad	
Thoracic anteroposterior diameter	Increased	
Risk of aspiration	Increased	
Respiratory rate	Slightly increases in the first trimester	
Oxygen consumption	Increased 15–20% at rest	
Blood gas		
pH	Unchanged	7.4–7.45
pCO$_2$	Decreased	27–32 mmHg
pO$_2$	Increased	100–108 mmHg
HCO$_3$	Decreased	18–21 mEq/l
Abdomen and genitourinary system		
Intraabdominal organs	Compartmentalization and cephalad displacement	
Gastrointestinal tract	Decreased gastric emptying; decreased motility; increased risk of aspiration	

(continued)

Table 17.1 (continued)

Conditions	Change during pregnancy	Normal pregnancy values
Peritoneum	Small amounts of intraperitoneal fluid normally present; desensitised to stretching	
Musculoskeletal system	Widened symphysis pubis and sacroiliacal joints	
Kidneys	Mild hydronephrosis (right > left)	
Renal blood flow	Increased 50–60%	700 ml/min
Glomerular filtration rate	Increased 60%	140 ml/min
Serum creatinine	Decreased	<0.8 mg/dl
Serum urea nitrogen	Deceased	<13 mg/dl

In the genitourinary system, there is gradual ascent of the uterus from the pelvis, where it is well protected, into the abdomen from the 12th week of gestation. Once the uterus becomes intra-abdominal, it is at greater risk of injury from blunt and penetrating trauma. The bladder is displaced anteriorly and superiorly. The renal pelvis and ureters become dilated due to the compressive effect of the uterus as well as the effect of circulating progesterone. The increased cardiac output and blood volume increases renal perfusion by up to 60% with a concomitant increase in the glomerular filtration rate. This leads to a significant reduction in the serum urea and creatinine levels [15].

17.3 Assessment of the Injured Pregnant Patient

17.3.1 General Assessment

The initial assessment and management of the injured pregnant patient follows the well-established routine of Advanced Trauma Life Support. The best initial treatment of the foetus is the provision of optimum resuscitation for the mother accompanied by foetal monitoring particularly when the foetus is viable. The safe and judicious assessment of the pregnant patient should be a multidisciplinary exercise with the early involvement of an obstetrician, a neonatologist, a radiologist and a trauma surgeon [11, 15, 16, 21, 22].

Pregnant trauma patients can be divided into four groups. The first group are women who are not aware that they are pregnant. Therefore, all female trauma patients of reproductive age should have a pregnancy test performed [23]. Identification of these patients is especially important because routine radiographic studies, performed in the trauma assessment, have the greatest teratogenic potential in early pregnancy. But this consideration should not interfere with life-saving investigations or interventions for the patient. Patients belonging to the second group are injured women of less than 26 weeks of gestation. In these patients, resuscitation is aimed primarily at the mother since the foetus is not yet independently viable. The third and perhaps the most challenging group consists of women with pregnancies of more than 26 weeks' gestation. At this stage, there are two patients to consider during the assessment and resuscitation. Finally, there are those patients who present in the perimortem stage. In these patients, early caesarean section may facilitate maternal resuscitation and preserve the life of the foetus [16].

After 20-weeks' gestation, nursing the pregnant patient in the supine position will induce supine hypotension syndrome as the gravid uterus compresses the vena cava, reducing the venous return and embarrassing maternal cardiac output by 30%. This can be alleviated by either displacing the uterus to the left side or, if possible, nursing the patient tilted left side down by 15°. Due to reduction in the mother's respiratory reserve, supplemental oxygen should be provided. Loss of up to 2,000 ml of blood is well tolerated, but this is at the expense of uterine blood supply. The use of vasopressors further compromises uterine blood flow and their use should be avoided unless it is a life-saving intervention. Monitoring of uterine activity and the assessment of the foetus is imperative and should continue for 2–6 h after an injury, even with relatively minor trauma [24, 25]. Signs of foetal distress may be the first signs of maternal hypovolaemia and haemodynamic compromise. The use of vasopressors should be avoided as they further embarrass uteroplacental perfusion. It is preferable to manage cardiac output and blood pressure by replacing volume.

In case of a positive Kleihauer-Betke test, indicating foetal blood in the maternal circulation, the rhesus-negative patients should receive anti-D antibody to prevent isoimmunisation [26–28].

As part of the secondary survey, a complete medical and obstetric history should be obtained, particularly details relating to pre-existing hypertension, eclampsia and diabetes. Information about the mechanism of injury, use of drugs and alcohol should be sought. Otherwise all limbs and body system should be examined in the usual manner. Radiological examination of all suspected fractures should be carried out with the involvement of a radiologist, as a close check needs to be kept on the cumulative dose of radiation received by the patient [22, 29–32].

An early vaginal examination must be conducted. Ideally, this should be performed with an obstetrician in attendance to assess cervical effacement and dilation, foetal position and the presence of amniotic fluid or blood. In the presence of vaginal bleeding, it is prudent to rule out a placenta previa prior to the formal examination of the cervix [31]. The bleeding may be due to placental abruption, labour or placenta previa. Other more traumatic causes such as uterine rupture and an open pelvic fracture must also be considered.

A focused assessment with sonography for trauma (FAST) scan is important to assess presence of intra-abdominal haemorrhage. An ultrasound examination of the foetus and placenta can be performed after the FAST scan or incorporated as part of the trauma scan. If a chest tube thoracostomy is needed, it has to be placed one or two intercostal spaces higher than usual to avoid diaphragmatic injury.

Tetanus prophylaxis is not contraindicated and should be administered according to standard protocols.

17.3.2 Radiological Assessment

17.3.2.1 General Considerations

Trauma in pregnancy represents a special situation as two patients are involved – the mother and the child. Radiographic and CT examinations of the pregnant patient irradiate the unborn and can cause severe harm. Intrauterine development consists of three phases, and radiation sensitivity is related to gestational age.

As a general guideline, the 'ALARA Principle' should be mentioned here – meaning, that radiation should be used 'as low as reasonably achievable' [33].

17.3.2.2 Basics of Radiation Protection

The following types of radiation have to be differentiated: α, β, γ and X-rays. For medical imaging, only γ-radiation (Nuclear Medicine) and X-rays are used.

Important Units for Radiation Benchmarking

Ion dose: measures radiation by the amount of the induced ionisation – the SI unit is R.

Absorbed dose: defines the absorbed dose/kg mass; the SI unit is Gray (Gy) = 1 J/kg.

Dose output: is dose/time; Gy/s represents the SI unit. Due to the inherently different properties of α-, β-, γ- and X-rays, they are converted into units that are representative of their varying biologic activity. This is achieved by multiplying the absorbed dose by a dimensionless radiation weighting factor (*WR*, prior *Q* – relative biological effectiveness). The result is the *dose equivalent*, which is measured in Sievert (Sv):

Sievert (Sv) = Gy × *WR* – the corresponding values can be found in Table 17.2.

Organ dose: represents the absorbed dose output of an organ, tissue or body part, which is multiplied by the radiation weighting factor – SI unit is again Sv.

Table 17.2 Weighting factor by radiation type [34]

Radiation type		Radiation weighting factor
Photons		1
Electrons, muons		1
Neutrons	<10 keV	5
	10–100 keV	10
	>100–2 MeV	20
	>2–20 MeV	10
	>20 MeV	5
Protons (Energy >2 MeV)		5
α–Radiation		20

Table 17.3 Tissue/organ weighting factor with due consideration of the differences in sensitivity of tissues/organs to radiation [35]

Tissue/organ	Weighting factor W_t
Gonads	0.20
Red bone marrow	0.12
Colon	0.12
Lung	0.12
Stomach	0.12
Urinary bladder	0.05
Chest	0.05
Liver	0.05
Oesophagus	0.05
Thyroid	0.05
Skin	0.01
Bone surface	0.01
Others	0.05

Table 17.4 Typical effective doses in imaging

Examination	Typical effective dose (mSv)	Number of chest X-rays leading to the comparable exposure
Chest (p.a.)	0.02	1.0
Extremities/joints	0.01	0.5
Skull	0.07	3.5
Thoracic vertebra	0.70	35.0
Hip	0.30	15.0
Pelvis	0.70	35.0
Mammography (bilateral, 2 planes)	0.50	25.0
Intravenous urography	2.50	125.0
Head CT	2.30	115.0
Chest CT	8.00	400.0
Abdomen/pelvis CT	10.00	500.0
Renal function scintigraphy	0.80	40.0
Thyroid scintigraphy	0.90	45.0
Lung perfusion scintigraphy	1.10	55.0
Skeletal scintigraphy	4.40	220.0
Myocardial perfusion scintigraphy	6.80	340.0
PET	7.20	360.0
Myocardial scintigraphy	17.00	865.0

Doses can vary due to technical factors (e.g., additional filtration) as well as adjustment of the exposure settings to body mass/size, age and several other factors [37]

Effective dose equivalent: considers the different radiation sensitivity for various human tissues by the so-called tissue/organ weighting factor (*WT* – Table 17.3). The effective dose equivalent is calculated by first multiplying the organ dose with the tissue/organ weighting factor, followed by adding all individual doses.

Natural Background Radiation

The source of natural background radiation falls into two broad categories – natural (from ground and space) and artificial (medicine, radioactive fallout, nuclear waste, consumer products, etc.). The cumulative dose is approximately 4 mSv. It is interesting to note that medical diagnostic imaging and nuclear medicine are responsible for about 79% of manmade radiation [36]. Typical radiation doses for medical imaging can be found in Table 17.4.

Deterministic Versus Stochastic Radiation Effects

In *deterministic effects*, there is a classical dose–effect relationship such as the LD50/30 (the dose of whole-body irradiation where 50% of subjects die within 30 days of exposure) [38] of ~4.0 Sv. After a 3.0 Sv there are severe skin burns, after 3.0-4.0 Sv cataracts occur – just to name some examples.

Stochastic effects are those that occur in a random manner, including cancer and genetic defects. These events cannot be related to a single dose, but the cumulative effect of multiple exposures may result in damage and, for this reason, the concept of the excess lifetime risk was introduced. The risk is higher for younger people, which can be partly explained by the higher sensitivity of dividing cells to radiation. The 'International Commission on Radiation Protection (ICRP)' suggests an excess rate of 5%/Sv for lower doses and 10% for higher ones.

An excess lifetime risk factor of 10% means that after exposing 10,000 individuals to 10 mSv dose of radiation, there will be about ten additional deaths due to leukaemia or cancer, but it is important to note that even without this radiation, there would be 2,500 cancer-related deaths [37].

Radiation Effects During Intrauterine Life

The following facts are based on the report of 'German Society for Medical Physics' and the 'German X-Ray Society' [39]. A summary of all effects can be found in Table 17.5.

The period of intrauterine life can be divided into three phases. These are the pre-implantation phase (until 10 days post conception), the phase of organogenesis (10 days to 8 weeks' gestation), and the foetal period (from 3 months' gestation to term). Exposure to radiation in each phase has characteristic effects.

Pre-implantation phase: High doses (>100 mSv) result in spontaneous abortion, which is often clinically silent, as pregnancy is not known yet. Birth defects are possible, with a risk coefficient of 0.1%/mSv.

Organogenesis: High doses (>100 mSv) cause organ malformations as well as growth retardation and functional disorders. The risk coefficient for organ malformations is 0.05%/mSv, which doubles at 200 mSv.

Foetal Period: The central nervous system is the most susceptible organ during this phase and radiation exposure has been linked to severe neuromotor development disorders, with a risk coefficient of 0.04%/mSv from the 8th to the 15th week of gestation and 0.01%/mSv from the 16th to the 25th week of gestation. Reduction in the 'Intelligent Quotient' (IQ) represents another known radiation effect, being more severe during early pregnancy: 30 IQ points for the 8th to the 15th week of gestation and 10 IQ points for the 16th to the 25th week.

Cancer Risk After Intrauterine Irradiation

A linear dose–effect relationship is presumed; however, there is no known threshold. It is assumed that doses of less than 100 mSv may pose a significant risk for the development of leukaemia and cancer. The risk coefficient is about 0.006%/mSv.

Genetic Effects After Irradiation

A linear dose–effect relationship is also assumed here. There are no data available from human studies; we have, however, extrapolated from some animal studies in Table 17.5.

17.3.2.3 Imaging of the Pregnant Patient

Radiographs of the extremities can be safely performed during all stages of pregnancy, but adequate shielding (Fig. 17.1) is a MUST and can reduce the radiation dose to the unborn by up to 30%. The generator settings should be on the lowest possible values

Table 17.5 Effects of irradiation during intrauterine life [36]

Effect	Gestational age	Lower threshold	Risk-coefficient
Death during pre-implantation phase	0–10 days	100 mSv	0.1%/mSv
Malformation	10 days–8 weeks	100 mSv	0.05%/mSv
Severe mental retardation	8–15 weeks	300 mSv	0.04%/mSv
	16–25 weeks	300 mSv	0.01%/mSv
IQ-reduction	8–15 weeks		0.03 IQ/mSv
	16–25 weeks		0.01 IQ/mSv
Cancer/leucemia			0.006%/mSv
Genetic defects			0.0003%/mSv male
			0.0001%/mSv female

Fig. 17.1 A 28-year-old woman was involved in a road traffic accident. She was 15 weeks pregnant and a front passenger in a car. On arrival in the emergency department, she was haemodynamically stable, but the left leg was internally rotated and in fixed adduction. A posterior dislocation of the left hip was immediately suspected. In order to protect the foetus, her lower abdomen was covered with a lead shield before obtaining the radiograph of the left hip (**a**). This demonstrated a subluxed femoral head with fracture of the posterior acetabular wall. She underwent an open reduction and internal fixation of her fracture. We did not utilise intraoperative imaging. In the post-operative radiograph (**b**), the gravid uterus was again protected with a lead shield. (**c**) AP radiograph of the pelvis 1 year post-operatively

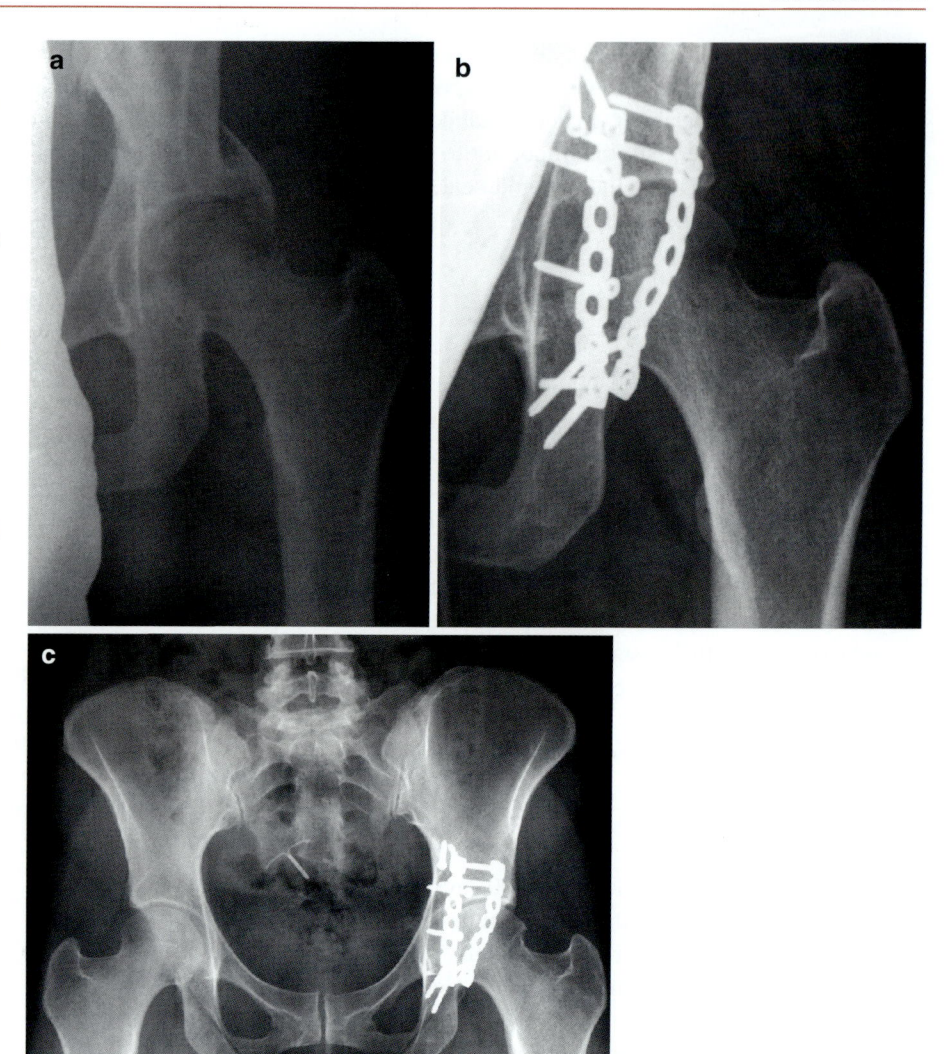

where diagnostic information can still be gleaned. This necessitates discussion and close collaboration with both radiologists and radiographers.

In stable patients with suspected ligamentous injuries (e.g., ankle), MRI is preferable over repeated stress radiographs.

In abdominal trauma or poly-trauma patients, ultrasound is the preferred first-line imaging modality – e.g., FAST scan in order to detect free, intraperitoneal fluid. It is imperative to include the foetus as well as the placenta in every sonographic evaluation of the abdomen and pelvis [40].

CT is the preferred modality in unstable patients or in patients with clinical/sonographic signs of injuries to chest, mediastinum, aorta, spine, retroperitoneum, bowel, bladder and pelvis. Intravenous iodine contrast may be administered as indicated clinically, but this may induce hypothyroidism in the unborn in addition to causing renal anomalies. Therefore, after delivery, follow-up investigations of thyroid and renal function are needed. CT should be performed with adapted dose values for the mother with considerations of her body habitus. It is important to note that with a 20% reduction in the ideal adjusted dose, there will be more image noise; however, the images will be of good enough quality to diagnose traumatic lesions. Other means of reducing the radiation dose with CT scans include the adjustment of the scanogram and appropriate reconstructions kernels. In newer CT systems, special attention to the image reconstruction kernel is needed, if automated exposure control systems are used.

In CT, a total radiation dose of more than 100 mSv should not be exceeded by a single examination using standard trauma protocols. Several significant differences exist between the various CT scanner generations. Old multidetector CT scanners suffer from 'Overbeaming', where the X-ray beam extends beyond the edge of detector rows, exposing the patient to a greater radiation dose. While the newer helical multi-detector-row CT systems 'Overrange' as the reconstruction algorithm requires additional raw data on both sides of the planned scan, extra rotations outside the planned length are needed for image reconstruction. This can be reduced by adequate tailoring of scan length. Nevertheless, calculations of the International Committee on Radiation Protection (IRCP) estimate that a foetal dose of 10 mGy will increase the risk of leukaemia or cancer considerably [41].

MRI is usually not an option in unstable pregnant patients, since the examinations are time consuming and not at all MRI scanners offer monitoring facilities.

Field strengths of up to 1.5 T are preferable as there are concerns about the heating effects of radiofrequency pulses as well as the effect of acoustic noise on the unborn. Gadolinium-based MRI contrast media have been shown to be teratogenic in animal studies if administered in doses two to seven times greater than normal. Gadolinium crosses the placenta and is excreted by the foetal kidney into the amniotic fluid. In the light of new insights in Gadolinium side effects including Nephrogenic Systemic Fibrosis (NSF), all statements regarding the use of Gadolinium have to be re-evaluated, especially in pregnant women. NSF occurs in people with severely impaired renal function, but as foetal kidneys are immature, the potential harm to the unborn is unquantifiable and extreme caution should be exercised [42].

It is the author's belief that if intravenous contrast is essential for clinical decision making, then CT should be considered, as the side effects of radiation and iodine contrast are known, whereas this is not the case with Gadolinium and MRI.

We recommend that departments where pregnant trauma patients are treated should have a management algorithm. This should address the use of imaging both for initial assessment of the patient (including dose settings for plane radiography and CT) as well as the subsequent clinical treatment (including intraoperative use of imaging or further imaging for follow-up).

Involvement of a radiologist from the outset of the management of the pregnant trauma patient is essential as imaging plays an integral role in all aspects of management and treatment of these patients.

17.4 Surgical Intervention

It is logical to postpone all elective procedures until after delivery [43, 44]. However, provision of optimum emergency surgical care should not be compromised. Surgical management of fractures is dictated by the bony and soft tissue injury and it may not be feasible to postpone these procedures [29]. Most can be safely carried out in the pregnant patient. Consideration specific to anaesthesia, intraoperative radiology and orthopaedics should be taken into account.

17.4.1 Anaesthesia

Pregnancy is not a contraindication to anaesthesia. No increase in stillbirths, birth defects [45] or neural tube defects [46] has been demonstrated as a result of pregnant women receiving anaesthesia.

The management of the airway can be a challenge in pregnant patients. The incidence of difficult intubations is 17-fold higher in advanced pregnancy. There is an increased risk of aspiration, and the risk of hypoxia is higher due to reduced functional reserve and increased oxygen consumption [47]. The combination of limited maternal reserve and a foetus sensitive to changes in maternal metabolism requires close monitoring and expedient action on the part of the anaesthetist. The goals of ventilation include a high PaO_2 and a $PaCO_2$ normal for the gestation [48]. Frequent measurements of blood gases may be invaluable in these circumstances.

Uterine and foetal monitoring are useful as foetal distress may be the first sign of maternal hypovolaemia. Monitoring volume status in pregnancy may be difficult as some data show poor correlation between central venous and left ventricular filling pressures. Some authors suggest insertion of a Sawn-Ganz catheter if accurate haemodynamic monitoring is required [49, 50].

17.4.2 Intraoperative Radiology

17.4.2.1 General Considerations

The following *hardware features* should be available:

Pulsed fluoroscopy: In cases where live imaging is required, 25 frames/s are used for fluoroscopy, but this temporal resolution is rarely needed in trauma surgery. Many machines allow a rate of 2 frames/s, which is often adequate in most circumstances.

Last image hold: The last fluoroscopy image stays on the screen and can be referred to, without further radiation.

Leaf Shutter: Allows the operator to control the size of the radiation field by coning onto the region of interest an example of dose distribution in dependence of the field of view can be seen in Fig. 17.2.

'Field of View (FOV)' (magnification): Using the system's zoom functions increases the dose e.g., Changing the FOV from 28 to 20 cm (usually one magnification step) doubles the dose [51].

Powerful generator: Primary rapid and steep increase in kV should be possible.

17.4.2.2 Intraoperative Imaging

During any operative procedure, the fluoroscopy unit should be handled by the radiographer. Exact placement of the primary beam, tight use of the shutter and lead shielding are mandatory – especially the uterus should be as far as possible from the primary beam. Lead shielding reduces the scatter from the unit itself and other outside sources, whereas scatter from the irradiated tissues cannot be reduced. Of course, irradiation time should be as short as possible and extensive use of the 'Last Image Hold' technique is mandatory. The same guidelines apply for intraoperative radiography; typical doses to the foetus can be found in Table 17.6. The dose output of C-arm systems can differ considerably between manufacturers. This makes it difficult to estimate an absolute tolerable time period for irradiation of the pregnant uterus. Using the data published by Schueler et al. [51], and assuming that the gravid uterus is directly in the X-ray beam, the threshold dose of 100 mSv will be reached in about 3 min at a FOV of 28 cm, but in only 1.5 min at a FOV of 20 cm.

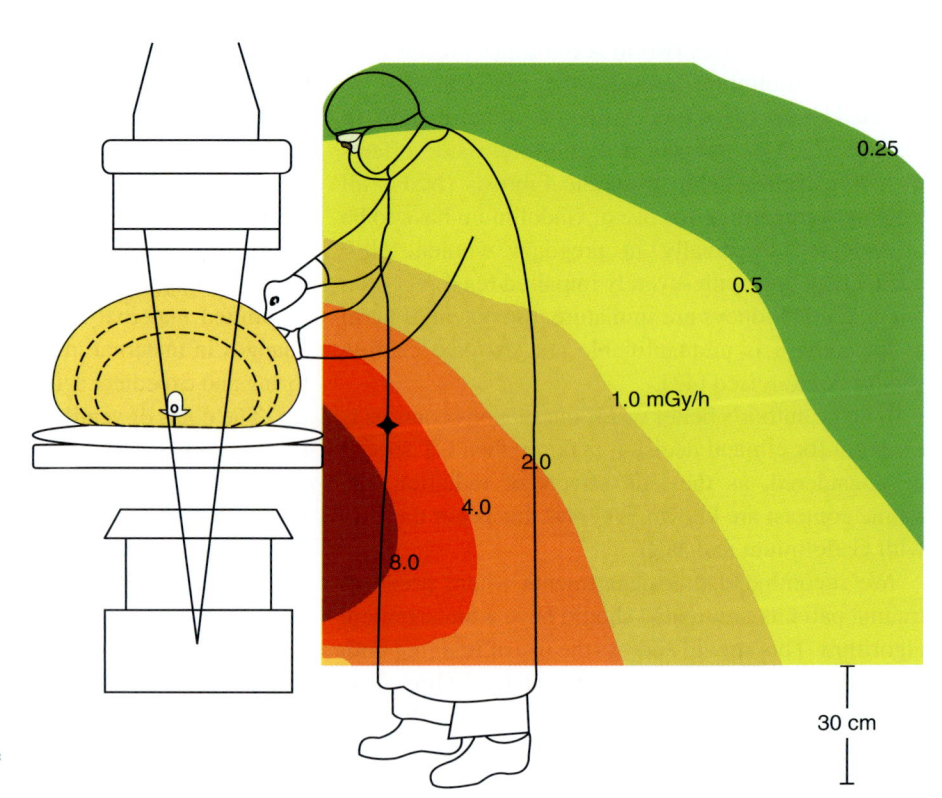

Fig. 17.2 *Isodose lines* during fluoroscopy – *colours* represent areas of almost same dose (Modified after [51])

Table 17.6 Estimated doses of ionising radiation to the foetus with relation to investigation

Examination	Typical foetal dose (mGy)
Cervical spine (AP, lat)	0.001
Extremities	0.001
Chest (PA, lat)	2
Thoracic spine (AP, lat)	3
Abdomen (AP)	0
21-cm patient thickness	1
33-cm patient thickness	3
Lumbar spine (AP, lat)	1
Limited IVP[a]	6
Small-bowel study[b]	7
Double-contrast barium enema study[c]	7

Source: From Wikipedia [52]
AP anteroposterior projection, *lat* lateral projection, *PA* posteroanterior projection

[a]Limited IVP is assumed to include four abdominopelvic images. A patient thickness of 21 cm is assumed
[b]A small-bowel study is assumed to include a 6-min fluoroscopic examination with the acquisition of 20 digital spot images
[c]A double-contrast barium enema study is assumed to include a 4-min fluoroscopic examination with the acquisition of 12 digital spot images

17.4.2.3 Take Home Points for Imaging

- Design of an algorithm for the management of the pregnant traumatised patient with particular attention to the early involvement of a radiologist and medical physicist. Detailed knowledge of the cumulative dose received by the patient is essential for ongoing management decisions.
- Ultrasound is the first modality of choice – this should be carried out with an obstetrician present.
- If a CT scan is necessary, the region scanned should be kept as small as possible. Utilise all inherent possibilities to reduce dose of ionising radiation including rigorous mAs lowering.
- If administration of intravenous iodine contrast is necessary, close monitoring of thyroid and renal function and referral to a paediatrician are essential for the child after birth.
- In non-acute imaging, detailed counselling of the mother is necessary if the foetal dose is likely to go beyond 1 mGy.
- Intraoperative Imaging – avoid direct irradiation the uterus.

17.4.3 Orthopaedic Surgical Management

There is a paucity of literature on the outcomes of orthopaedic injuries in pregnancy. In a study from New Orleans, only 4% of pregnant trauma patients had orthopaedic injuries [53]; this, however, may not be representative in other populations. Extremity fractures should be treated in much the same way as they would be in the non-pregnant patient. The pregnant patient tends to be young, and suboptimal surgical management of her fracture has profound long-term consequences. As long as direct irradiation of the uterus is avoided and adequate shielding employed, there are no contraindications to intraoperative imaging. This is of course not the case with pelvic and proximal femoral fracture fixation. Modifications of surgical technique may reduce the need of intraoperative imaging. Most minimally invasive techniques are highly dependent on intraoperative imaging and are not advocated in this situation. An open technique of fracture reduction and fixation reduces the need for imaging.

Pregnancy is a prothrombotic state, and prolonged immobilisation and bed rest should be avoided. The increased risk of venous thromboembolism (VTE) begins in the first trimester and has a tendency to occur in the left lower limb [54]. There is little data regarding VTE in pregnant women, and recommendations are based on expert opinion derived from evidence in non-pregnant populations [55]. Some specific risk factors that may relate to the traumatised pregnant patient include immobility [56], blood loss and transfusion [57] as well as having any surgical procedures. It appears that low-molecular-weight heparins are safe to use in these patients [58]. The decision to prescribe anticoagulation should be based on assessment of individual patients and after consideration of risk factors. Surgical treatment of an injury to get the patient to be mobile is clearly desirable, and the benefits outweigh the risks of the procedure.

Positioning the patient in the left lateral decubitus position (left side down) moves the gravid uterus away from the vena cava and avoids the development of supine hypotension syndrome. If it is not possible to position the patient in this way, the uterus should be manually displaced. Any blood loss should be directly communicated with the anaesthetist. Although the patient's haemodynamic parameters may remain within normal limits, this is at the expense of the blood flow to the uterus and foetus.

Fractures of the pelvis and acetabulum (Fig. 17.3) present a particular challenge in this patient cohort. The literature on this subject is restricted to mostly case reports [59–62], and there is a general trend towards conservative management of these fractures. A retrospective review from a major trauma centre of 24 years reported only seven pregnant patients with a pelvic fracture [21]. Of these patients, five mothers and three foetuses survived. This group represented severely traumatised patients, and their care needs to be undertaken in specialist units. Up to 9% of the women and 35% of foetuses died following these injuries [60]. The surgical management of these fractures can also be hazardous to the patient and the foetus, with maternal blood loss and risk of direct injury to the uterus or the foetus [61]. In these circumstances, a caesarean section could save the life of the mother and her unborn child [60, 61, 63]. The cumulative dose of ionising radiation to the foetus may be prohibitive in employing minimally invasive techniques for the fixation of pelvic and acetabular fractures. The issue of emergent external fixation of the pelvis in the pregnant patient has not been addressed in the literature. The gestational age is important as in the third trimester, the gravid uterus may interfere with the placement of both high and low anterior external fixator half pins.

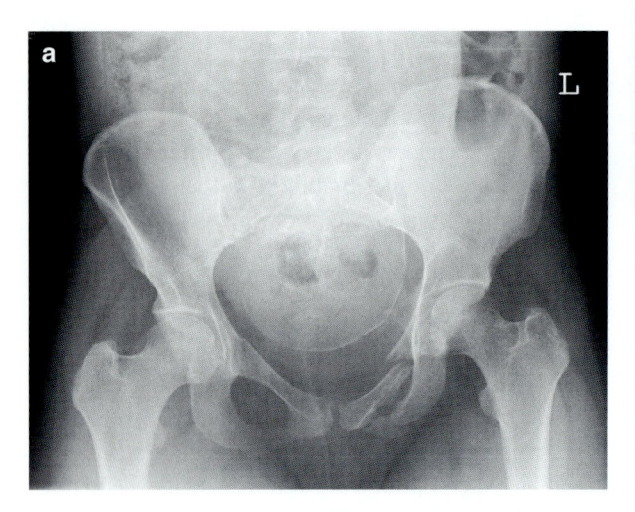

Fig. 17.3 This 32-year-old woman was involved in a road traffic accident. She was 34 weeks pregnant and was the front seat passenger wearing a seat belt. (a) The initial AP radiograph of the pelvis taken as part of the primary survey. It shows bilateral fractures of the inferior and superior pubic rami. The skeleton of the foetus with the head almost engaged in the pelvis is visible. (b) The 3D CT reconstruction of the pelvis also demonstrating an undisplaced type I left-sided sacral ala fracture. Due to haemodynamic instability and foetal distress, an emergent caesarean section was performed. Clinical examination of the pelvis only demonstrated rotational instability of the left hemi-pelvis. The definitive treatment of the pelvic fracture was with a low anterior external fixator as seen in (c) (Kindly provided by Dr Axel Gänsslen)

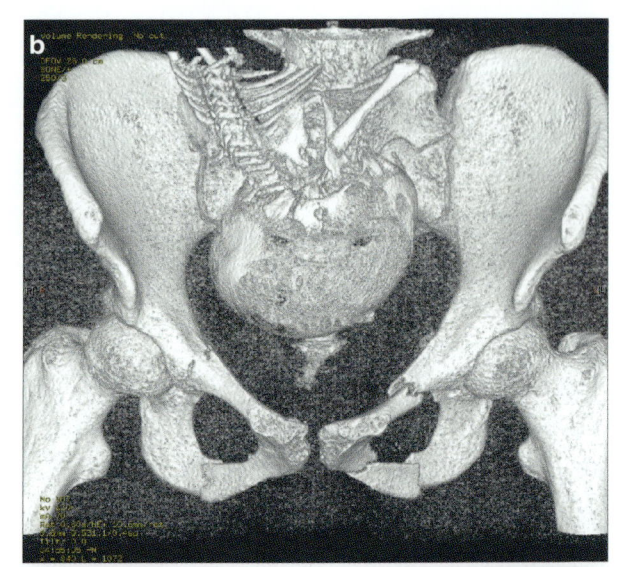

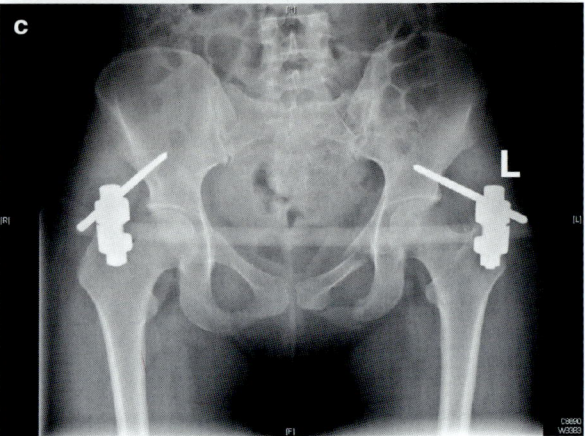

Fig. 17.3 (continued)

There are a few logical issues that must be considered to aid decision making in situations where operative intervention is required. These include foetal gestational age and viability, level of maternal and foetal compromise, the cumulative dose of ionising radiation and the necessities of fracture fixation. There simply are no easy answers and the treatment needs to be individually tailored to the patient.

17.5 Outcomes

Trauma puts both mother and the developing child at risk. This is well recognised, but quantification of the risks to the foetus and woman relies only on a few reports. This is a reflection of the unusual nature of injuries in the pregnant patient and the difficulties in collecting data on their outcome. Most of the data concentrates on the severely injured patient, but it should be borne in mind that even relatively minor trauma can lead to preterm labour and foetal loss. It has been estimated that between 4% and 61% of injured pregnant patients lose their foetuses [2].

In a study, Weiss et al. [64] reported on the causes of foetal death related to maternal injury. The data were collected from 16 states in the USA over a 3-year period. Motor vehicle accidents were by far the most common causes of foetal death (82%), with firearms (6%) and falls (3%) being far behind. The physiological diagnoses associated with foetal loss were placental abruption (42%) and maternal death (11%). They noted a trend between placental abruption accompanied by uterine rupture and advancing gestational age, but this was not a significant correlation.

As already detailed, maternal haemodynamic parameters are crude and do not provide reliable indications of the foetal status [65]. Some risk factors have been identified that herald the possibility of acute termination of pregnancy. Theodoru and colleagues [10] showed that an ISS ≥9 and a gestational age of ≤23 weeks are strong predictors of foetal loss. Other authors have demonstrated adverse foetal outcomes with increasing injury severity [66, 67], but it is interesting that even moderate maternal trauma can result in foetal death. The issue of gestational age is also contentious as some authors have not made this link [65, 67, 68]. The rates of preterm labour are increased in the presence of head injuries in patients who have a GCS ≤12, making them three times more likely to go into labour. This has not been related to increased foetal death [68].

In general, it is difficult to truly predict outcome. Indicators exist, but dramatic and devastating foetal outcomes are seen even in relatively minor trauma. It is therefore prudent to exercise caution. All pregnant patients with a viable foetus need to be closely monitored, and the early involvement of obstetricians is essential for the correct and judicious interpretation of foetal monitoring data.

References

1. El-Kady D, Gilbert WM, Anderson J, Danielsen B, Towner D, Smith LH. Trauma during pregnancy: an analysis of maternal and fetal outcomes in a large population. Am J Obstet Gynecol. 2004;190(6):1661–8.
2. Esposito TJ. Trauma during pregnancy. Emerg Med Clin North Am. 1994;12(1):167–99.
3. Rosenfeld JA. Abdominal trauma in pregnancy. When is fetal monitoring necessary? Postgrad Med. 1990;88(6):89–91. 94.
4. Vaizey CJ, Jacobson MJ, Cross FW. Trauma in pregnancy. Br J Surg. 1994;81(10):1406–15.
5. Lavin Jr JP, Polsky SS. Abdominal trauma during pregnancy. Clin Perinatol. 1983;10(2):423–38.
6. Connolly AM, Katz VL, Bash KL, McMahon MJ, Hansen WF. Trauma and pregnancy. Am J Perinatol. 1997;14(6):331–6.
7. Shah AJ, Kilcline BA. Trauma in pregnancy. Emerg Med Clin North Am. 2003;21(3):615–29.
8. Shah KH, Simons RK, Holbrook T, Fortlage D, Winchell RJ, Hoyt DB. Trauma in pregnancy: maternal and fetal outcomes. J Trauma. 1998;45(1):83–6.
9. Chang J, Berg CJ, Saltzman LE, Herndon J. Homicide: a leading cause of injury deaths among pregnant and postpartum women in the United States, 1991-1999. Am J Public Health. 2005;95(3):471–7.
10. Theodorou DA, Velmahos GC, Souter I, Chan LS, Vassiliu P, Tatevossian R, et al. Fetal death after trauma in pregnancy. Am Surg. 2000;66(9):809–12.
11. Hill CC. Trauma in the obstetrical patient. Womens Health (Lond Engl). 2009;5(3):269–83.
12. Ikossi DG, Lazar AA, Morabito D, Fildes J, Knudson MM. Profile of mothers at risk: an analysis of injury and pregnancy loss in 1,195 trauma patients. J Am Coll Surg. 2005;200(1):49–56.
13. Aynaci O, Kerimoglu S, Ozturk C, Saracoglu M. Bilateral non-traumatic acetabular and femoral neck fractures due to pregnancy-associated osteoporosis. Arch Orthop Trauma Surg. 2008;128(3):313–6.
14. Willis-Owen CA, Daurka JS, Chen A, Lewis A. Bilateral femoral neck fractures due to transient osteoporosis of pregnancy: a case report. Cases J. 2008;1(1):120.

15. Muench MV, Canterino JC. Trauma in pregnancy. Obstet Gynecol Clin North Am. 2007;34(3):555–83. xiii.
16. Tsuei BJ. Assessment of the pregnant trauma patient. Injury. 2006;37(5):367–73.
17. Greiss Jr FC. Uterine vascular response to hemorrhage during pregnancy, with observations on therapy. Obstet Gynecol. 1966;27(4):549–54.
18. Jouppila R, Jouppila P, Hollmen A. Laryngeal oedema as an obstetric anaesthesia complication: case reports. Acta Anaesthesiol Scand. 1980;24(2):97–8.
19. Kuczkowski KM, Reisner LS, Benumof JL. Airway problems and new solutions for the obstetric patient. J Clin Anesth. 2003;15(7):552–63.
20. Vanner RG. Mechanisms of regurgitation and its prevention with cricoid pressure. Int J Obstet Anesth. 1993;2(4):207–15.
21. Pape HC, Pohlemann T, Gansslen A, Simon R, Koch C, Tscherne H. Pelvic fractures in pregnant multiple trauma patients. J Orthop Trauma. 2000;14(4):238–44.
22. Petrone P, Asensio JA. Trauma in pregnancy: assessment and treatment. Scand J Surg. 2006;95(1):4–10.
23. Hirsh HL. Routine pregnancy testing: is it a standard of care? South Med J. 1980;73(10):1365–6.
24. Chames MC, Pearlman MD. Trauma during pregnancy: outcomes and clinical management. Clin Obstet Gynecol. 2008;51(2):398–408.
25. Sperry JL, Casey BM, McIntire DD, Minei JP, Gentilello LM, Shafi S. Long-term fetal outcomes in pregnant trauma patients. Am J Surg. 2006;192(6):715–21.
26. Eager R, Sutton J, Spedding R, Wallis R. Use of anti-D immunoglobulin in maternal trauma. Emerg Med J. 2003;20(5):498.
27. Huggon AM, Watson DP. Use of anti-D in an accident and emergency department. Arch Emerg Med. 1993;10(4):306–9.
28. Weinberg L. Use of anti-D immunoglobulin in the treatment of threatened miscarriage in the accident and emergency department. Emerg Med J. 2001;18(6):444–7.
29. Flik K, Kloen P, Toro JB, Urmey W, Nijhuis JG, Helfet DL. Orthopaedic trauma in the pregnant patient. J Am Acad Orthop Surg. 2006;14(3):175–82.
30. Lowe SA. Diagnostic radiography in pregnancy: risks and reality. Aust N Z J Obstet Gynaecol. 2004;44(3):191–6.
31. Mattox KL, Goetzl L. Trauma in pregnancy. Crit Care Med. 2005;33(10 Suppl):S385–9.
32. Patel SJ, Reede DL, Katz DS, Subramaniam R, Amorosa JK. Imaging the pregnant patient for nonobstetric conditions: algorithms and radiation dose considerations. Radiographics. 2007;27(6):1705–22.
33. Sardanelli F, Hunink MG, Gilbert FJ, Di LG, Krestin GP. Evidence-based radiology: why and how? Eur Radiol. 2010;20(1):1–15.
34. Wikipedia. Strahlungswichtungsfaktor. http://de.wikipedia.org/wiki/Strahlenwichtungsfaktor (2010). Accessed 14 Mar 2010.
35. Wikipedia. Effektive Dosis. http://de.wikipedia.org/wiki/Effektive_Dosis (2010). Accessed 13 Apr 2010.
36. Committee to Assess Health Risks from Exposure to Low Levels of Ionizing Radiation, National Research Council. Health risks from exposure to low levels of ionizing radiation: BEIR VII phase 2. Washington, DC: National Academies; 2006.
37. Shannoun F, Blettner M, Schmidberger H, Zeeb H. Radiation protection in diagnostic radiology. Dtsch Arztebl Int. 2008;105(3):41–6.
38. The United States Nuclear Regulatory Commission. Lethal dose (LD). http://www nrc gov/reading-rm/basic-ref/glossary/lethal-dose-ld html [serial online] 2010. [cited 27 Apr 2010].
39. Dierker J, Eschner W, Gosch D, et al. Pränatale strahlenexposition aus medizinischer indikation. Dtsch Ges Med Phys. 2002:7
40. Ma OJ, Mateer JR, Ogata M, Kefer MP, Wittmann D, Aprahamian C. Prospective analysis of a rapid trauma ultrasound examination performed by emergency physicians. J Trauma. 1995;38(6):879–85.
41. Brenner D, Elliston C, Hall E, Berdon W. Estimated risks of radiation-induced fatal cancer from pediatric CT. AJR Am J Roentgenol. 2001;176(2):289–96.
42. European Society of Urogenital Radiology. Guidelines of the European Society of Urogenital Radiology. Guidelines of the European Society of Urogenital Radiology. http://www.esur.org/Contrast-media.51.0.html [serial online] 2010. [cited 27 Apr 2010].
43. Brodsky JB, Cohen EN, Brown Jr BW, Wu ML, Whitcher C. Surgery during pregnancy and fetal outcome. Am J Obstet Gynecol. 1980;138(8):1165–7.
44. Steinberg ES, Santos AC. Surgical anesthesia during pregnancy. Int Anesthesiol Clin. 1990;28(1):58–66.
45. Mazze RI, Kallen B. Reproductive outcome after anesthesia and operation during pregnancy: a registry study of 5405 cases. Am J Obstet Gynecol. 1989;161(5):1178–85.
46. Kallen B, Mazze RI. Neural tube defects and first trimester operations. Teratology. 1990;41(6):717–20.
47. Meroz Y, Elchalal U, Ginosar Y. Initial trauma management in advanced pregnancy. Anesthesiol Clin. 2007;25(1):117–29. x.
48. Cook PT. The influence on foetal outcome of maternal carbon dioxide tension at caesarean section under general anaesthesia. Anaesth Intensive Care. 1984;12(4): 296–302.
49. Visser W, Wallenburg HC. Central hemodynamic observations in untreated preeclamptic patients. Hypertension. 1991;17(6 Pt 2):1072–7.
50. Wallenburg HC. Invasive hemodynamic monitoring in pregnancy. Eur J Obstet Gynecol Reprod Biol. 1991;42(Suppl):S45–51.
51. Schueler BA, Vrieze TJ, Bjarnason H, Stanson AW. An investigation of operator exposure in interventional radiology. Radiographics. 2006;26(5):1533–41.
52. Wikipedia. Strahlenbelastung. http://de.wikipedia.org/wiki/Strahlenbelastung (2010). Accessed 14 Mar 2010.
53. Timberlake GA, McSwain Jr NE. Trauma in pregnancy. A 10-year perspective. Am Surg. 1989;55(3):151–3.
54. James AH, Tapson VF, Goldhaber SZ. Thrombosis during pregnancy and the postpartum period. Am J Obstet Gynecol. 2005;193(1):216–9.
55. Gates S, Brocklehurst P, Davis LJ. Prophylaxis for venous thromboembolic disease in pregnancy and the early postnatal period. Cochrane Database Syst Rev. 2002;(2):CD001689.
56. Jacobsen AF, Skjeldestad FE, Sandset PM. Ante- and postnatal risk factors of venous thrombosis: a hospital-based case-control study. J Thromb Haemost. 2008;6(6):905–12.
57. James AH, Jamison MG, Brancazio LR, Myers ER. Venous thromboembolism during pregnancy and the postpartum period: incidence, risk factors, and mortality. Am J Obstet Gynecol. 2006;194(5):1311–5.
58. Andersen AS, Berthelsen JG, Bergholt T. Venous thromboembolism in pregnancy: prophylaxis and treatment with low molecular weight heparin. Acta Obstet Gynecol Scand. 2010;89(1):15–21.

59. Dunlop DJ, McCahill JP, Blakemore ME. Internal fixation of an acetabular fracture during pregnancy. Injury. 1997;28(7):481–2.
60. Leggon RE, Wood GC, Indeck MC. Pelvic fractures in pregnancy: factors influencing maternal and fetal outcomes. J Trauma. 2002;53(4):796–804.
61. Loegters T, Briem D, Gatzka C, Linhart W, Begemann PG, Rueger JM, et al. Treatment of unstable fractures of the pelvic ring in pregnancy. Arch Orthop Trauma Surg. 2005;125(3):204–8.
62. Yosipovitch Z, Goldberg I, Ventura E, Neri A. Open reduction of acetabular fracture in pregnancy. A case report. Clin Orthop Relat Res. 1992;282:229–32.
63. Prokop A, Swol-Ben J, Helling HJ, Neuhaus W, Rehm KE. Trauma in the last trimester of pregnancy. Unfallchirurg. 1996;99(6):450–3.
64. Weiss HB, Songer TJ, Fabio A. Fetal deaths related to maternal injury. JAMA. 2001;286(15):1863–8.
65. Esposito TJ, Gens DR, Smith LG, Scorpio R, Buchman T. Trauma during pregnancy. A review of 79 cases. Arch Surg. 1991;126(9):1073–8.
66. Rogers FB, Rozycki GS, Osler TM, Shackford SR, Jalbert J, Kirton O, et al. A multi-institutional study of factors associated with fetal death in injured pregnant patients. Arch Surg. 1999;134(11):1274–7.
67. Scorpio RJ, Esposito TJ, Smith LG, Gens DR. Blunt trauma during pregnancy: factors affecting fetal outcome. J Trauma. 1992;32(2):213–6.
68. Kissinger DP, Rozycki GS, Morris Jr JA, Knudson MM, Copes WS, Bass SM, et al. Trauma in pregnancy. Predicting pregnancy outcome. Arch Surg. 1991;126(9):1079–86.

Open Fractures: Initial Management

Robert Victor Cantu and Kenneth J. Koval

Contents

18.1	Introduction	205
18.2	History of Open Fracture Management	205
18.3	Initial Management and Treatment of Open Fractures	206
18.3.1	Diagnosis	206
18.3.2	Treatment	206
18.3.3	Antibiotic Treatment	207
18.3.4	Debridement and Irrigation	208
18.3.5	Timing of Wound Closure/Coverage	208
18.3.6	Type of Fracture Stabilization	209
18.3.7	Reconstruction Versus Amputation	211
18.3.8	Bone Morphogenic Proteins/Bone Grafting	211
18.3.9	Other Adjuncts to the Treatment of Open Fractures	212
18.4	Summary	213
References		213

18.1 Introduction

Each year, there are approximately 250,000 open fractures in the United States, representing 3–4% of all fractures [1, 2]. Ramon Gustilo stated that "the primary objective in the management of an open fracture is union with the prevention or eradication of wound sepsis" [3]. Treatment is focused on obtaining healthy soft-tissue coverage around the fracture. Gustilo added that "the degree to which that can be effectively managed may well determine the ultimate outcome for the bone" [3].

The initial treatment of open fractures includes administration of appropriate antibiotics and tetanus prophylaxis, debridement of nonviable tissue, followed by fracture stabilization and either primary or delayed wound closure, skin grafting, or flap coverage. Treatment of open fractures has evolved both in regard to the type of fracture stabilization and the type and timing of soft-tissue coverage. This chapter addresses some of the controversies in the initial management of open fractures with particular attention to the timing of soft-tissue coverage.

18.2 History of Open Fracture Management

The concept of surgically removing nonviable tissue from open fractures has a long history. In the 1500s, the idea of removing non-vital tissue from wounds that were not healing properly was advocated by Brunschwig and Botello [4]. In the eighteenth century, Pierre Joseph de Sault coined the term "debridement," although he was referring to the incision of wounds

R.V. Cantu (✉) and K.J. Koval
Orthopaedic Surgery, Dartmouth-Hitchcock Medical Center,
One Medical Center Drive, Lebanon, NH 03755, USA
e-mail: Robert.V.Cantu@Hitchcock.org

that were already infected to release purulence [4]. A pupil of de Sault named Dominique Jean Larrey extended the principles of debridement to include removal of nonviable tissue as soon as possible after an open wound, which is the basis of open fracture care today [4].

The concept of adding various substances to wounds to limit infection also has an extensive history. During the time of Lister, the mortality from open fractures was estimated at 40%. He introduced the idea of placing dressings soaked in carbolic acid over open wounds in an effort to decrease that rate [4]. Since that time, multiple substances have been advocated to help remove bacteria from open fractures, including soaps, antibiotics, alcohol, hydrogen peroxide, benzalkonium chloride, silver, and others. Interestingly, the use of soap in irrigation was common practice for open fractures in the early twentieth century, prior to the use of antibiotics, and recent studies have suggested that it may be superior to antibiotics used in irrigation such as bacitracin [5].

The idea of leaving wounds open after debridement of open fractures also has historical roots. In the Spanish Civil War, Trueta reportedly had excellent results when he debrided 1,073 open fractures and left all the wounds open [6]. The practice was further established in World War II, when open fractures were debrided and left open. Sulfa drugs were also used locally in wounds during World War II. The main reason the wounds were left open was the fear of clostridial infection and gas gangrene. Fractures were often covered with plaster casts and gangrene could progress undetected until the cast was removed leading to high rates of amputation and death.

The grading of open fractures took a step forward in the 1970s with the commonly used classification developed by Gustilo and Anderson [3] (See Table 18.1). Although the interobserver reliability has been questioned, the grading system has been shown to correlate with the risk of infection [7, 8].

18.3 Initial Management and Treatment of Open Fractures

18.3.1 Diagnosis

The first step in the management and treatment of open fractures is proper diagnosis. It has been said that "if there is any suspicion at all that a wound may communicate with an adjacent fracture it should be dealt with formally" [9]. For high-energy open fractures, the diagnosis is obvious, but for some low-energy grade I injuries, it may be more subtle. Indications that a wound is communicating with a nearby fracture include ongoing bleeding with fat droplets (from bone marrow) and air on X-rays or CT scan around the fracture. Some have recommended using a sterile probe to see if a wound connects with an underlying fracture. In general, however, it is best to assume any wound near a fracture communicates with the bone and treat it accordingly.

18.3.2 Treatment

In 1982, Patzakis wrote that "it is imperative that every patient with an open fracture, irrespective of the severity or type of soft-tissue wound, undergo formal surgical irrigation and debridement in an operating room setting" [10]. One exception to this rule is an open fracture resulting from a low-velocity gun shot. The dividing line between low- and high-velocity gun shots is a muzzle velocity of 2,000 ft/s. Low-velocity missiles have a muzzle velocity below 2,000 ft/s and include most civilian hand guns and a .22 rifle. High-velocity missiles have a muzzle velocity equal to or greater than 2,000 ft/s and include civilian rifles other than .22 and all military rifles. Low-velocity gun shots causing extra-articular fracture are one exception to

Table 18.1 Gustilo and Anderson classification of open fractures grades I, II, IIIA, IIIB, IIIC

Grade I	Grade II	Grade III
Low-energy fracture, laceration < 1 cm	Larger wound (1–10 cm) with minimal or moderate contamination	*IIIA* – High-energy fracture with extensive soft-tissue wound and moderate contamination but enough soft tissue to allow coverage of all bony surfaces
		IIIB – More severe soft-tissue loss necessitating flap coverage
		IIIC – Open fracture with vascular injury that requires repair

the rule of debridement and irrigation for all open fractures. In a prospective, randomized trial, Knapp et al. found that there was no difference in the infection rates between patients receiving intravenous or oral antibiotics for fractures caused by low-velocity gun shots [11]. In contrast, high-velocity gun shots are treated, like other open fractures, with surgical debridement and intravenous antibiotics. High-velocity bullets produce a shock wave as they pass through tissues and cause cavitation, resulting in a path of necrotic tissue. For this reason, the path of the bullet must be debrided to prevent residual necrotic tissue around the fracture.

18.3.3 Antibiotic Treatment

In open fractures, perhaps the area of least controversy is whether to administer antibiotics. Studies have shown that at least 70% of open fractures are contaminated with bacteria at the time of injury [3, 12]. Prior studies showed that *Staphylococcus aureus* was the most common organism causing infection in open fractures [3, 12, 13]. More recent studies have shown that gram-negative species, especially enteric organisms such as *Pseudomonas aeruginosa* and *E. coli*, are becoming more common [14, 15]. Concern also exists due to the growing rate of bacteria that are resistant to antibiotic therapy such as Methicillin-resistant *Staphylococcus aureus* and Vancomycin-resistant *Enterococcus faecium* (See Fig. 18.1). Patzakis et al. performed a prospective study on antibiotic use following an open fracture [15]. They found the lowest infection rate with cephalothin (2.4%) compared to either no antibiotics (13.9%) or penicillin and streptomycin (9.8%). The antibiotics were given before surgical debridement.

Controversy does exist regarding the type and duration of antibiotic therapy. Infection rates have been shown to correlate with the severity of injury. For Gustilo type-I fractures, infection rates range from 0 to 2%; for type-II fractures, the range is 2–10%; and for type-III fractures, the range is 10–50% [16]. Some have recommended single antibiotic therapy for type-I and type-II fractures, usually consisting of Cefazolin [14]. Others have argued that the final grading of open fractures is best done in the operating room and, therefore, even what initially appears to be a grade-I fracture should receive both gram-positive and gram-negative antibiotic coverage in the Emergency Department, usually with the addition of an aminoglycoside such as Gentamycin [17]. Alternatives to aminoglycosides include quinolones, aztreonam, or third-generation cephalosporins. There is more consensus that type-III fractures should be treated with both gram-positive and gram-negative coverage and that wounds contaminated with barn-yard debris should also receive penicillin to decrease the risk of anaerobic infection such as clostridial myonecrosis (gas gangrene) [18–20].

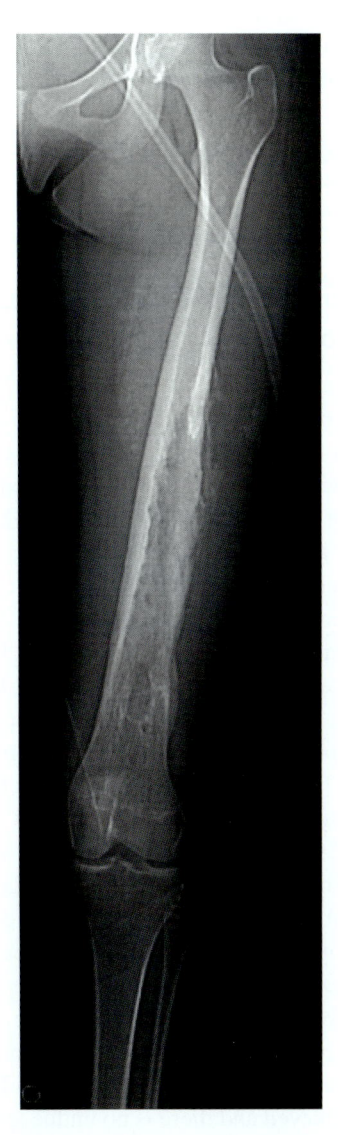

Fig. 18.1 Patient with chronic osteomyelitis of the left femur with culture positive for Vancomycin-resistant *Enterococcus faecium* following a prolonged hospitalization with an open thigh wound

18.3.4 Debridement and Irrigation

Surgical debridement of contaminated and nonviable tissue is the cornerstone of open fracture management. If dead or contaminated tissue or debris is left behind, it can serve as a nidus for bacterial growth and serve as a barrier to the normal immune response. Debridement should be performed in the operating room with appropriate anesthesia. Smaller wounds seen with Gustilo type I and type II fractures typically require extension to allow thorough debridement of the subcutaneous tissues and fracture ends. Thorough debridement of dead fat, muscle, and fascia should be performed and extra-articular bone fragments with no soft-tissue attachments removed. Exceptions to the debridement rule are large articular fragments, provided the joint can be reconstructed.

18.3.5 Timing of Wound Closure/Coverage

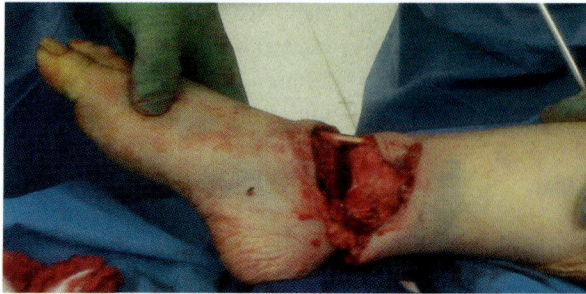

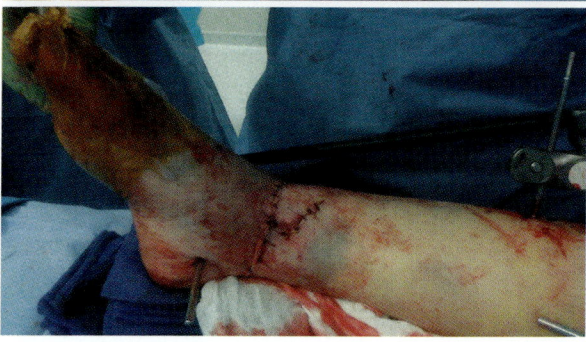

Fig. 18.2 Grade IIIA open ankle fracture treated with I+D and primary closure

Whether to close the open fracture wound at the initial surgery is a matter of debate. Historically, it has been recommended that the wound be left open and repeat debridement planned in 24–48 h [21–23]. As Weitz-Marshall et al. have reported, this practice dates back to the pre-antibiotic era when gas gangrene was a common problem. During the Spanish Civil War, it was common practice to cover the wound and fracture in a plaster cast and keep it in place "unless it became wet and soft, or there was an intolerable stench, or the patient's condition showed that some complication had developed" [24]. With current surgical techniques and antibiotics, gas gangrene is rare and it is much more common to see a late infection develop, with culture demonstrating nosocomial bacteria. Leaving the wound open carries the risk of colonizing the tissues and bone with hospital-acquired bacteria such as *Pseudomonas* or Methicillin-resistant *Staphylococcus aureus*, which can be difficult to eradicate.

More recently, some have recommended closing wounds after initial debridement, provided a clean wound is achieved and there is no undue tension of the tissues (See Fig. 18.2). Delong et al. reviewed 119 open fractures wounds treated with techniques that included: immediate closure after debridement, second look surgery at 48–72 h after primary closure with repeat closure, delayed primary closure, delayed skin grafts, delayed flaps, and primary amputation [25]. They found that the primary closure of wounds was performed for 88% of grade I, 86% of grade II, and 75% of grade IIIA fractures. This approach resulted in a 7% overall infection rate and a 16% delayed or nonunion rate. There was no significant difference in infection or nonunion rates between immediate and delayed closures. The authors concluded that primary closure is a "viable option" [25].

Primary closure of open fractures in children has been studied as well. Cullen et al. reviewed their results of primary closure in 24 grade I, 40 grade II, and 19 Grade III fractures [26]. Of the 57 fractures, 2 (3.5%) went on to superficial infection. Both of these wounds were grossly contaminated initially and according to the authors "in retrospect, not suitable for primary wound closure" [26]. There were no cases of deep infection or osteomyelitis.

When extensive soft-tissue damage occurs as in grade IIIB fractures, soft-tissue reconstruction should be performed early, ideally within the first 7 days. Delaying soft-tissue reconstruction beyond 7–10 days has been associated with increased flap complications and increased risk of infection [27, 28]. In an article entitled, "Fix and flap: the radical orthopedic and plastic treatment of severe open fractures of the tibia," Gopal et al. reviewed the results in 84 patients with grade IIIB or IIIC tibial fractures. They found a deep infection rate of 6% (4/63) for fractures covered within 72 h, and an infection rate of 29% (6/21) for fractures covered after 72 h [29]. In 33 of the patients, the debridement, fracture stabilization, and soft-tissue reconstruction was performed in a single procedure. A total of 9 pedicle flaps and 75 free muscle flaps were used in the reconstructions. The overall rate of flap failure was 3.5%. The authors concluded that provided an adequate debridement has been performed, "immediate internal fixation and healthy soft-tissue cover with a muscle flap is safe" [29].

Godina was one of the first to recommend early microvascular flap coverage for grade IIIB fractures [30]. In his article published over 20 years ago, he argued for immediate flap coverage when possible, reporting flap failures in less than 1% (1/134) when it was performed less than 72 h after injury compared to 12% (20/167) when done between 4 and 90 days. The early group had an infection rate of 1.5% (2/134) compared to 17.5% (29/167) in the late group. He argued that his technique of an immediate vascularized muscle flap quickly and reliably converted an open into a closed fracture in a single stage and allowed for the appropriate implant for the fracture from the outset.

18.3.6 Type of Fracture Stabilization

Fracture stabilization is an important step in treating open fractures. Secure stabilization limits further damage to the soft tissues, improves access to wound care, and aids in mobilization of patients. Type of fracture fixation depends on multiple factors, such as location of fracture (both which bone and where in the bone), degree of soft-tissue disruption, and age of the patient (i.e., open physes or not). Depending on these factors, fixation may involve intramedullary nails, external fixation, plates and screws, percutaneous pinning, or a combination of approaches.

For open fractures involving the diaphyseal region of long bones in the lower extremities, intramedullary nailing offers several advantages over other techniques. Intramedullary nails provide secure fixation and allow easy access to the surrounding tissues for continued wound care. Compared to external fixation, intramedullary nails have a lower rate of malunion [31]. For open femur fractures, reamed IM nails have proven effective. In 62 type I, II, and IIIA open femur fractures, Brumback et al. reported no cases of deep infection following fixation with a reamed IM nail.

They did have an 11% infection rate when reamed IM nails were used for type IIIB open femur fractures [32]. Infection rates are higher after IM nailing of open tibia fractures. Some authors have recommended unreamed tibial nails for open tibia fractures, while others have shown no difference in infection rates comparing reamed to unreamed nails [8, 33, 34]. Finkemeier et al. performed a prospective, randomized study of reamed versus unreamed nailing for open tibia fractures and found no difference in infection rates. They did find a lower incidence of screw failures in the reamed group [35]. Recently, the Study to Prospectively evaluate Reamed Intramedullary Nails in Tibial fractures (SPRINT) evaluated over 1,300 patients randomized to either reamed or unreamed tibial nails, including 400 open fractures [36]. In the open fracture group, there was a 27% risk of revision surgery. There was no statistically significant difference in need for revision comparing reamed to unreamed groups.

External fixation of open fractures can be used for either temporary or definitive treatment of fractures. One indication for temporary external fixation is the physiologically unstable patient who may not initially tolerate prolonged surgery (damage control). Another indication is a type IIIB wound that is not amenable to immediate flap coverage (See Fig. 18.3). Grossly

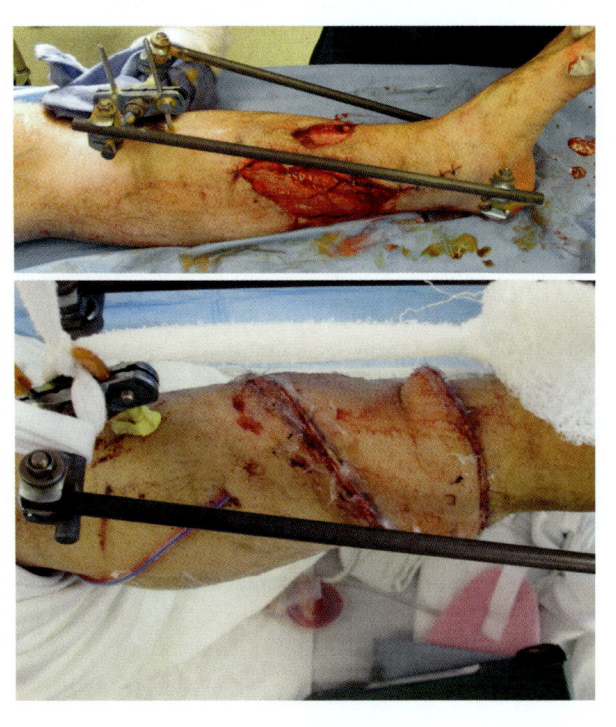

Fig. 18.3 Type IIIB open tibia fracture treated with initial spanning external fixation followed by reverse sural flap coverage

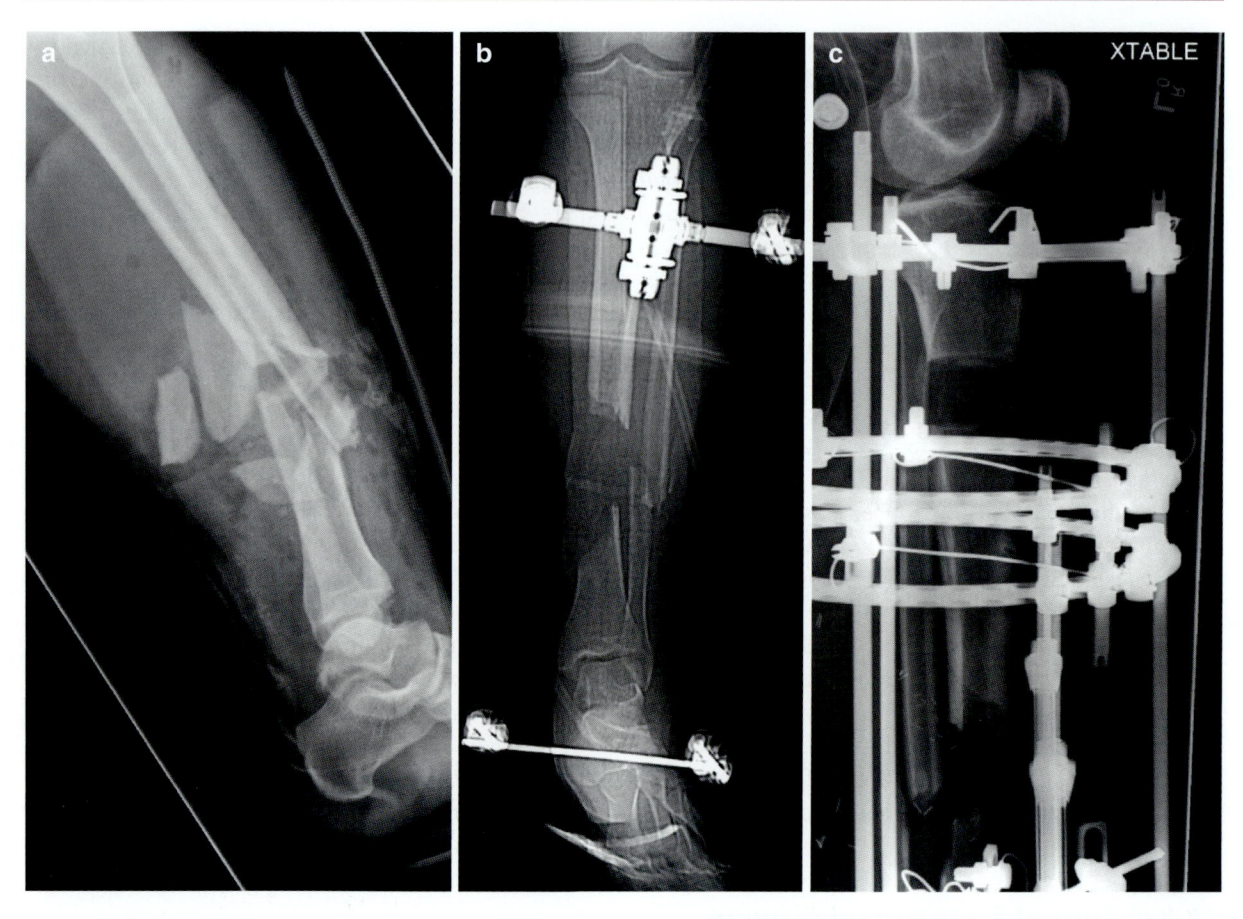

Fig. 18.4 Example of: (**a**) radiographs of grade IIIB tibia fracture with segmental bone comminution; (**b**) treated with debridement of avascular bone fragments and initial spanning external fixator; (**c**) followed by conversion to ring fixator and bone transport

contaminated fractures, especially those with farm yard debris, pond water, or fecal contamination, are often best treated, at least initially, with external fixation. External fixation can also be used for definitive treatment. Marsh et al. reported on 101 type II and type III fractures treated with external fixation. The union rate was 95% (96/101) and with a total of six deep infections [37]. Of the fractures that healed, 95% did so with less than 10° of angulation in any plane.

When external fixation is used as temporary fixation, the timing of conversion to other fixation is important (See Fig. 18.4). In a review of 54 multiply injured patients who underwent conversion of a femoral external fixator to a locked intramedullary nail on average 7 days after fixator placement, Nowotarski et al. reported a union rate of 97% at 6 months and an infection rate of only 1.7% [38]. Nineteen of the fractures in the study were open. The authors concluded that "immediate external fixation followed by early closed intramedullary nailing is a safe treatment method for fractures of the shaft of the femur" [38]. In the tibia, conversion from an external fixator to an intramedullary nail has been associated with higher infection rates, especially if the conversion is delayed. McGraw et al. reported their results after converting external fixators to intramedullary rods after open tibia fractures [39]. The average duration of the fixator was 8.5 weeks, and the average interval between removal of the fixator and nailing was 3 weeks. The overall incidence of nonunion was 50%, and the deep infection rate was 44%. They concluded that "alternative treatment options should be carefully considered before electing this sequential method of fixation" [39]. A more recent study by Blachut et al. found that if conversion of a fixator to a nail is done earlier (mean 17 days) and provided there are no pin tract infections, the infection rate is substantially lower (5%) [40].

Plate fixation is useful for open periarticular fractures in the lower extremities, provided soft-tissue coverage is possible. In the upper extremities, plate fixation is often used for open diaphyseal fractures as well. Plate fixation for open tibial fractures, however, has been shown to have a high incidence of infection and hardware failure [41, 42]. In a randomized trial, Bach et al. reported a 35% (9/26) infection rate following plating of open type II and type III tibial fractures [41]. They found a 12% (3/26) rate of fixation failure. Similarly, Clifford et al. found that four of nine type III open tibia fractures treated with plate fixation resulted in infection [42].

18.3.7 Reconstruction Versus Amputation

Technological advances have made it possible to salvage extremities that previously would have been treated only with amputation. One of the primary questions the treating physicians must answer is whether a mangled extremity with a grade IIIB or IIIC injury has the potential to recover function if successfully salvaged. If the answer to this question is no, then the multiple reconstructive surgeries required to salvage the leg, the time, expense, and duration of pain for the patient would be done in vain. Georgiadis et al. performed a retrospective review of 34 patients with grade IIIB or IIIC tibia fractures who were treated with either amputation or attempted reconstruction [43]. They found that early below the knee amputation and prosthetic fitting resulted in a faster recovery and a lower long-term disability compared to limb salvage for severely mangled extremities. Patients who had a "successful" limb salvage took more time to achieve full weight bearing, were less willing or able to work, and had higher hospital charges compared to the early amputation group. These findings are somewhat contradicted by the results of the Lower Extremity Assessment Project (LEAP) trial which found that at 2 and 7 years after severe lower extremity trauma, there was no difference in functional outcome between patients who underwent limb salvage compared to those who underwent amputation [44]. Overall outcomes were poor in both groups with only one in three patients at 7 years reporting outcome scores typical of the general population. The LEAP trial found that the factors that had the highest impact on the surgeon's decision to amputate were severe muscle injury followed by loss of plantar sensation. Follow-up work by Bosse et al. has questioned the value of the insensate foot in deciding to amputate or not [45]. They found that more than half the patients who initially had an insensate foot and underwent limb salvage regained sensation by 2 years.

18.3.8 Bone Morphogenic Proteins/Bone Grafting

Nonunion is substantially higher following open fractures compared to closed fractures. Open fractures release the fracture hematoma through the wound, thereby losing many of the factors involved in early fracture repair. What remains of the initial hematoma is removed at the time of irrigation and debridement. In an animal study, repeated irrigations of a fracture were shown to result in higher rates of delayed union and atrophic nonunion [46]. Because of the higher rate of nonunion, studies have looked at adding factors to promote fracture repair. The BMP-2 Evaluation in Surgery for Tibia Trauma (BESTT) study was a prospective, randomized trial involving 450 open tibia fractures treated with a tibial nail and either no BMP, 6 mg of rhBMP-2, or 12 mg of rhBMP-2 at the time of wound closure [47]. The 12 mg rhBMP-2 group had a 44% reduction in the risk of failure and significantly fewer invasive interventions (i.e., bone graft, nail exchange) than the control group. Interestingly, there were also fewer infections in the type III open tibia fractures in the rh-BMP group compared to controls.

Several studies have looked at early prophylactic bone grafting for treatment of open fractures [48–50]. In one retrospective review of 20 patients with grade III open tibial fractures who underwent initial debridement, external fixation, and autogenous bone grafting, the mean time to union was 28 weeks and there was only one (5%) deep infection [49]. The authors concluded that "primary prophylactic bone grafting performed at the same time reduces the rate of delayed union, shortens the time to union, and does not increase infection" [49]. This is contrary to other studies that have recommended waiting at least 2–6 weeks after soft-tissue coverage before bone grafting [48, 51]. The SPRINT trial did not allow for any reoperations to promote healing within 6 months of the initial surgery [36]. Although the study found a 27% increased risk of revision surgery for open fractures, this number would likely have been substantially higher if reoperations had been allowed during the first 6 months.

18.3.9 Other Adjuncts to the Treatment of Open Fractures

Whether to use high-pressure or low-pressure irrigation in treating open fractures has been the subject of investigation [52–55]. In vitro studies have shown that high-pressure lavage is more effective at removing bacteria [52, 53]. In an in vitro model performed by Bhandari et al., low- and high-pressure irrigation resulted in a similar reduction in bacteria following a delay of 3 h after inoculation, but only high-pressure lavage was effective in removing bacteria when the delay was 6 h [52]. The high-pressure lavage, however, did result in a greater degree of macroscopic bone damage. Whether the improved bacterial clearance at the expense of increased bone damage with high-pressure lavage is beneficial in vivo is still not fully resolved. Interestingly, an international survey of surgeons found that 71% favored low-pressure irrigation in the treatment of open fractures [56].

The type of irrigation fluid to use is also a matter of debate. The same international survey found that 70.5% of surgeons typically used normal saline as their irrigation [56]. Multiple studies have looked at the effects of adding various substances to the irrigant [57–60]. Animal and hardware studies have suggested that addition of castile soap to the irrigation may reduce the bacterial count compared to irrigation with normal saline alone [58, 61]. Soaps act as surface active agents or surfactants, theoretically disrupting the bonds between the bacteria and the underlying tissue. In a prospective, randomized clinical trial, 458 open fractures were randomized to either irrigation with saline and bacitracin or irrigation with saline and castile soap [59]. The infection rate in the bacitracin group was 18% while the infection rate in the castile soap group was 13%; however, this difference did not reach statistical significance. The bacitracin group did have a higher incidence of wound healing problems (9.5% vs. 4%, $p=0.03$). Many other additives have been tried in the irrigant including povidone-iodine, chlorhexidine, phenoxyethanol, Dakin's solution, hydrogen peroxide, and benzalkonium chloride. Some of these solutions do seem to be more effective at removing bacteria, but they may do so at the expense of toxicity to normal tissue [62–67].

For open fractures not amenable to initial wound closure or coverage, one option is the use of an antibiotic bead pouch. In a series of 1,085 open fractures, Ostermann et al demonstrated a reduction in the infection rate from 12% to 3.7% when local use of aminoglycoside-impregnated polymethylmethacrylate (PMMA) beads were placed in the wound compared to use of intravenous antibiotics alone [68]. More recently, there has been an increased use of vacuum-assisted wound closure (VAC) for severe soft-tissue wounds (See Fig. 18.5). In a retrospective review of 16 type III open pediatric tibia fractures, the use of subatmospheric pressure dressings after initial debridement was felt to decrease the need for free tissue transfer by 50% [69]. Another review of 43 open fractures found that delayed flap coverage after use of vacuum-assisted wound closure had favorable results, with loss of only three pedicle flaps and one microvascular flap [70]. Flap reconstruction was performed on average 28 days after injury (range 3–106) and the authors concluded that their flap survival results were similar to those of Gopal and Godina when flap reconstruction was performed within 72 h [70].

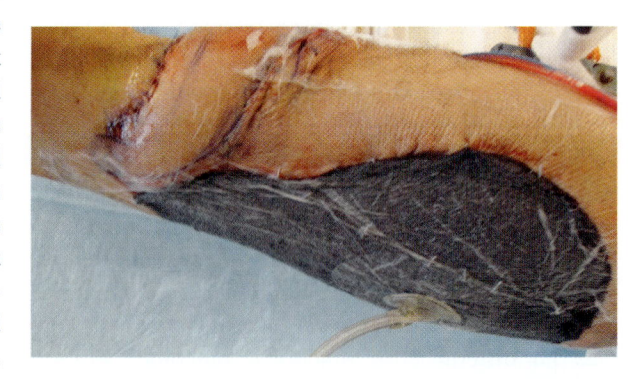

Fig. 18.5 Wound vacuum dressing to assist with closure/coverage of open femur fracture

18.4 Summary

Open fractures require a systematic approach for optimal evaluation and treatment. Early initiation of antibiotic therapy, thorough debridement and irrigation of the wound, followed by stable fixation and wound closure/coverage are the essential steps in the treatment. With grade IIIB fractures, debridement of nonviable tissue achieving a clean wound can allow for early flap coverage with successful results. Some recent tools that have been added to the treatment options include vacuum-assisted dressings and use of bone morphogenic protein for severe open fractures. With a systematic approach, the goals of preventing infection, achieving osseous union, and restoring function can be realised for these challenging fractures.

References

1. Meling T, Harboe K, Soreide K. Incidence of traumatic long-bone fractures requiring in-hospital management: a prospective age- and gender-specific analysis of 4890 fractures. Injury. 2009;40(11):1212–9.
2. Petrisor B, Jeray K, Schemitsch E, Hanson B, Sprague S, Sanders D, et al. Fluid lavage in patients with open fracture wounds (FLOW): an international survey of 984 surgeons. BMC Musculoskelet Disord. 2008;9:7.
3. Gustilo RB, Anderson JT. Prevention of infection in the treatment of one thousand and twenty-five open fractures of long bones: retrospective and prospective analyses. J Bone Joint Surg Am. 1976;58(4):453–8.
4. Anderson LB. Treatment of open fractures: a review. Va Med. 1978;105(9):648–57.
5. Anglen JO, Gainor BJ, Simpson WA, Christensen G. The use of detergent irrigation for musculoskeletal wounds. Int Orthop. 2003;27(1):40–6.
6. Hampton Jr OP. Surgery in World War II. In: Col Coates Jr JB, editor. Orthpedic surgery in the Mediterranean theater of operations. Washington: Office of the Surgeon General, Department of the Army; 1957. p. 53–7.
7. Horn BD, Rettig ME. Interobserver reliability in the Gustilo and Anderson classification of open fractures. J Orthop Trauma. 1993;7(4):357–60.
8. Henley MB, Chapman JR, Agel J, Harvey EJ, Whorton AM, Swiontkowski MF. Treatment of type II, cxxIIIA, and IIIB open fractures of the tibial shaft: a prospective comparison of unreamed interlocking intramedullary nails and half-pin external fixators. J Orthop Trauma. 1998;12(1):1–7.
9. Gregory CF. Open fractures. In: Rockwood Jr CH, Green DP, editors. Fractures. Philadelphia: J.B. Lippincott; 1975. p. 119–55.
10. Patzakis MJ. Management of open fractures and complications. Instr Course Lect. 1982;31:62–4.
11. Knapp TP, Patzakis MJ, Lee J, et al. Comparison of intravenous and oral antibiotic therapy in the treatment of fractures caused by low-velocity gun shots. A prospective, randomized study of infection rates. J Bone Joint Surg. 1996;78:1167–71.
12. Patzakis MJ, Harvey Jr JP, Ivler D. The role of antibiotics in the management of open fractures. J Bone Joint Surg. 1974;56A:532–41.
13. Patzakis MJ, Wilkins J, Moore TM. Use of antibiotics in open tibial fractures. Clin Orthop. 1983;178:31–5.
14. Templeman DC, Gulli B, Tsukayama DT, et al. Update on the management of open fractures of the tibial shaft. Clin Orthop Relat Res. 1998;350:18–25.
15. Patzakis MJ, Bains RS, Lee J, et al. Prospective, randomized, double-blind study comparing single-agent antibiotic therapy, ciprofloxacin, to combination antibiotic therapy in open fracture wounds. J Orthop Trauma. 2000;14:529–33.
16. Patzakis MJ, Wilkins J. Factors influencing infection rate in open fracture wounds. Clin Orthop. 1989;243:36–40.
17. Zalavras CG, Patzakis MJ. Open fractures: evaluation and management. J Am Acad Orthop Surg. 2003;11(3):212–9.
18. Cross WW, Swiontkowski MF. Treatment principles in the management of open fractures. Indian J Orthop. 2008;42(4):377–86.
19. Zalavras CG, Marcus RE, Levin LS, et al. Management of open fractures and subsequent complications. J Bone Joint Surg. 2007;89-A(4):884–95.
20. Zalavras CG, Patzakis MJ, Holtom PD, et al. Management of open fractures. Infect Dis Clin North Am. 2005;19:915–29.
21. Dabezies EJ, D'Ambrosia R. Fracture treatment for the multiply injured patient. Instr Course Lect. 1986;35:13–21.
22. Goldner JL, Hardaker Jr WT, Mabrey JD. Open fractures of the extremities: the case for open treatment. Postgrad Med. 1985;78:199–214.
23. Russell GG, Henderson R, Arnett G. Primary or delayed closure for open tibial fractures. J Bone Joint Surg Br. 1990;72:125–8.
24. Trueta J. "Closed" treatment of war fractures. Lancet. 1939;1:1452–5.
25. Delong Jr WG, Born CT, Wei SY, et al. Aggressive treatment of 119 open fracture wounds. J Trauma. 1999;46:1049–54.
26. Cullen MC, Roy DR, Crawford AH, et al. Open fracture of the tibia in children. J Bone Joint Surg Am. 1996;46:1039–47.
27. Fischer MD, Gustilo RB, Varecka TF. The timing of flap coverage, bone-grafting, and intramedullary nailing in patients who have a fracture of the tibial shaft with extensive soft-tissue injury. J Bone Joint Surg Am. 1991;73:1316–22.
28. Cierny III G, Byrd HS, Jones RE. Primary versus delayed soft tissue coverage for severe open tibial fractures. A comparison of results. Clin Orthop Relat Res. 1983;178:54–63.
29. Gopal S, Majumder S, Batchelor AG, et al. Fix and flap: the radical orthopaedic and plastic treatment of severe open fractures of the tibia. J Bone Joint Surg Br. 2000;82:959–66.
30. Godina M. Early microsurgical reconstruction of complex trauma of the extremities. Plast Reconstr Surg. 1986;78:285–92.
31. Tornetta III P, Bergman M, Watnik N, et al. Treatment of grade IIIb open tibial fractures: a prospective randomised

31. comparison of external fixation and non-reamed locked nailing. J Bone Joint Surg Br. 1994;76:13–9.
32. Brumback RJ, Ellison Jr PS, Poka A, et al. Intramedullary nailing of open fractures of the femoral shaft. J Bone Joint Surg Am. 1989;71:1324–31.
33. Bhandari M, Guyatt GH, Swiotkowski MF, et al. Treatment of open fractures of the shaft of the tibia. J Bone Joint Surg Br. 2001;83:62–8.
34. Keating JF, O'Brien PJ, Blachut PA, et al. Locking intramedullary nailing with and without reaming for open fractures of the tibial shaft: a prospective, randomized study. J Bone Joint Surg Am. 1997;79:334–41.
35. Finkemeier CG, Schmidt AH, Kyle RF, et al. A prospective, randomized study of intramedullary nails inserted with and without reaming for the treatment of open and closed fractures of the tibial shaft. J Orthop Trauma. 2000;14:187–93.
36. Bhandari M, Guyatt G, Tornetta III P, et al. Study to prospectively evaluate reamed intramedullary nails in patients with tibial fractures (SPRINT): study rationale and design. BMC Musculoskelet Disord. 2008;9:91.
37. Marsh JL, Nepola JV, Wuest TK, et al. Unilateral external fixation until healing with the dynamic axial fixator for severe open tibial fractures. J Orthop Trauma. 1991;5:341–8.
38. Nowotarski PH, Turn CH, Brumback RJ, et al. Conversion of external fixation to intramedullary nailing for fractures of the shaft of the femur in multiply injured patients. J Bone Join Surg Am. 2000;82(6):781–8.
39. McGraw JM, Lim EV. Treatment of open tibial-shaft fractures: external fixation and secondary intramedullary nailing. J Bone Joint Surg Am. 1988;70:900–11.
40. Blachut PA, Meek RN, O'Brien PJ. External fixation and delayed intramedullary nailing of open fractures of the tibial shaft: a sequential protocol. J Bone Joint Surg Am. 1990;72:729–35.
41. Bach AW, Hansen Jr ST. Plates versus external fixation in severe open tibial shaft fractures: a randomized trial. Clin Orthop. 1989;241:89–94.
42. Clifford RP, Beauchamp CG, Kellam JF, et al. Plate fixation of open fractures of the tibia. J Bone Joint Surg Br. 1988;70:644–8.
43. Georgiadis GM, Behrens FF, Joyce MJ, et al. Open tibial fractures with severe soft-tissue loss. Limb salvage compared with below-the-knee amputation. J Bone Joint Surg Am. 1993;75:1431–41.
44. Mackenzie EJ, Bosse MJ. Factors influencing outcome following limb-threatening lower limb trauma: lessons learned from the Lower Extremity Assessment Project (LEAP). J Am Acad Orthop Surg. 2006;14(10 Spec No.):S205–10.
45. Bosse MJ, McCarthy ML, Jones AL, et al. The insensate foot following severe lower extremity trauma: an indication for amputation? J Bone Joint Surg Am. 2005;87:2601–8.
46. Park SH, Silva M, Bahk WJ, et al. Effect of irrigation and debridement on fracture healing in an animal model. J Orthop Res. 2006;20(6):1197–204.
47. Govender S, Csimma C, Genant HK, et al. Recombinant human bone morphogenetic protein-2 for treatment of open tibial fractures: a prospective, controlled, randomized study of four hundred and fifty patients. J Bone Joint Surg Am. 2002;84:2123–34.
48. Blick SS, Brumback RJ, Lakatos R, et al. Early prophylactic bone grafting of high-energy tibial fractures. Clin Orthop Relat Res. 1989;240:21–41.
49. Kesemenli CC, Kapukaya A, Subasi M, et al. Early prophylactic autogenous bone grafting in type III open tibial fractures. Acta Orthop Belg. 2004;70:327–31.
50. Kobbe P, Frink M, Overbeck R, et al. Treatment strategies for gunshot wounds of the extremities. Unfallchirurg. 2008;111:247–55.
51. Edwards CC, Simons SC, Browner BD, et al. Severe open tibial fractures. Results treating 202 injuries with external fixation. Clin Orthop Relat Res. 1988;230:98–115.
52. Bhandari M, Schemitsch EH, Adili A, et al. High and low pressure pulsatile lavage of contaminated tibial fractures: an in-vitro study of bacterial adherence and bone damage. J Orthop Trauma. 1999;13(8):526–33.
53. Bhandari M, Thompson K, Adili A, et al. High and low pressure irrigation in contaminated wounds with exposed bone. Int J Surg Investig. 2000;2(3):179–82.
54. Bhandari M, Adili A, Schemitsch EH. The efficacy of low-pressure lavage with different irrigating solutions to remove adherent bacteria from bone. J Bone Joint Surg Am. 2001; 83-A(3):412–9.
55. Dirschl DR, Duff GP, Dahners LE, et al. High pressure pulsatile lavage irrigation of intraarticular fractures: effects on fracture healing. J Orthop Trauma. 1998;12:460–3.
56. Petrisor B, Jeray K, Schemitsch E, et al. Fluid lavage in patients with open fracture wounds (FLOW): an international survey of 984 surgeons. BMC Musculoskelet Disord. 2008;9:7.
57. Tarbox BB, Conroy BP, Malicky ES, et al. Benzalkonium chloride. A potential disinfecting irrigation solution for orthopaedic wounds. Clin Orthop. 1998;346:255–61.
58. Anglen JO, Gainor BJ, Simpson WA, et al. The use of detergent irrigation for musculoskeletal wounds. Int Orthop. 2003;27:40–6.
59. Anglen JO. Comparison of soap and antibiotic solutions for irrigation of lower-limb open fracture wounds. A prospective, randomized study. J Bone Joint Surg Am. 2005; 87-A(7):1415–22.
60. Hutette DR, Simpson WA, Walsh R, et al. Eradication by surfactant irrigation of Staphylococcus aureus from infected complex wounds. Clin Orthop Relat Res. 2004;427:28–36.
61. Conroy BP, Anglen JO, Simpson WA, et al. Comparison of castile soap, benzalkonium chloride, and bacitracin as irrigation solutions for complex contaminated orthopaedic wounds. J Orthop Trauma. 1999;13(5):332–7.
62. Goldheim PD. An appraisal of povidone-iodine and wound healing. Postgrad Med J. 1993;69 Suppl 3:S97–105.
63. Platt J, Bucknall RA. An experimental evaluation of antiseptic wound irrigation. J Hosp Infect. 1984;5:181–8.
64. Mitchell P, Powles R, Rege K, et al. Phenoxyethanol is effective topical therapy of gram-negative cellulitis in neutropenic patients. J Hosp Infect. 1993;25:53–6.
65. McDonell KJ, Sculco TP. Dakin's solution revisited. Am J Orthop. 1997;26:471–3.
66. Museru LM, Kumar A, Ickler P. Comparison of isotonic saline, distilled water, and boiled water in irrigation of open fractures. Int Orthop. 1989;19:179–80.

67. Gainor GJ, Hockman DE, Anglen JO, et al. Benzalkonium chloride: a potential disinfecting irrigation solution. J Orthop Trauma. 1997;11:121–5.
68. Ostermann PA, Seligson D, Henry SL. Local antibiotic therapy for severe open fractures: a review of 1085 consecutive cases. J Bone Joint Surg Br. 1995;77:93–7.
69. Dedmond BT, Kortesis B, Punger K, et al. Subatmospheric pressure dressings in the temporary treatment of soft tissue injuries associated with type III open tibial shaft fractures in children. J Pediatr Orthop. 2006;26(6):728–32.
70. Steiert AE, Gohritz A, Schreiber TC, et al. Delayed flap coverage of open extremity fractures after previous vacuum-assisted closure (VAC) therapy – worse or worth? J Plast Reconstr Aesthet Surg. 2009;62(5):675–83.

Vascular Injuries: Indications for Stents, Timing for Vascular and Orthopaedic Injuries

Luke P.H. Leenen

Contents

19.1	Introduction	217
19.2	**Signs, Symptoms and Diagnostics**	217
19.2.1	Clinical Evaluation	217
19.2.2	Doppler Evaluation	219
19.2.3	Angiography	219
19.2.4	CT-Angiogram	220
19.2.5	Digital Subtraction Angiography	220
19.2.6	MR Angiography	220
19.3	**Treatment**	220
19.3.1	General Strategies	220
19.3.2	Specific Anatomic Considerations	223
19.4	**Conclusion**	226
References		226

L.P.H. Leenen
Department of Trauma, UMC Utrecht, Heidelberglaan 100,
3584 CX Utrecht, The Netherlands
e-mail: l.p.h.leenen@umcutrecht.nl

19.1 Introduction

Although rare, every orthopaedic trauma has the possibility of having an accompanying vascular injury. However, delay in recognition can lead to loss of limb [1]. The combination of fracture and arterial injury is associated with amputation rates as high as 10–40% [2]. Therefore, every effort should be made to exclude synchronous injury of the vascular system. Simple diagnostic methods can lead to early discovery of compromises to the vascular system. The real challenge of these combined injuries, however, is the timing and logistics throughout initial management and definitive care. Irreversible tissue damage may occur if more than 6 h passes before blood flow to the leg is restored [3]. The ultimate problem is the patient with multisystem injuries, a situation in which the preservation of life should prevail over the preservation of limb. These cases call for quick diagnosis and targeted, temporary treatment modalities. A simple algorithm for these challenging injuries is provided (Fig. 19.1). Specifics of management of the mangled extremity are dealt with elsewhere in this book.

19.2 Signs, Symptoms and Diagnostics

19.2.1 Clinical Evaluation

Immediate clinical evaluation is of utmost importance in the evaluation of a patient with fracture or dislocation of some part of the musculoskeletal system. Hard signs of vascular injury are presented in Table 19.1. Paleness of the extremity distal to the supposed lesion

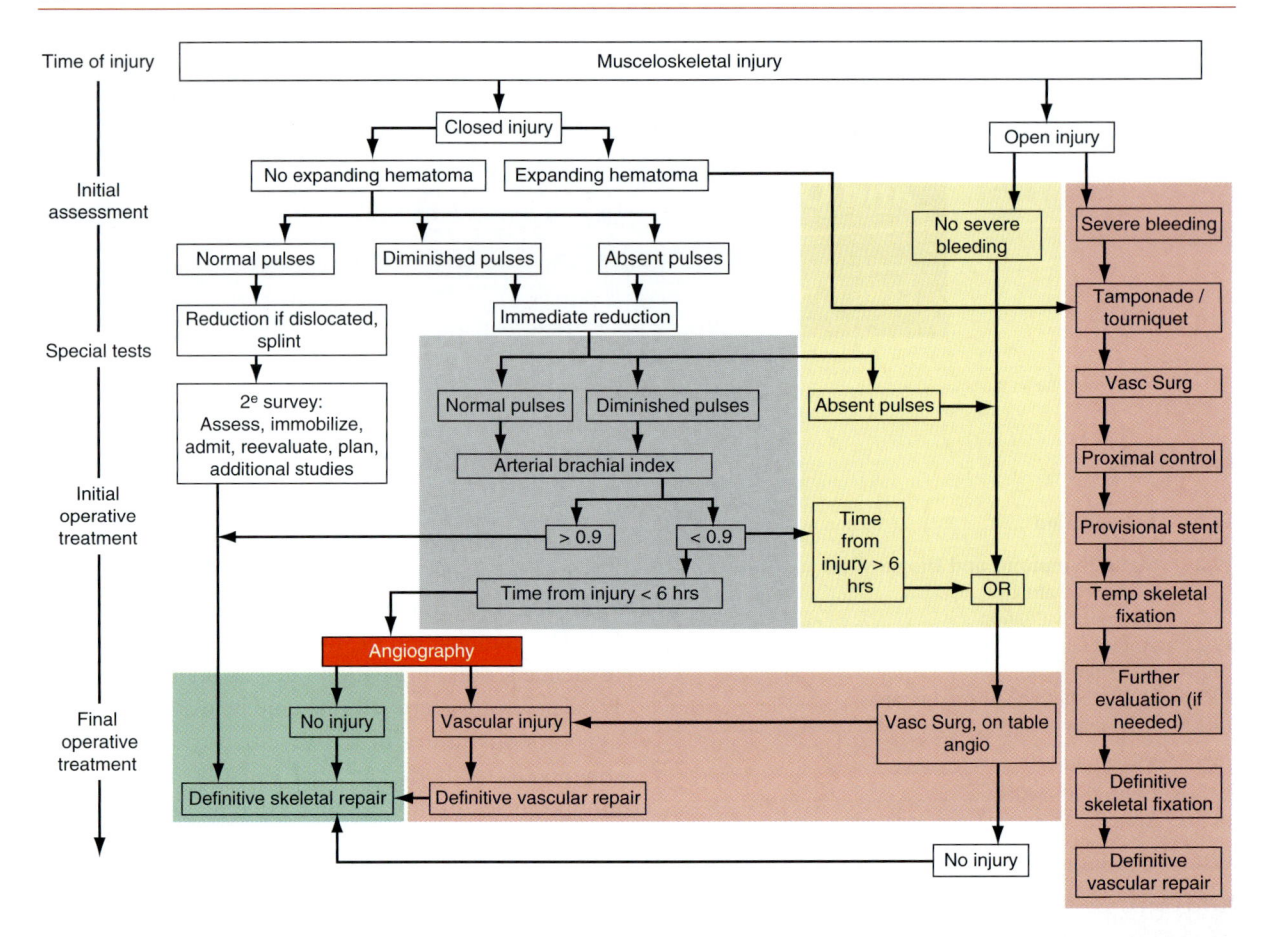

Fig. 19.1 Treatment algorithm: Algorithm of the UMC Utrecht, Department of Trauma and Vascular Surgery for the treatment of musculoskeletal injury with supposed vascular compromise

Table 19.1 Hard signs of vascular injury

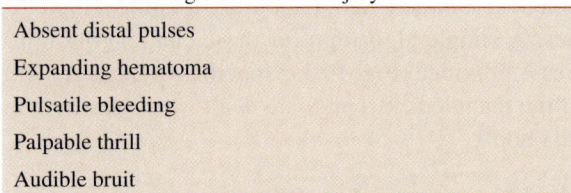

Absent distal pulses
Expanding hematoma
Pulsatile bleeding
Palpable thrill
Audible bruit

is a warning sign of vascular compromise if the patient is hemodynamically normal. Palpation of the peripheral pulses serves as a guide for further evaluation. If there is no palpable pulse in a patient without additional hemodynamic problems, then further evaluation is needed. Reduction of fractures and dislocations should be performed, after which another evaluation should take place. If there is still no palpable pulse, urgent further evaluation is warranted, preferably by angiography. A palpable thrill or an audible bruit are also indicators of a serious injury to the vascular system.

In rare cases, such as an expanding hematoma in an extremity, no further evaluation should take place and the patient should be taken to the operating room to stop the bleeding, preferably by proximal control or direct exploration. If free pulsatile bleeding is obvious from the open fracture, tamponade is done as quickly as possible and a tourniquet should be considered. Recent experiences in the Iraq and Afghanistan conflict show good results in these devastating events [4, 5].

19.2.2 Doppler Evaluation

In many cases a Doppler evaluation is performed to further evaluate the vascular system. However, the Doppler evaluation is a valuable tool only if it is accompanied by a Doppler guided pressure reading and an Ankle-Brachial Index evaluation. The Ankle-Brachial Index should read above 90% to exclude vascular injury [6]. A positive Doppler signal does not necessarily exclude a major vascular compromise, as in most cases a signal is obtained from collaterals, though insignificant in terms of the survival of the extremity. Only very experienced vascular surgeons or vascular technicians can evaluate the spectrum of the Doppler signal in such cases, although they mostly rely on a formal spectral analysis.

19.2.3 Angiography

The gold standard of vascular evaluation is the angiography (Fig. 19.2) [7]. Depending on the urgency or complexity of the case, this may be done either in the angio suite, which is in many cases preferable due to the extensive and high quality radiological possibilities, or in the OR, many times with less sophisticated equipment. The OR environment, however, is favorable for patients with multisystem injuries or in damage control situations [8]. A simple one-shot angiogram through a proximal arterial puncture generally gives a very adequate overview of the vascular system and the level of the problem.

The advantage of the arteriography is the possibility of an angio embolization. In cases of severe arterial bleeding, e.g., in pelvic fractures, angio embolization can be an important adjunct in the treatment of these severely injured patients after initial mechanical stabilization and packing. Intraluminal manipulation when performing an angiogram also provides the possibility of using intraluminal stents. These stents can be utilized for bridging defects, occluded trajectories, and coverage of traumatic pseudoaneurysm [9]. Using large amounts of intra-venous contrast carries the disadvantage of possible contrast nephropathy or allergic reaction. In emergency cases, the chance of local vessel injury is also relevant.

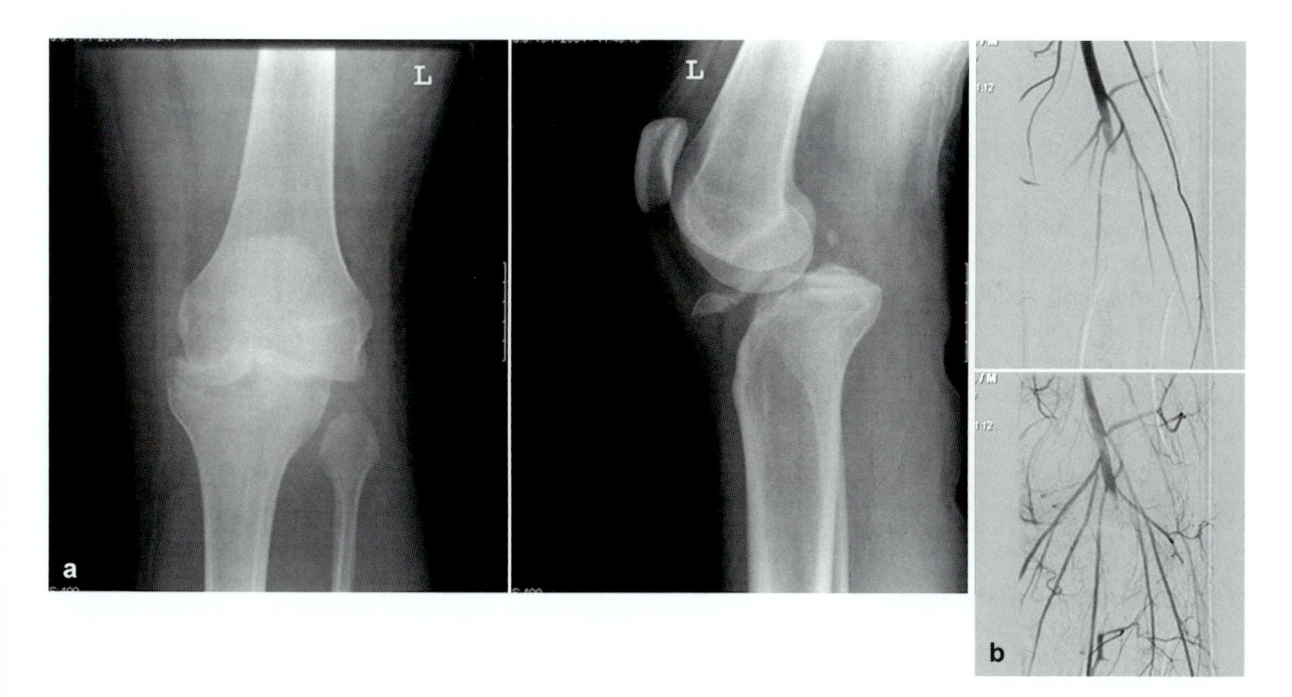

Fig. 19.2 (a) Patient with a knee dislocation. (b) Subsequent arteriography demonstrated at the popliteal artery

19.2.4 CT-Angiogram

Just as CT is very often used in current practice for evaluation of the trauma patient, CT angiography is an option for further evaluation of the vascular status of the trauma patient. A specific protocol and timing should be utilized for optimal result. This modality is less invasive as compared to the classic angiogram; however, contrast related problems may also occur with this technique. CT angiography has largely replaced the invasive angiography for initial diagnostics in the trauma setting as it is readily available [10].

19.2.5 Digital Subtraction Angiography

Intravenous digital subtraction arteriography (DSA) may be used in select cases, although it produces inferior image quality and requires a trip to the radiology department. In children, however, this can be a viable option, as their vascular system is less easy to catheterize (Fig. 19.3). The disadvantage of this technique is the relatively high dose of contrast that must be given.

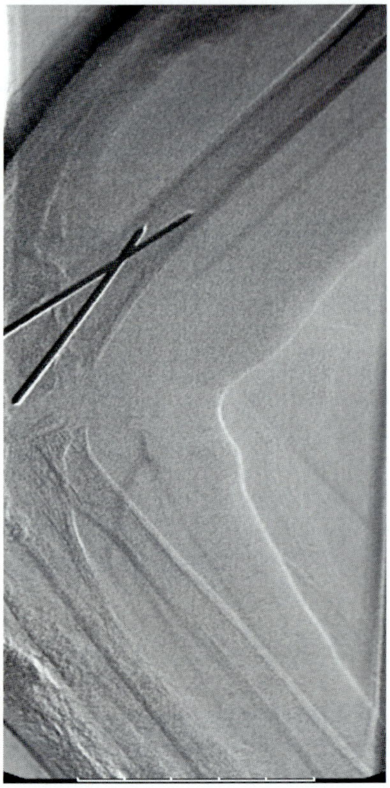

Fig. 19.3 Digital intravenous subtraction angiography in a child with a supracondylar humeral fracture. Disruption of the brachial artery in the area of the fracture fixed with two K-wires

19.2.6 MR Angiography

Increasingly popular in vascular surgery is the use of MR angiography. However, due to the very specific requirements and situation of the multiply injured patient who is often on ventilation, this modality has been until now infrequently used in the early evaluation of the trauma patient [7].

19.3 Treatment

19.3.1 General Strategies

Several tactics may be chosen once the diagnosis is obvious. For severe open wounds with heavy bleeding, tamponade is the treatment of choice. This may be done manually. Recent incidents in the Iraq and Afghanistan conflicts showed a renewed interest and good result from the application of tourniquets, as mentioned above.

After the prehospital and initial resuscitation phase, gaining proximal control is of the utmost importance. Thereafter, revascularization is accomplished as soon as possible. In the case of complex combined vascular and musculoskeletal injuries, regaining perfusion in the distal part of the extremity is very important. Nevertheless vascular procedures should not compromise the possibilities for orthopaedic intervention, and neither should the orthopaedic intervention make an adequate vascular procedure impossible. Although 6 h of ischemia time is tolerable in an injured leg, as little ischemia time as possible should be allowed. The longer the ischemia time in an injured leg, the higher the coagulation disposition will be. An adequate option is to use a shunt (Fig. 19.4) to bridge the time to definitive care using a well perfused distal part of the extremity.

From the orthopaedic standpoint, temporary stabilization of the fracture with an external fixator is a good option. It shortens the time to vascular reconstruction as well as reperfusion, and leaves open the opportunity

Fig. 19.4 (**a**) Shunt in situ in the superficial femoral artery in a patient with a femoral fracture and severe head injury. After hemorrhage control, restoration of flow by (**b**) a shunt, (**c**) temporary external fixation, and (**d**) ultimate plate fixation of the femur

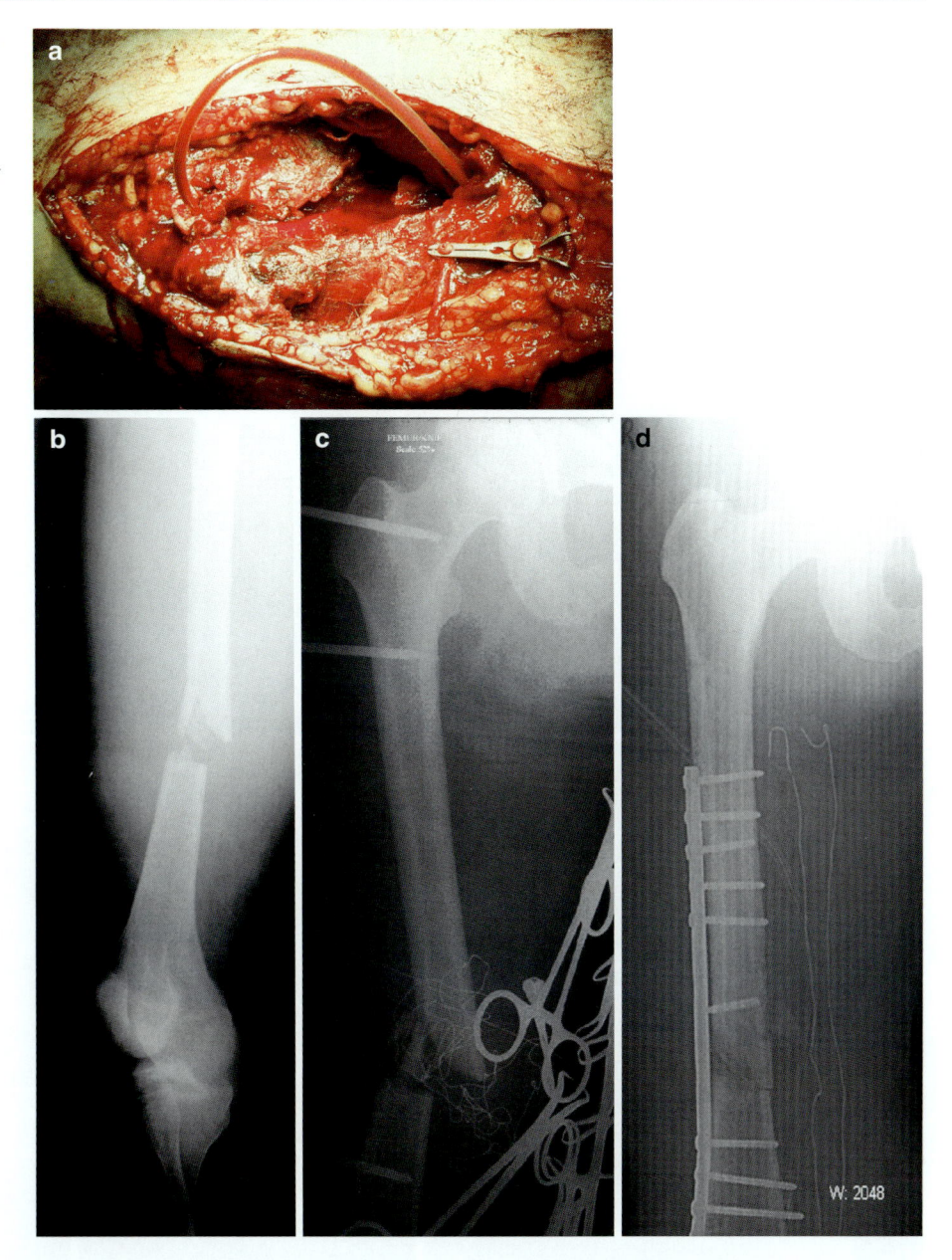

for extensive reconstruction after vascular continuity is restored. Care should be taken to restore adequate length so that the definitive reconstruction of the bone may be done without major shortening or lengthening of the extremity, as this can compromise the vascular conduit later.

Because of immunological properties, an interposition vein graft is mainly used [11] for repair. A PTFE conduit may be used, but this is the less preferable option for open fractures and contaminated wounds. Direct repair may be used in select cases; however, in order to prevent a relevant stenosis after direct repair a vein patch is often used instead [12].

In the case of an incomplete occlusion of an artery, often times based on a stretching mechanism and resulting in an intimal tear, several options are available [13]. Anti-platelet therapy has been advised for such cases, e.g., for carotid artery lesions after cervical fractures [14]. Other authors advocate the use of a wall stent placed with radiological intervention (Fig. 19.5). Stents have been used for a variety of vascular problems such as aneurysms, dissections, and hematoma [15].

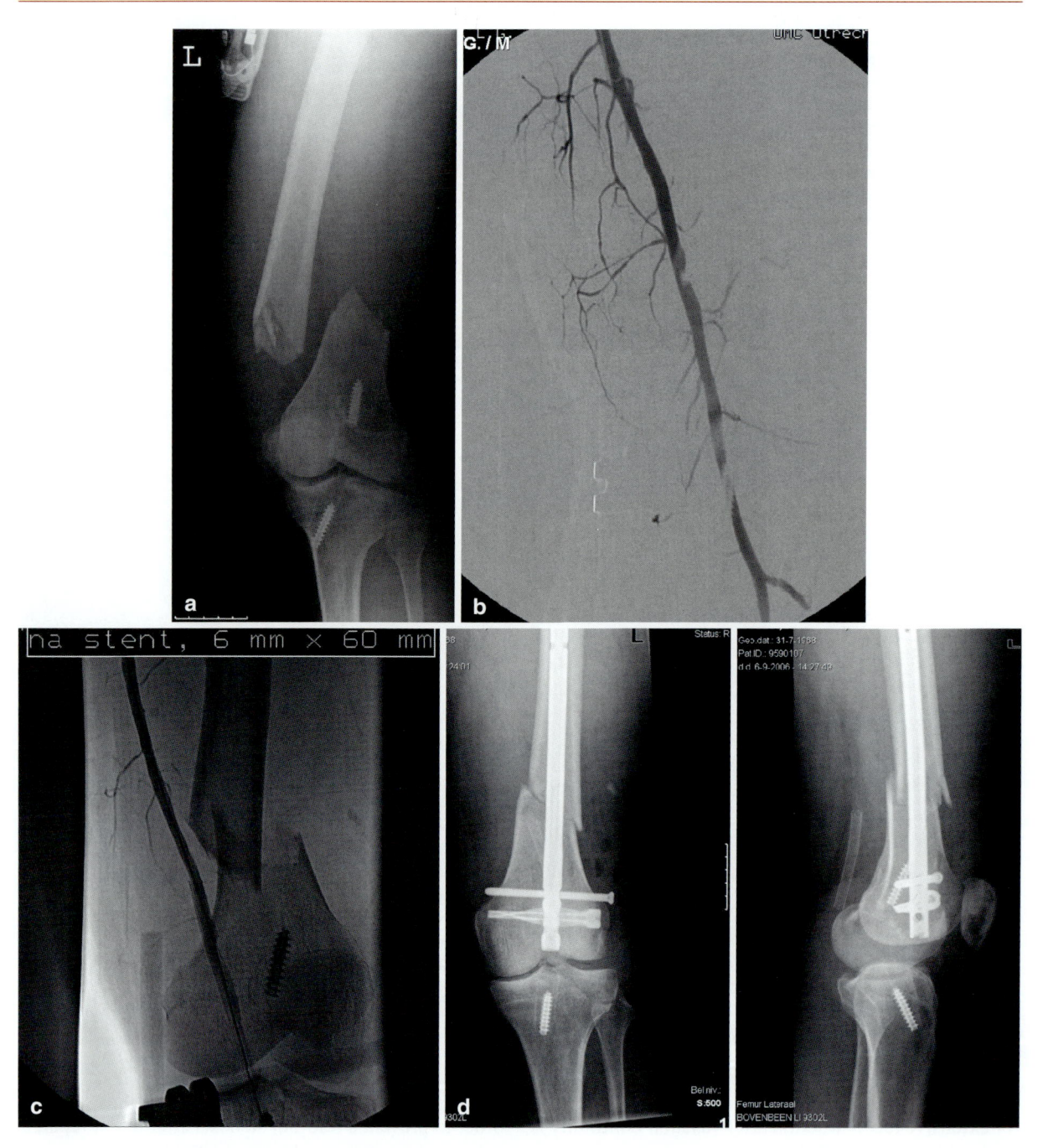

Fig. 19.5 (a) Distal shaft fracture of the femur, with an intimal lesion of the superficial femoral artery, as shown by (b) arteriography, treated with (c) a wall stent after initial external fixator, with (d) a distal femoral nail

19.3.2 Specific Anatomic Considerations

19.3.2.1 The Neck

As mentioned previously, patients with a stretch to the neck, signified for instance by fractures of the cervical spine [16], must be evaluated by plain angiography or CT angiography [17]. A 16 slice CT scan is appropriate [17]. This should be a separate sequence done after evaluating the neck for other traumatic injuries. In the case of an intimal lesion (Fig. 19.6), anti-platelet therapy is currently the treatment of choice [14].

19.3.2.2 Upper Extremity

Fractures of the proximal humerus are also known for accompanying vascular compromise, as shown in Fig. 19.7. This area is not easily approached surgically, and may be managed with recanalization and stents as shown here. Castelli and coworkers [18] used stents in this area successfully without major complications.

In cases of severe bleeding in the area of the subclavian artery, gaining proximal control is very difficult. However, with catheterization and subsequent use of intraluminal detachable balloons control can be obtained, as described by Scalea and Sclafani [19].

The highest incidence of vascular compromise in upper extremity injuries is found in distal humeral supracondylar fractures during childhood. The type of extension is mainly related to the vascular injuries (Fig. 19.3). Vascular problems in the area of the elbow should be repaired, as the brachial artery is the principle end artery for the lower part of the arm. A short bypass is generally the treatment of choice in this area.

Because of the duplicate pursuance of the vasculature below the level of the elbow, major problems generally do not occur there. In cases of severe bleeding the vessel may be tied off if its counterpart is open. Sufficient flow is generally available through the arc of the hand to the area downstream of the lower arm.

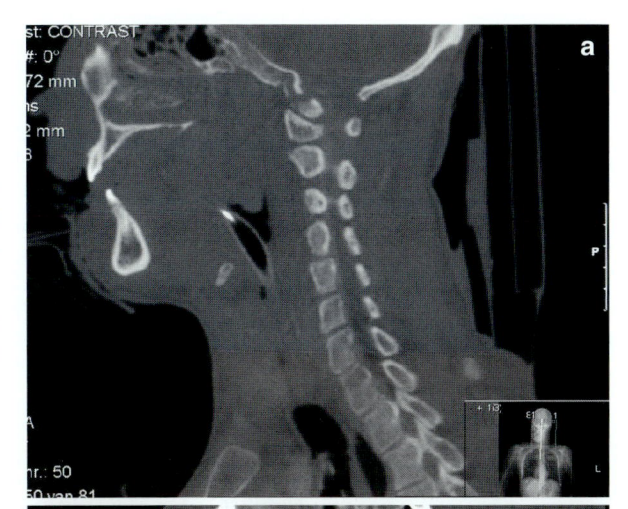

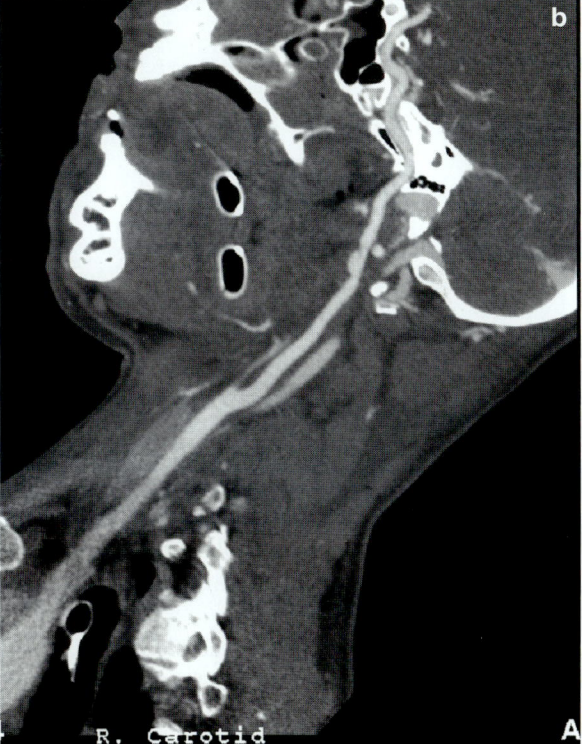

Fig. 19.6 (a) Fracture of the foraminal condyel after a motor vehicle accident with head-on collision. (b) Routine evaluation with CT Angio demonstrated an intimal flap. The patient was treated with anti platelet medication with good outcome

19.3.2.3 Pelvic Bleeding

Exsanguination after pelvic fractures remains a major challenge. After initial stabilization and packing, angio embolization should be contemplated [20]. However, local circumstances dictate whether this method is safe and can be accomplished in timely fashion. A vascular interventional radiology team should be readily available around the clock. Intricacies of pelvic trauma are dealt with elsewhere in this book.

Fig. 19.7 (**a**) Proximal humeral fracture, with (**b**) vascular compromise of the axillary artery. (**c**) Good patency after a Dotter procedure and stent placement

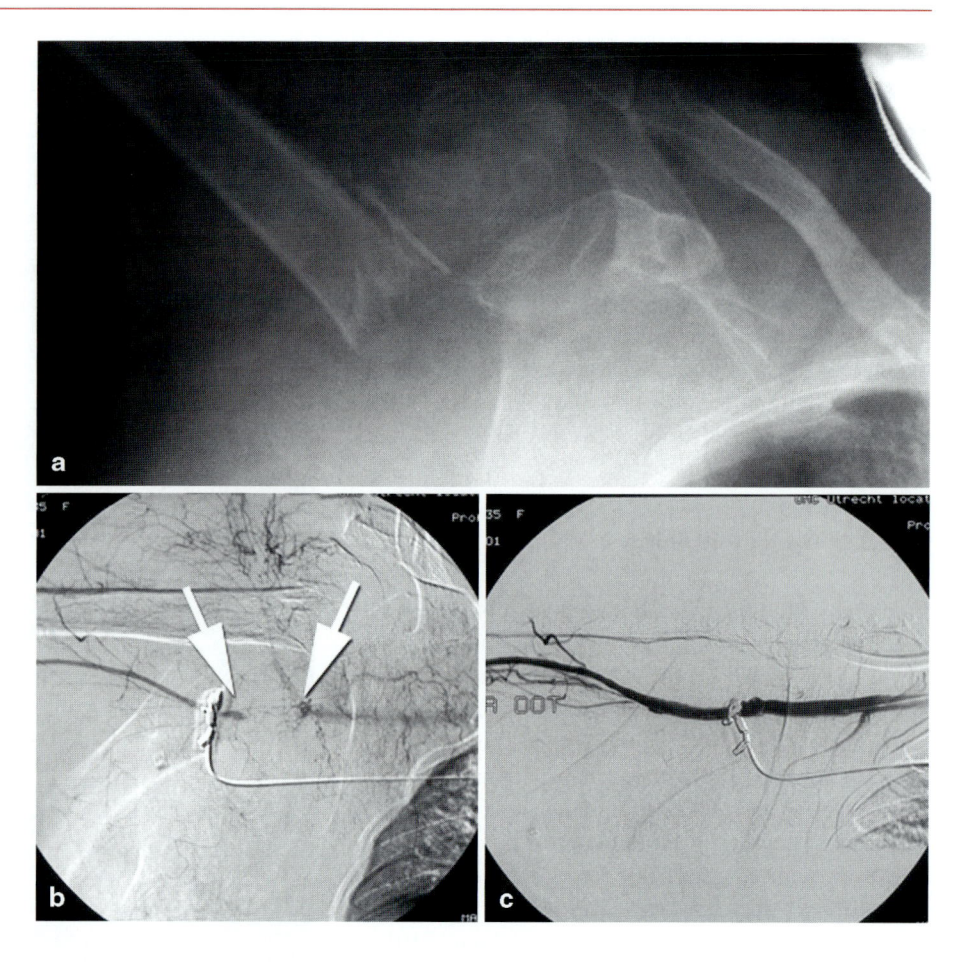

In addition, after the initial resuscitation pelvic bleeding may still remain a challenge, as smaller vessels can demonstrate continued bleeding, as shown in Fig. 19.8. Interventional radiology is an elegant way of approaching this problem.

In pelvic cases, evaluation of the bleeding vascular injury precedes evaluation of the degree of vascular compromise. Thereafter, an exact evaluation of the integrity of the iliac arteries should be performed. In cases in which a vascular and a nervous injury exist together with disruption of the SI joint and symphysis, an internal hemipelvectomy should be suspected. In these lesions a crossover bypass is one possible strategy; however, care should be taken to shut down the proximal side to preclude bleeding after revascularization.

19.3.2.4 Lower Extremity

Tourniquets are currently gaining popularity, based on experiences with severe open exsanguinating extremity wounds from the Iraq war. Revascularization should be performed as early as possible, taking into account, however, the general condition of the patient and the status of the vital functions.

Temporary stents have been of value for acute revascularization (Fig. 19.4), as has been discussed above, followed by a venous bypass, preferably with the great saphenous vein from the contralateral side (Fig. 19.9). The use of the homolateral saphenous vein is contraindicated, as it may be damaged, and together with concomitant injury of the deep veins, the swelling of the homolateral leg can compromise venous return altogether [7].

Huynh evaluated skeletal injuries of the lower extremity and found that tibia and fibula fractures are most associated with arterial injury [12], followed by knee dislocations (Fig. 19.2). The popliteal artery below the knee and the distal superficial femoral artery are most often involved. They recommend the reconstruction of the vascular injury, and afterwards the repair of the bone, which they did in 63% of cases. In general they do not use shunting in this area. Their protocol calls for a medial approach to

19 Vascular Injuries: Indications for Stents, Timing for Vascular and Orthopaedic Injuries 225

Fig. 19.8 (**a**) Pelvic fracture, with pelvic ring and acetabular involvement. (**b**) Further evaluation of persistent blood loss showed arterial bleeding. (**c**) Treatment with embolization with good result

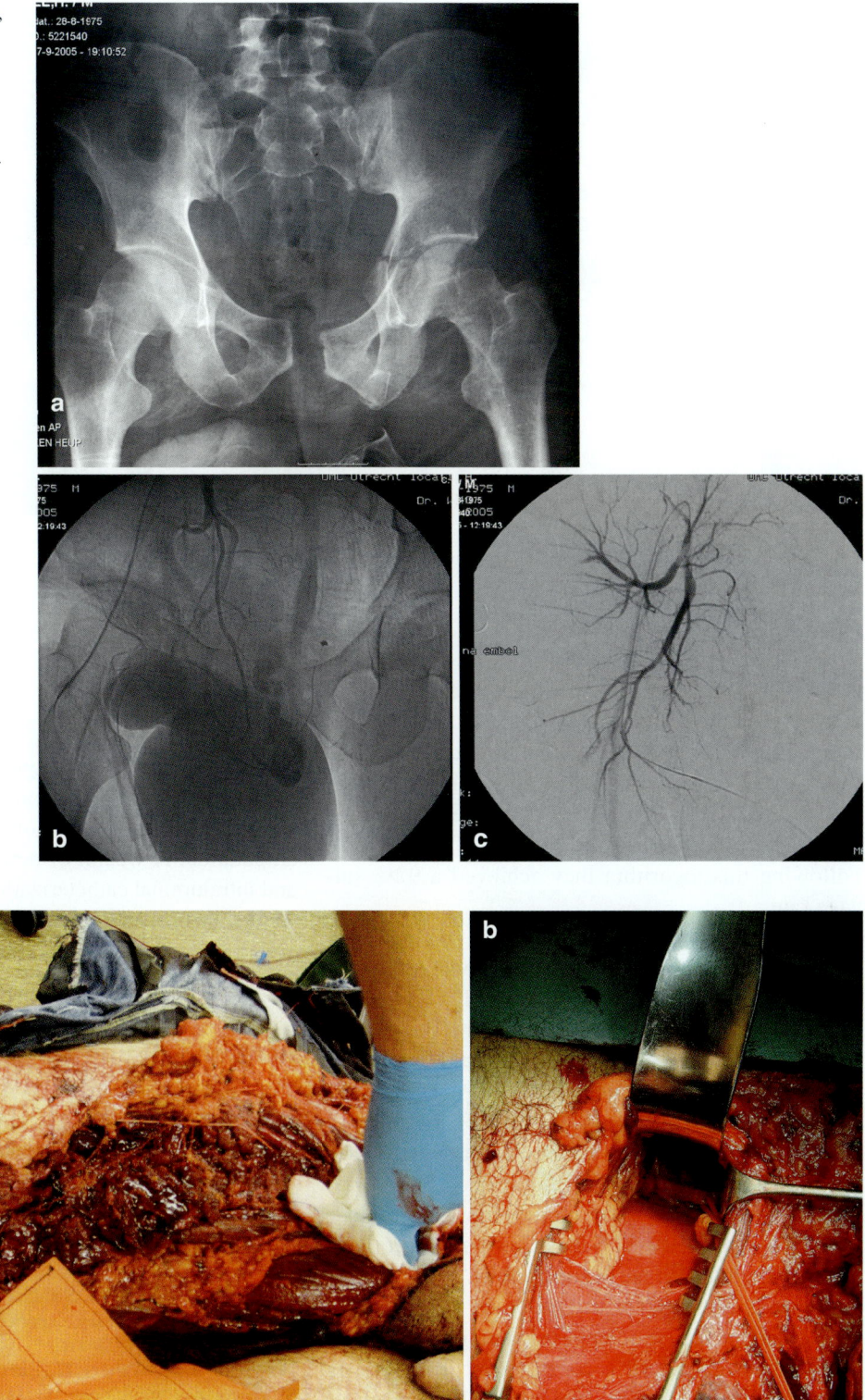

Fig. 19.9 (**a**) Severe open injury of right leg and pelvic region. Direct manual tamponade of the arterial bleeding. Head of the patient is to the right. (**b**) Proximal control of external iliac artery through an incision above the iliac crest and retroperitoneal approach. (**c**) Vascular lesion of the femoral artery. (**d**) Postoperative CT with volume rendering technique of pelvic region with pelvic fracture after vascular repair with interposition vein graft

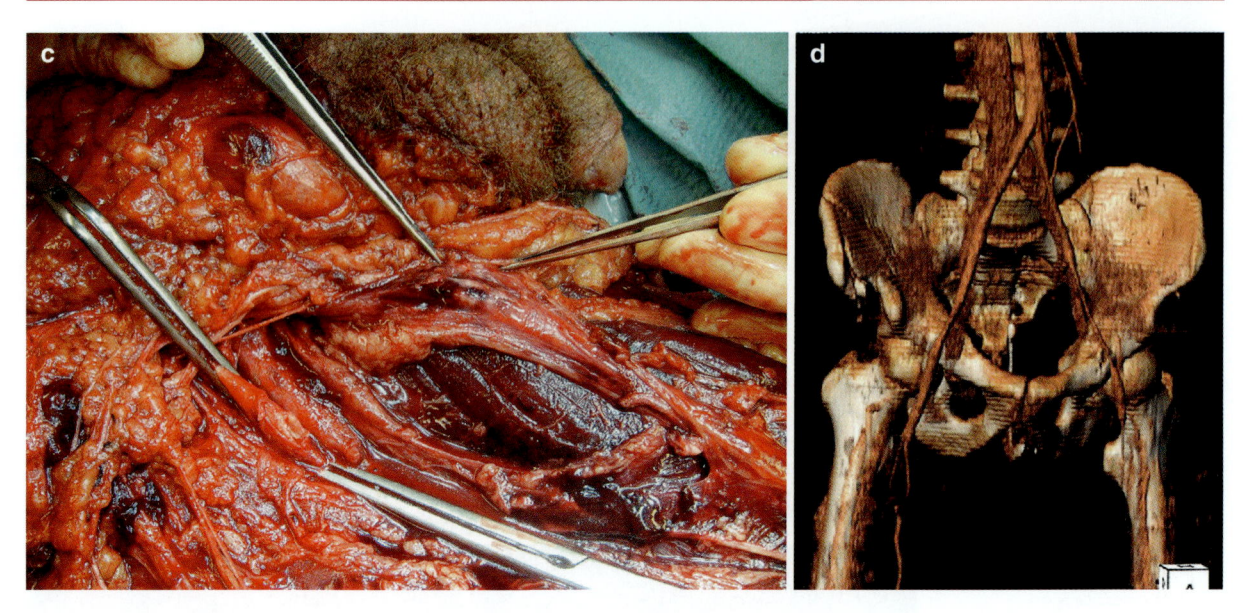

Fig. 19.9 (continued)

the vessel; debridement of the injured segment; heparinisation; embolectomy if needed; and reconstruction with graft, venous patch, and, in the minority of cases, direct repair. They also recommend using a low threshold for fasciotomy to prevent compartment syndrome, as they did in 60% of their cases. Following this algorithm they achieved a 92% salvage rate.

Lesions below the trifurcation are generally not amenable to repair. Usually one artery will suffice for adequate perfusion [21]. Brinker et al. [22] evaluated the opinions of 200 vascular surgeons on the various lesions in this area, but no consensus could be reached on the treatment of these injuries. Hafez et al. [23] evaluated a total series of 550 vascular injuries, the majority of which were penetrating injuries, and reported fairly good results for the repair of crural arteries. Segal evaluated 18 patients with lower limb injuries and vascular repair. They, as well as al-Salman [11], used a contralateral vein graft with fairly good results. Nevertheless, the last authors report that these lower limb injuries carry a high incidence of amputation of up to 30%.

The development of a compartment syndrome is generally recognized as a major complication of an orthopaedic injury with concomitant vascular injury. Therefore, it is generally agreed that a fasciotomy should be performed after revascularization.

19.4 Conclusion

Vascular injury accompanying skeletal trauma is relatively rare. However, prompt diagnosis and expeditious repair are the prerequisites for the prevention of amputation. A wealth of new techniques, such as CT and intraluminal catheterization, has become available for diagnostics and repair. When treated early the general prognosis for such injuries is good.

References

1. Andrikopoulos V, Antoniou I, Panoussis P. Arterial injuries associated with lower-extremity fractures. Cardiovasc Surg. 1995;3:15–8.
2. Bishara RA, Pasch AR, Douglas DD, Schuler JJ, Lim LT, Flanigan DP. The necessity of mandatory exploration of penetrating zone II neck injuries. Surgery. 1986;100: 655–60.
3. Persad IJ, Reddy RS, Saunders MA, Patel J. Gunshot injuries to the extremities: experience of a U.K. trauma centre. Injury. 2005;36:407–11.
4. Kragh Jr JF, Walters TJ, Baer DG, et al. Practical use of emergency tourniquets to stop bleeding in major limb trauma. J Trauma. 2008;64:S38–49.
5. Kragh JF, Jr, Littrel ML, Jones JA, et al. Battle casualty survival with emergency tourniquet use to stop limb bleeding. J Emerg Med. 2009.

6. Lynch K, Johansen K. Can Doppler pressure measurement replace "exclusion" arteriography in the diagnosis of occult extremity arterial trauma? Ann Surg. 1991;214:737–41.
7. Doody O, Given MF, Lyon SM. Extremities – indications and techniques for treatment of extremity vascular injuries. Injury. 2008;39:1295–303.
8. Leenen L, Moll FL. Vascular Injuries in polytrauma patients. In: Pape HC, Peitzman AB, Schwab CW, editors. Damage control management in the polytrauma patient. New York: Springer; 2009. p. 315–30.
9. Onal B, Ilgit ET, Kosar S, Akkan K, Gumus T, Akpek S. Endovascular treatment of peripheral vascular lesions with stent-grafts. Diagn Interv Radiol. 2005;11:170–4.
10. Fleiter TR, Mervis S. The role of 3D-CTA in the assessment of peripheral vascular lesions in trauma patients. Eur J Radiol. 2007;64:92–102.
11. al-Salman MM, al-Khawashki H, Sindigki A, Rabee H, al-Saif A, Al-Salman FF. Vascular injuries associated with limb fractures. Injury. 1997;28:103–7.
12. Huynh TT, Pham M, Griffin LW, et al. Management of distal femoral and popliteal arterial injuries: an update. Am J Surg. 2006;192:773–8.
13. Frykberg ER, Vines FS, Alexander RH. The natural history of clinically occult arterial injuries: a prospective evaluation. J Trauma. 1989;29:577–83.
14. Cothren CC, Moore EE, Biffl WL, et al. Anticoagulation is the gold standard therapy for blunt carotid injuries to reduce stroke rate. Arch Surg. 2004;139:540–5.
15. Piffaretti G, Tozzi M, Lomazzi C, et al. Endovascular treatment for traumatic injuries of the peripheral arteries following blunt trauma. Injury. 2007;38:1091–7.
16. Cothren CC, Moore EE, Biffl WL, et al. Cervical spine fracture patterns predictive of blunt vertebral artery injury. J Trauma. 2003;55:811–3.
17. Biffl WL, Egglin T, Benedetto B, Gibbs F, Cioffi WG. Sixteen-slice computed tomographic angiography is a reliable noninvasive screening test for clinically significant blunt cerebrovascular injuries. J Trauma. 2006;60: 745–51.
18. Castelli P, Caronno R, Piffaretti G, et al. Endovascular repair of traumatic injuries of the subclavian and axillary arteries. Injury. 2005;36:778–82.
19. Scalea TM, Sclafani SJ. Angiographically placed balloons for arterial control: a description of a technique. J Trauma. 1991;31:1671–7.
20. Leenen LPH. Pelvic fractures: soft tissue trauma. Eur J Trauma Emerg Surg. 2010;35:117–23.
21. Segal D, Brenner M, Gorczyca J. Tibial fractures with infrapopliteal arterial injuries. J Orthop Trauma. 1987;1:160–9.
22. Brinker MR, Caines MA, Kerstein MD, Elliott MN. Tibial shaft fractures with an associated infrapopliteal arterial injury: a survey of vascular surgeons opinions on the need for vascular repair. J Orthop Trauma. 2000;14:194–8.
23. Hafez HM, Woolgar J, Robbs JV. Lower extremity arterial injury: results of 550 cases and review of risk factors associated with limb loss. J Vasc Surg. 2001;33:1212–9.

Management of Articular Fractures

Frankie Leung and Tak-Wing Lau

Contents

20.1	Introduction	229
20.1.1	Types of Articular Injuries	229
20.2	Assessment	230
20.3	Strategy of Management of Articular Fractures in Polytrauma Patients	230
20.4	Floating Joint Injuries	231
20.4.1	Floating Knee Injury	231
20.4.2	Floating Shoulder Injuries	234
20.4.3	Floating Elbow	237
20.5	Traumatic Knee Dislocation	238
20.5.1	Classification	238
20.5.2	Associated Injuries	238
20.5.3	Evaluation and Assessment	239
20.5.4	Management	239
20.5.5	Rehabilitation	240
20.5.6	Outcome and Complications	240
20.6	Conclusions	240
References		241

F. Leung (✉) and T.-W. Lau
5/F, Professorial Block, Department of Orthopaedics and Traumatology, Queen Mary Hospital,
102 Pokfulam Road, Hong Kong
e-mail: klleunga@hkucc.hku.hk;
catcherlau@yahoo.com.hk

20.1 Introduction

Articular injuries are common in polytraumatized patients and will cause significant disability if not appropriately treated. One should also remember that polytrauma is a systemic surgical condition that requires an efficient resuscitation and a well-timed plan of surgical management including initial damage control measures and later definitive fixation. The fundamental goal of treatment is patient's survival, to be followed by limb viability. In this regard, most articular fractures will not be life threatening, and some conditions are limb threatening. As a result, the treating surgeon should not just focus on individual fracture or injury, but rather formulate an overall plan that takes the trauma pathophysiology into account. Hence, although treatment planning for individual fracture can be considered separately to achieve the optimal result, the effect of that treatment must be considered in the light of the overall patient condition and injury status.

20.1.1 Types of Articular Injuries

The joint can be affected in one of the following ways. Firstly, the high energy trauma causes a fracture that involves the articular surface. Such intra-articular fractures can cause severe disability to the patient if they are not treated appropriately. Accurate joint reconstruction with stable fixation allowing early mobilization of the joint is important for good cartilage healing and good joint motion recovery. The surgical reconstruction will require careful preoperative planning and should be done later as definitive fixation.

Floating joint injuries refer to the fractures occurring both proximal and distal to the joint, resulting in a total lack of bony support of the affected joint. The fractures may not extend to the articular surface. Since nerves and blood vessels are commonly in close vicinity to the joint, the risk of neurovascular complication is usually much higher in the presence of a floating joint.

Major joint dislocations or fracture dislocations are orthopaedic emergencies. These conditions must be recognized promptly in the emergency room during secondary survey. Reduction should be achieved with appropriate analgesics or anesthesia as soon as possible. If the dislocations are left unattended, there will be a high chance of vascular or neurological complications.

20.2 Assessment

In the emergency room, resuscitation should follow the ATLS protocol. After the primary survey, a thorough secondary survey should be performed and the whole body should be examined for other injuries. The presence of any open fracture or compartment syndrome should not be missed. Floating joint injuries or major joint dislocations have to be recognized based on the deformity of the limbs. However, the treating doctor should not be distracted by the obvious deformity and overlooks other associated complications. The distal circulation of the limb must be checked and if the patient is conscious, a quick motor and sensory examination should be recorded as a baseline for further reference appropriate splints must be applied. Radiographs in two planes, including the full length of the long bones, must be obtained to confirm the diagnosis.

20.3 Strategy of Management of Articular Fractures in Polytrauma Patients

Complex fractures around joints remain challenges in the management of polytraumatized patients and they are associated with an increased risk of complications. During decision making to formulate the plan of management, the surgeon must take into account any

Table 20.1 Surgical priorities in the treatment of complex articular fractures in polytrauma

A. Primary surgical procedures in the emergency setting
 1. Limb-saving procedures:
    - Reduction of large joints, such as hip, knee, by close or open means with temporary stabilization by splint or traction
    - Bony stabilization with urgent vascular surgery for acute damage to vascular supply
    - Debridement and spanning external fixation for open articular fractures together with appropriate intravenous antibiotics
    - Fasciotomy and spanning external fixation for articular fractures complicated by compartment syndrome
 2. Spanning transarticular external fixation as a damage control procedure
    - To stabilize floating joint injuries or unstable joint dislocation after reduction in unstable patients
    - To stabilize periarticular fractures with unfavorable local soft tissue conditions

B. Secondary surgical procedures that should be done when the general condition of the patient is stabilized or the soft tissue condition has improved
 1. Definitive fixation of intra-articular fractures with initially unfavorable soft tissue conditions
 2. Definitive fixation of unstable fracture dislocations, e.g., shoulder, acetabulum
 3. Definitive fixation of floating joint injuries that are initially treated with spanning external fixation
 4. Soft tissue coverage and definitive fixation of open intra-articular fractures

associated injuries to other major internal organs and body parts (Table 20.1). At the same time the local soft tissue condition around the joint must be carefully assessed. These two factors will affect the timing of the fracture fixation and the method of fracture fixation [1].

In general, complex fractures around the joints are better managed with a staged strategy [2, 3]. First, the soft tissue condition around the injured joint, especially the knee and the ankle, is usually in an unfavorable condition. There are usually severe edema and blisters, thus rendering primary fracture fixation very risky with high complication rates. Secondly, intra-articular fractures are complex injuries. In order to achieve a good outcome, the articular surface should be reconstructed anatomically, the limb axis should be restored correctly, and a stable fixation connecting the articular block to the metaphysis and diaphysis should be obtained to allow for early joint motion. This often necessitates a good preoperative assessment of the fracture including good quality radiographs, CT scans

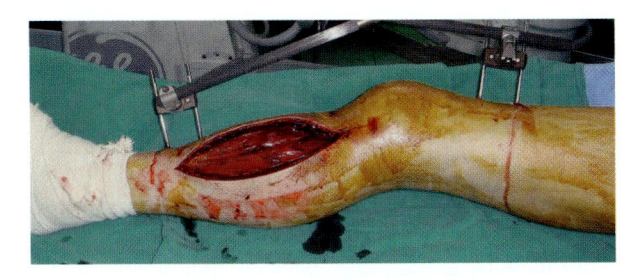

Fig. 20.1 Temporary knee-spanning external fixation in a 34-year-old polytrauma victim with comminuted proximal tibial fracture complicated by compartment syndrome. Emergency fasciotomy was performed. Vacuum-assisted closure was applied and wound closure was performed on day 10 after injury. The definitive fixation was then carried out on day 14

with reconstruction, and, in indicated cases, MRI. Good and accurate surgical planning and meticulous surgical skills are crucial in achieving a good fixation. Hence, these difficult, definitive reconstructions should not be performed in the setting of emergency surgery in a polytraumatized patient.

Generally speaking, the management of articular fractures in polytrauma patients should include a primary spanning external fixation applied in the emergency setting (Fig. 20.1). The configuration should be simple and allow easy access to the soft tissue during subsequent surgeries. The surgeon applying the external fixation should preferably be the surgeon who will fix the fracture definitively. Definitive fixation should be carried out when both the general condition of the patient and the local soft tissue condition are optimized. In recent years, there are some reports showing the benefit of vacuum-assisted closure (VAC) therapy in managing large soft tissue defects and in assisting wound closure [4–6].

Sometimes in high energy articular fractures, the stability of the joint is affected, resulting in a fracture-dislocation. In principle, a major joint dislocation that causes significant deformity should be reduced as soon as possible or the distal circulation will be affected. In the case of posterior hip dislocation that commonly occurs with posterior wall fracture of the acetabulum, reduction can usually be done quickly with closed manipulation once the patient is anesthetized. Fixation of the posterior wall fracture should be done at a later stage after thorough assessment with CT scan. Similarly, fracture dislocation involving the ankle should be reduced urgently to avoid complication of the soft tissue envelope and the distal circulation.

20.4 Floating Joint Injuries

20.4.1 Floating Knee Injury

A floating knee refers to the injury when the ipsilateral femur and tibia are both fractured. A significant force must be needed in order to break these two bones and therefore this injury frequently implies a more substantial mechanism of injury. The patients are commonly hemodynamically unstable and may have significant injuries of other organs and the other extremities. This injury is also associated with complications that carry an increased risk of morbidity and mortality.

Fraser et al. classified floating knee injuries by whether there is joint involvement [7] (Fig. 20.2).

- Type I is the injury with extra-articular fractures of both bones.
- Type II is subdivided into three groups, as follows:
  – Type IIa involves femoral shaft and tibial plateau fractures.

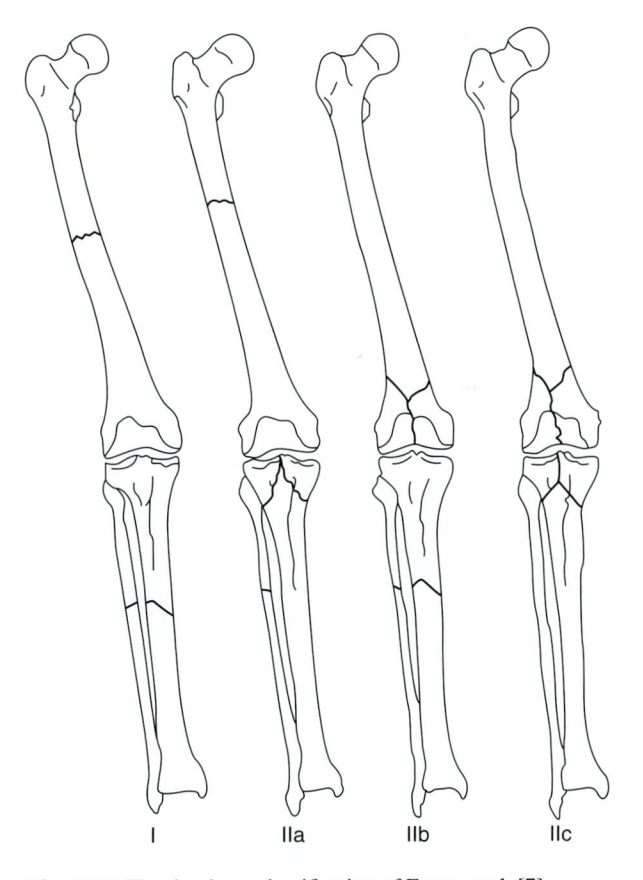

Fig. 20.2 Floating knee classification of Fraser et al. [7]

- Type IIb includes fractures of the distal femur and the shaft of the tibia.
- Type IIc indicates fractures of the distal femur and tibial plateau.

This is the commonest classification system for floating knee injury and is of prognostic value since type I fractures have better functional outcome than type II with various extent of intra-articular involvement.

20.4.1.1 Management of Fractures in Floating Knee Injury

Historically, floating knee injuries were totally treated or partially treated non-operatively. However, the results were unsatisfactory [7]. The current recommended treatment of the bony injuries is surgical fixation of both the femoral and the tibial fractures [8]. There is no single ideal method of fixation. The surgeon should take into consideration the extent of soft tissue injury, the location and pattern of the fractures, and the associated injuries.

Isolated floating knee injury without significant articular involvement should be treated acutely if the patient is hemodynamically stable. If both fractures occur in the diaphysis, then both the femoral shaft and tibial shaft should be treated with intramedullary nailing. There is still a controversy as to whether antegrade or retrograde femoral nailing should be used. Rethnam [9] suggested that antegrade nailing should be done. Advocates for retrograde femoral nailing suggested that the quickest surgical procedure is to perform a retrograde intramedullary nailing of the femur with an intramedullary nailing of the tibia using a single incision over the knee. Alternatively, the tibia fracture is temporarily splinted with a cast and an antegrade femoral nailing is done first, followed by the tibial nailing. If either one or both fractures involve the epi-metaphyseal region, then the appropriate periarticular plate fixation should be performed according to the location. In case of severe soft tissue swelling as in tibial plateau or plafond fractures, the definitive fixation may be delayed until the soft tissue condition improves resulting in a lower chance of soft tissue complications. In case of complex articular involvement with significant fracture comminution, such as tibial plateau fracture, then one can also elect to apply an external fixator temporarily and the definitive fixation done at a later stage when the required surgical expertise is available (Fig. 20.3).

On the other hand, in unstable patients or those in extremis, life threatening injuries such as hemothorax, pneumothorax, intraabdominal hemorrhage, and intracranial hematoma must be managed as the first priority. Under these circumstances, temporary stabilization with a spanning external fixator should be performed, following the principles of damage control orthopaedic surgery. Once the patient's physiological status is stabilized, conversion to internal fixation and definitive surgery can then be performed.

In the post-operative period, range of motion of the knee joint should be started early. Continuous passive motion can be used until satisfactory knee motion has been achieved. The patient should do partial weight bearing walking if both fractures are extra-articular. If one or both fractures involve the knee joint articular surface, then weight bearing should be delayed for 6–8 weeks.

20.4.1.2 Associated Injuries in Floating Knee Injuries

Vascular injuries of the affected limb can occur in a floating knee injury. The reported incidence ranges from 21% to 29% [10, 11]. Limb ischemia may occur if the popliteal or posterior tibial arteries are injured. As a result, a thorough vascular assessment is crucial in early detection of this injury. Preoperatively, the peripheral pulses should be assessed with palpation and hand-held Doppler in all floating knee injuries. If arterial injury is suspected, an intraoperative arteriogram should be performed vascular repair should be performed together with the bony stabilization.

The incidence of open fractures in a floating knee injury can be as high as 50–70% [11]. The commonest pattern is a closed femoral fracture with an open tibial fracture. Paul et al. [11] reported that 17 of 21 patients had open fractures of one or more bones and 76% of these were either grade II or grade III. In general, the management of open fractures associated with floating knee injuries should follow the principles of open fracture management. This should include adequate debridement and stabilization of the fractures with either

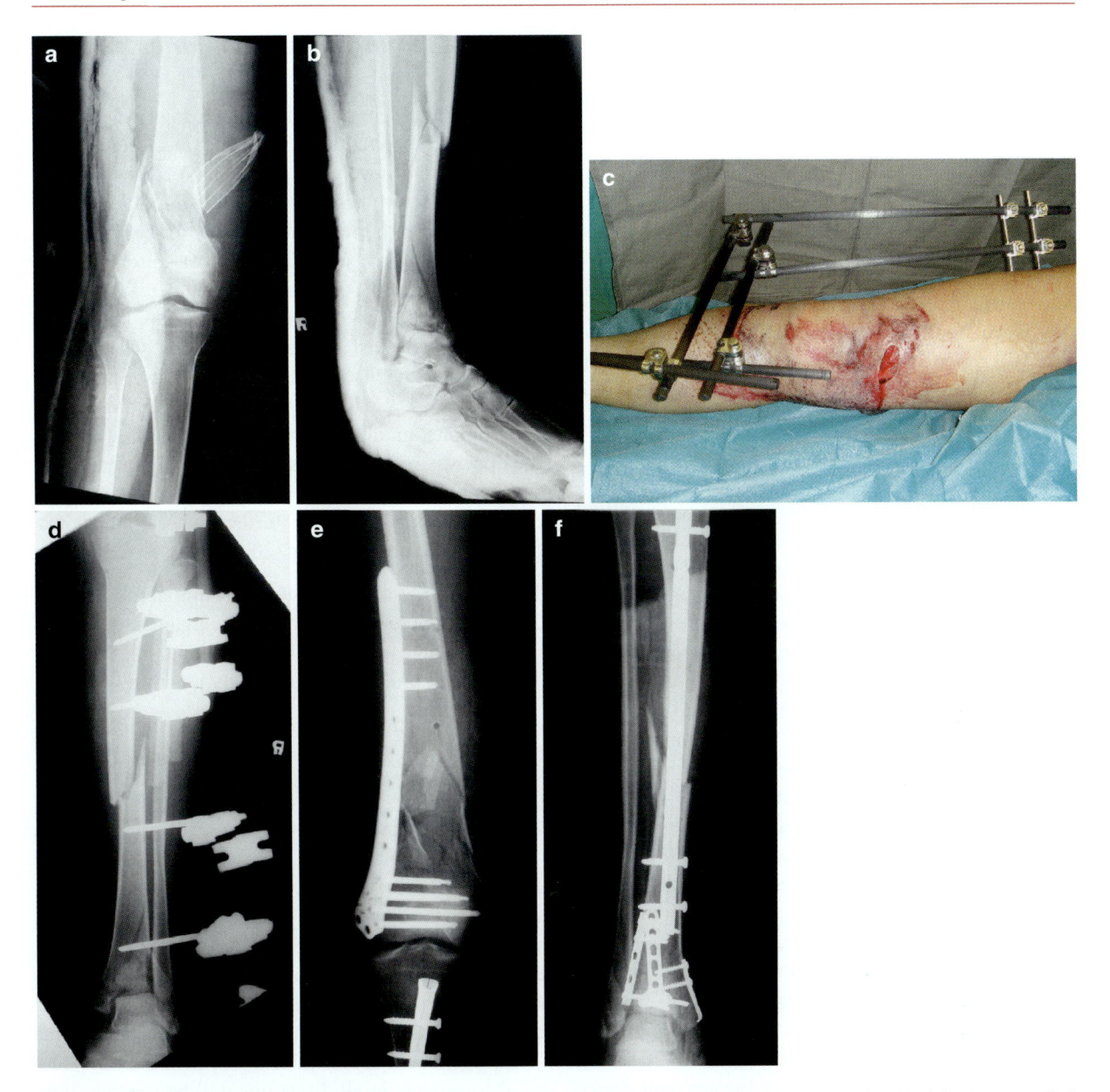

Fig. 20.3 (**a, b**) Twenty-one-year-old man was injured by a fallen heavy object and sustained a type I floating knee injury and ipsilateral pilon fracture. On admission, he had a low hemoglobin of 6.9 g/dL. (**c**) The femur fracture was a grade II open injury occurring at the distal femur metaphysis. During the emergency surgery, the thigh wound was debrided. (**d**) Spanning external fixation across the knee and ankle joints was applied. Six units of blood were given in total. (**e, f**) As the patient's condition improved, definitive fixation was performed with bridging locking plate fixation for distal femur, intramedullary nailing for the tibial shaft, and open reduction and plate fixation for the pilon fracture

external fixation or intramedullary nailing depending on the grading of the open fractures. It is expected that multiple surgical procedures are usually required, and in patients with severey mangled limbs and unstable general conditions, amputation should be considered [11].

Associated ipsilateral knee ligament injuries are common in the floating knee injury [12]. Anterolateral rotatory instability is the commonest instability pattern. However, there is a diagnostic difficulty as the floating joint cannot be tested for ligamentous injuries. Hence, after stabilization of the fractures, stress testing of the knee ligaments must be performed. If a ligamentous injury is suspected, then an acute arthroscopy can be performed and the injured ligaments can be repaired acutely or at a later stage.

20.4.1.3 Complications

The management of the fractures in floating knee injuries is challenging to orthopaedic surgeons. Fraser et al. [7] reported 35% of patients with floating knee injuries required late surgery for delayed union or nonunion, osteomyelitis, refracture, and malunion. There are several explanations to this high rate of complications. The first reason is that most of the fracture fixation surgeries are performed in the emergency setting. The level of surgical expertise available is a crucial factor to the success of the surgery since sometimes a good fixation can be difficult for the average surgeon. Moreover, the floating knee segment presents great difficulty in achieving an accurate reduction of either fracture. Hence, floating knee injuries are prone to delayed union or non-union. Rotational mal-alignment can also be difficult to detect intra-operatively. The overall leg length should be checked at the end of the surgery and in the early post-operative period. If the patient's general condition allows, any mal-reduction should be corrected within the first few weeks before hard bone is formed, necessitating an osteotomy surgery (Fig. 20.4).

Fat embolism can occur in a floating knee injury. Karlstrom and Olerud [13] reported 6 out of 31 patients with fat embolism syndrome. Veith et al. [14] reported 13% incidence of fat embolism syndrome in 54 patients of floating knee injuries. The diagnosis is made if the patient has pyrexia, tachycardia, tachypnea, and altered sensorium within 48 h of admission. To confirm the diagnosis, an arterial blood gas test should be done and will reveal hypoxia. The patient should be managed in an intensive care unit with mechanical ventilation. The fractures should also be provisionally stabilized to minimize further hemorrhage and the chance of the fatty bone marrow entering the circulation. Hence, a spanning external fixator should be applied in the emergency surgery. Definitive fixation of the fractures should be delayed until the patient's condition improves which usually take place after 1 week of supportive care.

20.4.2 Floating Shoulder Injuries

Floating shoulder is an uncommon injury with both clavicle and scapular neck fractured, resulting in gross instability and severe displacement of the shoulder girdle. The term floating shoulder is initially describing the inherent bony instability as described similarly in elbow and knee joints. Later Goss introduced the important concept of superior shoulder suspensory complex [15, 16]. It is a ring of complex soft tissue structures that exist between two struts. The middle third of the clavicle acts as the superior strut while the scapular body and spine serves as the inferior strut. The complex maintains a normal relationship between the upper extremity and axial skeleton. The scapula is suspended to the clavicle by ligaments and acromioclavicular joint. It can be further sub-classified into three components [16] (Fig. 20.5):

1. The clavicle-acromioclavicular joint-acromial strut
2. The clavicle–coracoclavicular ligamentous-coracoid linkage
3. The three process-scapular body junction

A single disruption of the ring is a stable injury. A double disruption will result in an unstable injury [16, 17].

20.4.2.1 Clinical Presentation and Diagnosis

The clinical presentation of floating shoulder injuries varies with the associated injuries. When there are other serious injuries, the condition is often overlooked. During secondary survey, one can notice that the shoulder is usually grossly swollen and tender. A displaced clavicle fracture or in prominent lateral clavicular end in an acromioclavicular joint dislocation may be visible. Movements in all directions will be severely limited. Rib fractures are not uncommon. Shortly after the injury, a detailed neurovascular examination around the shoulder may be difficult. Nevertheless, the distal neurovascular status should still be checked as the nearby brachial plexus and axillary vessels may be injured. This is one of the most important prognostic factors with regards to final clinical outcome [18]. Open injuries are not uncommon.

Radiological examination including anteroposterior view and the transcapular lateral view of the scapula is usually most informative. Important factors include the

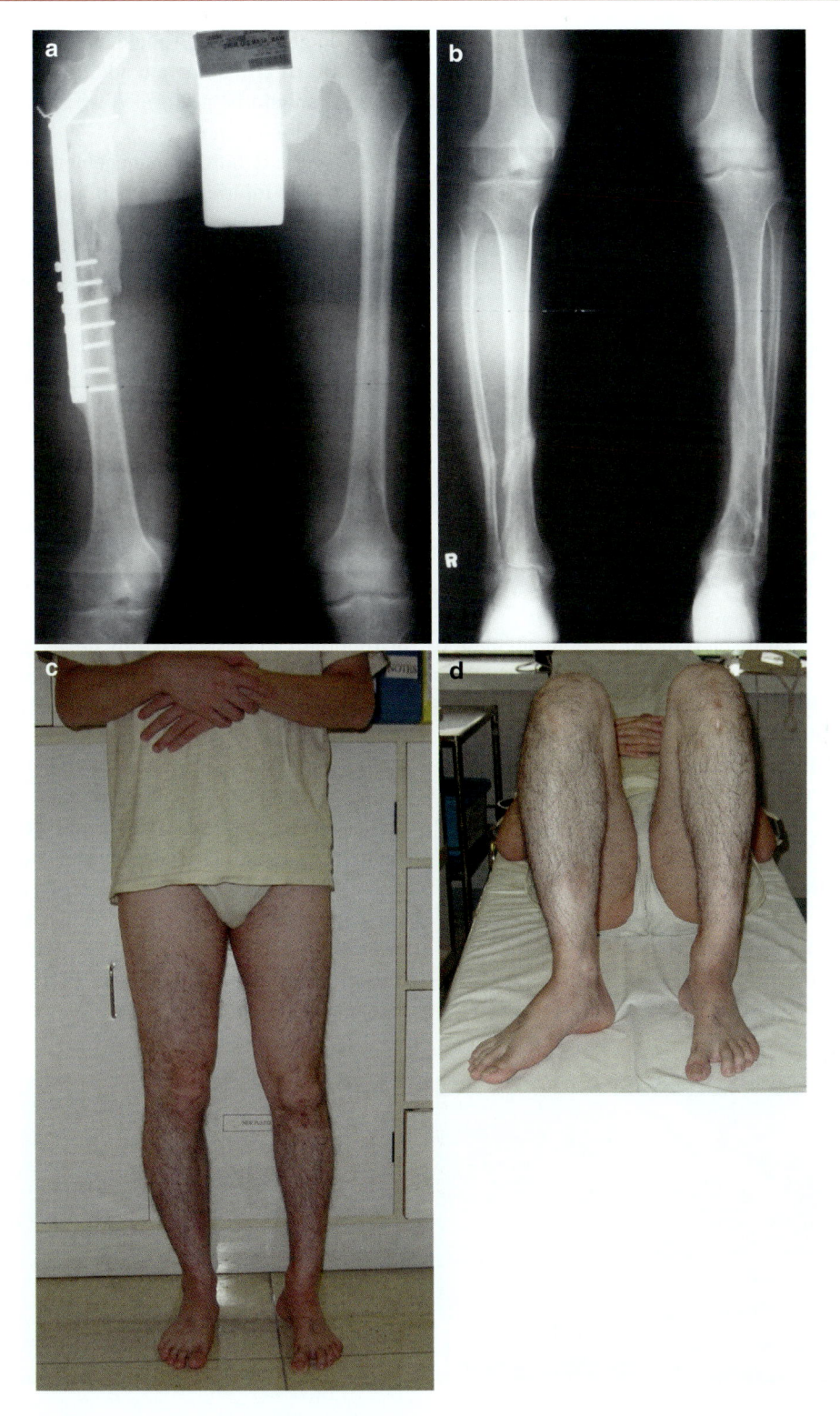

Fig. 20.4 (**a**, **b**) A 24-year-old man sustained multiple injuries during a motor vehicle accident, including head injury, pelvic fracture, left distal tibial fracture and a floating knee injury on the right side. The right proximal femur fracture was treated with plating and both tibial fractures were treated with casting. (**c**, **d**) However, the right floating knee segment was internally rotated resulting in a rotational malunion of 30°. Subsequently, correctional de-rotational osteotomies were performed for both the right femur and tibia. He also received left foot reconstructive surgery for post-traumatic deformity

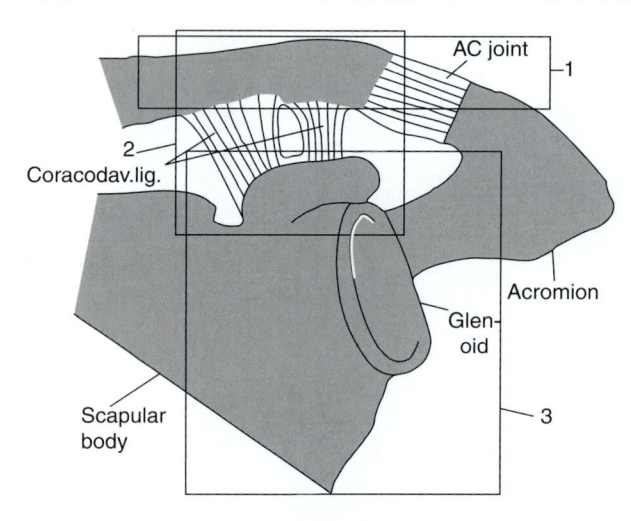

Fig. 20.5 The superior shoulder suspensory complex has three components: *1* – the acromioclavicular joint-aromial strut, *2* – the clavicular–coracoclavicular ligamentous-coracoid linkage, *3* – the three process–scapular body junction

amount of clavicular displacement, glenoid angulation and medialization, the extent of intra-articular involvement, and the extent of comminntion [19]. If the patient is physiologically stable, further evaluation with CT scan and three dimensional reconstructions can help to better delineate the fracture pattern.

20.4.2.2 Management

Floating shoulder injuries normally do not require emergency management, unless there is an associated open clavicular fracture that needs urgent debridement. Once diagnosed, the shoulder should be supported with a broad arm sling and additional evaluation with CT scan should be performed when the patient's general condition is stable.

As for the definitive management of isolated floating shoulder injuries, in general, there is no hitherto consensus of the best treatment method because of the small patient number and heterogeneity of all the studies. Based on current literature review, the treatment options are now evenly divided into nonsurgical treatment and open reduction and internal fixation [19]. The degree of displacement of both clavicle and scapular neck fractures plays an important role in deciding the stability of the fractures.

Nonsurgical management has its popularity because of its noninvasiveness and low morbidity [20, 21]. It includes a period of immobilization and pain management, followed by gradual mobilization exercise and strengthening exercise in 4–6 weeks time. Minimally displaced fractures with no sign of significant ligament disruptions can be successfully treated by conservative means [19]. It is also indicated when the multiply injured patient is in a hemodynamically unstable condition or in extremis.

In a multiply injured patient with a floating shoulder injury, surgical intervention should be considered because the unstable shoulder girdle presents great difficulty for nursing, especially in the intensive care unit where they require breathing exercises and chest physiotherapy. Hence, once the patient is stable hemodynamically, one should consider fixing the clavicle fracture alone, which can indirectly reduce and stabilize the glenoid fracture (Fig. 20.6). The patient is allowed

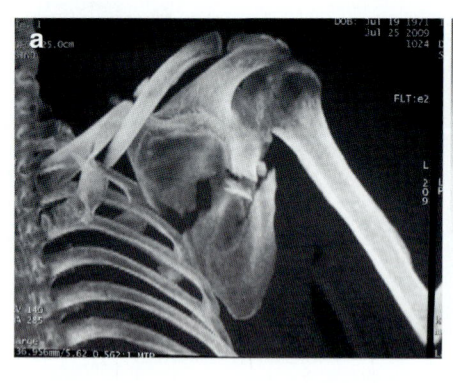

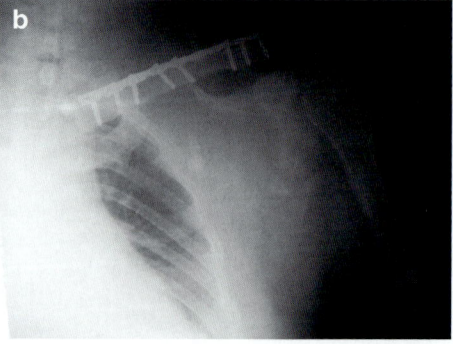

Fig. 20.6 (**a**) A 38-year-old man fell from 20 ft during work and sustained head concussion, fractures of right fourth to sixth ribs and left second and sixth ribs, fracture left clavicle and left scapula fracture with comminution over the scapular body and an undisplaced glenoid neck fracture. CT thorax revealed bilateral small apical pneumothorax. (**b**) In order to improve the ventilatory effort and to facilitate nursing processes in intensive care unit, plate fixation of left clavicle was performed

to perform earlier supervised mobilization exercise. This has the benefit of reducing pain and minimizes the chance of frozen shoulder. Hashiguchi and Ito reported successful treatment in five patients with floating shoulder injuries by clavicular fixation alone [22].

If significant displacement of glenoid remains after clavicle fixation, reduction and fixation of the glenoid may be indicated because of the theoretical restoration of the rotator cuff lever arm [19, 23]. However, surgical fixation of the scapular neck needs surgical expertise. It usually involves a posterior skin incision in a prone position which is not good especially for a chest injured patient. This will also lead to an inevitable increase in surgical trauma with more intraoperative blood loss and more post-operative pain. Hence the scapular fixation may be performed later as a second stage procedure.

20.4.2.3 Complications

In the setting of untreated or neglected floating shoulder, the weight of the arm and the contraction of the biceps, triceps, and coracobrachialis will result in downward pull of the distal fragment, with resultant change of the shoulder contour, the "drooping shoulder." This shortening will cause loss of mechanical advantage of the rotator cuff muscles [18, 24]. The increase in displacement of the fracture will result in complication of malunion, non-union, post-traumatic arthritis, subacromial impingement or chronic brachial plexopathy [25–28].

20.4.3 Floating Elbow

Ipsilateral diaphyseal factures of the humerus and the forearm are termed as floating elbow. These injuries are rare and they can happen in both adult and children. Usually, these injuries are the results of high energy trauma, such as road traffic accident, industrial accident or fell from height. As a result, open injuries are common. Nevertheless, with the advance of modern plating and nailing, debridement and antibiotics, there is a major improvement in the outcome of this severe injury compared with two decades ago [29–33].

There is no special classification for floating elbow injury. The fracture pattern of humerus and forearm are classified individually using the traditional ways, e.g., AO/OTA classification.

20.4.3.1 Associated Injuries

Floating elbow is generally the consequence after high energy trauma. As a result, this injury is usually associated with conditions such as open fractures, nerve injuries, vessels injuries, compartment syndrome, and multisystem injuries [30, 33–35]. In the literature, the incidence of open fracture is more than 50% [33]. In many cases, the soft tissue injury is so severe that multiple staged operations are required for soft tissue coverage before the fracture fixation. Uncommonly, the elbow joint itself can also be dislocated [36].

20.4.3.2 Management

With the advance of modern fracture fixation and soft tissue management, this injury is much better managed than before. The protocol of ATLS when dealing with multisystem injuries should be employed. Grossly contaminated wound should be thoroughly debrided. External fixator in open humeral fractures is applied in case of grossly contaminated wound or when rapid skeletal stabilization is required for urgent revascularization.

After good soft tissue coverage achieved, the humeral fractures can be fixed with either plating or nailing. The use of different implants and techniques depends on the local soft tissue condition and individual surgeon experience. At present, there is no clear advantage of whether plate or nail fixation is better in the setting of floating elbow [31]. The forearm fracture is treated like an isolated one. Stable plate fixation is the standard with attention paid to the alignment, rotation and the interosseous distance.

20.4.3.3 Outcome

Although excellent and good functions can be achieved after surgical treatment in up to 67% of patients, the presence of brachial plexus injury and peripheral nerve injury seems to have an adverse effect in functional outcome [32, 33]. Timing of surgery, the existence of open fractures, multisystem injuries and presence of neurovascular injuries are all not significantly related to poor functional outcome. These patients' functional outcome falls into a bimodal distribution. One group of patients recovers at around 1 year time and behaves similar to those with an isolated fracture. However, another group of patients have significant problem afterwards and remains disabled for long period of time.

20.4.3.4 Complications

Despite all the improvement in management, floating elbow is a complex injury and prone to have complications. The incidence of non-union, malunion, infection, and myositis ossificans are exceptionally high [30, 35, 36]. Another common problem is loss of elbow flexion and extension movement. Supination and pronation problem is less frequent but it is usually associated with high energy trauma to the forearm [31].

20.5 Traumatic Knee Dislocation

Traumatic knee dislocation is an uncommon problem. It accounts for <0.02% of all orthopaedic problems [37, 38]. However, this may be an underestimation of the real situation because a high percentage of the knee is spontaneously reduced at the scene [39]. Besides fall from height and motor vehicle accidents, people involved in high speed sport activities also have a chance of getting knee dislocation. They present with multiligamentous disruption, but vascular and nerve injuries are common as well. The historical way of conservative treatment using simple immobilization resulting in variable outcome [40, 41] has evolved to the present principles of early surgical ligaments repair and reconstruction together with early mobilization [39].

20.5.1 Classification

Classification can be done according to the time of injury. Injury happens in less than 3 weeks is classified as acute and chronic after this [42]. Anatomical classification, proposed by Kennedy is 1963, is more commonly used [38]. The classification is based on the direction of tibia displacement in relation to the femur, i.e., anterior, posterior, medial, or lateral. The fifth type, rotatory dislocation, is the combination of the multidirectional displacement. Among these, anterior dislocation is the commonest type as a result of hyperextension injury. It comprises 40% of all knee dislocations. The second commonest one is posterior dislocation, which is usually due to "dash-board" type injury in motor vehicle. It comprises another one-third of cases [43]. Rotatory dislocation is the least common type, roughly about 5%. It is further subdivided into anteromedial, posteromedial, anterolateral, and posterolateral, in which posterolateral is the commonest with a high incidence of irreducibility [44]. However, the major drawback of this classification is the difficulty of application when the knee is spontaneously reduced. Another more recent classification, proposed by Schenck in 1994 [45], is based on the status of the ligamentous disruptions and any associated intra-articular fractures. It tries to help providing more information on the nature and severity of the problem which guides to specific management.

20.5.2 Associated Injuries

Traumatic knee dislocation often associates with other concomitant injuries. Vascular injury, mainly popliteal artery injury, which may result in disastrous consequence, is quite common. The reported incidence can be up to 65% [46]. There is a great discrepancy in the incidence reported. One of the reasons is that there is a spectrum of degree of damage to vessels, ranging from minor intimal damage to complete transaction. Besides, there may be a lot of occult injury not being diagnosed. The degree of suspicion and the use of arteriography greatly affect the pick-up rate of any vascular compromise.

Another commonly associated injury is common peroneal nerve damage, which happens in about 20% of cases [47]. The incidence is much higher in posterolateral dislocation or involvement of the posterolateral complex. The reported incidence can be up to 45% [48]. Tibial nerve injury can also occur but it is much less common.

Fractures, especially avulsion fractures, are often encountered. The usual sites are origins of PCL or lateral tibial plateau in the form of Segond fracture. Fractures of the distal femur or proximal tibia are not uncommon as well.

20.5.3 Evaluation and Assessment

In emergency setting, a brief history is all one needs, which includes the time and mode of injury. Then the examination should be directed to neurovascular examination since the consequence of missing the vascular injury is disastrous. The dislocated knee is usually presented with tremendous pain and effusion with lots of lower limb swelling. A pitfall in diagnosis would be those spontaneously reduced knee dislocations which may look benign on presentation. Since most of the time the joint capsules and ligaments are severely disrupted, a spontaneously reduced knee is presented with severe and extensive bruising on medial and lateral side of the leg because of the uncontained hemarthrosis. In addition, the presence of multiple ligamentous laxity is another clue to spontaneously reduced dislocated knee.

The current trend of vascular assessment is now based on both clinical assessment and imaging, with clinical evaluation as the more important aspect. Selective arteriography in patients with abnormal physical abnormalities is practiced nowadays. The manual palpation of the pulses of dorsalis pedis and posterior tibialis is sufficient to detect any clinically significant vascular injury. Although minor intimal injuries are not detected by clinical examination, these non-flow-limiting intimal injuries rarely progressed to occlusive lesion [49]. Nevertheless, repeated serial careful vascular examination within the first 48 h is important. Whenever there is an abnormal clinical finding, one should proceed to urgent arteriography without delay. Ankle-brachial index (ABI) is a useful and non-invasive adjunct to detect vascular compromise. It is the ratio of Doppler systolic pressure in injured limb (ankle) to the Doppler systolic pressure in uninjured limb (brachial). The presence of ABI <0.9 indicates immediate further investigation of the arterial status, usually an arteriography [50]. However, the result can be inaccurate in patients with peripheral vascular disease.

A complete neurological examination should be obtained. The degree of damage can be as minor as neuropraxia to complete neuronotmesis. Like vascular assessment, serial neurological reassessment should also be done, as the development of deteriorate neurological deficit can be a sign of developing compartment syndrome or ischemia.

The evaluation of the knee stability should be done after the lower limb is cleared of any impending vascular damage. The examination is usually difficult because of intense pain, muscle spasm, and gross swelling. It should be done as gently as possible to minimize the chance of iatrogenic damage. The ACL is best tested by Lachman test and the PCL by posterior drawer test. The presence of valgus and varus instability signifies medial and lateral collateral ligaments disruptions [39].

The radiological assessment must include plain radiographs during injury and after the reduction. Besides confirmation of the reduction of joint, they also give details on any associated fractures and avulsions. Nevertheless, these investigations should not delay the vascular assessment and intervention. Angiography should be done when there is suspicion of vascular compromise. Magnetic resonance imaging is useful in evaluation of the type and extent of ligamentous injuries as well as cartilage and meniscal damage.

20.5.4 Management

20.5.4.1 Acute

In acute dislocation, the vascular status should be checked first. The joint should be reduced gently by gentle traction and manipulation under conscious sedation. The direction of reduction should be guided by the direction of dislocation. The reduced knee joint is then temporarily held with a long leg splint.

Once the reduction is done, the vascular status should be reassessed clinically immediately. If pulses are absent or ABI is <0.9, urgent angiography should be obtained and vascular surgeon opinion is sought. When the site of vascular injury is confirmed, urgent revascularization, using bypass grafting of the popliteal artery or repair using a reverse saphenous vein graft, is required [47]. Fasciotomy is usually performed after revascularization. The knee is preferably immobilized by a knee-spanning external fixator to protect the vascular repair and the knee from re-dislocation. The use of the joint spanning external fixator is also indicated in open injury and joint that failed to maintain reduction in a splint.

In case of knee dislocation necessitating vascular repair, concomitant repair of the torn medial or lateral collateral ligaments can be attempted, but the use of sutures and magnitude of the procedure should be kept to minimal. On the other hand, a late repair of these ligaments in a few days time is also a good option [39]. The delay in repair can help the surgeon to monitor the vascular status of the limb in the next 48 h after the repair. It also allows further imaging study for better preoperative planning and delineation of the extent of ligamentous injuries. In open injuries, all ligamentous procedure should be delayed until the wound is well covered and clean.

20.5.4.2 Definitive

The definitive management of multiligamentous knee injuries is controversial. However, there are more and more well designed studies which provide guidelines for the management of this difficult problem [39, 51–53].

Nowadays, surgical treatment is the treatment of choice unless the patient is surgically unfit. Some conditions are absolute indications for surgical treatment, including irreducible knees, dysvascular limbs, and open injuries. Studies have shown that the surgically treated dislocated knees usually have better range of movement, higher level of activities and better knee scores [40, 51–54].

Another important issue is the timing of ligamentous repair and reconstruction. Meanwhile, there is no consensus on the right timing of surgery. Although many studies showed that the range of movement, knee stability, knee scores (Lysholm score and International Knee Documentation Committee [IKDC] score), and level of activities are better in patients managed within 3 weeks of injury [51–53], there is evidence showing no significant difference between the early and late management groups [55]. The delay of surgery in 3–6 weeks time may allow the healing of the capsule to facilitate the use of arthroscopic repair. In fact, the timing of the definite ligamentous repair is affected by many other factors, especially the vascular status, swelling of the knee, soft tissue coverage, and the presence of concomitant fractures.

20.5.5 Rehabilitation

The general principle of rehabilitation in multiligamentous injured knee is to restore the knee range of movement followed by progressive strengthening exercise. The reconstructed knee should be protected by a hinged knee brace or a mobile hinged external fixator. The knee was immobilized for first 3 weeks followed by passive mobilization exercise in brace in the next 3 weeks. Starting from seventh week, the patient is allowed to start gradual weight bearing training till full-weight-bearing walking. Range of movement and strengthening exercise are practiced up to 3 months and then followed by further training to allow patients to reintegrate into his/her previous activities of daily living [39, 47].

20.5.6 Outcome and Complications

Acute traumatic knee dislocation is a severe injury with multiple ligamentous disruption and a high incidence of neurovascular damage. The most disastrous local consequence is probably amputation. The chance of it in failed revascularization within first 8 h can be up to 86% [43]. Return to normal function is rare. Using the IKDC score, about 39% of patients are nearly normal, 40% are abnormal, and the remaining 21% are severely abnormal [51, 52, 56]. The most common complications are joint stiffness and failure of some of the component of ligamentous reconstruction. Post-traumatic osteoarthritis can be up to 50% [57]. Common peroneal nerve injuries are common. Many of them are neuropraxia and they are managed by observation. Unfortunately, spontaneous full recovery is only about 20% [52].

20.6 Conclusions

The timing of surgical treatment of articular injuries in polytrauma patients must be based on priorities and be integrated into the optimal management of the overall patient. Open fractures and associated neurovascular injuries are common and often require urgent treatment in the emergency setting. On the other hand, the complex fractures will require careful preoperative planning and preparation. Although primary definitive fracture fixation can be performed in selected patients, a spanning transarticular external fixation should be used most of the time as an initial immobilization method while the patient's physiological status is being stabilized or the soft tissue injury is optimal. In general, the overall injury severity and the extent of soft tissue injury will dictate the timing of definitive fracture fixation.

References

1. Kobbe P, Lichte P, Pape HC. Complex extremity fractures following high energy injuries: the limited value of existing classifications and a proposal for a treatment-guide. Injury. 2009;40(S4):S69–74.
2. Mills WJ, Nork SE. Open reduction and internal fixation of high-energy tibial plateau fractures. Orthop Clin North Am. 2002;33(1):177–98.
3. Sirkin M, Sanders R, DiPasquale T, Herscovici Jr D. A staged protocol for soft tissue management in the treatment of complex pilon fractures. J Orthop Trauma. 2004;18(8 Suppl):S32–8.
4. Argenta LC, Morykwas MJ. Vacuum-assisted closure: a new method for wound control and treatment: clinical experience. Ann Plast Surg. 1997;38:563–76.
5. Lee HJ, Kim JW, Oh CW, Min WK, Shon OJ, Oh JK, et al. Negative pressure wound therapy for soft tissue injuries around the foot and ankle. J Orthop Surg Res. 2009;4:14.
6. Webb LX. New techniques in wound management: vacuum-assisted wound closure. J Am Acad Orthop Surg. 2002;10:303–11.
7. Fraser RD, Hunter GA, Waddell JP. Ipsilateral fracture of the femur and tibia. J Bone Joint Surg Br. 1978;60-B(4):510–5.
8. Lundy DW, Johnson KD. "Floating knee" injuries: ipsilateral fractures of the femur and tibia. J Am Acad Orthop Surg. 2001;9:238–45.
9. Rethnam U, Yesupalan RS, Nair R. Impact of associated injuries in the floating knee: a retrospective study. BMC Musculoskelet Disord. 2009;10:7.
10. Adamson GJ, Wiss DA, Lowery GL, Peters CL. Type II floating knee: ipsilateral femoral and tibial fractures with intraarticular extension into the knee joint. J Orthop Trauma. 1992;6:333–9.
11. Paul GR, Sawka MW, Whitelaw GP. Fractures of the ipsilateral femur and tibia: emphasis on intra-articular and soft tissue injury. J Orthop Trauma. 1990;4:309–14.
12. Szalay MJ, Hosking OR, Annear P. Injury of knee ligament associated with ipsilateral femoral shaft fractures and with ipsilateral femoral and tibial shaft fractures. Injury. 1990; 21:398–400.
13. Karlström G, Olerud S. Ipsilateral fracture of the femur and tibia. J Bone Joint Surg Am. 1977;59(2):240–3.
14. Veith RG, Winquist RA, Hansen Jr ST. Ipsilateral fractures of the femur and tibia. A report of fifty-seven consecutive cases. J Bone Joint Surg Am. 1984;66(7):991–1002.
15. Goss TP. Double disruptions of the superior shoulder suspensory complex. J Orthop Trauma. 1993;7:99–106.
16. Goss TP. Scapular fractures and dislocations: diagnosis and treatment. J Am Acad Orthop Surg. 1995;3:22–33.
17. Williams Jr GR, Narania J, Klimkiewicz J, Karduna A, Iannotti JP, Ramsey M. The floating shoulder: a biomechanical basis for classification and management. J Bone Joint Surg Am. 2001;83:1182–7.
18. van Noort A, van der Weken C. The floating shoulder. Injury. 2006;37(3):218–27.
19. DeFranco MJ, Patterson BM. The floating shoulder. J Am Acad Orthop Surg. 2006;14(8):499–509.
20. Edwards SG, Whittle AP, Wood II GW, et al. Nonoperative treatment of ipsilateral fractures of the scapula and clavicle. J Bone Joint Surg Am. 2001;83A:1188–94.
21. Ramos L, Mencia R, Alonso A, Fernandez L. Conservative treatment of ipsilateral fractures of the scapula and clavicle. J Trauma. 1997;42:239–42.
22. Hashiguchi H, Ito H. Clinical outcome of the treatment of floating shoulder by osteosynthesis for clavicular fracture alone. J Shoulder Elbow Surg. 2003;12:589–91.
23. Owens BD, Goss TP. The floating shoulder. J Bone Joint Surg Br. 2006;88(11):1419–24.
24. Obremskey WT, Lyman JR. A modified Judet approach to the scapula. J Orthop Trauma. 2004;18:696–9.
25. Egol KA, Connor PM, Karunakar MA, Sims SH, Bosses MJ, Kellam JF. The floating shoulder: clinical and functional results. J Bone Joint Surg Am. 2001;83:1188–94.
26. Hardegger FH, Simpson LA, Weber BG. The operative treatment of scapular fractures. J Bone Joint Surg. 1984; 668:725–31.
27. Rikli D, Regazzoni P, Renner N. The unstable shoulder girdle: early functional treatment utilizing open reduction and internal fixation. J Orthop Trauma. 1995;9:93–7.
28. van Noort A, eSlaa RL, Marti RK, van der Werken C. The floating shoulder: a multicentre study. J Bone Joint Surg. 2001;83:795–8.
29. Lange RH, Foster RJ. Skeletal management of humeral shaft fractures associated with forearm fractures. Clin Orthop Relat Res. 1985;195:173–7.
30. Rogers JF, Bennett JB, Tullos HS. Management of concomitant ipsilateral fractures of the humerus and forearm. J Bone Joint Surg Am. 1984;66(4):552–6.
31. Simpson NS, Jupiter JB. Complex fracture patterns of the upper extremity. Clin Orthop Relat Res. 1995;318:43–53. Review.
32. Solomon HB, Zadnik M, Eglseder WA. A review of outcomes in 18 patients with floating elbow. J Orthop Trauma. 2003;17(8):563–70.
33. Yokoyama K, Itoman M, Kobayashi A, Shindo M, Futami T. Functional outcomes of "floating elbow" injuries in adult patients. J Orthop Trauma. 1998;12(4):284–90.
34. Levin LS, Goldner RD, Urbaniak JR, et al. Management of severe musculoskeletal injuries of the upper extremity. J Orthop Trauma. 1990;4:432–40.
35. Pierce RO, Hodorski DF. Fractures of the humerus, radius and ulna in the same extremity. J Trauma. 1979;19:182–5.

36. Viegas SF, Gogan W, Riley S. Floating dislocated elbow: case report and review of the literature. J Trauma. 1989;29:886–8.
37. Hoover N. Injuries of the popliteal artery associated with dislocation of the knee. Surg Clin North Am. 1961;41:1099–112.
38. Kennedy JC. Complete dislocation of the knee joint. J Bone Joint Surg Am. 1963;45:889–903.
39. Rihn JA, Groff YJ, Harner CD, Cha PS. The acutely dislocated knee: evaluation and management. J Am Acad Orthop Surg. 2004;12(5):334–46.
40. Richter M, Bosch U, Wippermann B, Hofmann A, Krettek C. Comparison of surgical repair of reconstruction of cruciate ligaments versus nonsurgical treatment in patients with traumatic knee dislocations. Am J Sports Med. 2002;30:718–27.
41. Taylor AR, Arden GP, Rainey HA. Traumatic dislocation of the knee. A report of forty-three cases with special reference to conservative treatment. J Bone Joint Surg Br. 1972;54:96–102.
42. Palmar I. On the injuries of the ligaments of the knee joint: a clinical study. Acta Chir Scand. 1938;53:1–28.
43. Green NE, Allen BL. Vascular injuries associated with dislocation of the knee. J Bone Joint Surg Am. 1977;59:236–9.
44. Quinlan AG. Irreducible posterolateral dislocation of the knee with buttonholing of the medial femoral condyle. J Bone Joint Surg Am. 1966;48:1619–21.
45. Schenok RC. The dislocated knee. Instr Course Lect. 1994;43:127–36.
46. Meyers MH, Harvey Jr JP. Traumatic dislocation of the knee joint: a study of eighteen cases. J Bone Joint Surg Am. 1971;53-A:16–29.
47. Robertson A, Nutton RW, Keating JF. Dislocation of the knee. J Bone Joint Surg Br. 2006;88(6):706–11.
48. Niall DM, Nutton RW, Keating JF. Palsy of the common peroneal nerve after traumatic dislocation of the knee. J Bone Joint Surg Br. 2005;87-B:664–7.
49. Stain SC, Yellin AE, Weaver FA, Pentecost KN. Selective management of nonocclusive arterial injuries. Arch Surg. 1989;124:1136–40.
50. Mills WJ, Barei DP, Mc Nair P. The value of the ankle-brachial index for diagnostic arterial injury after knee dislocation: a prospective study. J Trauma. 2004;56:1261–5.
51. Harner CD, Waltrip RIL, Bennett CH, Francis KA, Cole B, Irrgang JJ. Surgical management of knee dislocations. J Bone Joint Surg Am. 2004;86:262–73.
52. Liow RY, McNicholas MJ, Keating JF, Nutton RW. Ligament repair and reconstruction in traumatic dislocation of the knee. J Bone Joint Surg Br. 2003;85:845–51.
53. Tzurbakis M, Diamantopoulos A, Xenakis T, Gergoulis A. Surgical treatment of multiple knee ligament injuries in 44 patients: 2–8 years follow-up results. Knee Surg Sports Traumatol Arthrosc. 2006;14:739–49.
54. Dedmond BT, Almekinders LC. Operative versus nonoperative treatment of knee dislocations: a meta-analysis. Am J Knee Surg. 2001;14:33–8.
55. Fanelli C, Giannotti BF, Edson CJ. Arthroscopically assisted combined posterior cruciate ligament/posterior lateral complex reconstruction. Arthroscopy. 1996;12:521–30.
56. Wascher DC, Dvirnak PC, DeCoster TA. Knee dislocation: initial assessment and implications for treatment. J Orthop Trauma. 1997;11:525–9.
57. Werier J, Keating JF, Meek RN. Complete dislocation of the knee: the long-term results of ligamentous reconstruction. Knee. 1998;5:255–60.

21 Techniques of Soft Tissue Coverage in Open Fractures

Norbert Pallua and Ahmet Bozkurt

Contents

21.1 General Principles: Surgical Decision Making ... 243

21.2 Classification of Flaps 244
21.2.1 Cutaneous Flaps 245
21.2.2 Muscle Flaps 246
21.2.3 Osseus Flaps 246

21.3 "Fix and Flap": Early Soft Tissue Coverage in Open Fractures 246

21.4 Anatomy and Techniques 250
21.4.1 Lateral Arm Flap 250
21.4.2 Radial Forearm Flap 250
21.4.3 Anterior Lateral Thigh Flap 250
21.4.4 Gracilis Flap 251
21.4.5 Fibula Flap 253
21.4.6 Gastrocnemius Flap 253
21.4.7 Scapular and Parascapular Flap 253
21.4.8 Latissimus Dorsi Flap 255

References 263

21.1 General Principles: Surgical Decision Making

Preservation of life and limb salvage with restoration of form and function are the primary goals of reconstructive plastic surgery. The concept of the "Reconstructive Ladder" [1] describes a possible guide in selecting the appropriate surgical technique, which is based on the complexity of the technique and defect requirements for safe wound closure. In ascending order the reconstructive ladder starts with simple techniques such as wound closure or skin grafts and continues with more complex procedures like distant (pedicled) flaps or free microvascular tissue transfer (Fig. 21.1).

Although still relevant, it is thought that the reconstructive ladder may not always provide optimal results regarding form, function, and safety, since more complex techniques can often achieve better results. Depending on surgical skills and the complexity of the defect, form and function can be improved by microvascular techniques. Therefore, the reconstructive ladder has widely been replaced by the "Reconstructive Triangle" (Fig. 21.2). This reconstructive triangle represents the basis for a systematic approach to patient care through the key phases of management:

1. Evaluation and treatment of organ system derangements
2. Defect analysis
3. Timing
4. Assessment of surgical options
5. Identification of reconstructive goals
6. Execution of the operative procedure

First, the defect has to be evaluated with a concomitant evaluation of the medical and functional status of the

N. Pallua (✉) and A. Bozkurt
Department of Plastic Surgery, Hand Surgery – Burns Unit,
RWTH Aachen University, Pauwelsstraße 30,
52074 Aachen, Germany
e-mail: npallua@ukaachen.de; abozkurt77@gmx.de

H.-C. Pape et al. (eds.), *The Poly-Traumatized Patient with Fractures*,
DOI: 10.1007/978-3-642-17986-0_21, © Springer-Verlag Berlin Heidelberg 2011

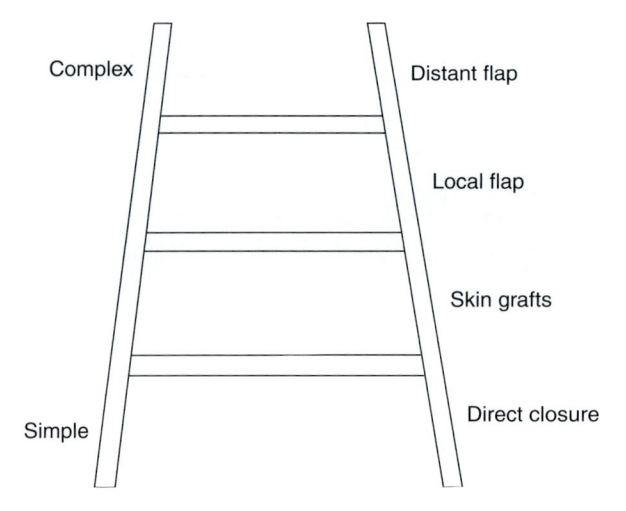

Fig. 21.1 Reconstructive ladder [1]

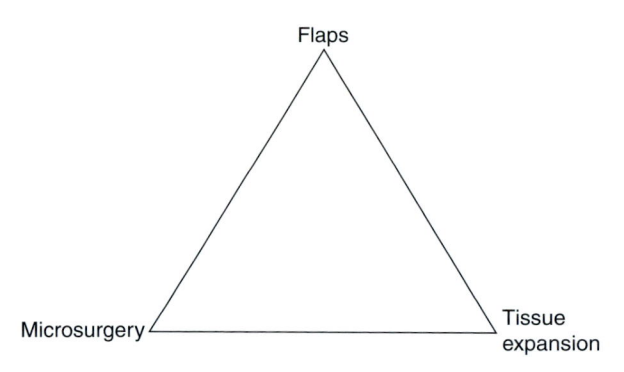

Fig. 21.2 Reconstructive triangle (microsurgery-flaps-tissue expansion) [1]

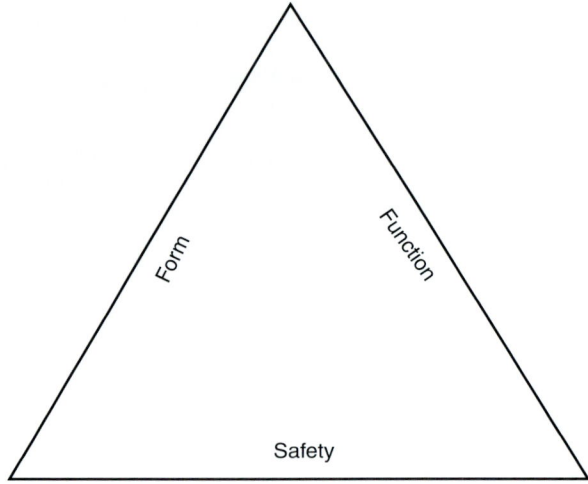

Fig. 21.3 Reconstructive triangle (form-function-safety) [1]

patient. Then, the defect has to be analyzed with its impact on patients' survival and quality of life. Treatment of vital organ systems takes absolute precedence over defect reconstruction ("life before limb"). Second, wound analysis has to be accomplished regarding location, size, and defect components (skin, subcutaneous tissue, muscle, vessels, nerves, cartilage, bone etc.). Third, timing of the surgical procedure has to be determined. For example, temporary wound coverage after stabilization of vital organ systems and control of acute infections. Definitive defect closure may have to be delayed after stabilization of the patient. Fourth, surgical options need to be assessed. This includes temporary wound coverage or definitive wound coverage using skin grafts, local flaps, distant flaps, or free microvascular flaps. Fifth, reconstructive goals need to be defined. According to Mathes and Nahai [1] this includes selection of an appropriate technique assuring safe and successful reconstruction of form and function (Fig. 21.3).

21.2 Classification of Flaps

The timeline of flap surgery goes back to Sushruta Samhita in 600 BC and Tagliacozzi in 1597 with attempts of nasal reconstruction [2]. The application of flap surgery could be extended on the basis of anatomical studies. The concept of anatomic skin territories supplied by consistent blood vessels was studied by Carl Manchot in 1889 [3].

Over the last decades, microvascular plastic surgery has advanced due to the combination of (a) anatomical expertise as a result of detailed anatomical dissection studies [4–6] and (b) continuous technical progress (i.e., development of special operating microscopes, magnifying loupes, microinstruments, etc.). Since the 1970s [2], an exponential increase of new flaps, concepts, and classifications could be observed and has revolutionized the field of plastic surgery.

In general, flaps can be defined as mobilized tissues on the basis of their vascular anatomy with the optional combination of skin, fat, fascia, muscle, bone, tendons, and nerves. Flaps can be differentiated according to their form (e.g., bilobed, rhomboid, etc.), their destination with local versus distant (pedicled flap or free

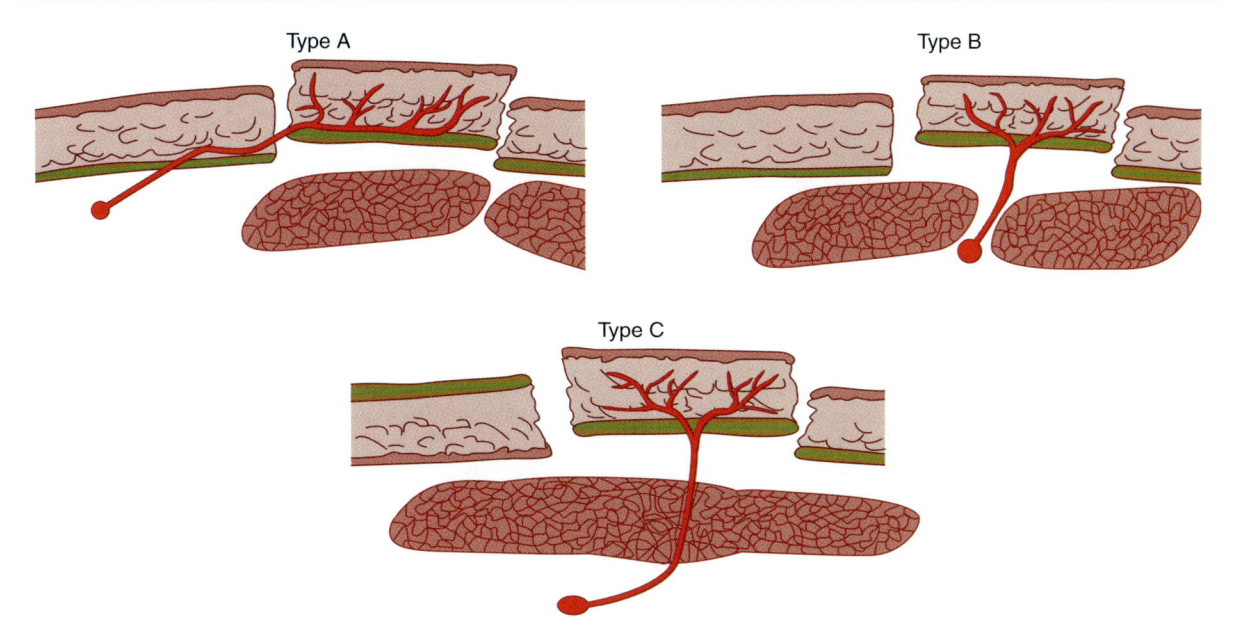

Fig. 21.4 Cutaneous flaps [1]

flap) or their special preparation (e.g., delay, tissue expansion etc.) [7]. However, there is no system that perfectly categorizes all types of flaps. Cormack and Lamberty [8, 9] tried to give a broad classification of pedicled and free flaps by introducing their "6 Cs":

1. *Circulation* (blood supply): direct vessels (axial, septocutaneous, endosteal) versus indirect vessels (myocutaneous, periosteal)
2. *Constituents* (composition): fasciocutaneous, muscle/myocutaneous, visceral, nerve, bone, cartilage, etc.
3. *Contiguity* (destination): local, regional, distant (pedicled flap)
4. *Construction* (flow): uni-/bipedicled, ortho-/retrograde flow, turbo-/supercharged
5. *Conditioning* (preparation): delay, tissue expansion, prefabrication
6. *Conformation* (geometry): combined flaps

For practical reasons, we will give only a short overview of the most common classifications.

21.2.1 Cutaneous Flaps

Similar to Cormack and Lamberty's tripartite system [10], Mathes and Nahai [1] subcategorize fasciocutaneous flaps on the basis of the type of deep fascial perforators into (Fig. 21.4):

1. Type A: direct cutaneous
2. Type B: septocutaneous
3. Type C: musculocutaneous.

Over the last years, further refinements in flap surgery have led to a new genre of so-called perforator flaps (Fig. 21.5) as a new form of cutaneous flaps. Perforator flaps have evolved from musculocutaneous and fasciocutaneous flaps. It has been shown that neither a muscle nor the underlying fascial plexus of vessels is necessary [11, 12].

The great advantage is the decrease of donor-site morbidity due to preservation of the innervation, vascularity, and function of the donor muscle. Relatively large and thin skin flaps can be harvested without postoperative muscle atrophy as seen in myocutaneous flaps, the presence of long vascular pedicles, and the possibility of harvesting sensory nerves with the flap [11]. Disadvantages are the meticulous dissection for perforator vessel isolation with increased operation time, variability in the position and size of perforator vessels, and the ease with which the vessels can be damaged [2].

According to Blondeel and colleagues [11], a perforator is a vessel that has its origin in one of the axial

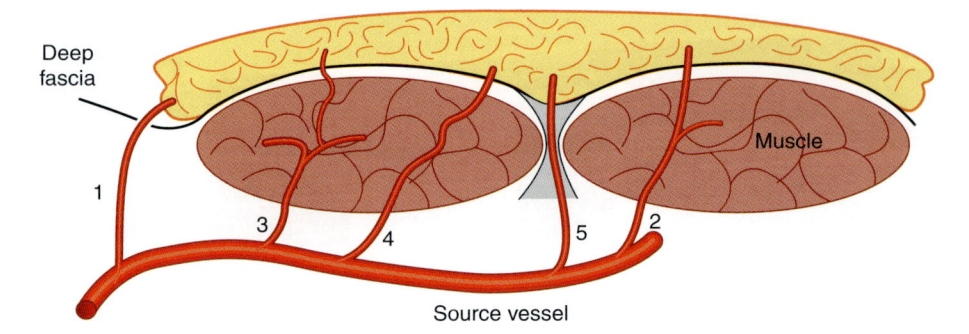

Fig. 21.5 Perforator vessels according to the "Gent" consensus on perforator flap terminology [11]. Schematic drawing of the different types of direct and indirect perforator vessels with regard to their surgical importance. *1* – Direct perforators perforate the deep fascia only; *2* – indirect muscle perforators predominantly supply the subcutaneous tissues; *3* – indirect muscle perforators predominantly supply the muscle but have secondary branches to the subcutaneous tissues; *4* – indirect perimysial perforators travel within the perimysium between muscle fibers before piercing deep fascia; *5* – indirect septal perforators travel through the intermuscular septum before piercing the deep fascia

vessels of the body and that passes through certain structural elements of the body, besides interstitial connective tissue and fat, before reaching the subcutaneous fat layer. They differentiated five different perforators (Fig. 21.5):

1. Direct perforators perforate the deep fascia.
2. Indirect muscle perforators predominantly supply subcutaneous tissue.
3. Indirect muscle perforators predominantly supply the muscle with secondary branches to the subcutaneous tissue.
4. Indirect perimysial perforators travel within the perimysium between muscle fibers before piercing the deep fascia.
5. Indirect septal perforators travel through the intermuscular septum before piercing the deep fascia.

Thus, Blondeel and colleagues [11] defined a perforator flap as a flap that consists of skin and/or subcutaneous fat and differentiated between muscle perforator flaps vascularized by muscle perforators and septal perforator flaps vascularized by septal perforators. The perforator flaps are named after the nutrient vessels and not after the underlying muscle (Table 21.1).

21.2.2 Muscle Flaps

In contrast to the cutaneous flaps, the classification of muscle flaps (Fig. 21.6), as introduced by Mathes and Nahai [13], experienced far less discussions and received a relatively broad acceptance:

1. Type I: Single vascular pedicle
2. Type II: Dominant vascular pedicle(s) and minor vascular pedicle(s)
3. Type III: Two dominant pedicles
4. Type IV: Segmental vascular pedicles
5. Type V: Single dominant vascular pedicle and secondary segmental pedicles

According to Mathes and Nahai [13], a dominant pedicle is a source of artery and vein that represents the flap circulation maintaining tissue viability. A secondary pedicle is smaller in relation to the dominant pedicle but will reliably maintain tissue viability after division of the dominant pedicle. In contrast, a minor pedicle is smaller in relation to the dominant vascular pedicle of a flap but may not reliably maintain tissue viability after division of the dominant pedicle.

21.2.3 Osseus Flaps

In accordance to Serafin [14] vascularized bone flaps can be classified as either endosteal with direct blood supply (usually via the nutrient foramen) or periosteal with indirect blood supply (within the periosteum).

21.3 "Fix and Flap": Early Soft Tissue Coverage in Open Fractures

A conservative and established management of complex open fractures consists of initial wound debridement and lavage, stabilization of the fracture, and

21 Techniques of Soft Tissue Coverage in Open Fractures

Table 21.1 Abbreviations and terminology of muscular and septal perforator flaps [11]

Flap/abbreviation	Flap/full name	Nutrient artery
Muscle perforator flaps		
DIEAP	Deep inferior epigastric artery perforator	Deep inferior epigastric vessels
TAP	Thoracodorsal artery perforator	Thoracodorsal vessels
SGAP	Superior gluteal artery perforator	Superior gluteal vessels
IGAP	Inferior gluteal artery perforator	Inferior gluteal vessels
IMAP	Internal mammary artery perforator	Internal mammary vessels
ICAP	Intercostal perforator	Intercostal vessels
PLP	Paralumbar perforator	Paralumbar perforating vessels
GP	Gracilis perforator	Medial circumflex femoral vessels
TFLP	Tensor fasciae latae perforator	Transverse branch of the lateral circumflex femoral vessels
ALTP	Anterolateral thigh perforator	Descending branch of the lateral circumflex femoral vessels
AMTP	Anteromedial thigh perforator	Innominate branch of the descending branch of the lateral circumflex femoral vessels
SAP	Sural artery perforator	Sural vessels
PTAP	Posterior tibial artery perforator	Posterior tibial vessels
ATAP	Anterior tibial artery perforator	Anterior tibial vessels
Septal perforator flaps		
RAP	Radial artery perforator	Radial vessels
AP	Adductor perforator	Medial circumflex femoral vessels
ALTP	Anterolateral thigh perforator	Descending branch of the circumflex femoral lateral vessels
AMTP	Anteromedial thigh perforator	Innominate branch of the descending branch of the lateral circumflex femoral vessels (if perforator runs only in septum)

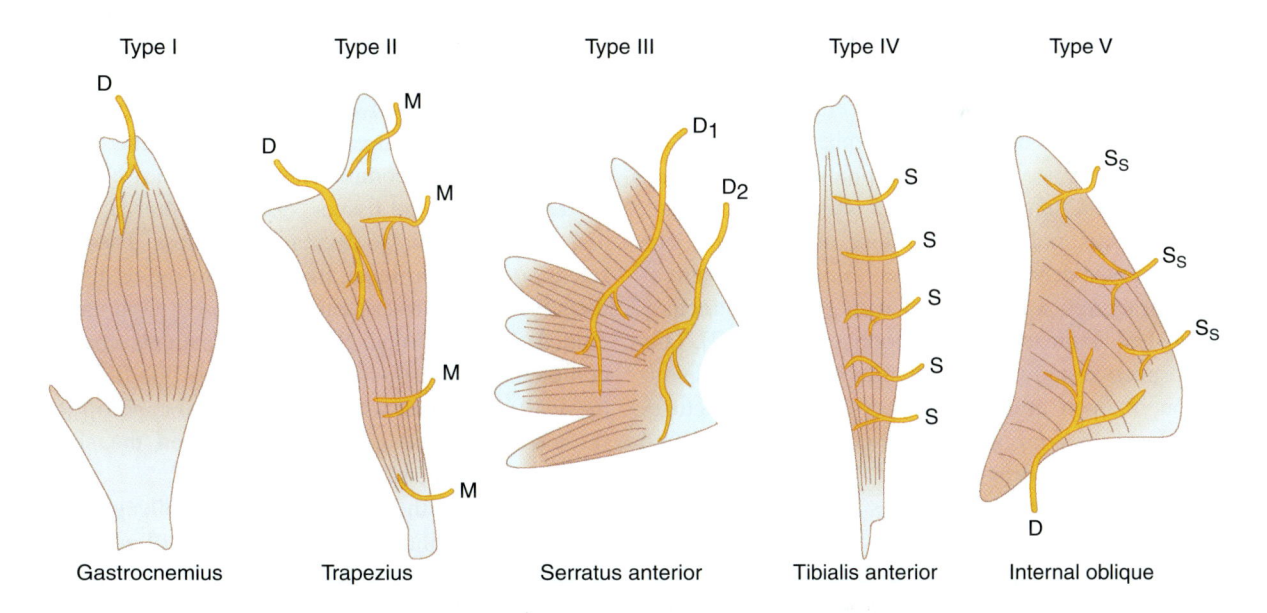

Type I — Gastrocnemius
Type II — Trapezius
Type III — Serratus anterior
Type IV — Tibialis anterior
Type V — Internal oblique

Fig. 21.6 Muscle flaps. Patterns of vascular anatomy of muscle: type I, one vascular pedicle; type II, dominant pedicle(s) plus minor pedicles; type III, two dominant pedicles; type IV, segmental vascular pedicles; type V, dominant pedicle plus secondary segmental pedicles. *D* dominant pedicle, *M* minor, *SS* Secondary segmental, *S* segmental

delayed wound closure. Bone stabilization is often performed by an external fixator due to concerns of implanting metal into contaminated tissue. Soft tissue coverage is delayed to allow both a second-look debridement and for reduction of tissue swelling [15].

A coordinated team of orthopaedic and plastic surgeons in a large trauma center has a number of advantages. However, the optimal timing for soft-tissue coverage of open fractures has become a matter of controversial debate. Advocates for a staged or delayed procedure propagate the need for second or multiple debridements to allow more adequate excision of traumatized tissue. Supporters of early reconstruction postulate a reduction and prevention of nosocomial contamination and secondary tissue necrosis [16].

The concept of immediate or early bone fixation and soft tissue coverage of open fractures is frequently referred to as "fix and flap" [17, 18]. This paradigm change in the management of open fractures goes mainly back to the mid 1980s with the landmark publications of Byrd et al. [19] and Godina [17]. Their concept included aggressive initial debridement, early definitive internal bone fixation and soft tissue coverage with muscle flaps in the lower extremity. This has led to a debate between surgeons about the ideal timing of defect closure including a discussion about the correct nomenclature: primary/immediate/early or secondary/delayed/late.

In 1985, Byrd and colleagues [19] presented a prospective study about the management of open tibial fractures with pedicled and free muscle flaps. Using three categories (acute = 1–5 days, subacute = 1–6 weeks, chronic = >6 weeks) they found better results in the acute group. This included less number of surgical procedures, lower accumulative hospital time, lower average time to union, and fewer complications (i.e., osteomyelitis, non-union, flap loss, amputations). The controversial debate of early versus delayed closure of open fractures was launched with the posthumously published landmark paper of Godina in 1986 [17]. This retrospective study about free microvascular transplantation in open upper and lower extremity fractures compared three groups: (a) early (<72 h), (b) delayed (>72 h, <3 months), and (c) late reconstruction (>3 months, <12.6 years). In this large series with 532 patients, best results were achieved in the early group with a lower postoperative infection rate, shorter hospitalization, less number of anesthesias, decreased time for bone healing, and lower incidence of flap failure.

In this landmark paper, the clear and determined operative strategy by Godina and coworkers becomes clear. For instance, Godina attributed his lower free-flap failure rate in the early group to the absence of fibrosis that affected arteries (vasospasm), nerves, and veins (constriction of the lumen, tear-resistance). In particular, the veins are strongly affected by the posttraumatic fibrosis leading to the fact that the venous microanastomosis is the critical point of free microvascular surgery in the delayed or late phase. According to Godina, the higher postoperative infection rate is based on superficial infection of granulation tissue, left over necrotic tissue in the wound pocket, and immature and poorly perfused scars. Especially remaining desiccated bone devoid of periosteum may lead to postoperative infection and sequestration. So the initial wound debridement is of critical interest. Godina postulated that debridement at later time points becomes technically more difficult due to edema and fibrotic changes. He hypothesizes that many surgeons may doubt the efficacy of the first debridement and that superficial infections may mask the appearance of normal tissue. Therefore, the use of free flaps may have two advantages. First, their relatively large dimensions compensate the large defects of initial radical debridement and, second, they eliminate dead space and enable skin closure without tension diminishing the risk of infection. Since the initial wound debridement is the crucial part impacting on the final result, Godina gave recommendations how to differentiate between unhealthy tissue (contused, crushed, devitalized) and healthy tissue. He discouraged debridement without tourniquet control, because blood may cover the operating field hiding the necrotic areas and deeper extensions of the wound. Instead, he first recommended starting in a bloodless field to evaluate the tissues, eliminate foreign bodies, and, for hemostasis, to decrease blood loss. Then, with release of the tourniquet, the quality of the tissues and their bleeding surfaces can be assessed. Godina concluded that more than 80% of the patients could be completely reconstructed at the time of the first anesthesia, if the patient was in good general condition and if there was good cooperation between the skilled orthopedic and plastic surgeons [17].

At the end of the 1990s, Hertel and colleagues [16] presented a similar study on the timing of soft tissue reconstruction of lower leg open fractures with local or free muscle flaps. They compared immediate reconstruction with delayed (day 1–9) reconstruction using local or free muscle flaps. They found better results in the group with immediate reconstruction regarding time to full weight-bearing, definitive bone union, number of operations, and bone infections. They assumed that the shorter time for bone union in the immediate group was related to the lower incidence of bone infections. Vice versa, they hypothesized that the higher number of bone infections was due to the lengthy exposure of the fracture to nosocomial contamination, secondary damage of exposed tissue, and "necessarily incomplete nature of second-look debridements, particularly in an around a reduced fracture" [16]. An interesting aspect, as already mentioned by Godina [17], is the logistical aspect. Hertel and colleagues described that only 3 out of 15 patients with delayed reconstruction were delayed for medical reasons. Instead, the organization and logistics played a major role in providing 24 h availability of skilled plastic and orthopaedic surgeons, medical staff, and operating room time [16].

Another widely noticed study was published by Gopal and colleagues [20]. They examined soft tissue reconstruction using pedicled muscle flaps (gastrocnemius, soleus) or free muscle flaps (latissimus dorsi, gracilis, rectus abdominis). Gopal and colleagues differentiated between immediate (<24 h), early (<72 h) and late reconstruction (>72 h). Both superficial (skin) infection and deep (bone) infection were lowest in the immediate group, followed by the early group with the highest rates in the late group. Again, they hypothesized that the lower rate of infection in the immediate and early groups was associated with the adequacy of the debridement, skeletal stabilization, and the obliteration of the dead space by well-vascularized muscle flaps [20].

Breugem and Stracke [21] performed a Medline research and reviewed the literature regarding (a) timing of soft tissue coverage and (b) incidence of complications. From the reviewed literature it was suggested that the time of surgery has no or little influence on flap failure, but indicated that "early" soft tissue coverage within 3–5 days reduced osteomyelitis and delayed bone union [21].

However, despite these studies with convincing datasets and almost more than 20 years since Godina's study [17] the management of open fractures remained largely the same and the "fix and flap" procedure is not the mainstream thinking [22]. Levin analyzed this in his publication [22] and gave his personal preference, which is performing early (<72 h) but not emergency closure of open fractures. He argues that within the early group (<72 h) of Godina in 1986 there was no difference in infection rates between patients with immediate coverage or coverage at day 3. However, Levin put forward seven possible reasons why the "fix and flap" procedure still does not represent mainstream thinking in all trauma centers. First, fewer and fewer orthopaedic surgeons are skilled or are willing to perform microvascular free tissue transfer. Second, many orthopaedic surgeons may suggest that microsurgical techniques are not necessary due to alternatives like dermal substitutes and wound VACS. Third, Levin appreciated the work and enthusiasm of Godina and coworkers, but emphasize that the health care systems have since changed around the world. Godina had a tireless and highly motivated crew working around the clock in teams, but part of their motivation to perform emergency free flap was the fact that these cases had to be treated immediately because more cases would be presented later on. Levin says that there is no reason not to do emergency free transfer if a skilled replant or microvascular team including trained nursing staff is available around the clock. This also includes a team which is available for the treatment of postoperative complications (i.e., microvascular thrombosis). But in the reality there is not always such a team available. It is wiser to transfer a patient to another trauma center or to perform a delayed closure instead of performing immediate coverage with an inexperienced team with doubtful outcomes. Fourth, demarcation is important between vital or healthy and unviable or unhealthy tissues. Especially in open fractures with vascular injuries it is wise to wait till viability is proven within the first 72 h. Fifth, the decision between amputation or limb salvage and reconstruction may represent a rationale for "delayed coverage". Decision making may take a few days, as well as the agreement between the patient (i.e., patient, family) and the trauma team. Sixth, it might be helpful to wait few days for edema resolution since the tissue and extremities are usually too swollen immediately after the injury. Initial radical debridement in combination with procedures to reduce edema (elevated position, cooling, etc.) may be advantageous. Seventh, another reason is that many patients are polytrauma patients that have severe systemic or general problems which are not appropriate for such a time-consuming procedure like free microvascular transfer [22].

21.4 Anatomy and Techniques

The following section comprises a brief overview on frequently performed distant (pedicled) or free flaps. This outline includes text information supplemented with clinical examples.

21.4.1 Lateral Arm Flap

The lateral arm flap is a relatively thin septofasciocutaneous flap of type-B according to Mathes and Nahai (Fig. 21.4). It is located over the distal half of the lateral upper arm and the proximal third of the forearm. It can be used as a free flap (e.g., coverage of the hand), as a distally based reversed pedicled flap at the level of the lateral condyle (e.g., for the coverage of elbow defects), or as a proximally based pedicled flap (e.g., for the coverage of shoulder defects). Typically, the lateral arm flap can be harvested as a neurosensory flap innervated by the lower lateral cutaneous nerve of the arm.

The lateral arm flap receives its vascular supply by the radial collateral artery of the deep brachial artery in the lateral intermuscular septum of the upper arm between the brachialis and the lateral head of the triceps muscle. During flap elevation identification and preservation of the radial nerve is required [1, 23].

21.4.2 Radial Forearm Flap

The radial forearm flap (Figs. 21.7–21.8) is a large and thin fasciocutaneus flap of type-B according to Mathes and Nahai (Fig. 21.4) with an extensive skin territory extending from the antecubital fossa to the wrist. The donor site is usually closed with split-thickness skin grafts. Care must be taken not to injure the paratenon which covers the tendons of the long finger flexors, brachioradialis, and flexor carpi radialis muscles.

It receives its vascular supply by the radial artery. To ensure sufficient perfusion of the hand through the ulnar artery after elevation of the radial forearm flap, it is absolutely necessary to perform preoperative Doppler probe or Allen's test. If in doubt, the radial artery can be reconstructed using vein grafts (e.g., great saphenous vein).

The radial forearm flap can be used as a proximally based pedicled flap (e.g., for the coverage of elbow or distal upper arm defects), as a distally based pedicled flap (e.g., for the coverage of hand defects), or as a free flap, characterized by its very long vascular pedicle. As a free flap, the radial forearm flap can be harvested with bone, tendons, fascia, or nerves as an osteocutaneous flap (vascularized bone of the radius), tendinocutaneous flap (e.g., tendinous portion of the flexor carpi radialis), fascia flap (preserving skin and subcutaneous tissue), neurosensory flap (lateral or medial antebrachial cutaneous nerve), and as a flow-through flap with microvascular anastomosis of the proximal and distal end of the radial artery in the respective defect site [1, 23].

21.4.3 Anterior Lateral Thigh Flap

The anterolateral thigh (ALT) (Figs. 21.9–21.10) flap has become very popular in the last few years for general reconstructive procedures. The ALT can be used as a pedicled island flap or as a free flap [1]. The skin territory of the ALT is located over the anterolateral area of the thigh [23]. The ALT flap has its vascular supply by the deep femoral artery with the subsequent transverse or descending branch of the lateral circumflex femoral artery (LCFA). There are different variations in terms of the cutaneous blood supply, but schematically, 84% are myocutaneous and 16% are septocutaneous perforator vessels. These are mainly located in a circle with a 3 cm radius located at a midpoint between the superolateral edge of the patella and the anterior superior iliac spine [23].

The ALT flap has two major advantages: an extensive territory of pliable and relatively thin skin in combination with a long vascular pedicle characterized by large vessel diameters [23]. Furthermore, similar to the radial artery flap, the ALT can be used as a "flow-through" flap, since the distal end of the LCFA can be used as interpositional graft. By using the distal end of the descending branch for anastomosis with the vessels in an ischemic portion of the respective extremity, the ALT can help to revascularize and, thus, salvage the respective extremity [23].

Furthermore, the ALT can be used as a "chimeric" flap. This term is derived from the word "Chimera," which is, according to Greek myth, a fire-breathing monster with the head of a lion, body of a goat, and tail of a serpent. In reconstructive surgery, a chimeric flap is compounded from multiple different flaps, which are usually supplied by different branches from the same source vessel. Without microsurgical anastomosis, the

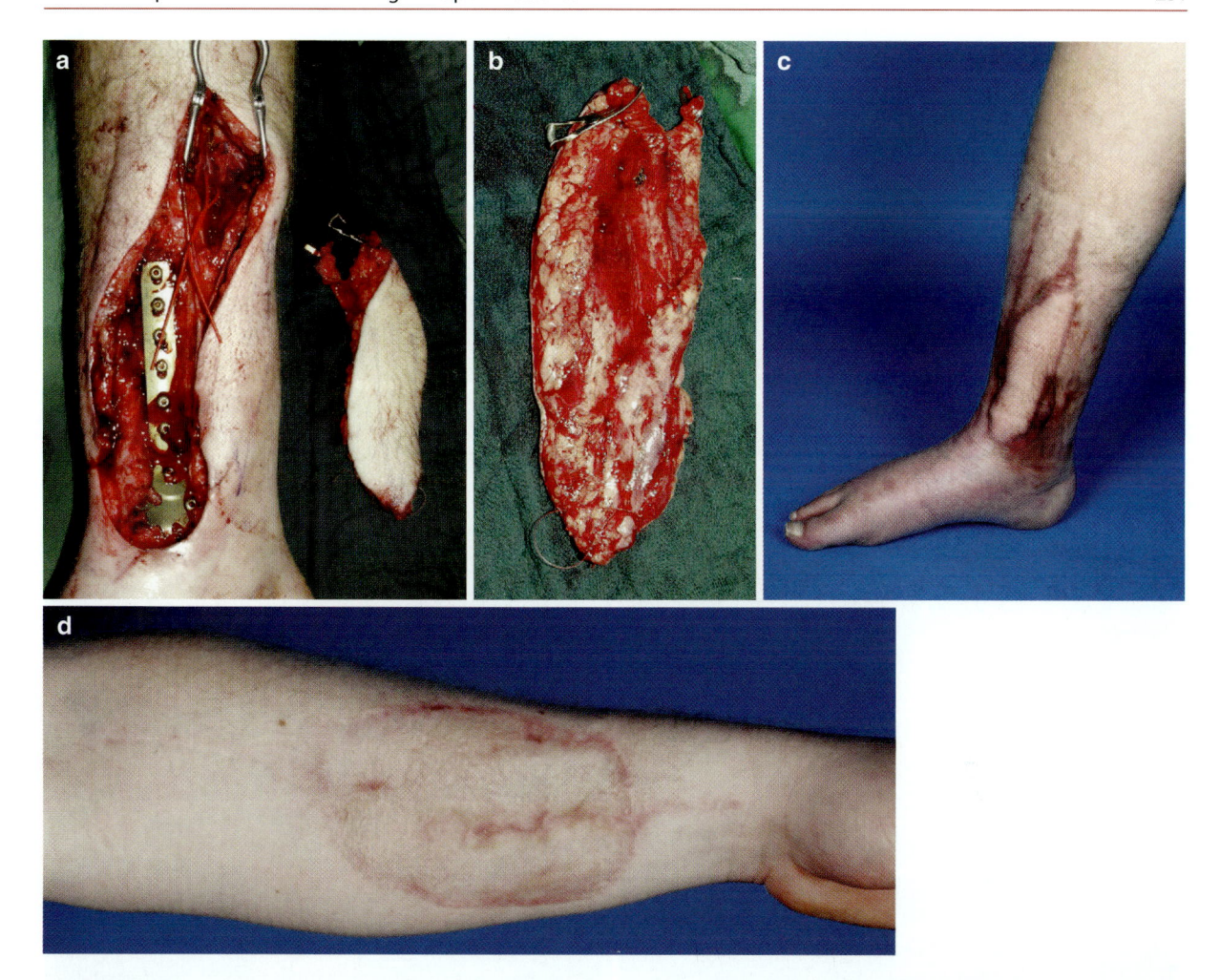

Fig. 21.7 Free microvascular transfer of the radial forearm flap. (**a**) Intraoperative view of a soft tissue defect of the right distal tibia after fracture with subsequent plate osteosynthesis. (**b**) Undersurface of a harvested free radial forearm flap. (**c**) Postoperative view of the recipient site (right lower leg). (**d**) Postoperative view of the donor site (left forearm) after split-thickness skin grafting

ALT can be combined with the "Tensior Fasciae Latae" flap (TFL) from the lateral area of the thigh. In addition, using microvascular techniques, the ALT flap can be used as a chimeric flap with a variety of other tissues. As an example, the ALT flap can be combined with a vascularized fibula [23].

21.4.4 Gracilis Flap

The gracilis muscle is the most superficial muscle on the medial side of the thigh. It is a relatively thin muscle, which is broad proximally and narrow or tapering distally. The gracilis muscle arises from the pubic symphysis and inserts at the medial tibial condyle via the pes anserinus [23].

The gracilis is widely used as a pedicled or free (Fig. 21.11) microsurgical muscle flap in reconstructive plastic surgery. The donor-site morbidity is relatively low; the donor defect can usually be closed primarily and loss of the gracilis muscle does not produce any obvious dysfunction since the adductor longus and adductor magnus muscles are preserved as thigh adductors.

It is classified as a type-II muscle flap (Fig. 21.6) [13]. It receives its dominant blood supply from the profunda femoris vessels approximately 8–10 cm below the pubic tubercle. If used as myocutaneous flap sufficient blood supply is usually only reliable for the proximal two-thirds of the overlying skin island.

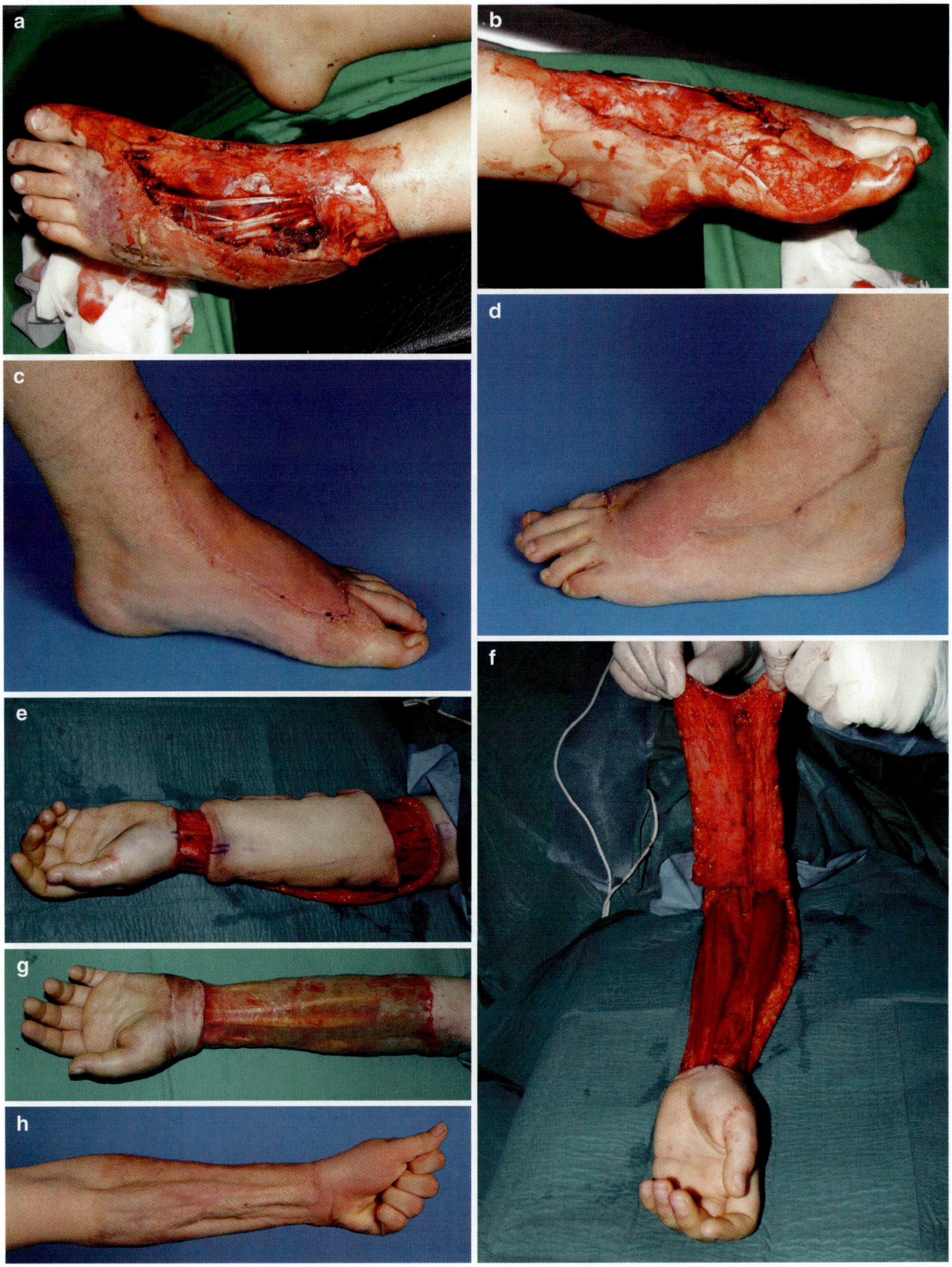

21.4.5 Fibula Flap

The fibula flap (Fig. 21.12) can be harvested as a vascularized bone graft or osseus flap with a muscle cuff to preserve periosteal vessels, as osteocutaneous flap, or osteomuscular flap (including lateral half of the soleus muscle). It can be used for long-segment defects of the long bones of the upper and lower extremities.

The dominant vessels (nutrient vessels) are derived from the peroneal vessels entering the fibula posterior to the interosseus membrane in the middle third of the fibula. Furthermore, periosteal and muscular branches from the peroneal vessels serve as a minor pedicle.

The fibula flap can be used as a free flap and as a proximally based pedicled osseus flap. In the latter case, the fibula can be used for the reconstruction of proximal tibia defects as a vascularized bone graft. Although harvesting of the fibula usually does not result in functional morbidity, the distal 7 cm should be preserved to avoid any possible instability of the ankle joint [1, 23].

21.4.6 Gastrocnemius Flap

The gastrocnemius muscle consists of two separate heads, which originate from the medial and lateral condyles of the femur, respectively. They join the tendon of the soleus and insert into the calcaneus via the Achilles tendon. If the soleus muscle is functioning, either one or both heads of the gastrocnemius muscle can be used [1].

Each head has its independent blood supply via the medial or lateral sural artery (level of the fibular head) arising from the popliteal artery (approximately 3–4 cm above the head of the fibula).Therefore, the gastrocnemius muscle can be harvested as a medial (Fig. 21.13) or lateral muscle or musculocutaneous flap with a type I circulation pattern (Fig. 21.6) according to Mathes and Nahai [1].

For coverage of the distal thigh, the knee joint or upper tibia, the medial gastrocnemius muscle flap (Fig. 21.13) is used in preference to the lateral counterpart in order to avoid possible injuries to the peroneal nerve. This may occur during the elevation of the tunnel for lateral gastrocnemius transposition.

Release of the origin from the medial or lateral condyle of the femur will extend the arc of rotation allowing a more effective coverage of the distal thigh and knee region.

Free muscle transfer is not widely established because of the short pedicle length. Since the transfer of a myocutaneous flap leads to a considerable contour deformity both in the donor and recipient site, a muscle flap in combination with split-thickness skin grafts is widely preferred [23].

21.4.7 Scapular and Parascapular Flap

The scapular and parascapular (Fig. 21.14) flaps are located between the posterior axillary line and the posterior midline centered over the scapula. They are fasciocutaneous flaps of type B (Fig. 21.14) according to Nahai and Mathes [1]. The circumflex scapular vessels are the dominant pedicle arising from the triangular space, which is formed by the teres major, teres minor, and long head of the triceps muscle. The scapular flap is located horizontally (horizontal branch of the circumflex scapular vessels), while the parascapular flap (Fig. 21.14) is located vertically at the lateral margin of the scapula (vertical branch of the circumflex scapular vessels). The pedicled parascapular flap can be used for coverage of the shoulder, axilla, and lateral thoracic wall.

Fig. 21.8 Free microvascular transfer of the radial forearm flap. (**a–b**) Preoperative view: soft tissue defect of the back of the left foot after decollement and fracture of the distal fibula as well as metatarsal and tarsal bones. (**c–d**) Postoperative result after reconstruction with a free radial forearm flap. (**e–f**) Intraoperative view: Elevation of the radial forearm flap. (**g**) Coverage of the donor site using Integra® Dermal Regeneration Template. (**h**) Postoperative result of the donor site after Integra® Dermal Regeneration Template in combination with split-thickness skin grafting

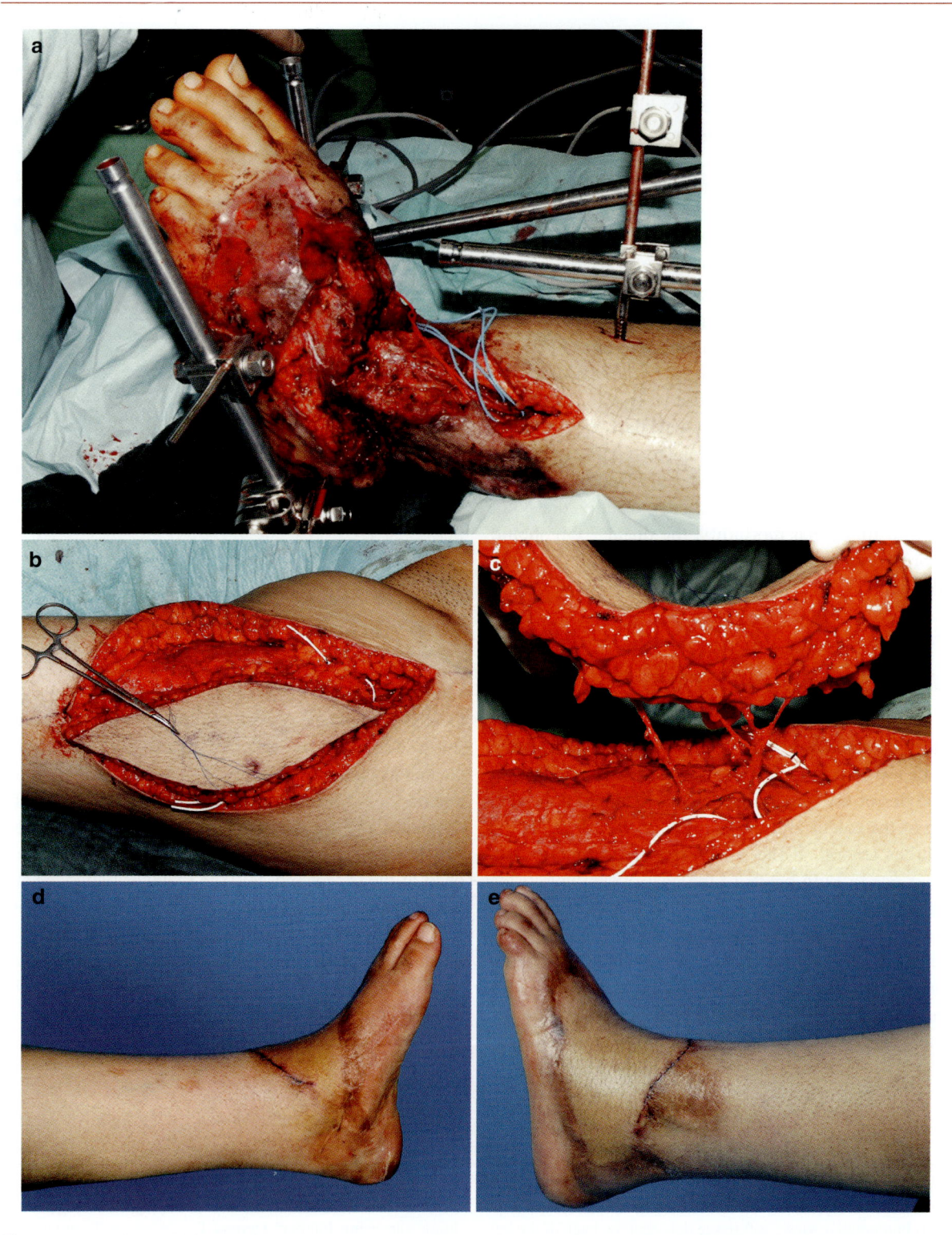

Fig. 21.9 Free microvascular transfer of the anterior lateral thigh perforator flap (ALTP). (**a**) Preoperative view: soft tissue defect of the back of the left foot and left distal lower leg after decollement and fracture of the distal tibial, distal fibula as well as metatarsal and tarsal bones. (**b–c**) Intraoperative view: Elevation of the ALTP from the left thigh. (**d–e**) Postoperative result of the recipient site (left foot and distal lower leg). (**f**) Postoperative result of the donor site site (left thigh)

(Fig. 21.6) with the thoracodorsal vessels serving as the dominant pedicle with branches of the posterior intercostal vessels as well as lumbar vessels serving as secondary segmental pedicles. In open fractures or areas of exposed hardware, the standard pedicled flap (vascularization: thoracodorsal vessels) can be used for coverage of the cranium, spinal column, clavicula, sternum, or upper arm. The point of rotation is located at the posterior axilla where the thoracodorsal vessels enter the muscle. As a reverse pedicled flap (vascularization: secondary segmental vessels), after dividing the insertion in the axilla, this flap may reach the midthoracic, inferior thoracic, and lumbar vertebral regions.

For free microvascular transplantation, the LDM flap is one of the most widely used free flaps with a large amount of soft tissue. It is reliable and characterized by its constant and long pedicle with a large diameter. It can be used for distant coverage in the head and neck region, trunk, and upper and lower extremity [1, 23]. The LDM can also be harvested as osteomyocutaneous free flap for the reconstruction of bony defects of the tibia or femur. The LDM can either be combined with ribs (ninth or tenth rib) or the lower lateral portion of the scapula [1, 23].

A disadvantage is the bulkiness; this can be avoided by using the LDM as a split free muscle flap (medial or lateral branches of the thoracodorsal vessels) or as a muscle flap without a skin island but with a skin graft. Furthermore, muscle atrophy of up to 50% will decrease the volume. Another technique to overcome the bulkiness and avoid donor-site morbidity is to use a perforator flap based on the thoracodorsal vessels preserving both the LDM and the thoracodorsal nerve. This perforator flap is called the "Thoracodorsal artery perforator (TAP) flap."

Similar to the ALT flap, the LDM can also be used as a chimeric flap. Based on the thoracodorsal vessels, the LDM can be combined with the serratus anterior muscle [23].

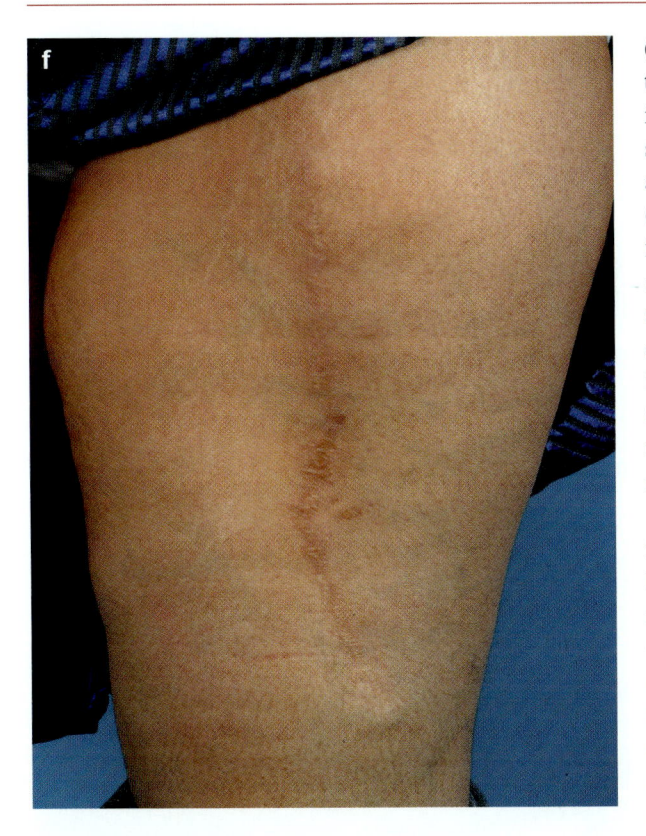

Fig. 21.9 (continued)

21.4.8 Latissimus Dorsi Flap

The latissimus dorsi muscle (LDM) is a flat and large triangular muscle. It originates from the spinous processes T7 to L5, the sacrum, posterior part of the iliac crest, and external surface of the four inferior ribs. Its insertion is the intertubercular groove of the humerus. The LDM is an expendable muscle if the synergistic shoulder girdle muscles (teres major, pectoralis major) are intact.

It can be harvested as a muscle or musculocutaneous (Fig. 21.15) flap. According to the Mathes and Nahai classification [13], it is a type-V muscle flap

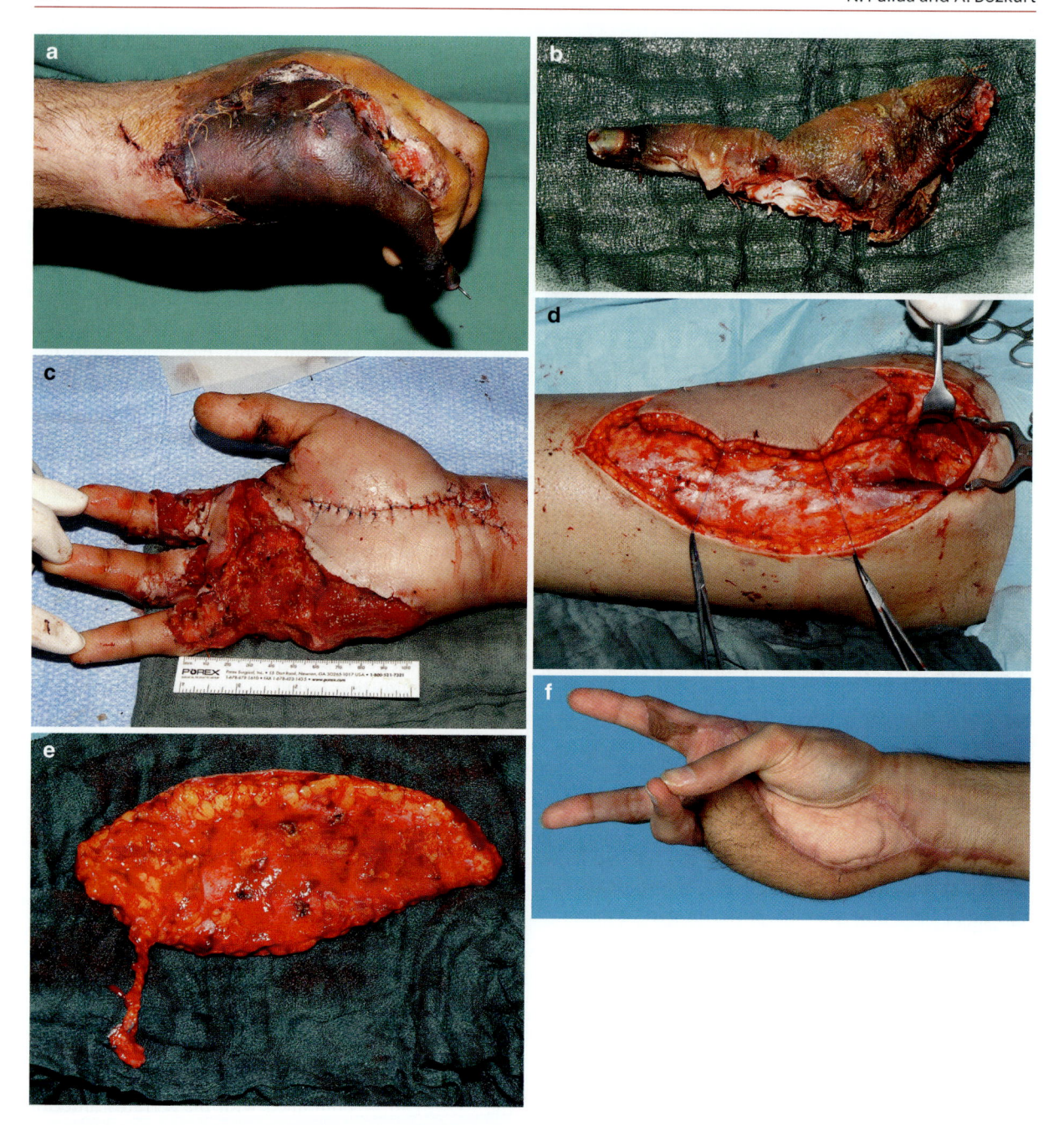

Fig. 21.10 Free microvascular transfer of the anterior lateral thigh perforator flap (ALTP) (**a–c**) Preoperative view: defect of the ulno-volar region of the right hand after car accident. (**d**) Intraoperative view: Elevation of the ALTP from the left thigh. (**e**) Undersurface of a harvested free ALTP flap. (**f**) Postoperative result of the recipient site (right hand)

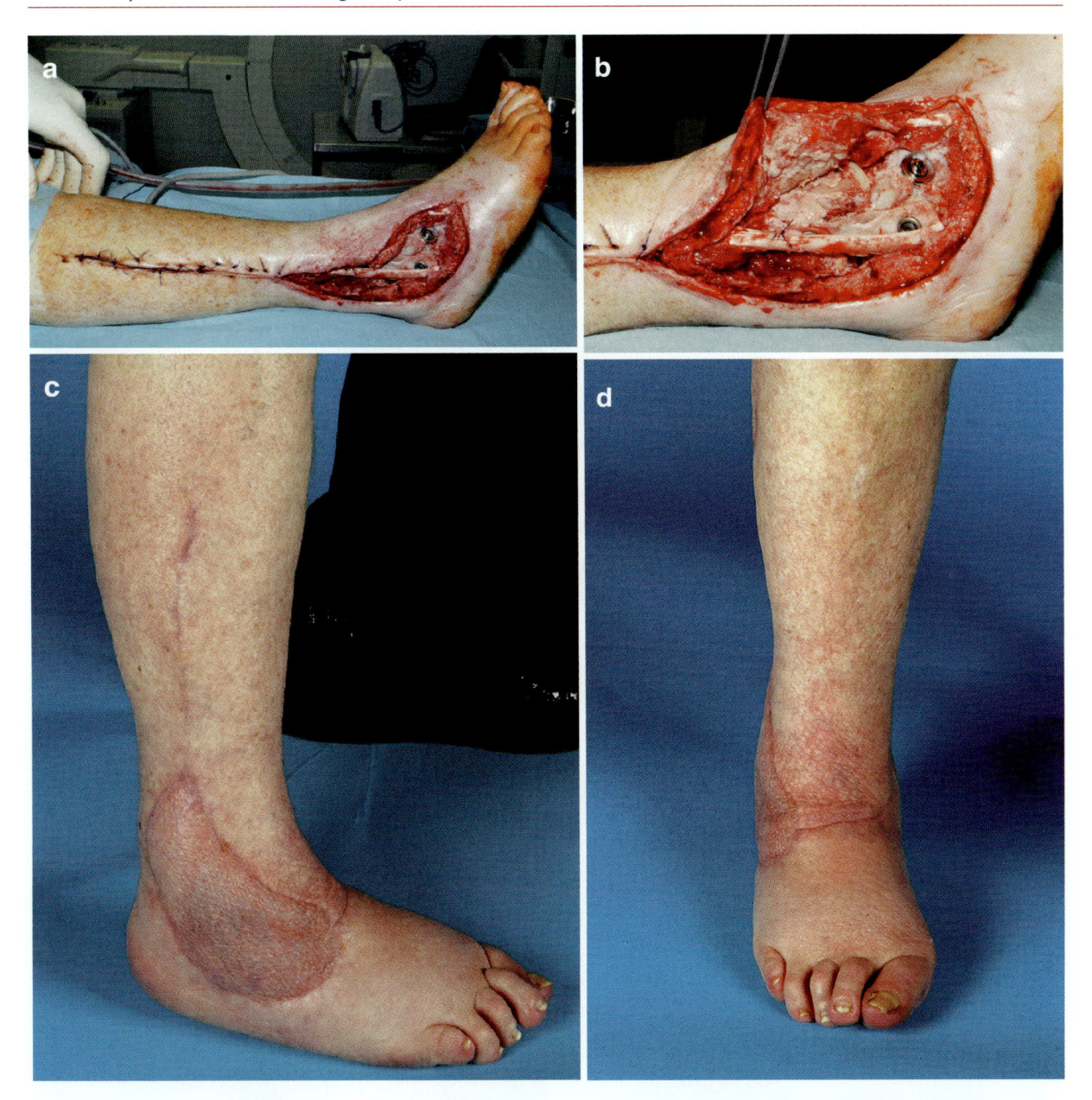

Fig. 21.11 Free microvascular transfer of the gracilis muscle flap. (**a–b**) Preoperative view: soft tissue defect of the right lateral ankle after arthrodesis with exposed material. (**c–d**) Postoperative result after reconstruction with a free gracilis muscle in combination with split-thickness skin grafting

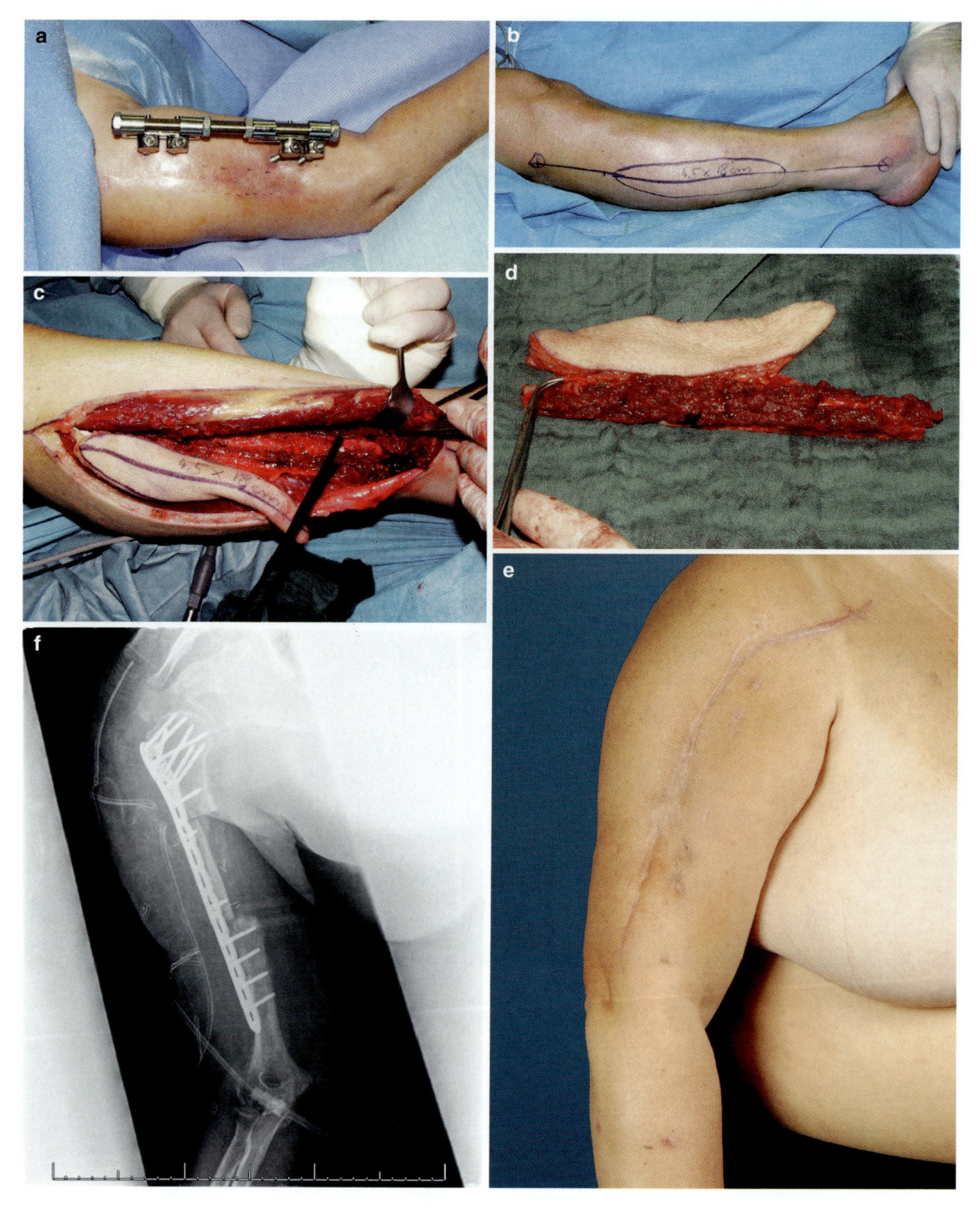

Fig. 21.12 Free microvascular transfer of a free osteocutaneous fibula flap. (**a**) Pseudarthrosis of the right upper arm stabilized with an external fixator. (**b**) Intraoperative planning at the outer surface of the right lower leg. (**c–d**) Intraoperative view: Harvesting of the free osteocutaneous fibula flap with muscle cuff. (**e–f**) Postoperative result at the recipient site. (**g–h**) Postoperative result at the donor site

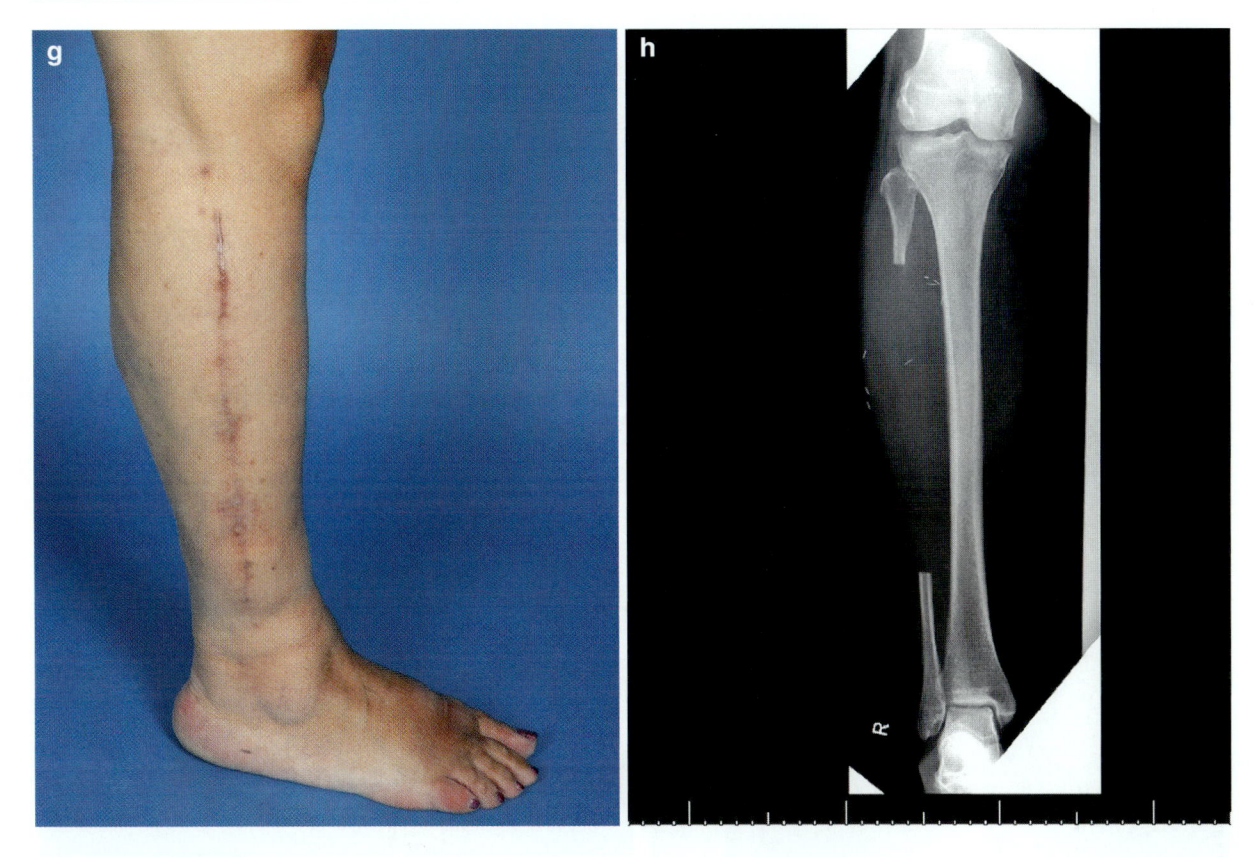

Fig. 21.12 (continued)

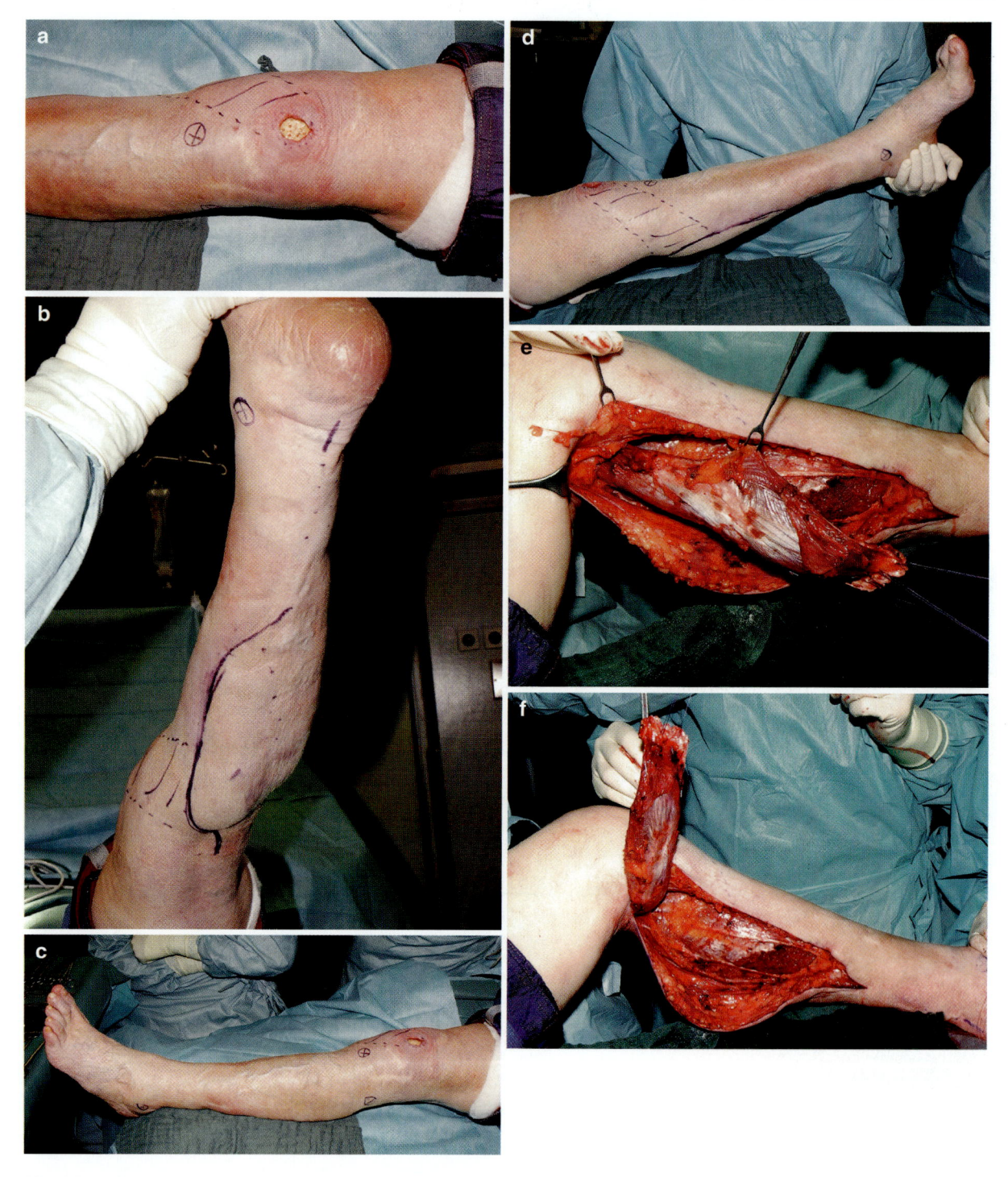

Fig. 21.13 Pedicled medial gastrcocnemius muscle flap (**a**) Preoperative view: soft tissue defect of the left knee region with exposed patella after drilling of small holes (Pridie Drilling). (**b–d**) Intraoperative planning of a proximally based medial gastrocnemius muscle flap. (**e–f**) Intraoperative view: Elevation of a proximally based medial gastrocnemius flap. (**g–h**) Intraoperative view: Subcutaneous tunneling of the gastrocnemius flap with coverage of the patella

21   Techniques of Soft Tissue Coverage in Open Fractures

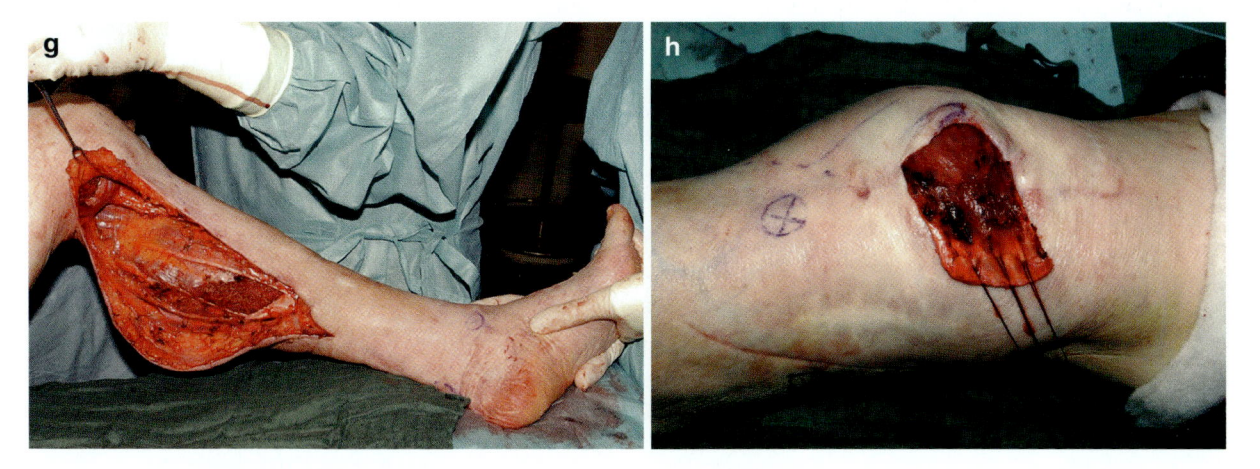

Fig. 21.13 (continued)

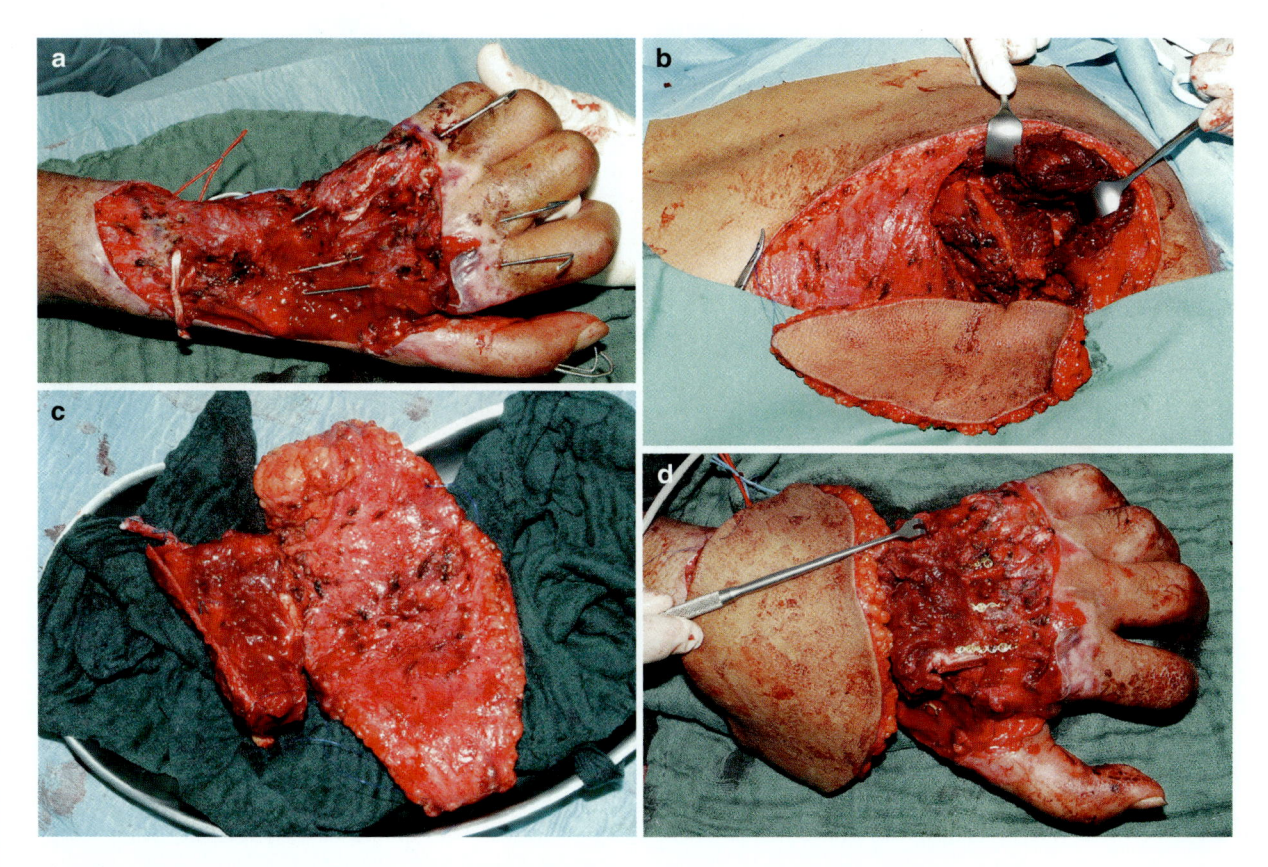

Fig. 21.14 Free osteocutaneous Parascapular flap. (**a**) Bone and soft tissue defect of the left hand. (**b–d**) Elevation and free microvascular transfer of an osteocutaneous parascapular flap. (**e**) X-ray control after plate osteosynthesis. (**f**) Postoperative result after soft tissue coverage

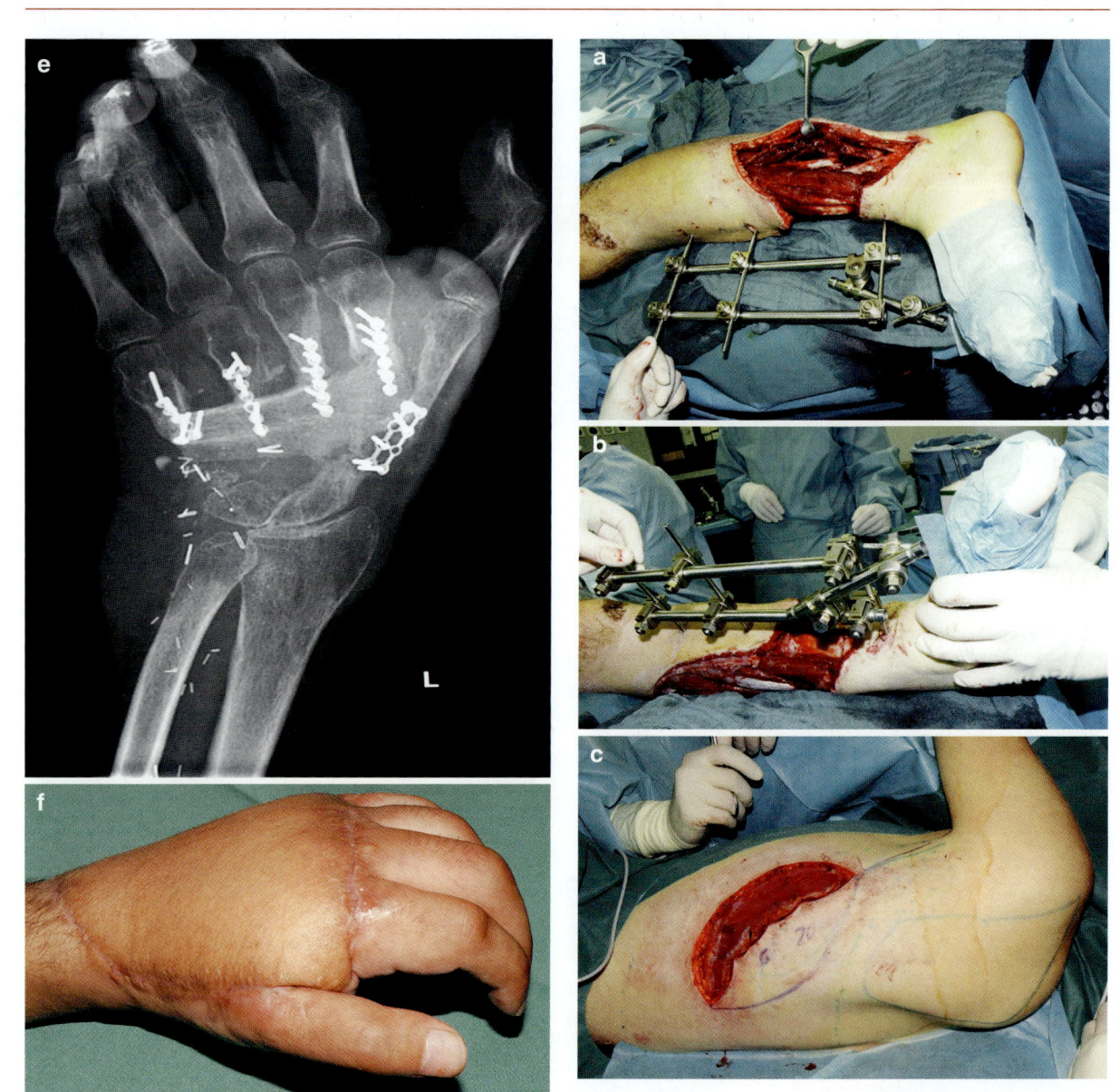

Fig. 21.14 (continued)

Fig. 21.15 Free latissimus dorsi muscle flap (**a–b**) Extensive soft tissue defect of the left lower leg after third-degree open fracture of the left tibia and fibula stabilized with an external fixator. (**c**) Intraoperative view of planning and elevation of a free latissimus dorsi muscle flap from the left back. (**d–f**) Postoperative results after free latissimus dorsi muscle transfer with end-to-end anastomosis to the anterior tibial artery and vein

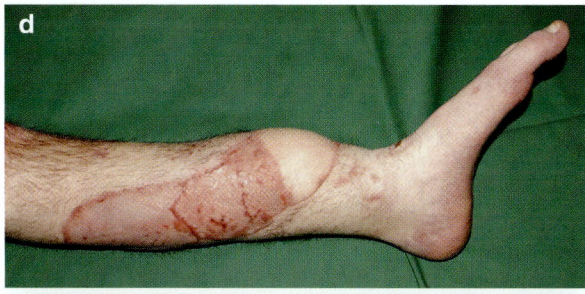

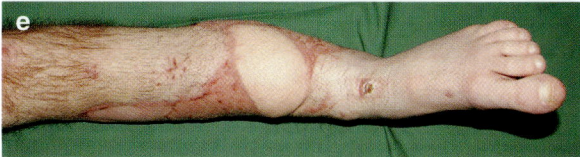

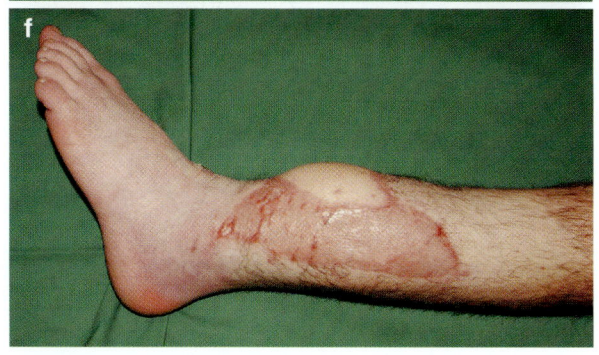

Fig. 21.15 (continued)

References

1. Mathes S, Nahai F. Reconstructive surgery – principles, anatomy & technique. Oxford: Elsevier; 1997.
2. Mathes SJ, Hansen SL. Classification and applications. In: Mathes SJ, editor. Plastic surgery, vol. I. Philadelphia: Saunders; 2006. p. 365–483.
3. Manchot C. Die Hautarterien des menschlichen Körpers. Leipzig: Vogel; 1889.
4. O'Dey D, Prescher A, Pallua N. Vascular reliability of nipple-areola complex-bearing pedicles: an anatomical microdissection study. Plast Reconstr Surg. 2007;119(4): 1167–77.
5. O'Dey DM, Heimburg DV, Prescher A, Pallua N. The arterial vascularisation of the abdominal wall with special regard to the umbilicus. Br J Plast Surg. 2004;57(5):392–7.
6. O'Dey DM, Okafor CA, Bozkurt A, Prescher A, Pallua N. Perforator vessel anatomy of the papilla umbilicalis: topography and importance for reconstructive abdominal wall surgery. Langenbecks Arch Surg. 2010;395(8):1121–7.
7. Tolhurst DE. A comprehensive classification of flaps: the atomic system. Plast Reconstr Surg. 1987;80(4):608–9.
8. Cormack G, Lamberty B. The anatomical basis for fasciocutaneous flaps. In: Hauock GG, editor. Fasciocutaneous flaps. Cambridge, MA: Blackwell Scientific; 1992. p. 13–24.
9. Lamberty BGH, Healy C. Flaps: physiology, principles of design, and pitfalls. In: Cohen M, editor. Mastery of plastic and reconstructive surgery, vol. 1. Boston: Little, Brown & Co; 1994. p. 56–70.
10. Cormack G, Lamberty B. A classification of fascio-cutaneous flaps according to their patterns of vascularisation. Br J Plast Surg. 1984;37:80–7.
11. Blondeel PN, Van Landuyt KH, Monstrey SJ, Hamdi M, Matton GE, Allen RJ, et al. The "Gent" consensus on perforator flap terminology: preliminary definitions. Plast Reconstr Surg. 2003;112(5):1378–83; quiz 1383, 1516; discussion 1384-1377.
12. Koshima I, Soeda S. Inferior epigastric artery skin flaps without rectus abdominis muscle. Br J Plast Surg. 1989; 42(6):645–8.
13. Mathes SJ, Nahai F. Classification of the vascular anatomy of muscles: experimental and clinical correlation. Plast Reconstr Surg. 1981;67(2):177–87.
14. Serafin D. Atlas of microsurgical composite tissue transplantation. Philadelphia: W.B. Saunders; 1996.
15. Gustilo RB, Merkow RL, Templeman D. The management of open fractures. J Bone Joint Surg Am. 1990;72(2):299–304.
16. Hertel R, Lambert SM, Muller S, Ballmer FT, Ganz R. On the timing of soft-tissue reconstruction for open fractures of the lower leg. Arch Orthop Trauma Surg. 1999;119(1–2):7–12.
17. Godina M. Early microsurgical reconstruction of complex trauma of the extremities. Plast Reconstr Surg. 1986;78(3): 285–92.
18. Stannard JP, Singanamala N, Volgas DA. Fix and flap in the era of vacuum suction devices: what do we know in terms of evidence based medicine? Injury. 2010;41(8):780–6.
19. Byrd HS, Spicer TE, Cierney III G. Management of open tibial fractures. Plast Reconstr Surg. 1985;76(5):719–30.
20. Gopal S, Majumder S, Batchelor AG, Knight SL, De Boer P, Smith RM. Fix and flap: the radical orthopaedic and plastic treatment of severe open fractures of the tibia. J Bone Joint Surg Br. 2000;82(7):959–66.
21. Breugem CC, Strackee SD. Is there evidence-based guidance for timing of soft tissue coverage of grade III B tibia fractures? Int J Low Extrem Wounds. 2006;5(4):261–70.
22. Levin LS. Early versus delayed closure of open fractures. Injury. 2007;38(8):896–9.
23. Strauch B, Yu H-L. Atlas of microvascular surgery: anatomy and operative techniques. New York: Thieme Medical Publishers; 2006.

22 Outcome and Management of Primary Amputations, Subtotal Amputation Injuries, and Severe Open Fractures with Nerve Injuries

William W. Cross III and Marc F. Swiontkowski

Contents

22.1	Introduction	265
22.2	**Traumatic Primary Amputations: Considerations and Completions**	266
22.2.1	Outcome of Traumatic Primary Amputations	267
22.3	**The Subtotal Amputation Injury: Limb-Salvage or Amputation**	268
22.3.1	Factors Influencing Initial Salvage Decisions	268
22.3.2	Lower-Extremity Injury-Severity Scales and Scores: Tools for Assisting Surgeons with Salvage or Amputation Decisions	273
22.3.3	Lower-Extremity Injury-Severity Scales and Scores: Predicting Functional Outcomes of Salvaged Limbs After Limb-Threatening Trauma	274
22.3.4	Lower-Extremity Injury-Severity Scales and Scores: Summary	275
22.3.5	Outcomes in Patients Undergoing Limb-Salvage or Amputation for Limb-Threatening Injuries	275
22.3.6	Complications in the Treatment of Severe Lower-Extremity Trauma	276
22.3.7	Psychological Distress in Patients with Severely Injured Lower Extremities	276
22.3.8	Societal Costs Associated with Limb-Salvage and Amputation	277
22.4	**The Open Fracture with Severe Nerve Injury**	277
22.5	**Summary**	278
References		278

W.W. Cross III
Mayo Medical School, Rochester, MN, USA and
Department of Orthopaedic Surgery, Mayo Clinic,
Rochester, MN, USA

M.F. Swiontkowski (✉)
Department of Orthopaedic Surgery, University
of Minnesota and TRIA Orthopaedic Center
University of Minnesota, Minneapolis, MN, USA and
University of Minnesota Medical School, Minneapolis, MN, USA
e-mail: swion001@umn.edu

22.1 Introduction

More than three out of five accidental injuries in the USA are to the musculoskeletal system. Costs associated with the care of these injuries have been estimated to be $849 billion or 7.7% of the US gross domestic product (GDP) in the year 2004. Musculoskeletal disease and injury continue to account for the majority of both lost wages and hospital bed days in the USA [1]. We must improve the care of these injuries so that we may help patients rehabilitate from injury and prevent future morbidity.

A small but resource-heavy subset is the high-energy trauma patient with a mangled extremity [2]. The evaluation and subsequent management of this patient group can be a great source of stress for both the patient and the treating surgical team. The decision-making processes are difficult, can be controversial, and the clinical evidence for these decisions has been largely based upon small case series and historical Level V evidence [3]. These data have influenced the treatment of limb-threatening trauma and have potentially led to large numbers of limb amputations with severe lower-extremity trauma where limb-salvage may have been technically possible but not recommended [4, 5]. As medical and surgical technology, skills, procedures, and concepts have evolved, so has our ability to salvage limbs previously thought to be unsalvageable. Particular areas of advancement include soft-tissue handling, less-invasive fracture management, microvascular repair, and soft-tissue coverage [6–13]. Limb-salvage protocols have been evaluated and many of them have influenced our current treatment strategies [14, 15]. These studies and others reviewing complicated limb trauma have suggested that early amputation may be preferable due to the mental and physical toll that limb-salvage can levy on patients [16–18]. Most studies have included small numbers of patients, and their results have correspondingly not yielded definitive results [9, 10, 16, 19].

In an effort to provide evidence for clinicians to rely upon when making amputation versus salvage decisions, a large multicenter, prospective, observational study was undertaken entitled the Lower Extremity Assessment Project (LEAP) [20–22]. Utilizing data from this project, several areas of the amputation – limb-salvage debate have been explored. Evidence from this trial and others are presented in the following chapter to assist treatment teams in these difficult and complex situations. The goals of this chapter are to present the data from this study and provide a framework for surgical treatment teams to employ when evaluating the high-energy trauma patient with a mangled extremity.

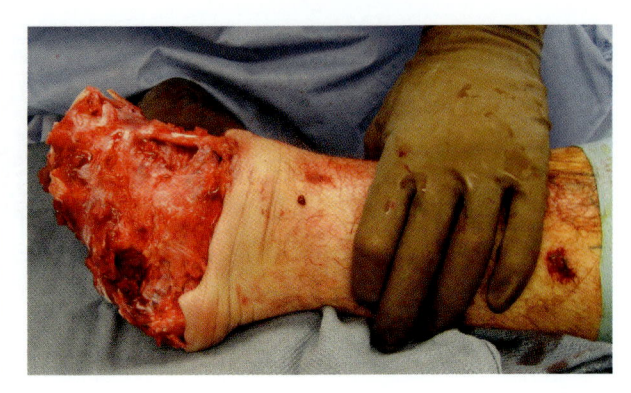

Fig. 22.1 This 28 year-old male was involved in a high-speed motorcycle crash and sustained significant forefoot and midfoot trauma. As often occurs with significant foot and lower-extremity trauma, his heel pad was severely damaged making reconstructive efforts difficult with amputation levels below the midsection of the tibia (i.e., Syme amputations)

22.2 Traumatic Primary Amputations: Considerations and Completions

The patient presenting with a complete or near-complete traumatic amputation as the result of high-energy trauma requires an evaluation consistent with the latest recommendations of the American College of Surgeons and the principles of Advanced Trauma Life Support [23–25]. Once the patient's life-threatening issues have been stabilized, attention can then be focused on the injured extremity. It is perhaps best to have the orthopaedic surgeon present prior to any surgical intervention. It is typically this surgeon who will follow the patient through subsequent recovery and functional gain with the affected extremity. In addition, any further surgical interventions are likely to be performed by an orthopaedic surgeon.

Standard open wound protocols should be followed in accordance with open fracture principles surrounding the acute zone of injury (see Chap. 20). Once the patient is physiologically stable, the zone of injury on the affected limb is defined in the surgical suite, and the limb is deemed appropriate for definitive amputation, appropriate surgical steps are taken according to the desired amputation level and planned technique (i.e., bone cut lengths, muscle flap coverage, myodesis planning).

In the orthopaedic trauma setting, there are three primary lower-extremity amputations that we consider appropriate: below-the-knee, above-the-knee, and in some select cases – through-the-knee. In the high-energy trauma patient, more often than not, the heal pad has been traumatized over the hind foot making the Syme amputation less optimal and a rarely used option (see Fig. 22.1). The hip disarticulation is also rarely used except for the most severe proximal injuries. This usually includes those with massive soft-tissue injury and/or an obvious vascular and complete sciatic nerve transection. The indications and techniques for the above three primary amputations have been well described [26] and are not the focus of this chapter. However, when contemplating an amputation through-the-knee, the surgeon must critically evaluate the soft-tissue envelope around this tenuous area. If there is any evidence that the zone of injury includes this area, most especially the proximal gastroc-soleus musculature, then there should be strong consideration to proceed with an amputation level above-the-knee. Data from the LEAP study [21, 22, 27] has suggested that through-the-knee amputations do not perform as well as above-the-knee amputations in the mangled extremity patient. This finding was most likely attributed to the condition of the soft-tissue envelope in their patient cohort and to difficulties with prosthetic fitting. In the absence of compromised soft tissues in this area and in the properly selected patient with experienced prosthetics support, a through-the-knee amputation has been shown to provide good muscular balance and has a low risk for the late development of joint contractures [28].

Severe upper extremity injuries, which present as complete or near-complete amputations, warrant special consideration and evaluation by a surgeon who is familiar with reconstruction procedures in this area. The decision-making process in the mangled upper extremity can be challenging, especially when limb-salvage becomes an option [29]. Primary amputation may not be in the best interest of some patients as it has been suggested that a sensate hand with minimal prehensile function can outperform a prosthesis [30]. Standard principles of wound care should be employed until appropriate consultation can be obtained. When definitive surgical intervention is required, preservation of length is critical and can decrease the energy needed for patients to suspend their prosthesis (see Fig. 22.2). Furthermore, the increased surface area of the limb can help with load distribution, prosthesis propulsion in space, and counterpressure with task performance [26].

Table 22.1 Primary amputation guidelines

Absolute indications	1. Presentation with complete or near-complete limb amputation
	2. Complete sciatic OR tibial nerve transection in an adult
Relative indications	1. Concurrent ipsilateral severe foot injury
	2. Large intercalary soft-tissue or bone loss
	3. Warm ischemia time of >6 h
	4. Severe concurrent multiple injuries

Absolute indications for primary limb amputation have been suggested in the literature with varying algorithms. Generally, these indications have included a patient presenting with a total or near-total leg amputation or complete tibial or sciatic nerve transection in an adult [15, 31, 32]. Relative indications have included two or more of the following: concurrent severe ipsilateral foot injury, large intercalary soft-tissue or bone loss, warm ischemia time of greater than 6 hours, and severe concurrent multiple injuries (see Table 22.1) [7, 14, 31, 33–35]. Uniformly, however, these studies indicate that the clinician's judgment at the time of initial evaluation is critical; amputation decision making should employ a multitude of factors. We also advise seeking multi-specialty input with this difficult decision (i.e., orthopedics, plastic surgery, general surgery). In one study, a combined approach led to 89% of patients achieving a successful viable limb, and only 11% went on to secondary amputation [31].

22.2.1 Outcome of Traumatic Primary Amputations

There is little in the literature reporting the long-term outcome of traumatic amputations. Recently, Dougherty published a study evaluating the outcomes of 123 transtibial amputees from the Vietnam War – 65% of which were victims of land mines and booby traps. He found that with isolated amputations, these patients led relatively normal lives. However, when concomitant injuries were sustained by these patients, their SF-36 scores lowered and their incidence of psychological illness increased [36]. Smith et al. [37]

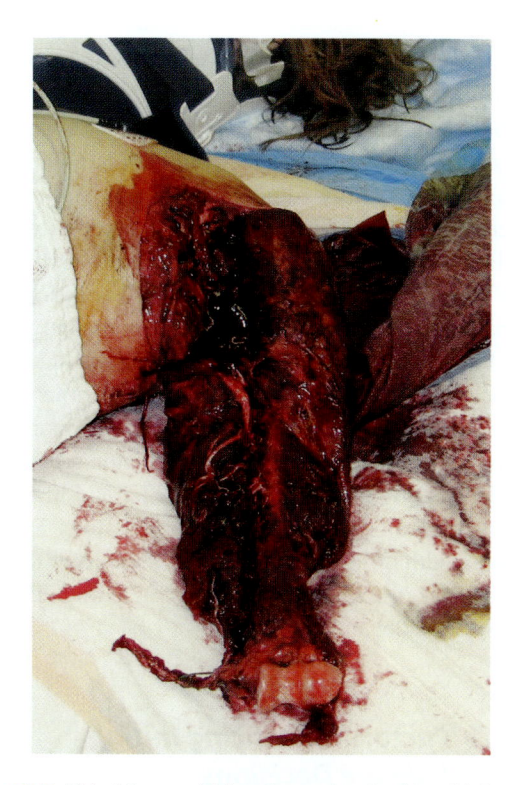

Fig. 22.2 This 16 year-old female was involved in a high-speed motor-vehicle crash in which the vehicle rolled multiple times. She sustained a traumatic amputation of the forearm including the entire radius and ulna. The proximal soft-tissue involvement was extensive, and she underwent a proximal amputation leaving 14 cm of residual humerus. She was ultimately fit with a myoelectric hand

published a descriptive study describing outcomes of 20 patients with unilateral transtibial amputations. They found that SF-36 scores were lower than normal age-matched scores in the categories of physical function and role limitations because of physical health problems and pain. Aside from those two sections, scores from the normal population were not significantly different. Lerner et al. [38, 39] evaluated three groups of patients: post-traumatic fracture nonunion, chronic refractory osteomyelitis, and lower-extremity amputation. In their group of 109 patients, they found that the chronic osteomyelitis patients were the most adversely affected among the three groups. Interestingly, 85% of the amputee patients believed they had been "mentally scarred" by their orthopaedic problem, but despite that complaint, they had minimal restriction in lifestyle and activity – a direct contrast to the poorer functioning osteomyelitis group.

In 2004, a study was published which reviewed 161 trauma-related amputation patients that were participants in the LEAP study [27]. This study found no differences in outcomes between the above-the-knee amputees and the below-the-knee amputees. The exception to this finding was with walking speeds in which the below-the-knee group performed better. A key finding in this study was the significantly poorer outcomes of patients who had undergone a through-the-knee amputation. The poorer outcome was associated with worse walking speeds and also less physician-measured satisfaction in terms of clinical, functional, and cosmetic recoveries of their patients. As we noted earlier, we believe the surgeon must critically evaluate the zone of injury prior to proceeding with a through-the-knee amputation.

The outcome of isolated traumatic lower-extremity amputations is mixed but can generally be associated with residual disability and lower outcome scores than the general population. While Dougherty's [40] study of transtibial amputations demonstrated relatively normal scores with a select population with an isolated lower-extremity injury, other studies indicate substantially poorer outcomes. In another study by Dougherty examining more proximal trans-femoral amputations, substantial disability was found in patient follow-up [36]. Smith et al. [37] and the LEAP study [27] also identified significant disability with traumatic amputations in follow-up. These studies indicate that when lower-extremity injuries are among a constellation of traumatic injuries, which they often are, outcomes demonstrate increased disability. An extensive rehabilitation program offered at the treating US Army hospital may have influenced the better outcomes identified in Dougherty's transtibial amputation study. This finding and those of the LEAP study underscore the need to have high-energy traumatic amputation patients closely followed and managed by a multidisciplinary team, including surgeons, rehabilitation physicians, nurses, prosthetists, and therapists. It is also the surgeon's responsibility to inform patients of expected outcomes and ensure that unrealistic expectations are not confusing patients during their recovery. These discussions can allay patient fears and allow both the patient, their families, and support networks to adjust to the trauma and plan ahead for expected changes.

22.3 The Subtotal Amputation Injury: Limb-Salvage or Amputation

The high-energy trauma patient with a subtotal amputation to an extremity presents immediate challenges to the trauma team. The Lower Extremity Assessment Project (LEAP) was a prospective cohort study of 601 patients who had been admitted to eight Level I trauma centers for the treatment of severe lower-extremity injuries below the distal part of the femur [20]. This study sought to provide evidence for clinicians to use when faced with this dilemma and has recently published 7 year follow-up data [22]. The LEAP study has produced multiple projects investigating various facets of the lower-extremity injured patient and many are discussed in the ensuing sections. Inclusion criteria for the LEAP study are listed in Table 22.2 and highlight the severity of trauma evaluated in this study as well as the breadth of injuries included. Please refer to case 1 in Figs. 22.3–22.5, case 2 in Figs. 22.6 and 22.7 for limb-salvage debate examples.

22.3.1 Factors Influencing Initial Salvage Decisions

Initial decisions for the acute trauma patient with a severely injured lower extremity include immediate amputation (i.e., within the first 24 h) or delayed (i.e., secondary procedure with the first hospitalization)

Table 22.2 Inclusion criteria of the LEAP[a] study [21]

1. Traumatic amputations below the distal femur
2. Gustilo type IIIA Fracture *with*
    (a) Length of hospital stay >4 days *and*
    (b) Two or more surgical limb procedures *and*
    (c) Two of more of the following: (i) severe muscle damage (>50% loss of one or more major muscle groups or associated compartment syndrome with myonecrosis); (ii) associated nerve injury (posterior tibial or peroneal deficit); (iii) major bone loss or bone injury (associated fibula fracture, and >50% displacement, comminution, and segmental type fracture, and >75% probability of requiring bone graft/transport)
3. Gustilo type IIIB tibia fracture
4. Gustilo type IIIC tibia fracture
5. Dysvascular injuries below distal femur excluding foot including: knee dislocations, closed tibia fractures, and penetrating wounds with vascular injury documented from arteriogram, surgery, or ultrasound
6. Major soft-tissue injuries below distal femur excluding foot including:
    (a) AO[b] type IC3-IC5 degloving injuries
    (b) Severe soft-tissue crush/avulsion injuries with muscle disruption or compartment syndrome
    (c) Compartment syndrome resulting in myonecrosis and requiring partial or full muscle unit resection
7. Severe foot injuries including:
    (a) Type IIIB open ankle fractures
    (b) Sever open hindfoot or midfoot injury (i.e., either insensate plantar surfaces, devascularization, major degloving injury, or open soft-tissue injury requiring coverage)
    (c) Open type III pilon fractures

[a]Lower Extremity Assessment Project
[b]Arbeitgemienschaft Fur Osteosynthesfragen

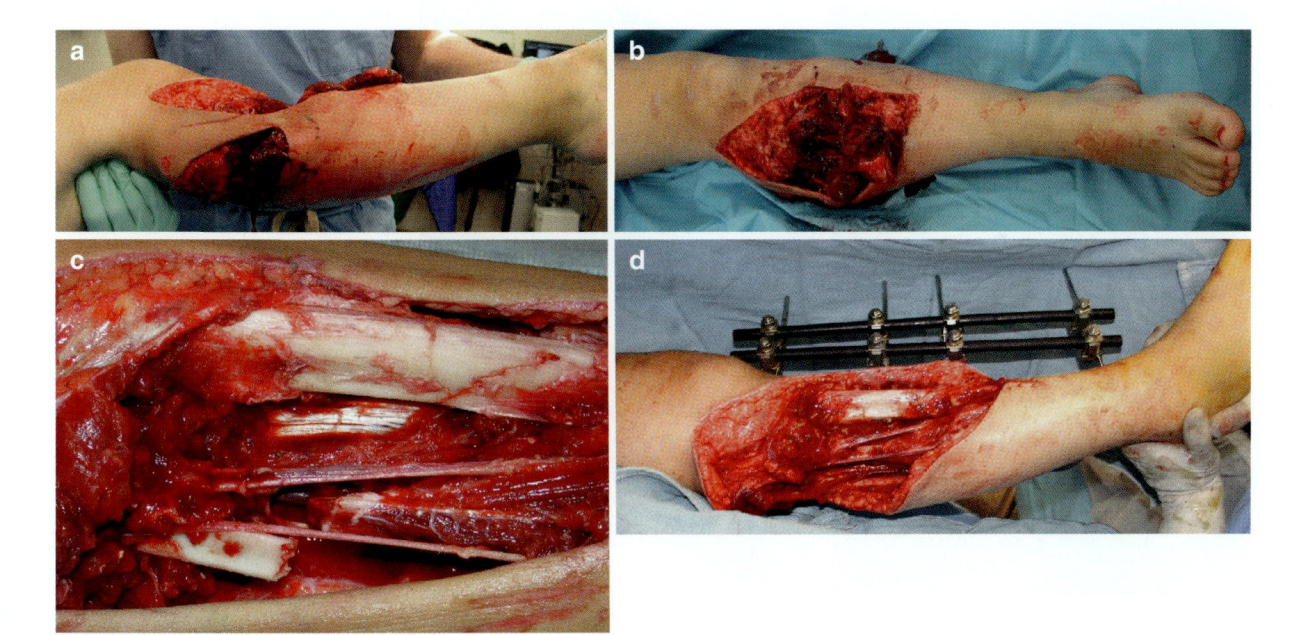

Fig. 22.3 This 20 year-old female sustained severe right-lower-leg trauma after being run over by a personal watercraft. (**a–d**) Initial surgical evaluation and debridement with subsequent external fixation. (**c**) Extensive soft-tissue loss and intact neurovascular bundle posterior to the tibia fracture. At this time, we confirmed our decision to salvage the limb. This wound had a vacuum-assisted closure device until the plastic surgery team could evaluate and ultimately place a soft-tissue flap over the wound (Case and photographs courtesy of David P. Barei, M.D.)

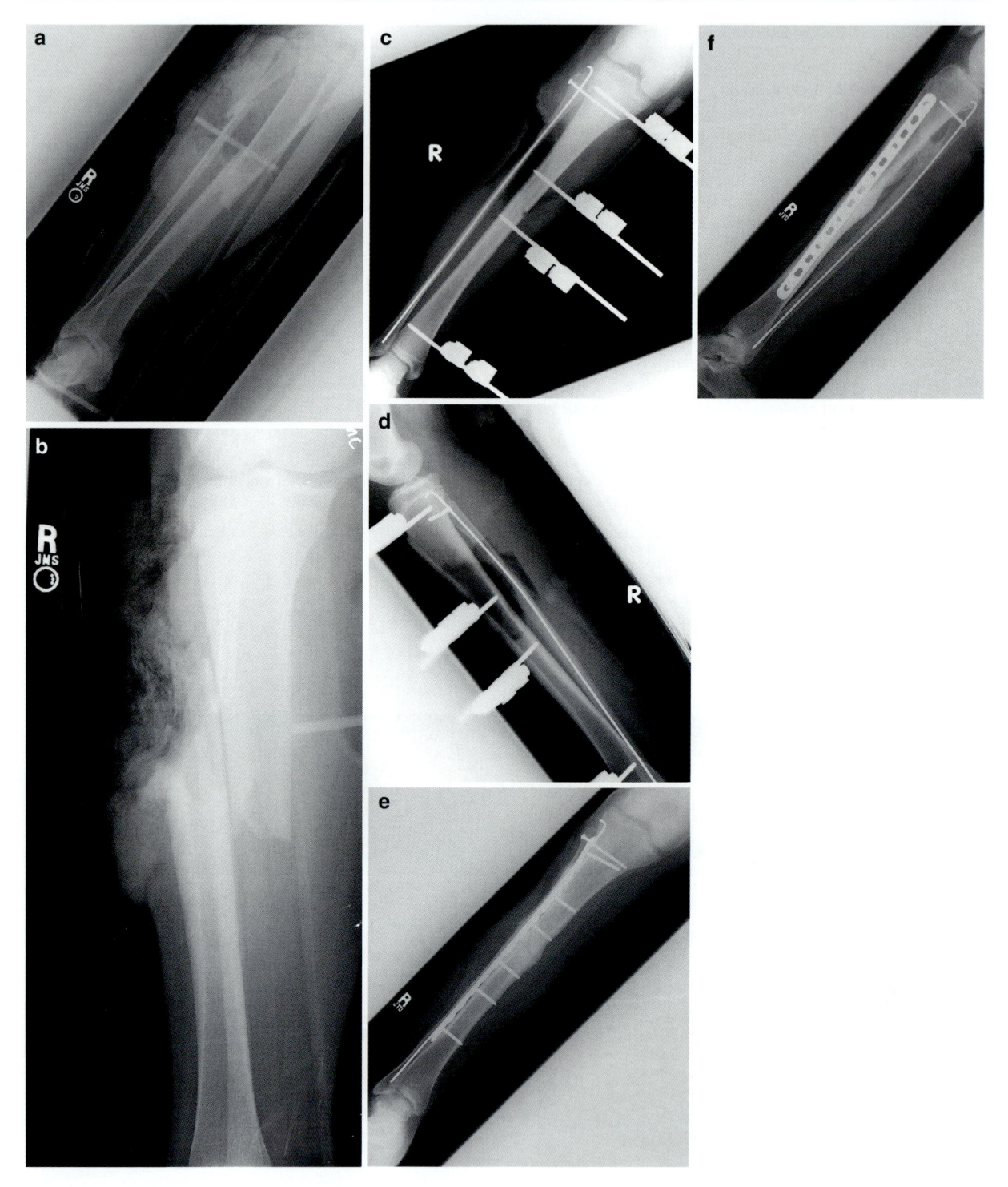

Fig. 22.4 (**a**, **b**) Anterior–posterior and lateral radiographic views of the injured lower extremity. Note significant soft-tissue shadow highlighting the extensive damage. This patient was fortunate and did not sustain substantial bone loss. (**c**, **d**) Provisional external fixation was employed to restore length, alignment, and rotation to the injured limb. (**e**, **f**) One year post-injury radiographs demonstrating complete union of both the tibia and fibula (Case and photographs courtesy of David P. Barei, M.D.)

Fig. 22.5 (**a–c**) Clinical follow-up demonstrating good result of limb-salvage with this patient. She was able to gain excellent range of motion and had an outstanding support network aiding her in the recovery process (Case and photographs courtesy of David P. Barei, M.D.)

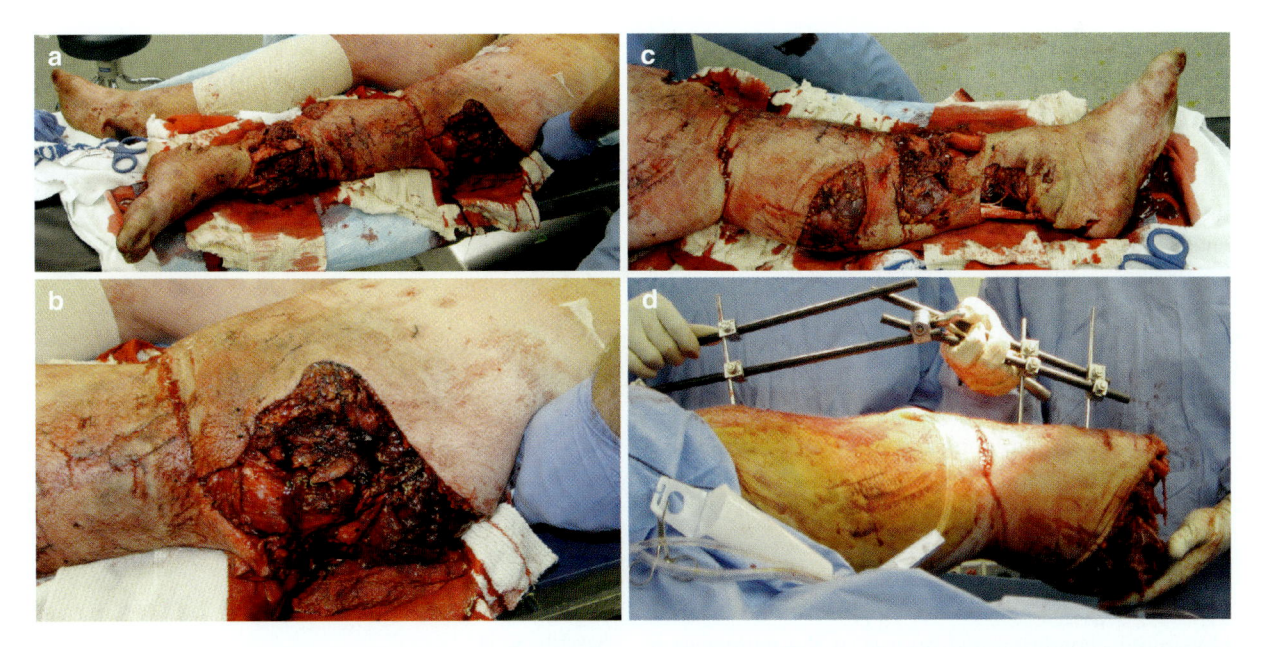

Fig. 22.6 This 27 year-old male was involved in a severe motor-vehicle crash. (**a–c**) Profound soft-tissue and osseous damage sustained. Emergency Department evaluation demonstrated the foot to be avascular. The patient underwent emergent operative intervention and initially had a below-the-knee amputation (**d**). The next day, he returned to the operating suite and had the amputation level moved proximally to above-the-knee due to worsening laboratory values, including increasing myoglobinuria. Intraoperative evaluation at that time revealed muscle damage to the most proximal margins of the quadriceps and hamstring musculature. It could be argued that this patient would have benefited from the above-the-knee amputation at the initial operative intervention. Radiographs for this patient are shown in Fig. 22.7a and b

Fig. 22.7 (a, b) Anterior–operative intervention of the patient depicted in Figure 22.6

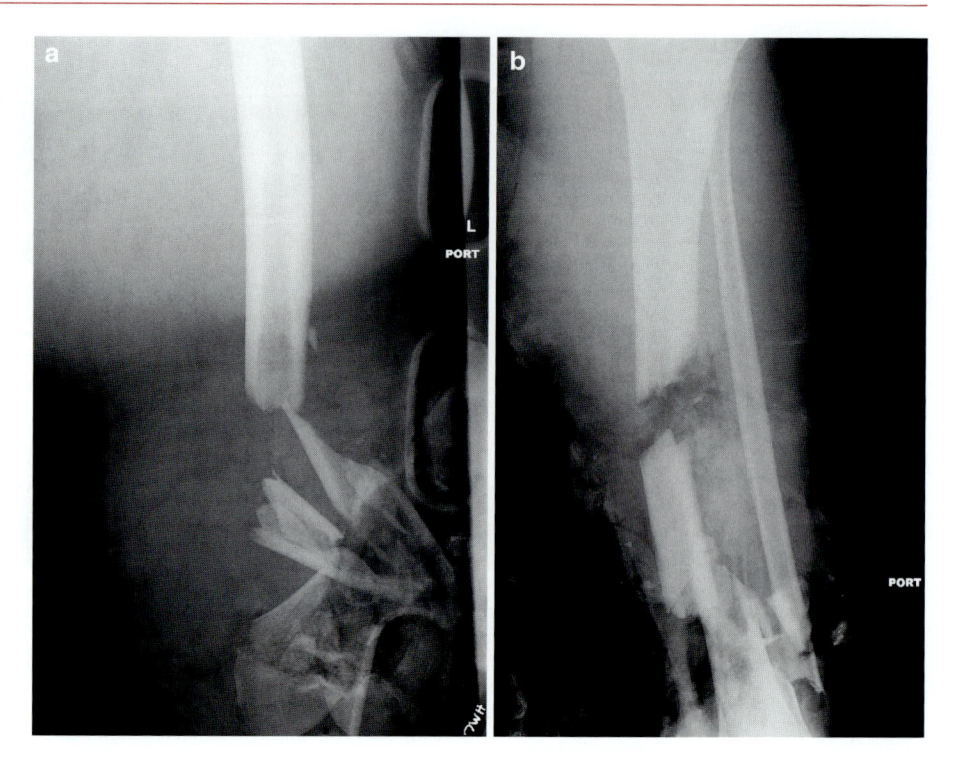

[7, 14, 15, 17, 41, 42]. There are a multitude of factors influencing this decision: those related directly to the leg injury itself, the extent and severity of associated injuries, the physiologic reserve of the patient, and their social support network. The training and experience of the attending surgeon may also play a role in the decision-making process [43].

MacKenzie et al. published the results of a survey pertaining to surgeons and their decision to amputate or reconstruct traumatized lower extremities. This study highlighted various factors that different specialties (general surgeons and orthopedic surgeons) deemed most important to consider in the critical decision of amputation versus salvage (see Table 22.3). Interesting perspectives representative of specialty-specific training and goals were identified. Namely, the general surgeons tended to emphasize the overall physiologic condition and reserve of the patient as a whole (the injury-severity scale, limb ischemia), whereas the orthopedic surgeon emphasized functional outcome prognosis (nerve integrity, soft-tissue coverage, limb ischemia). The study conclusions suggest that the main factor influencing surgeons on the

Table 22.3 Percent distribution of most important factor typically considered in decision to amputate vs. reconstruct by specialty

Factor	Total (%)	General surgeons (%)	Orthopaedic surgeons (%)
Nerve integrity/ plantar sensation	32	21	38
Limb ischemia	20	27	15
Soft-tissue coverage	14	9	17
Muscle damage	7	6	8
Neurovascular damage	3	0	6
Fracture pattern/ bone loss	4	0	6
High Injury Severity Scale (ISS)	12	31	0
Patient characteristics	2	0	4
Other	6	6	6

Source: Adapted from MacKenzie et al. [43]

question of salvageable limbs is apparent soft-tissue damage: muscle injury, absence of sensation, arterial injury, and vein injury. Patient factors were found to play much less of a role, although alcohol consumption and socioeconomic status were noted to be of some influence [43].

22.3.2 Lower-Extremity Injury-Severity Scales and Scores: Tools for Assisting Surgeons with Salvage or Amputation Decisions

Lower-extremity injury-severity scores were developed by clinicians to assist surgical teams in making the often difficult initial decision of whether to attempt limb-salvage or amputate a severely traumatized extremity. Surgeons have hypothesized that patients who undergo initial salvage attempts but subsequently require later amputation have worse outcomes than those who have early amputation. This makes intuitive sense and was shown to be correct in the LEAP study [18] and highlights the importance of early and accurate selection on which patients should proceed with a limb amputation during their first hospitalization.

Several studies [31, 33, 44–46] have examined the application of high-energy lower-extremity trauma scoring systems to patients with severe lower-extremity trauma. The LEAP study [20] contained the largest patient cohort of 565 prospectively evaluated high-energy lower-extremity injured patients. Each patient in this study had five well known injury-severity scoring systems applied to their case in an effort to determine the clinical utility of each system [44]. The five systems evaluated were the Mangled Extremity Severity Score (MESS) [29, 47], the Limb Salvage Index (LSI) [32], the Predictive Salvage Index (PSI) [34], the Nerve injury, Ischemia, Soft-tissue injury, Skeletal, Shock, and Age of patient score (NISSSA) [48], and the Hanover Fracture Scale (HFS-97) [49]. Table 22.4 represents the components of each injury-severity scale

Table 22.4 Components of Lower-Extremity Injury-Severity Scoring systems

Severity scale factors	Lower-Extremity Injury-Severity Scales					
	MESS	LSI	PSI	NISSSA	HFS-97	GHOISS
Age	X			X		X
Shock	X			X	X	X
Warm ischemia time	X	X	X	X	X	X
Bone injury		X	X		X	
Muscle injury		X	X			X
Skin injury		X			X	X
Nerve injury		X		X	X	X
Deep-vein injury		X				
Skeletal/soft-tissue injury	X			X		
Contamination				X	X	X
Time-to-treatment			X			
Comorbidities						X
Score-predicting amputation	≥7	≥6	≥8	≥11	≥9	≥17 (14–17 gray zone)

Source: Adapted from Bosse et al. [44] and Rajasekaran [51]

Mangled Extremity Severity Score (MESS) [29, 47], the Limb Salvage Index (LSI) [32], the Predictive Salvage Index (PSI) [34], the Nerve Injury, Ischemia, Soft-Tissue Injury, Shock, and Age of Patient score (NISSSA) [48], the Hanover Fracture Scale (HFS-97) [49], Ganga Hospital Open Injury Severity Scale (GHOISS) [50] with the addition of a newer scale that was developed in India to predict hospital days required, flap requirements, rate of infection, and the number of secondary procedures required. This scale also incorporates patient comorbidities, but emphasized primarily the evaluation of Type IIIB open tibia fractures [50]. It was not assessed in the LEAP trial, but is included for the sake of completeness.

When reviewing the initial studies for each of these instruments, reports indicated both high sensitivity and specificity for their respective scores [29, 32, 34, 47, 48]. However, when these scoring instruments have been evaluated subsequently by other clinicians, the initial results have been unable to be reproduced (see Table 22.5) with widely varying sensitivity and specificity values. The differences among these instruments (typically a higher specificity) demonstrate that they may be more helpful to treatment teams in determining which injuries may support entry of the injured extremity into a limb-salvage pathway [44] and not to which extremities should undergo immediate amputation. The sensitivities were generally low in the LEAP study demonstrating that their accuracy at predicting which extremities may eventually require amputation is poor and certainly should not be relied upon to make acute treatment decisions. Furthermore, in the face of low test sensitivity, placing too much emphasis upon these scores may delay an inevitable amputation risking complications in patient care potentially resulting in sepsis and even death [41].

Bosse et al. [44] were unable to recommend any scale for independent use in determining the fate of an injured limb. With the initial presentation of a trauma patient, they concluded that lower-extremity injury-severity scales have limited usefulness and that scores at or above respective amputation thresholds should be used cautiously in decision making with high-energy trauma patients. Their utility is in providing a list of the factors to consider when making the clinical decision.

22.3.3 Lower-Extremity Injury-Severity Scales and Scores: Predicting Functional Outcomes of Salvaged Limbs After Limb-Threatening Trauma

It has been hypothesized that lower-extremity injury-severity scores may have utility in the accurate prediction of functional outcome in limbs that underwent salvage after severe trauma. This important and useful question has been studied recently in a number of studies [33, 45, 52, 53]. Ly et al. [53] evaluated the clinical and functional outcomes of the patient cohort in the LEAP study as determined by the Sickness Impact Profile [54, 55] and the patients' scores on the MESS, PSI, and LSI lower-extremity injury-severity scores. They found no correlation amongst these instruments with patient clinical or functional outcomes. A unique point this study investigated was the specific evaluation of functional scores on patients in whom the injury-severity threshold-scores had recommended an amputation, but the patients had undergone limb-salvage instead. Very interestingly, these "amputation recommended" patients had outcome scores that were *no worse* than those patients who had salvaged limbs and had injury-severity scores indicating that amputation was not recommended. Durham et al. [45] studied 30 limbs that had undergone limb-salvage and had similar findings as Ly et al. Based upon phone interviews and clinic visits where return-to-work, impairment, and disability were assessed, they also concluded that none of the extremity injury scales could predict functional outcome.

Table 22.5 Independent analyses of Lower-Extremity Injury-Severity Scales

	MESS	PSI	LSI	NISSSA	HFS-97
Bosse et al. [44]					
Sensitivity	0.45	0.47	0.51	0.33	0.37
Specificity	0.93	0.84	0.97	0.98	0.98
Bonanni et al. [33]					
Sensitivity	0.22	0.33	0.61		
Specificity	0.53	0.70	0.43		
Durham et al. [45]					
Sensitivity	0.79	0.96	0.83		
Specificity	0.83	0.50	0.83		
Dagum et al. [31]					
Sensitivity	0.40	0.60	0.60		
Specificity	0.89	0.94	0.83		

Evaluating Gustilo type III fractures, including immediate amputations

22.3.4 Lower-Extremity Injury-Severity Scales and Scores: Summary

Whenever evaluating patients and deciding upon optimal care for their injured limb, due caution should be exercised when interpreting the lower-extremity injury-severity scales. This holds true with both initial management and extrapolating ultimate functional outcomes with patients. It is the author's opinion that these lower-extremity scoring systems should still play a role in the management decisions for some patients, but should simply be used as one data point among many in the complex processes surrounding the care of the high-energy trauma patient.

22.3.5 Outcomes in Patients Undergoing Limb-Salvage or Amputation for Limb-Threatening Injuries

In 2002, Bosse et al. [20] and LEAP study group published their initial report on a prospective cohort of 569 patients that had sustained high-energy lower-extremity trauma from March 1994 to June 1997. The patients in this study had either undergone limb-salvage or amputation and were followed prospectively for 24 months and then reported on again at 7 years follow-up [22].

The initial report demonstrated that patients had similar functional outcomes regardless of whether they underwent limb reconstruction/salvage or amputation. The results also indicated that although the outcomes were similar, both groups had substantial levels of disability and only half had returned to work at 2 years post-injury. Indeed, patients in both groups were able to show significant improvement over the study period, but an important overreaching finding of the study was the profound disability and persistently low psychosocial-functioning subscale [55, 56].

This study was also able to enlighten surgeons on particular factors not related to the injury itself that may predispose some trauma patients to a poorer or less than optimal outcome. These included a lower level of education, poverty, lack of private health insurance, smoking, and involvement with disability-compensation litigation [20]. The elucidation of these factors provides areas for treatment teams to intervene and assist patients in achieving a better outcome. We advocate for the early involvement and intervention by psychosocial and vocational rehabilitation specialists. Their function in the patient's recovery we believe is imperative and a key component for a better functional outcome. With their expertise, they can directly address the variables listed above and change or even prevent adverse outcomes.

In addition to the listed factors above, self-efficacy and an involved social support network are important determinants of outcome and should be emphasized in rehabilitation [57–59]. The orthopaedic surgeon evaluating this patient in the outpatient setting can be instrumental in this area and help empower the social support network to assist the patient through both the difficult physical and mental recovery. The orthopaedist is also likely the only clinician who can help determine the activity level of the patient in the postoperative timeframe and, with this knowledge and assistance from the social workers and disability specialists, help make vocational retraining possible. Both of the above functions should help facilitate the patient's return to work as excessive delay in this area could potentially lead to poorer outcomes [60, 61].

Longer-term follow-up on the LEAP patient cohort was published at 7 years post-injury [22]. Perhaps unexpectedly, one-half of the patients in the LEAP study remained "severely" disabled, and one-quarter were "very severely" disabled [54, 55]. Only one-third of the patients had outcome scores similar to the general population. As found in the initial LEAP 2-year results, there were no significant differences identified among limb-salvage and amputation groups. This follow-up study confirmed and added other factors that were found to be predictive of poor outcomes in the LEAP patient cohort: older age, female gender, non-white race, lower education level, living in a poor household, current or previous smoking history [62], low self-efficacy, poor self-reported health status before the injury, and involvement with the legal system in an effort to obtain disability payments. Conclusions drawn from this study warrant attention from treatment teams and do not necessarily involve the acute surgical management of this traumatized population. The optimization of recovery in these patients should emphasize the involvement of professionals who can address certain areas of recovery beyond the operating theater – namely, job retraining, intensive rehabilitative therapy, and education [63–65].

Furthermore, educating patients and their families on realistic and typical expected outcomes is important, as many patients will foster unrealistic expectations. The presence and mental fixation on these unrealistic expectations may predispose patients to poorer outcomes and generalized dissatisfaction with their condition and care [22, 60, 61].

22.3.6 Complications in the Treatment of Severe Lower-Extremity Trauma

The management of limb-threatening trauma is challenging and complications can be significant. Harris et al. [66] reported that among the 149 amputations performed among the LEAP patients, there was a 5.4% amputation revision rate. There was an overall 24% complication rate with most of these being reported at 3 months post-injury. The most common complications were wound infection (34%) followed by wound dehiscence (13%). In the 371 limb-salvage patients, 3.9% required a late amputation, which was defined as a limb undergoing amputation after the initial hospitalization. Most complications were noted at 6 months post-injury and included a total of 37.7% of this group. Similar to the amputation group, the most common complication noted was wound infection (23.2%). The complications of osteomyelitis and nonunions were, not surprisingly, seen predominantly in the salvage group and entailed 8.6% and 31%, respectively.

Soft-tissue coverage associated with limb-salvage and reconstruction is also associated with significant complications and has been reported to occur in 53% of flap procedures within the LEAP patient cohort. Operative intervention was required in 87% of these patients [67]. Rehospitalization, often a setback in recovery, occurred in one-third of LEAP study patients and involved the limb-salvage/reconstruction group more than amputation group.

Complications in the management of this severely injured group of patients are sadly unavoidable. It is in our and our patients best interest to understand the nature of the complications and how then to best avoid them. From the initial evaluation and subsequent follow-up of these patients, treatment teams should not underestimate the difficult nature of the recovery process and the potential for complications and secondary procedures.

22.3.7 Psychological Distress in Patients with Severely Injured Lower Extremities

Accompanying the significant challenges with physical recovery and impairment is an often under-appreciated source of morbidity with orthopaedic trauma patients – psychological distress and mental illness [68, 69]. This is especially evident in the high-energy lower-extremity trauma patient where limb-salvage and amputations are being debated and subsequent recoveries managed. During the course of the LEAP study, patients were evaluated for psychological distress [70] utilizing the Brief Symptom Inventory [71, 72]. At 2 years post-injury, 42% of the patients screened positive for a psychological disorder, yet only 22% had reported receiving any mental health services. Almost 20% of the study group reported severe phobic anxiety and/or depression. The authors of the study were able to identify factors that were likely to be associated with patients that had psychological distress. These included poorer physical function, younger age, nonwhite race, poverty, a likely drinking problem, neuroticism, a poor sense of self-efficacy, and limited social support. Interestingly, some of these same factors have been attributed to chronic pain syndromes which could certainly exacerbate any coexisting psychological distress these patients may be suffering from [73].

As emphasized previously, the orthopaedic surgeon is most likely going to be the primary coordinator of care with these patients in the postoperative period during their lengthy functional recoveries. Along with recognizing the physical dysfunction and instituting appropriate referrals for therapy and job retraining, the treating surgeon must also be astute enough to evaluate and screen these traumatized patients for psychological distress. If mental distress is suspected or identified, appropriate consultation or referral should be initiated to a provider trained in this area. Furthermore, by understanding and recognizing potential risk factors for psychological distress and thus poorer outcomes with this patient population (i.e., drinking problems, poor social support network or poor self-efficacy), prophylactic referrals can be made early in the patient's recovery. Ultimately, for patients to be given the best chance for the most favorable outcome, the physical and psychological needs of this population should be addressed simultaneously [70].

22.3.8 Societal Costs Associated with Limb-Salvage and Amputation

An argument we have heard and understand is that of the cost of limb-salvage and its toll on society in comparison to a "quick amputation and be done with it" attitude… "let the patient get on with their life." The cost burden of the limb-salvage and amputation debate was recently reported [2], and the results directly counter what many have argued in the past. At 2 years of follow-up, both groups had essentially the same healthcare costs. However, projected lifetime costs were $509,000 for amputees and $163,000 for limb-salvage patients (2002 US Dollar figures) – over a threefold difference. The difference was mainly attributed to the repair and replacement costs associated with prostheses for the amputation population, which had an estimated 40–45 years of life remaining. In regards to complications, they found a 46% increase in costs if patients had required a rehospitalization – a finding that underscores the importance of clinicians having a solid understanding of risk factors for both complications and poorer outcomes.

22.4 The Open Fracture with Severe Nerve Injury

The management of severe limb-threatening injuries is challenging and often requires difficult decisions to be made acutely. Predicting the outcome of patients with this type of trauma (see Table 22.2) has proved challenging, and the utility of limb-salvage predictive scores has been shown to be limited. A repetitive and concerning theme in the scientific literature surrounding limb-salvage and amputation is the severe open fracture with associated nerve injury and purported poor results of 60–100% disability with this type of injury [74–76]. This scenario represents a unique conundrum in the decision-making process.

The loss of foot plantar sensation has been ingrained into the trauma surgeon's psyche as a major, if not sometimes the primary predictor of acute amputation. In fact, MacKenzie et al. [43] showed that nearly 40% of orthopedic surgeons place nerve integrity and plantar sensation as the primary determinant in the decision to amputate or reconstruct (see Table 22.3). Often, this decision is made based on initial emergency room evaluation, even though this sometimes rudimentary exam has been shown to be unpredictable [35]. The influence of nerve integrity on the trauma community has been borne out by its direct and independent inclusion into three of the major limb-salvage prediction scales: the LSI, NISSSA, and HFS-97 (see Table 22.4).

The insensate foot was recently evaluated amongst a 55 patient cohort of the LEAP study [77]. This group presented to the emergency department with an insensate foot and underwent either amputation (26 patients) or limb-salvage (29 patients). The insensate-salvage group was also matched and compared with a sensate-salvage group as a control group in the study. The authors identified some interesting and important findings directly impacting commonly held beliefs pertaining to limb-salvage versus amputation debates and predicted outcomes. First and foremost, patients that had absent plantar sensation demonstrated substantial impairment at final follow-up. However, their outcomes were similar and appeared to be unaffected whether undergoing amputation or limb-salvage. Second and perhaps most interesting, the patients with the insensate foot on presentation that underwent limb-salvage did not have worse outcomes than the matched cohort with intact sensation that underwent limb-salvage. This included no differences in final plantar sensation or the need for late amputation. In fact, 67% of the patients in the insensate foot group regained normal foot sensation over the study period – a highlight that supports increased diligence in treatment decisions utilizing emergency department nerve exams. Ultimately, the 2 year outcome of patients that had undergone limb-salvage with an insensate foot did not appear to be influenced or adversely affected by the presence or absence of plantar sensation [77].

The decisions in this analysis and others are often based upon emergency department evaluation and not upon direct surgical observation. The initial evaluation demonstrating a loss of plantar sensation can easily be attributed to a transient neurapraxia from compression or stretch and/or temporary ischemia, which can be reversible. The intraoperative finding of complete nerve transection or segmental neural element loss could be suggestive of an absolute indication for primary limb amputation, especially in light of an associated vascular injury or other severe injuries. However, it is important to note that often clinicians treat patients with insensate feet in the clinical setting, namely, in the diabetic and spinal cord injury patient populations

[77]. In the surgical suite, we do not advocate invasive surgical exploration of nerve structures in the lower extremity when they are not already exposed secondary to the trauma itself. This practice is associated with unwarranted tissue damage and should be avoided. With evidence to support return of plantar sensation during recovery, the reliance upon plantar sensation in the initial physical exam finding should be avoided in the amputation decision-making process.

22.5 Summary

The high-energy lower-extremity trauma patient presents many challenges to treatment teams. Past literature has not been overly supportive of limb-salvage and often makes the point that early amputation is advantageous to save patients from lengthy suffering [14, 17]. However, as technology and surgical concepts have evolved, so have our abilities to salvage limbs previously thought to be candidates only for amputation. These salvaged limbs, although demonstrating generally poor outcomes, have been shown to have equivalent results to limbs treated with primary amputation [20–22] and entail equivalent 2-year healthcare costs and substantial savings over the long term.

Often, given the option of limb-salvage or amputation, most patients opt to save their extremity rather than undergo an amputation. While data presented here and in the LEAP data show equivalent results among the salvage/amputation groups, it should be noted that most of the data were derived from care patients had received at Level I trauma centers. It has been argued that these centers, with their experienced trauma staff, may impart different outcomes than patients treated elsewhere [78].

We believe that limb-salvage is a reasonable goal for clinicians and patients at experienced Level I trauma centers. The LEAP data and other studies present sufficient evidence to support this conclusion. The early involvement of post-acute-care services, such as therapists, rehabilitation specialists, psychologists, and many others, is imperative for the optimization of patient outcomes and potentially hold the highest value in recovery efforts. Diligent, thoughtful care and presenting realistic expectations will allow these traumatized patients to achieve their best recovery and functional outcomes.

References

1. American Association of Orthopaedic Surgeons. The burden of musculoskeletal diseases in the United States: prevalence, societal and economic cost. Rosemont: American Academy of Orthopaedic Surgeons; 2008.
2. MacKenzie EJ, Jones AS, Bosse MJ, et al. Health-care costs associated with amputation or reconstruction of a limb-threatening injury. J Bone Joint Surg Am. 2007;89:1685–92.
3. Wright JG. A practical guide to assigning levels of evidence. J Bone Joint Surg Am. 2007;89:1128–30.
4. Dillingham TR, Pezzin LE, MacKenzie EJ. Incidence, acute care length of stay, and discharge to rehabilitation of traumatic amputee patients: an epidemiologic study. Arch Phys Med Rehabil. 1998;79:279–87.
5. Dillingham TR, Pezzin LE, MacKenzie EJ. Limb amputation and limb deficiency: epidemiology and recent trends in the United States. South Med J. 2002;95:875–83.
6. Anglen J, Kyle RF, Marsh JL, et al. Locking plates for extremity fractures. J Am Acad Orthop Surg. 2009;17:465–72.
7. Caudle RJ, Stern PJ. Severe open fractures of the tibia. J Bone Joint Surg Am. 1987;69:801–7.
8. Collinge CA, Sanders RW. Percutaneous plating in the lower extremity. J Am Acad Orthop Surg. 2000;8:211–6.
9. Francel TJ, Vander Kolk CA, Hoopes JE, et al. Microvascular soft-tissue transplantation for reconstruction of acute open tibial fractures: timing of coverage and long-term functional results. Plast Reconstr Surg. 1992;89:478–87; discussion 488-9.
10. Godina M. Early microsurgical reconstruction of complex trauma of the extremities. Plast Reconstr Surg. 1986;78:285–92.
11. Gorman PW, Barnes CL, Fischer TJ, et al. Soft-tissue reconstruction in severe lower extremity trauma. A review. Clin Orthop Relat Res. 1989;243:57–64.
12. Haidukewych GJ. Innovations in locking plate technology. J Am Acad Orthop Surg. 2004;12:205–12.
13. Haidukewych GJ, Ricci W. Locked plating in orthopaedic trauma: a clinical update. J Am Acad Orthop Surg. 2008;16:347–55.
14. Hansen Jr ST. The type-IIIC tibial fracture. Salvage or amputation. J Bone Joint Surg Am. 1987;69:799–800.
15. Lange RH. Limb reconstruction versus amputation decision making in massive lower extremity trauma. Clin Orthop Relat Res. 1989;243:92–9.
16. Georgiadis GM, Behrens FF, Joyce MJ, et al. Open tibial fractures with severe soft-tissue loss. Limb salvage compared with below-the-knee amputation. J Bone Joint Surg Am. 1993;75:1431–41.
17. Hansen Jr ST. Overview of the severely traumatized lower limb. Reconstruction versus amputation. Clin Orthop Relat Res. 1989;243:17–9.
18. Smith DG, Castillo R, MacKenzie E, et al. Functional outcomes of patients who have late amputation after trauma is significantly worse than for those who have early amputation in Orthopaedic Trauma Association. Annual meeting, Salt Lake City; 2003.
19. Francel TJ. Improving reemployment rates after limb salvage of acute severe tibial fractures by microvascular soft-tissue reconstruction. Plast Reconstr Surg. 1994;93:1028–34.

20. Bosse MJ, MacKenzie EJ, Kellam JF, et al. An analysis of outcomes of reconstruction or amputation after leg-threatening injuries. N Engl J Med. 2002;347:1924–31.
21. MacKenzie EJ, Bosse MJ, Kellam JF, et al. Characterization of patients with high-energy lower extremity trauma. J Orthop Trauma. 2000;14:455–66.
22. MacKenzie EJ, Bosse MJ, Pollak AN, et al. Long-term persistence of disability following severe lower-limb trauma. Results of a seven-year follow-up. J Bone Joint Surg Am. 2005;87:1801–9.
23. Alexander RH, Proctor HJ, American College of Surgeons. Committee on Trauma. Advanced trauma life support program for physicians: ATLS. 5th ed. Chicago: American College of Surgeons; 1993.
24. American College of Surgeons Committee on Trauma. Advanced trauma life support for doctors: student course manual. 6th ed. Chicago: American College of Surgeons; 1997.
25. American College of Surgeons Committee on Trauma. Advanced trauma life support for doctors ATLS: manuals for coordinators and faculty. 8th ed. Chicago: American College of Surgeons; 2008.
26. Pinzur M. Amputations in trauma. In: Browner BD, Jupiter J, Levine A, et al., editors. Skeletal trauma: basic science, management, and reconstruction, 2 vols. Philadelphia: Saunders/Elsevier; 2009. p. xxv, 2882, I56.
27. MacKenzie EJ, Bosse MJ, Castillo RC, et al. Functional outcomes following trauma-related lower-extremity amputation. J Bone Joint Surg Am. 2004;86-A:1636–45.
28. Pinzur MS, Smith DG, Daluga DJ, et al. Selection of patients for through-the-knee amputation. J Bone Joint Surg Am. 1988;70:746–50.
29. Johansen K, Daines M, Howey T, et al. Objective criteria accurately predict amputation following lower extremity trauma. J Trauma. 1990;30:568–72; discussion 572-3.
30. Pinzur MS, Angelats J, Light TR, et al. Functional outcome following traumatic upper limb amputation and prosthetic limb fitting. J Hand Surg Am. 1994;19:836–9.
31. Dagum AB, Best AK, Schemitsch EH, et al. Salvage after severe lower-extremity trauma: are the outcomes worth the means? Plast Reconstr Surg. 1999;103:1212–20.
32. Russell WL, Sailors DM, Whittle TB, et al. Limb salvage versus traumatic amputation. A decision based on a seven-part predictive index. Ann Surg. 1991;213:473–80; discussion 480-1.
33. Bonanni F, Rhodes M, Lucke JF. The futility of predictive scoring of mangled lower extremities. J Trauma. 1993;34:99–104.
34. Howe Jr HR, Poole Jr GV, Hansen KJ, et al. Salvage of lower extremities following combined orthopedic and vascular trauma. A predictive salvage index. Am Surg. 1987;53:205–8.
35. Lange RH, Bach AW, Hansen Jr ST, et al. Open tibial fractures with associated vascular injuries: prognosis for limb salvage. J Trauma. 1985;25:203–8.
36. Dougherty PJ. Long-term follow-up of unilateral transfemoral amputees from the Vietnam war. J Trauma. 2003;54:718–23.
37. Smith DG, Horn P, Malchow D, et al. Prosthetic history, prosthetic charges, and functional outcome of the isolated, traumatic below-knee amputee. J Trauma. 1995;38:44–7.
38. Lerner RK, Esterhai Jr JL, Polomono RC, et al. Psychosocial, functional, and quality of life assessment of patients with posttraumatic fracture nonunion, chronic refractory osteomyelitis, and lower extremity amputation. Arch Phys Med Rehabil. 1991;72:122–6.
39. Lerner RK, Esterhai Jr JL, Polomano RC, et al. Quality of life assessment of patients with posttraumatic fracture nonunion chronic refractory osteomyelitis, and lower-extremity amputation. Clin Orthop Relat Res. 1993;295:28–36.
40. Dougherty PJ. Transtibial amputees from the Vietnam War. Twenty-eight-year follow-up. J Bone Joint Surg Am. 2001;83-A:383–9.
41. Bondurant FJ, Cotler HB, Buckle R, et al. The medical and economic impact of severely injured lower extremities. J Trauma. 1988;28:1270–3.
42. Dirschl DR, Dahners LE. The mangled extremity: when should it be amputated? J Am Acad Orthop Surg. 1996;4:182–90.
43. MacKenzie EJ, Bosse MJ, Kellam JF, et al. Factors influencing the decision to amputate or reconstruct after high-energy lower extremity trauma. J Trauma. 2002;52:641–9.
44. Bosse MJ, MacKenzie EJ, Kellam JF, et al. A prospective evaluation of the clinical utility of the lower-extremity injury-severity scores. J Bone Joint Surg Am. 2001;83-A:3–14.
45. Durham RM, Mistry BM, Mazuski JE, et al. Outcome and utility of scoring systems in the management of the mangled extremity. Am J Surg. 1996;172:569–73; discussion 573-4.
46. O'Sullivan ST, O'Sullivan M, Pasha N, et al. Is it possible to predict limb viability in complex Gustilo IIIB and IIIC tibial fractures? A comparison of two predictive indices. Injury. 1997;28:639–42.
47. Helfet DL, Howey T, Sanders R, et al. Limb salvage versus amputation. Preliminary results of the Mangled Extremity Severity Score. Clin Orthop Relat Res. 1990;256:80–6.
48. McNamara MG, Heckman JD, Corley FG. Severe open fractures of the lower extremity: a retrospective evaluation of the Mangled Extremity Severity Score (MESS). J Orthop Trauma. 1994;8:81–7.
49. Tscherne H, Gotzen L. Fractures with soft tissue injuries. Berlin/New York: Springer; 1984.
50. Rajasekaran S, Naresh Babu J, Dheenadhayalan J, et al. A score for predicting salvage and outcome in Gustilo type-IIIA and type-IIIB open tibial fractures. J Bone Joint Surg Br. 2006;88:1351–60.
51. Rajasekaran S. The utility of scores in the decision to salvage or amputation in severely limbs. Indian J Orthop. 2008;42(4):368–76.
52. Lin CH, Wei FC, Levin LS, et al. The functional outcome of lower-extremity fractures with vascular injury. J Trauma. 1997;43:480–5.
53. Ly TV, Travison TG, Castillo RC, et al. Ability of lower-extremity injury severity scores to predict functional outcome after limb salvage. J Bone Joint Surg Am. 2008;90:1738–43.
54. Bergner M, Bobbitt RA, Kressel S, et al. The sickness impact profile: conceptual formulation and methodology for the development of a health status measure. Int J Health Serv. 1976;6:393–415.
55. Bergner M, Bobbitt RA, Carter WB, et al. The sickness impact profile: development and final revision of a health status measure. Med Care. 1981;19:787–805.
56. de Bruin AF, de Witte LP, Stevens F, et al. Sickness impact profile: the state of the art of a generic functional status measure. Soc Sci Med. 1992;35:1003–14.

57. Berkman LF, Glass T. Social integration, social networks, social support, and health. In: Berkman LF, Kawachi I, editors. Social epidemiology. New York: Oxford University Press; 2000.
58. MacKenzie EJ, Morris Jr JA, Jurkovich GJ, et al. Return to work following injury: the role of economic, social, and job-related factors. Am J Public Health. 1998;88:1630–7.
59. MacKenzie EJ, Bosse MJ. Factors influencing outcome following limb-threatening lower limb trauma: lessons learned from the Lower Extremity Assessment Project (LEAP). J Am Acad Orthop Surg. 2006;14:S205–10.
60. O'Toole RV, Castillo RC, Pollak AN, et al. Determinants of patient satisfaction after severe lower-extremity injuries. J Bone Joint Surg Am. 2008;90:1206–11.
61. O'Toole RV, Castillo RC, Pollak AN, et al. Surgeons and their patients disagree regarding cosmetic and overall outcomes after surgery for high-energy lower extremity trauma. J Orthop Trauma. 2009;23:716–23.
62. Castillo RC, Bosse MJ, MacKenzie EJ, et al. Impact of smoking on fracture healing and risk of complications in limb-threatening open tibia fractures. J Orthop Trauma. 2005;19:151–7.
63. Archer KR, Castillo RC, Mackenzie EJ, et al. Gait symmetry and walking speed analysis following lower-extremity trauma. Phys Ther. 2006;86:1630–40.
64. Archer KR, MacKenzie EJ, Bosse MJ, et al. Factors associated with surgeon referral for physical therapy in patients with traumatic lower-extremity injury: results of a national survey of orthopedic trauma surgeons. Phys Ther. 2009;89: 893–905.
65. Castillo RC, MacKenzie EJ, Archer KR, et al. Evidence of beneficial effect of physical therapy after lower-extremity trauma. Arch Phys Med Rehabil. 2008;89:1873–9.
66. Harris AM, Althausen PL, Kellam J, et al. Complications following limb-threatening lower extremity trauma. J Orthop Trauma. 2009;23:1–6.
67. Pollak AN, McCarthy ML, Burgess AR. Short-term wound complications after application of flaps for coverage of traumatic soft-tissue defects about the tibia. The Lower Extremity Assessment Project (LEAP) study group. J Bone Joint Surg Am. 2000;82-A:1681–91.
68. Crichlow RJ, Andres PL, Morrison SM, et al. Depression in orthopaedic trauma patients. Prevalence and severity. J Bone Joint Surg Am. 2006;88:1927–33.
69. Singh G, Harkema JM, Mayberry AJ, et al. Severe depression of gut absorptive capacity in patients following trauma or sepsis. J Trauma. 1994;36:803–8; discussion 808-9.
70. McCarthy ML, MacKenzie EJ, Edwin D, et al. Psychological distress associated with severe lower-limb injury. J Bone Joint Surg Am. 2003;85-A:1689–97.
71. Derogatis LP. BSI: brief symptom inventory. 3rd ed. Minneapolis: National Computer Systems; 1993.
72. Derogatis LR, Melisaratos N. The brief symptom inventory: an introductory report. Psychol Med. 1983;13:595–605.
73. Castillo RC, MacKenzie EJ, Wegener ST, et al. Prevalence of chronic pain seven years following limb threatening lower extremity trauma. Pain. 2006;124:321–9.
74. Aldea PA, Shaw WW. Management of acute lower extremity nerve injuries. Foot Ankle. 1986;7:82–94.
75. Bateman JE. Trauma to nerves in limbs. Philadelphia: Saunders; 1962.
76. Lusskin R, Battista A. Evaluation and therapy after injury to peripheral nerves. Foot Ankle. 1986;7:71–81.
77. Bosse MJ, McCarthy ML, Jones AL, et al. The insensate foot following severe lower extremity trauma: an indication for amputation? J Bone Joint Surg Am. 2005;87:2601–8.
78. MacKenzie EJ, Rivara FP, Jurkovich GJ, et al. The impact of trauma-center care on functional outcomes following major lower-limb trauma. J Bone Joint Surg Am. 2008;90: 101–9.

High-Energy Injuries Caused by Penetrating Trauma

Yoram A. Weil and Rami Mosheiff

Contents

23.1	**Gunshot Ballistics and Injuries**	281
23.1.1	Mechanism of Injury	282
23.1.2	Vascular Injuries	282
23.1.3	Principles of Treatment	282
23.1.4	Fracture Care	283
23.2	**Blast Injuries**	285
23.2.1	Mechanisms of Blast Injury	288
23.3	**Triage and Primary Resuscitation**	289
23.4	**Treatment of Specific Injuries**	289
23.5	**Specific Considerations**	290
23.6	**Conclusions**	290
	References	291

As blunt trauma care involving orthopaedic injuries evolved over the years, penetrating orthopaedic trauma was vastly underrepresented in the literature, despite the recent rise in firearms related causality rate, especially in North America and other industrialized countries [1], as well as the surge in global terrorism [2]. Therefore, the practicing orthopaedic trauma surgeon is in need for more information regarding the recognition, management and preparation needed to cope with isolated or mass casualties with high-energy penetrating musculoskeletal injuries.

The topic of penetrating limb injuries is wide, but can be divided into two main subgroups: those inflicted by firearms both of high and low velocity, and those caused by blast or explosions. Both injuries had been long discussed in the military setting, but are now encountered in an alarming rate in the civilian setting.

The purpose of this chapter is to characterize both gunshot and blast-related extremity injuries, discuss their initial and definite management, and review some of the recent experience with emphasis on the civilian setting.

23.1 Gunshot Ballistics and Injuries

Many authors and surgeons have attempted to classify the injury pattern of gunshots based on the type of weapon, bullet, energy transfer, and velocity of the projectile [1, 3, 4]. Traditionally, projectiles were classified as either "low velocity" or "high velocity," with low-velocity weapons represented by handguns and high-velocity bullets the product of assault rifles. The cut-off point has been controversial, but it is widely accepted that most high-velocity injuries refer to a bullet travelling greater than 2,000 ft/s [1].

Y.A. Weil and R. Mosheiff (✉)
Department of Orthopedic Surgery,
Hadassah Hesrew University Medical Center,
Jerusalem, Israel
e-mail: ramim@cc.huji.ac.il

Since the kinetic energy is proportional to the square of the velocity, most modern guns have switched to smaller but faster ammunition. Both in vivo evidence in dogs [5], as well as in vitro simulation in gelatin blocks [1, 6] demonstrate a wider wound tract and tissue damage inflicted by faster ammunition. Early clinical reports from the Vietnam war describe the unusual injuries inflicted by the M-16 assault rifle at that time [7]. Despite the above, the distinction between high velocity and low velocity can at times become artificial. A 0.45 caliber pistol, firing what is usually considered a "low-velocity" bullet, can transmit 900 J of energy, equivalent to a 5 kg weight being dropped from a height of 20 m, which can cause severe musculoskeletal injury [8], while a military assault rifle, classified as high-velocity, can hit a thigh with a clean in-and-out wound without significant damage [1].

23.1.1 Mechanism of Injury

After the bullet leaves the firearm muzzle, it propagates in a compound movement pattern consisting of yaw and rotation. These together create a complex form of motion called nutation, and a well-designed bullet with a yaw of less than 3° will usually hit the target straight [9]. Upon striking its target, the bullet forms a temporary cavity due to the stretching forces and vacuum created by its passing. This temporary cavity is reported to be significantly larger as velocity increases to 2,000 ft/s or higher [1, 10, 11]. The cavitation process lasts only a few milliseconds, and the amount of tissue damage is dictated by the tissue elasticity and tolerance to stretch. For example, near-liquid organs such as the brain, liver, or spleen might be violently disrupted during this temporary cavity formation [1, 3]. In the limbs, however, muscle is damaged mainly within the close vicinity of the passing bullet, but can tolerate stretching quite well [12]. Major vessels are rarely injured by stretch. Nerves rarely tear due to cavitation, and typically nerve injury results only in neuropraxia. Therefore current practice is to not perform nerve exploration routinely in gunshot wounds [13].

Bone can be damaged incompletely or completely. Various fracture patterns have been described for both complete and incomplete fractures, but the clinical value of these classifications is questionable. However, it should be mentioned that bone fragments can be propelled to the area of temporary cavitation and can create damage in adjacent structures. This is not always obvious when looking at injury films since most bone fragments usually retract back to the original bone [1].

Virtually, all gunshot wounds are contaminated [1, 3]. In an experimental model, the number of organisms in a gunshot wound tend to multiply 10–100 times within 24 h, and all cultures from devitalized muscle are positive at the time of the initial injury [14]. Therefore, the time of wound excision is believed to be of a greater value if performed earlier in the course of treatment.

23.1.2 Vascular Injuries

Vascular injuries are not uncommon in high-energy gunshot wounds and potential vascular damage must be evaluated [1, 15]. Although physical examination is often sufficient to rule out major vascular injury [16], minor vascular injuries have been reported to appear late. Angiography, although very accurate, is not routinely warranted if the physical examination is normal [17]. On the other hand, in a hypo-perfused limb with a localized lesion and "hard" signs of vascular injury, the location of injury is obvious, and immediate exploration is indicated without further studies [1]. Angiography, performed in borderline cases when "hard" physical findings (an ischemic, pulseless limb, expanding hematoma or a bruit) are absent, is negative in many cases and demonstrates benign, non-threatening lesions in the other cases [18]. Therefore, arteriography should be reserved for only borderline cases when physical examination is difficult to perform or is unreliable. An example may be where multiple penetrating injuries in the same limb are present. Recently, high resolution multi-slice CT angiography has been used with a high accuracy rate approaching 94%[19]. This modality seems to be promising in the initial diagnosis of vascular extremity trauma.

23.1.3 Principles of Treatment

As with all high-grade open fractures, treatment goals should be stabilization of bone, adequate care of the soft tissue, wound coverage, and restoration of limb function. This is true both for diaphyseal as well as articular fractures [20].

Perhaps the most common known wound excision term has been "debridement" coined by Larrey in 1812. The original "debridement" implied incision and decompression of the wound [21], more likely to be a sort of fasciotomy [3] than the current mode of excisional surgery. While it is accepted that in many cases of low-velocity gunshots nonoperative treatment can succeed, most high-velocity (high-energy) wounds require some degree of surgical wound care. Whatever kind of excisional surgery is performed, it is now well accepted that the single most important factor in reducing the risk of infection is the timely administration of intravenous antibiotics [1, 3].

The degree of wound excision necessary for healing is highly controversial and remains one of the greatest challenges for the trauma surgeon. Although ideally, devitalized tissue should be removed in order to decrease the infection burden and to promote angiogenesis, it is clinically hard to judge which tissue warrants removal, especially in regards to muscle. In an experimental high energy gunshot model produced in pigs, extensive tract excision did not results in a better outcome than simple wound drainage and antibiotic treatment [11]. On the other hand, retaining devitalized tissue can result in necrosis and sepsis [22]. The four "Cs" – color, consistency, contractility and circulation – have served as a rough guideline for identification of dead muscle for generations of surgeons and are still valid today [10]. Attempts to correlate between gross findings associated with these "Cs" to microscopic findings yielded some inaccuracies (reference needed). This is related to temporary ischemia around the injury zone which resolves after a few hours [1]. Therefore, it is advised not to apply the *when in doubt, cut it out* regime, but rather to repeat wound exploration within 48–72 h, thus sparing more viable tissue [3]. Clearly, however, detached, devascularized, or contaminated tissue should be excised during the first session. Wounds traditionally are best left open initially, but closure should be considered early in order to improve joint motion and reduce stiffness, ideally not longer than 5–10 days after injury [10]. In case tension occurs, a primary skin graft should be used. Recently, vacuum assisted closure has become a powerful tool in reducing infection, promoting granulation, and expediting closure in war wounds, and is continuing to evolve rapidly [23]. This is especially helpful in situations where prolonged transport is expected, such as in remote war zones.

An increased rate of vascular injuries occurs in extremity fractures caused by gunshots [8]. Despite controversies about the sequence of fixation and vascular supply restoration, recent war experience demonstrates the advantage of immediate vascular temporary shunting, especially when prolonged and remote evacuation to a tertiary care center for definite treatment is expected [24].

23.1.4 Fracture Care

Most modern texts recommend treating gunshot-related fractures using the same surgical principles applied to open fractures caused by other mechanisms [1]. However, there are special considerations which are unique to these injuries and require alternative management strategies. Due to the limited scope of this chapter we will review only some of the important ones.

23.1.4.1 Long Bones

Traditionally, gunshot injuries were considered grossly contaminated and, therefore, external fixation was the mainstay of their treatment for many years. However, reports from the 1990s demonstrated the efficacy of immediate intramedullary nailing of femoral shaft fracture caused by low to mid-energy gunshot with acceptable clinical results [25]. These were supplanted with evidence that such treatment could be applied to higher-energy firearm trauma [26].

With femoral fractures, care should be taken to avoid rotational malalignment since comminution will often distort the anatomical landmarks such as the cortical step sign [27] used to judge femoral rotation (Fig. 23.1). Bone loss and tissue coverage are a major challenge for tibial fractures, especially involving the distal third, when soft tissue availability is scant. Due to these difficulties, our policy in high-energy gunshot wounds is to minimize bone debridement and preserve as much bone as possible. Treatment options then include rotational flaps, free tissue transfer, and immediate or late bone grafting [28–30]. All of these techniques can be used in conjunction with either internal

Fig. 23.1 (**a**) Gunshot fracture to a 25 years-old counter-terrorist fighter, caused by AK-47. (**b**) Three months following irrigation, debrident, and fixation with a proximal femoral nail (Synthes, Battlach, Switzerland) with no apparent wound complications. (**c**) Due to complaints of difficulty running and intoeing, a CT scanogram was performed and revealed almost a 40° internal rotation deformity. (**d**) Fracture revised by a derotation osteotomy and a reamed nail

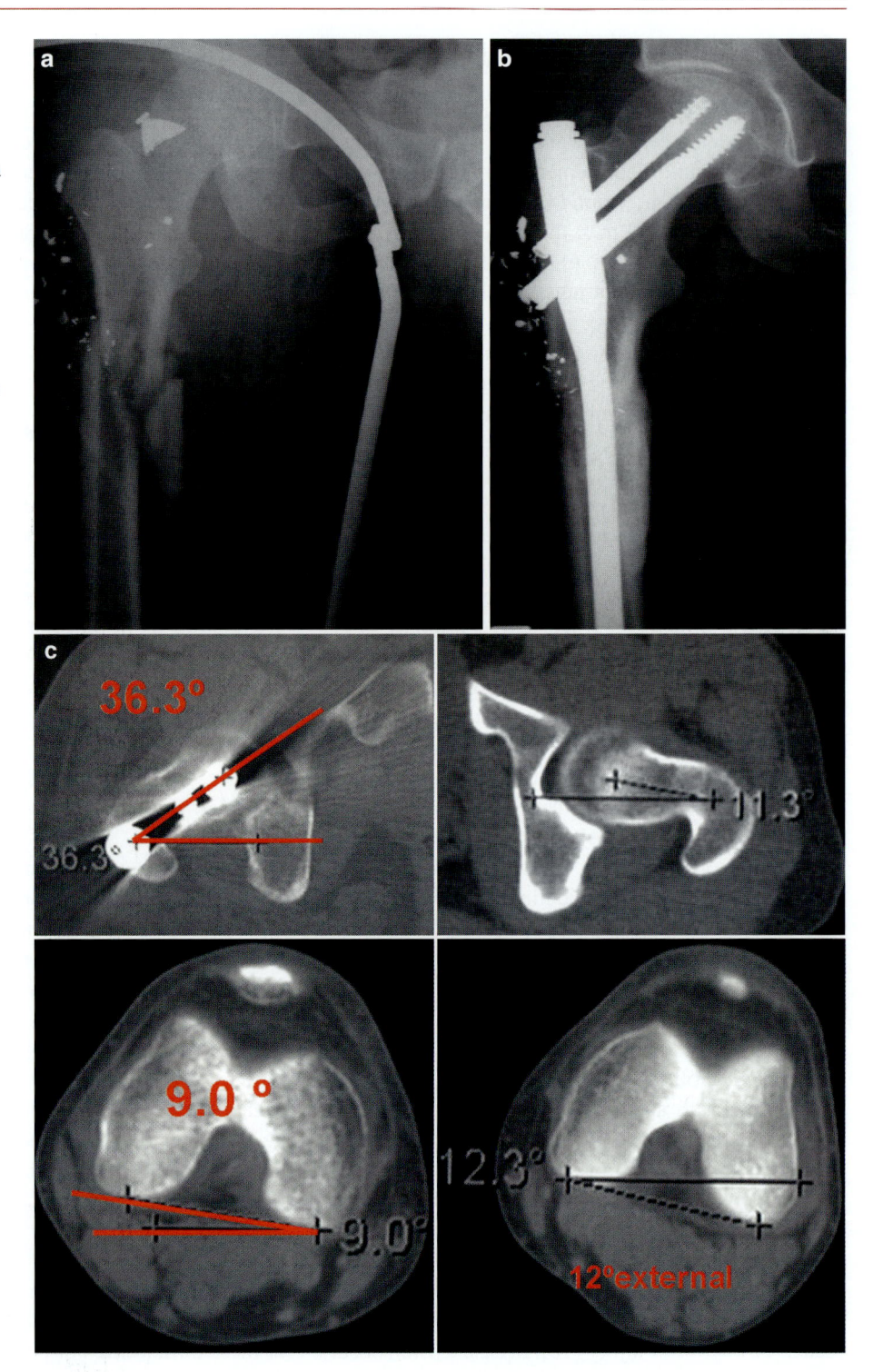

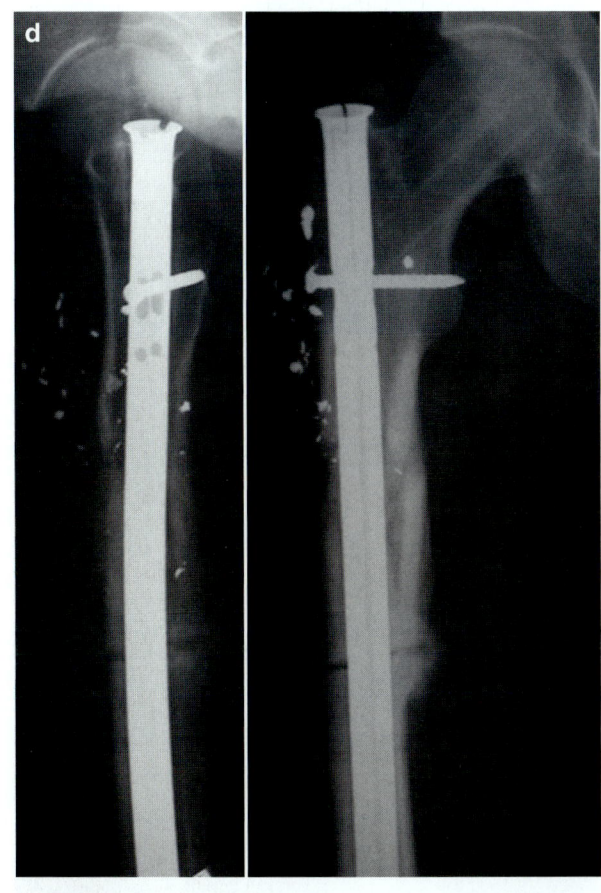

Fig. 23.1 (continued)

fixation or a circular frame for distraction osteogenesis (Fig. 23.2).

It should be noted, however, that even with a relatively high success rates when managing these fractures, the recovery period is excessive and associated with multiple reconstructive surgical procedures [31]. As with other mangled extremity injuries, the option for primary amputation should be considered. Increasingly, the bulk of modern reports, both civilian and military [32, 33], suggest that the use of "scoring systems" such as the MESS score, are inadequate. Most authorities now prefer to rely on the surgeon's experience and on the general condition of the gunshot victim as predictors for early amputation.

23.1.4.2 Joints

As with other articular fractures, joint reconstruction and stable fixation should become the primary goal of treatment. However, some unique considerations exist. First, due to the contaminated nature of the injury, either arthroscopic or open irrigation should be strongly considered even in cases where a joint space violation is only suspected [20]. A rare but a relevant example is the case where abdominal penetration occurred concomitant with pelvic or hip involvement. In these cases, contamination and joint sepsis would ultimately result in a catastrophic joint destruction.

Restoring metaphyseal comminution and building the articular block back to the shaft might be challenging in cases of severe comminution (Fig. 23.3), but efforts should be made to restore joint congruity in order to maintain function and early motion [20]. Finally, chronic retention of metallic foreign bodies can results either in a local reaction [34, 35], or in rare cases, in systemic toxicity, such as lead poisoning [36, 37]. These will mandate early removal even in asymptomatic patients.

23.2 Blast Injuries

The other penetrating trauma type relates to an explosion or blast. In the modern military setting, these are by far more common injuries than gunshot wounds [38]. Though not yet a leading etiological factor for civilian penetrating trauma in most industrialized countries, it is on a steady rise due to geopolitical reasons [39]. Despite the threat of chemical and biological warfare, conventional terrorism in the form of blasts is the most common form of attack, and results in a high causality rate [40]. Examples include the London subway attacks of 2005 [41], the Madrid train attacks of 2004 [42], as well as the succession of suicide bombing during the Palestinian uprising between 2000 and 2005 [43, 44].

Blast injuries are different from gunshots wounds mainly because of their multiple mechanisms of injury [15, 45, 46]. They tend to involve more body regions, and generally tend to be of higher severity scores, with increased overall potential for prolonged ICU stay and mortality [15, 47]. Although the surgical management of individual injuries may be similar to that of other types of trauma, the general management of these patients as individuals as well as in the context of mass-casualty event is worthy of consideration.

Fig. 23.2 (**a**) A 50-year old schizophrenic smoker was injured by an M-16 military assault rifle sustaining a grade III-B open distal tibial fracture. (**b**) After irrigation and debridment with attempt to preserve as much bone as possible, and immediate fixation with an unreamed tibial nail. (**c, d**) A year after a definite treatment that included further wound irrigation, latissimus dorsi free-flap, and iliac crest bone graft. Despite the imperfect ankle alignment, patient was doing clinically well and returned to function

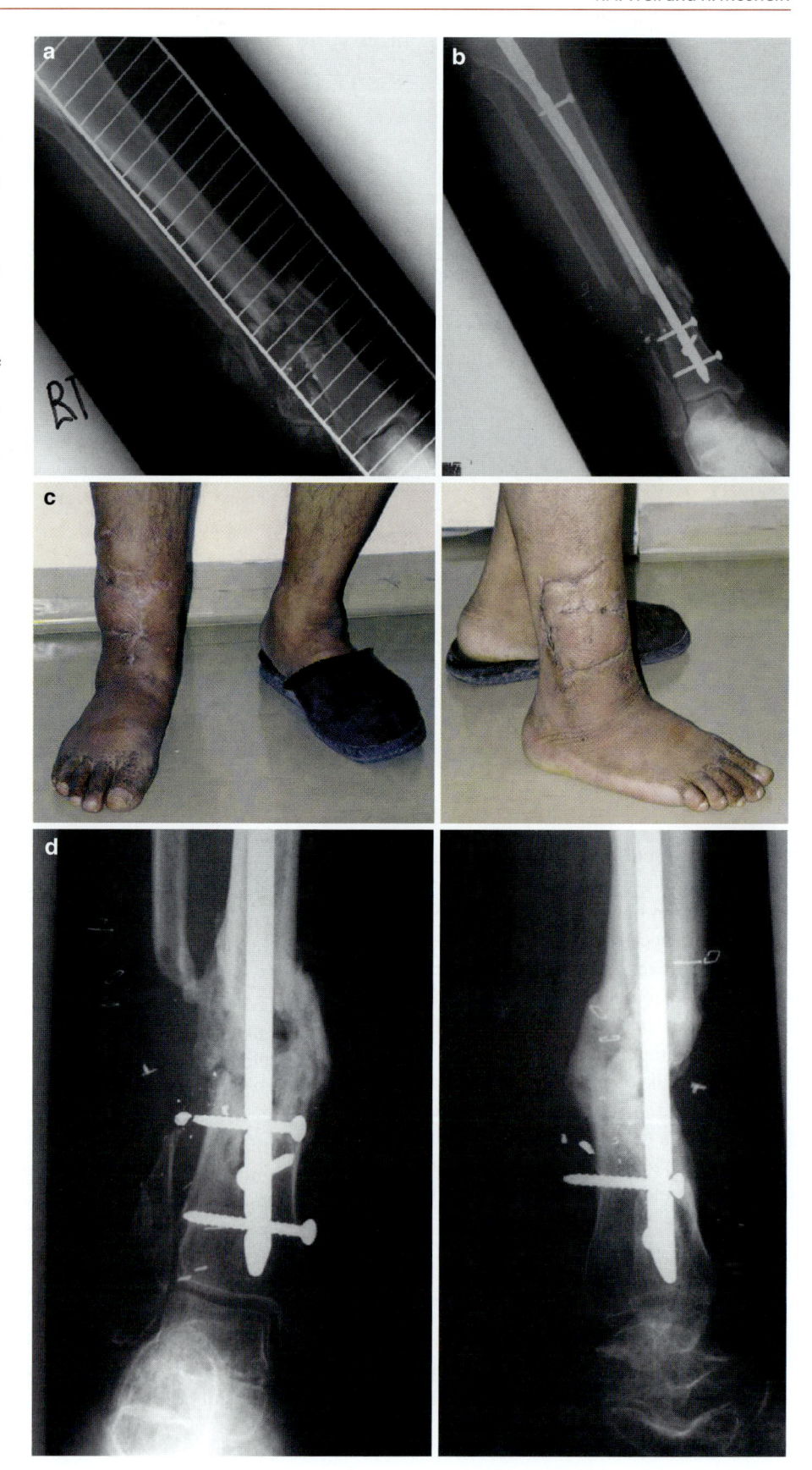

Fig. 23.3 (a) A 40-year old patient was shot in his left lower arm and treated elsewhere with an external fixator with attempted internal fixation and brought to us for evaluation. (b) A staged protocol was used – removal of external fixator and wound debridement, definite treatment using parallel locked 3.5 reconstruction plates and iliac crest bone graft. Eighteen months after injury, the fracture is solidly healed and the patient has a reasonable range of painless motion

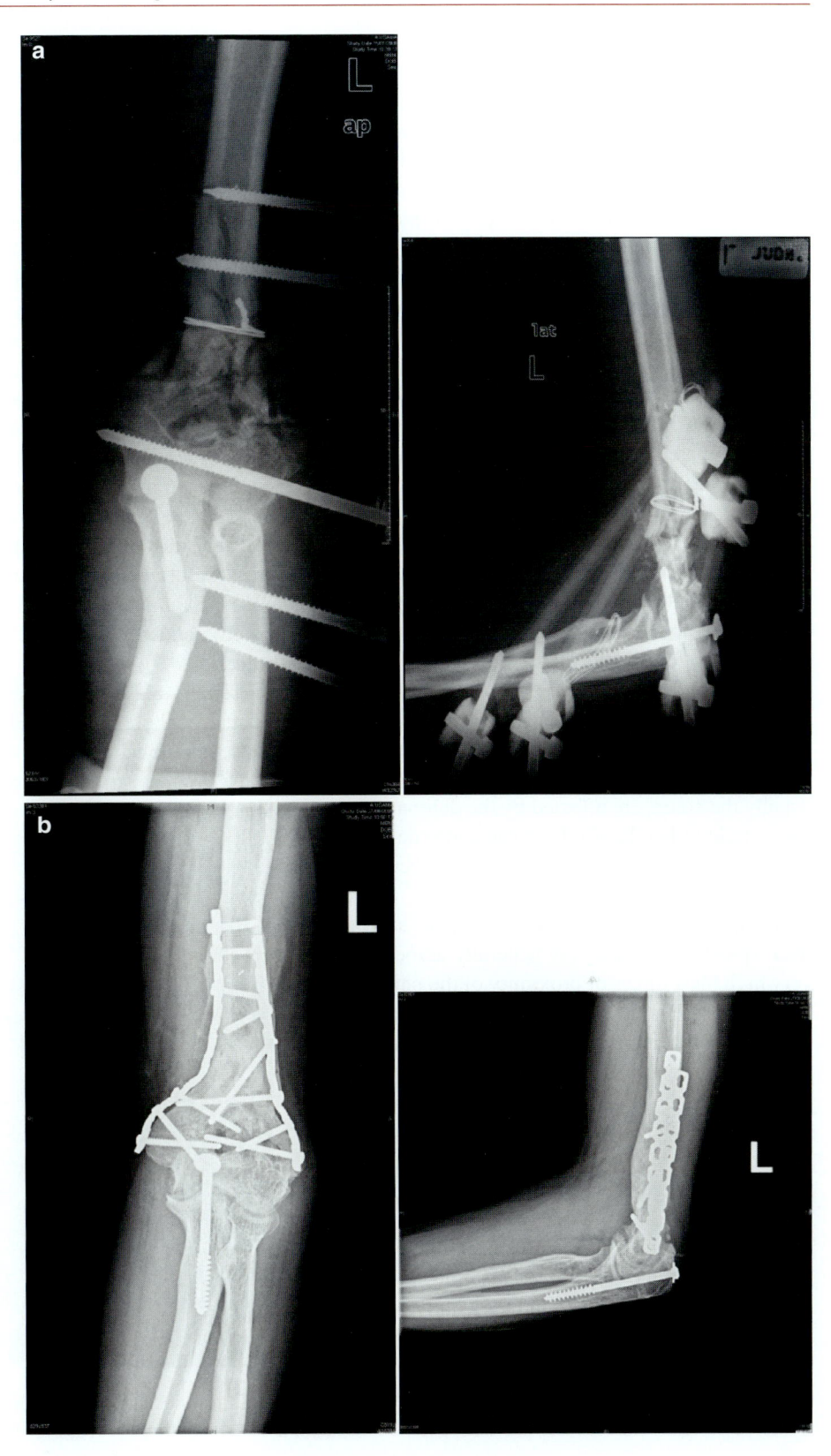

23.2.1 Mechanisms of Blast Injury

The primary blast effect is related to the rapid pressure wave created during the detonation of an explosive [48]. The scene location and type of explosive used have a direct effect on the severity of injuries. Blast wave energy tends to decrease rapidly in space and dissipate [49]. However, when the blast occurs in a closed or confined space, such in a bus or a room, the blast waves are reverberated from the walls instead of dissipating [49–51], thus inflicting more damage on human victims. In a series of suicide bombing in Israel occurring in buses during the years 1995–96, a threefold increase in primary blast injuries was observed when compared to those of open-space explosions, exemplifying this phenomenon [51].

When the pressure wave created by detonation encounters certain air-fluid interfaces, unique tissue damage may occur. The most common and perhaps the most life-threatening injury involve the lung. Pressure differentials across the alveolar-capillary interface can cause disruption, hemorrhage, pulmonary contusion, pneumothorax, hemothorax, pneumo-mediastinum, and subcutaneous emphysema [52].

The second most common type of primary blast injury is that to hollow viscera. The intestines, most usually the colon, are affected by the detonation wave. Mesenteric ischemia or infarct can cause delayed rupture of the large or the small intestine; these injuries are difficult to detect initially. Rupture, infarction, ischemia, and hemorrhage of solid organs such as the liver, spleen, and kidney are generally associated with very high blast forces or proximity of the patient to the blast center [53].

Tympanic membrane injury has been extensively discussed in the literature. It is the most common nonlethal injury caused by relatively low-pressure blast waves. Traditionally, its presence was used to predict severe primary blast injuries (such as the lung or bowel), yet it is now considered questionable and unreliable [54].

Limb injury due to a blast is rarely caused by the primary blast effect. Hull and Cooper studied primary blast effects on the extremities resulting in traumatic amputations in Northern Ireland [55]. Only 9 of 52 victims with traumatic amputations caused by primary blast survived, demonstrating the high level of energy needed to avulse a limb. Practically, a limb injury caused solely by the primary blast effect is a rare occurrence.

The secondary blast effects comprise the majority of orthopaedic injuries observed in both warfare [38, 56] and civilian terrorism [45, 57, 58]. Secondary blast effects are related to penetrating injuries caused by fragments ejected from the explosives and/or by foreign bodies impregnated within it. The extent of this effect depends on the subject's distance from the detonation center, the shape and size of the fragments, and the number of foreign bodies implanted or created by the explosive. In contrast to most war injuries, the improvised explosive devices (I.E.D.) used by terrorists have multiple added fragments, including screws, bolts, nails, and other objects, that may increase the damage caused by penetrating injuries (Fig. 23.4) [59]. Open fractures, severe soft tissue injuries, and multiorgan penetrating injury are the more common pattern seen in the severely injured victim [59, 60]. Unfortunately, these items are frequently coated in excrement before being inserted into the IED, and in many cases, flammable materials are applied as well. This has the added effect of severe burns as well as deep infections.

Tertiary blast injury refers to the blunt trauma component of the explosion. Flying or falling objects can cause additional traumatic elements to those described above. When structural collapse takes place, a high

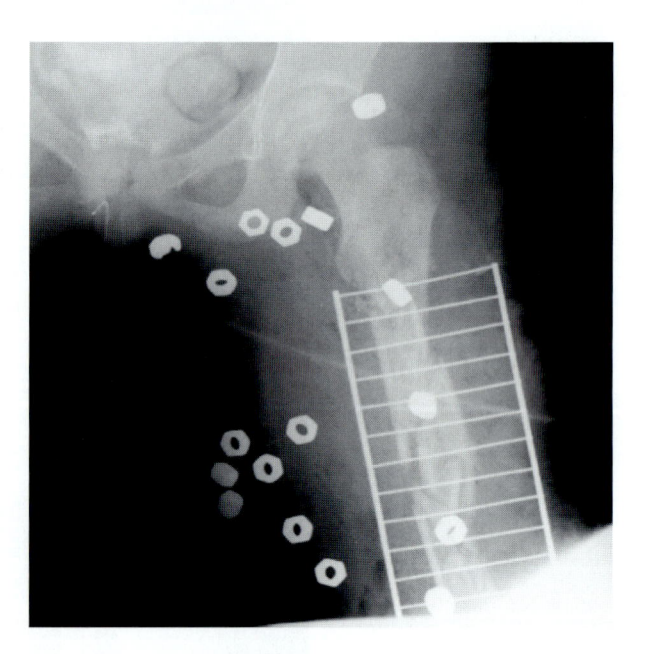

Fig. 23.4 A comminuted femoral fracture caused by secondary blast: note the numerous bolts implanted in the explosive

casualty and mortality event occurs [43]. Our experience in Israel in recent years did not demonstrate a significant proportion of additional blunt trauma, but reports from other parts of the world, such as those following the Oklahoma city explosion [61] or the Beirut Bombing in 1983 [62], state this as the primary mechanism of injury, as well as the cause of devastating results.

The quaternary blast effect is a recently added one, and includes the thermal and chemical damage caused by fire and noxious substances occurring at the vicinity of the explosion. Confined-space explosions significantly increase these types of injuries [51].

23.3 Triage and Primary Resuscitation

Perhaps the most significant difference between gunshots and the blast wounded, besides the individual injury pattern, is the "mass-casualty" effect caused by multiple military and civilian attacks. Instead of treating a single patient brought into the treating facility, the surgeons face a scenario of mass casualty and are required to simultaneously deal with multiple patients having multiple injuries. Hence, the initial effort should be to establish an orderly triage system and to allocate both the medical team and hospital resources even before the first patient arrives to the hospital [63, 64].

In the military setting, front medical teams using "damage-control" strategies and performing only emergency surgeries have recently been introduced, especially in the global war against terrorism [24]. Further procedures are then performed in secondary and tertiary centers after further triage and usually prolonged transportation. However, this is not the case in the civilian setting which is in the primary focus of this section.

At recent attacks, such in Jerusalem, Madrid, and London, evacuation time to a definite care facility ranged between 18 min and 1–2 h [46, 65, 66]. Some events, especially those on a large scale, described only a few severely injured patients in a majority of "walking wounded". The Middle East experience, such as in Jerusalem, paradoxically demonstrated that smaller bombing scenes resulted in overall less causalities, but a higher proportion of critically injured victims (four to eight per event) arriving in very short notice to treating facilities. These can significantly encumber the hospital resources available at that time point [43].

Logistics of Emergency Department management have a major impact on triage. We recommend evacuation of noncritical non-terror-related patients temporarily to the hospital floors, while the seriously ill patients can be treated in designated areas. The trauma bays are thus devoted solely to resuscitative efforts performed on critically ill patients, while the rest of the ED serves as an admitting area for the remainder of the patients. Each area is staffed with a surgeon-in-charge and other members of the treating team (surgical and orthopaedic residents, nurses, medical students, etc.). A surgeon-in- charge should be designated beforehand and should serve in critical junctions as suggested by Almogy et al. [65]. Triage at the initial admitting phase and in various treating cycles as well as diagnostics and direction of patients' flow until the general chaos is reduced must be accomplished. Every hospital should explore and identify the logistics mechanism required to provide the best and most efficient setting for disaster management under its capacity, should an actual disaster occur.

The next important principle in managing an event of this nature is to direct the flow of patients in an orderly fashion in a "one-way" system. Potential bottlenecks, such as in the CT scanner, ICUs, and limited number of available operating rooms, should be identified, and the patients should be directed to their proper destination only after the available resources of the hospital have been mapped and identified [43]. In many events, it was demonstrated that 50% of patients required either operative procedures or some sort of intensive care management in their initial or subsequent management [67]. Therefore, hospital management in such events should take these issues into consideration when preparing for a mass causality event involving blast injuries.

23.4 Treatment of Specific Injuries

Blast injuries to the extremities tend to be more varied and less predictable than gunshot wounds [15, 68]. The energy of the penetrating foreign body is extremely variable and greatly depends on the distance from the detonation center [38]. The existence of an extremity fracture, therefore, indicates a high-energy mechanism and has proven many times to implicate a polytrauma situation. This is in contrast to a gunshot patient, who can present with an extremity injury as a sole manifestation [15, 69]. In fact, one of the studies performed at our center correlated the mere existence of a fracture with life-risking conditions such as blast lung injury (BLI) [70]. Although more injuries are identified per patient with the blast injury as compared to a gunshot victim, the local injury pattern afflicted by the latter tends to be more severe, involve a higher rate of vascular injury, compartment syndrome, and higher-grade open fractures [15].

Despite the above, a recent study using a national database has shown that in most instances the treatment of individual blast injuries to the extremity is similar to gunshot wounds [71]. However, it should be stressed again that the overall care of patients is different.

In general, blast extremity injury involves multiple fracture sites as opposed to gunshot wounds, as well as a higher ISS and more associated life-threatening injuries [15, 71, 72]. In this context, the treatment plans and strategies of each patient should be meticulously defined. As more patients are simultaneously expedited to the operating room on an emergent basis, more orthopaedic teams should be available to undertake emergent procedures.

Damage control orthopaedic and soft-tissue strategies should generally be the rule in these cases since 70% of bone-injured blast patients have an ISS of >20 [68, 69] and are highly prone to prolonged ICU stay, respiratory failure, and coagulopathy [47, 72]. An orthopaedic surgeon-in-charge should direct the teams in decision making, but the first stage treatment plan should be limited since definitive reconstruction can occur in subsequent phases.

As in blunt polytrauma situations, tertiary surveys are extremely important in order to identify missed injuries, most of them of musculoskeletal in nature [73]. Significant number of fractures and foreign bodies requiring removal are identified during this process.

23.5 Specific Considerations

Most treatment principles described above are also true for blast injuries, especially regarding wound, vascular, and fracture treatment. However, specific considerations unique to blast injury in the civilian setting should also be applied. First, as mentioned above, a polytrauma situation dictates decision making in regard to staging of bone and soft-tissue treatment that is slightly different than that applied to the typical gunshot wounded victim (Fig. 23.5). Also, the metal load and the amount of foreign bodies in certain patients warrant removal, otherwise unnecessary in gunshot wounds. The mere removal can cause further soft tissue damage, thus mandating minimally invasive techniques. We reported the use of computerized navigation as well as metal detectors to attempt and minimize dissection involved in these removals [34, 74].

Lastly, the fact that more and more suicide bombers are involved in modern terrorism may increase the risk of biological contamination of the victims with tissues originating from the terrorists themselves, such as bone fragments [75]. Concerns of blood-borne infections such as Hepatitis B/C and HIV should be taken into consideration when dealing with suicide bombers [76].

23.6 Conclusions

As the new millennium begins, firearm and terror-related violence has not shown signs of decline, and instead, the world is facing a rise in casualties related to these mechanisms. Much has been learned during recent years regarding mechanisms of injury, scenarios of mass-casualty events, and treatment strategies. Despite this reality, the principles of treating an isolated penetrating injury, such as gunshot wound, and multiple penetrating limb injuries, such as blast, are not yet part of the standard medical education of the orthopaedic surgeon. Keeping in mind that no part of the world is immune at this point to these devastating injuries, research and investigation of outcome and treatment strategies are in strong need, as well as internalization of the current knowledge and principles among the orthopedic- and trauma-surgeons community.

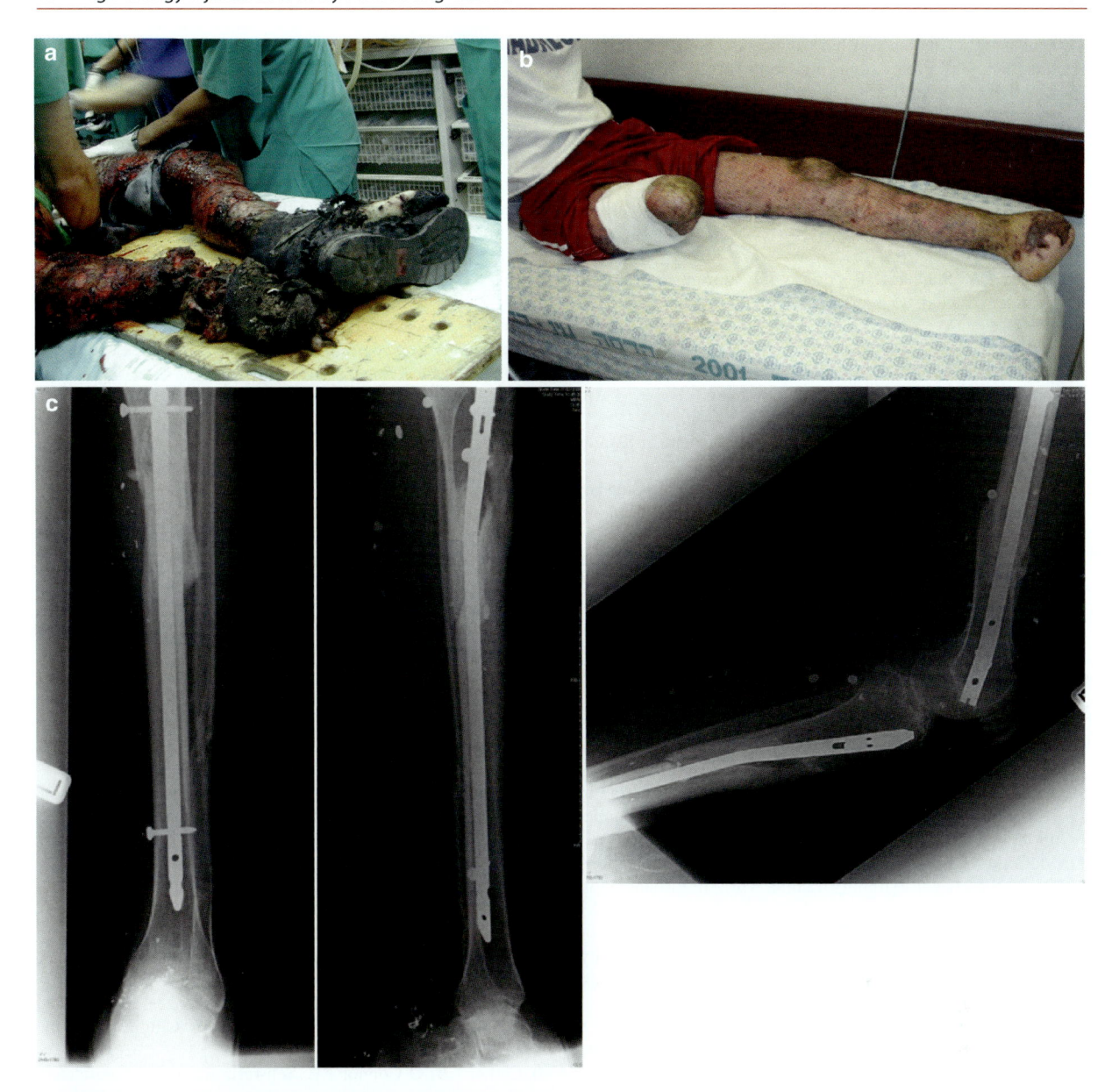

Fig. 23.5 (**a**) A 19-year old male standing next to a suicide bomber: injury resulted in traumatic above knee amputation on the right, distal femoral and tibial fractures on the left, as well as a lisfranc midfoot amputation at the left. (**b**) Soft tissues almost healed at 3 months post injury after numerous reconstructive attempts. (**c**) Healed tibial and femoral fractures on the left 2 years after initial injury

References

1. Bartlett CS. Clinical update: gunshot wound ballistics. Clin Orthop Relat Res. 2003;408:28–57.
2. Almogy G, Rivkind AI. Terror in the 21st century: milestones and prospects – part I. Curr Probl Surg. 2007;44:496–554.
3. Fackler ML. Gunshot wound review. Ann Emerg Med. 1996;28:194–203.

4. Fackler ML. Civilian gunshot wounds and ballistics: dispelling the myths. Emerg Med Clin North Am. 1998;16:17–28.
5. Liu YQ, Chen XY, Li SG, et al. Wounding effects of small fragments of different shapes at different velocities on soft tissues of dogs. J Trauma. 1988;28:S95–8.
6. Fackler ML, Malinowski JA. Ordnance gelatin for ballistic studies. Detrimental effect of excess heat used in gelatin preparation. Am J Forensic Med Pathol. 1988;9:218–9.
7. Dimond Jr FC, Rich NM. M-16 rifle wounds in Vietnam. J Trauma. 1967;7:619–25.
8. Volgas DA, Stannard JP, Alonso JE. Current orthopaedic treatment of ballistic injuries. Injury. 2005;36:380–6.
9. Hopkinson DA, Marshall TK. Firearm injuries. Br J Surg. 1967;54:344–53.
10. Bartlett CS, Helfet DL, Hausman MR, et al. Ballistics and gunshot wounds: effects on musculoskeletal tissues. J Am Acad Orthop Surg. 2000;8:21–36.
11. Fackler ML. Wound ballistics: the management of assault rifle injuries. Mil Med. 1990;155:222–5.
12. Hollerman JJ, Fackler ML, Coldwell DM, et al. Gunshot wounds: 1. Bullets, ballistics, and mechanisms of injury. AJR Am J Roentgenol. 1990;155:685–90.
13. Omer Jr GE. Injuries to nerves of the upper extremity. J Bone Joint Surg Am. 1974;56:1615–24.
14. Tian HM, Deng GG, Huang MJ, et al. Quantitative bacteriological study of the wound track. J Trauma. 1988;28: S215–6.
15. Weil YA, Petrov K, Liebergall M, et al. Long bone fractures caused by penetrating injuries in terrorists attacks. J Trauma. 2007;62:909–12.
16. Dennis JW, Frykberg ER, Veldenz HC, et al. Validation of nonoperative management of occult vascular injuries and accuracy of physical examination alone in penetrating extremity trauma: 5- to 10-year follow-up. J Trauma. 1998;44:243–52; discussion 242-243.
17. McCorkell SJ, Harley JD, Morishima MS, et al. Indications for angiography in extremity trauma. AJR Am J Roentgenol. 1985;145:1245–7.
18. Frykberg ER, Crump JM, Vines FS, et al. A reassessment of the role of arteriography in penetrating proximity extremity trauma: a prospective study. J Trauma. 1989;29:1041–50; discussion 1050-1042.
19. White PW, Gillespie DL, Feurstein I, et al. Sixty-four slice multidetector computed tomographic angiography in the evaluation of vascular trauma. J Trauma. 2010;68:96–102.
20. Dougherty PJ, Vaidya R, Silverton CD, et al. Joint and long-bone gunshot injuries. J Bone Joint Surg Am. 2009;91:980–97.
21. Cleveland M, Manning JG, Stewart WJ. Care of battle casualties and injuries involving bones and joints. J Bone Joint Surg Am. 1951;33-A:517–27.
22. Mendelson JA. The relationship between mechanisms of wounding and principles of treatment of missile wounds. J Trauma. 1991;31:1181–202.
23. ET P. The role of negative pressure wound therapy with reticulated open cell foam in the treatment of war wounds. J Orthop Trauma. 2008;22:S138–41.
24. Gifford SM, Aidinian G, Clouse WD, et al. Effect of temporary shunting on extremity vascular injury: an outcome analysis from the Global War on Terror vascular injury initiative. J Vasc Surg. 2009;50:549–55; discussion 555-546.
25. Nowotarski P, Brumback RJ. Immediate interlocking nailing of fractures of the femur caused by low- to mid-velocity gunshots. J Orthop Trauma. 1994;8:134–41.
26. Nicholas RM, McCoy GF. Immediate intramedullary nailing of femoral shaft fractures due to gunshots. Injury. 1995;26: 257–9.
27. Langer JS, Gardner MJ, Ricci WM. The cortical step sign as a tool for assessing and correcting rotational deformity in femoral shaft fractures. J Orthop Trauma. 2010;24:82–8.
28. Atesalp AS, Yildiz C, Basbozkurt M, et al. Treatment of type IIIa open fractures with Ilizarov fixation and delayed primary closure in high-velocity gunshot wounds. Mil Med. 2002;167:56–62.
29. Tropet Y, Garbuio P, Obert L, et al. One-stage emergency treatment of open grade IIIB tibial shaft fractures with bone loss. Ann Plast Surg. 2001;46:113–9.
30. Hutson Jr JJ, Dayicioglu D, Oeltjen JC, et al. The treatment of Gustilo grade IIIB tibia fractures with application of antibiotic spacer, flap, and sequential distraction osteogenesis. Ann Plast Surg. 2010;64:541–52.
31. Celikoz B, Sengezer M, Isik S, et al. Subacute reconstruction of lower leg and foot defects due to high velocity-high energy injuries caused by gunshots, missiles, and land mines. Microsurgery. 2005;25:3–14; discussion 15.
32. Bosse MJ, MacKenzie EJ, Kellam JF, et al. A prospective evaluation of the clinical utility of the lower-extremity injury-severity scores. J Bone Joint Surg Am. 2001;83-A:3–14.
33. Brown KV, Ramasamy A, McLeod J, et al. Predicting the need for early amputation in ballistic mangled extremity injuries. J Trauma. 2009;66:S93–7; discussion S97-98.
34. Peyser A, Khoury A, Liebergall M. Shrapnel management. J Am Acad Orthop Surg. 2006;14:S66–70.
35. Eylon S, Mosheiff R, Liebergall M, et al. Delayed reaction to shrapnel retained in soft tissue. Injury. 2005;36:275–81.
36. Peh WC, Reinus WR. Lead arthropathy: a cause of delayed onset lead poisoning. Skeletal Radiol. 1995;24:357–60.
37. Linden MA, Manton WI, Stewart RM, et al. Lead poisoning from retained bullets. Pathogenesis, diagnosis, and management. Ann Surg. 1982;195:305–13.
38. Covey DC. Blast and fragment injuries of the musculoskeletal system. J Bone Joint Surg Am. 2002;84-A:1221.
39. Stein M, Hirshberg A. Medical consequences of terrorism. The conventional weapon threat. Surg Clin North Am. 1999;79:1537–52.
40. Lerner EB, O'Connor RE, Schwartz R, et al. Blast-related injuries from terrorism: an international perspective. Prehosp Emerg Care. 2007;11:137–53.
41. Aylwin CJ, Konig TC, Brennan NW, et al. Reduction in critical mortality in urban mass casualty incidents: analysis of triage, surge, and resource use after the London bombings on July 7, 2005. Lancet. 2006;368:2219–25.
42. Gutierrez de Ceballos JP, Turegano Fuentes F, Perez Diaz D, et al. Casualties treated at the closest hospital in the Madrid, March 11, terrorist bombings. Crit Care Med. 2005;33:S107–12.
43. Shamir MY, Rivkind A, Weissman C, et al. Conventional terrorist bomb incidents and the intensive care unit. Curr Opin Crit Care. 2005;11:580–4.
44. Shapira SC, Adatto-Levi R, Avitzour M, et al. Mortality in terrorist attacks: a unique modal of temporal death distribution. World J Surg. 2006;30:2071–7; discussion 2078-2079.

45. Peleg K, Aharonson-Daniel L. Blast injuries. N Engl J Med. 2005;352:2651–3; author reply 2651-2653.
46. Peleg K, Aharonson-Daniel L, Michael M, et al. Patterns of injury in hospitalized terrorist victims. Am J Emerg Med. 2003;21:258–62.
47. Kluger Y, Peleg K, Daniel-Aharonson L, et al. The special injury pattern in terrorist bombings. J Am Coll Surg. 2004;199:875–9.
48. Wightman JM, Gladish SL. Explosions and blast injuries. Ann Emerg Med. 2001;37:664–78.
49. Arnold JL, Halpern P, Tsai MC, et al. Mass casualty terrorist bombings: a comparison of outcomes by bombing type. Ann Emerg Med. 2004;43:263–73.
50. DePalma RG, Burris DG, Champion HR, et al. Blast injuries. N Engl J Med. 2005;352:1335–42.
51. Leibovici D, Gofrit ON, Stein M, et al. Blast injuries: bus versus open-air bombings – a comparative study of injuries in survivors of open-air versus confined-space explosions. J Trauma. 1996;41:1030–5.
52. Mellor SG, Cooper GJ. Analysis of 828 servicemen killed or injured by explosion in Northern Ireland 1970–84: the Hostile Action Casualty System. Br J Surg. 1989;76:1006–10.
53. Almogy G, Mintz Y, Zamir G, et al. Suicide bombing attacks: can external signs predict internal injuries? Ann Surg. 2006;243:541–6.
54. Leibovici D, Gofrit ON, Shapira SC. Eardrum perforation in explosion survivors: is it a marker of pulmonary blast injury? Ann Emerg Med. 1999;34:168–72.
55. Hull JB, Cooper GJ. Pattern and mechanism of traumatic amputation by explosive blast. J Trauma. 1996;40:S198–205.
56. Covey DC. Combat orthopaedics: a view from the trenches. J Am Acad Orthop Surg. 2006;14:S10–7.
57. Barham M. Blast injuries. N Engl J Med. 2005;352:2651–3; author reply 2651-2653.
58. Ashkenazi I, Olsha O, Alfici R. Blast injuries. N Engl J Med. 2005;352:2651–3; author reply 2651-2653.
59. Ad-El DD, Eldad A, Mintz Y, et al. Suicide bombing injuries: the Jerusalem experience of exceptional tissue damage posing a new challenge for the reconstructive surgeon. Plast Reconstr Surg. 2006;118:383–7; discussion 388-389.
60. Aharonson-Daniel L, Klein Y, Peleg K. Suicide bombers form a new injury profile. Ann Surg. 2006;244:1018–23.
61. Teague DC. Mass casualties in the Oklahoma City bombing. Clin Orthop Relat Res. 2004;422:77–81.
62. Scott BA, Fletcher JR, Pulliam MW, et al. The Beirut terrorist bombing. Neurosurgery. 1986;18:107–10.
63. Hirshberg A, Scott BG, Granchi T, et al. How does casualty load affect trauma care in urban bombing incidents? A quantitative analysis. J Trauma. 2005;58:686–93. discussion 694–685.
64. Hirshberg A, Stein M, Walden R. Surgical resource utilization in urban terrorist bombing: a computer simulation. J Trauma. 1999;47:545–50.
65. Almogy G, Belzberg H, Mintz Y, et al. Suicide bombing attacks: update and modifications to the protocol. Ann Surg. 2004;239:295–303.
66. Einav S, Feigenberg Z, Weissman C, et al. Evacuation priorities in mass casualty terror-related events: implications for contingency planning. Ann Surg. 2004;239:304–10.
67. de Ceballos JP, Turegano-Fuentes F, Perez-Diaz D, et al. 11 March 2004: The terrorist bomb explosions in Madrid, Spain – an analysis of the logistics, injuries sustained and clinical management of casualties treated at the closest hospital. Crit Care. 2005;9:104–11.
68. Weil YA, Mosheiff R, Liebergall M. Blast and penetrating fragment injuries to the extremities. J Am Acad Orthop Surg. 2006;14:S136–9.
69. Weil YA, Peleg K, Givon A, et al. Musculoskeletal injuries in terrorist attacks – a comparison between the injuries sustained and those related to motor vehicle accidents, based on a national registry database. Injury. 2008;39:1359–64.
70. Almogy G, Luria T, Richter E, et al. Can external signs of trauma guide management?: Lessons learned from suicide bombing attacks in Israel. Arch Surg. 2005;140:390–3.
71. Weil Y, Peleg K, Givon A, ITG, Mosheiff R. Penetrating and orthopaedic trauma from blast vs. gunshots caused by terrorism – Israel's National experience. J Orthop Trauma. 2011, Mar 25(3);145-9.
72. Peleg K, Aharonson-Daniel L, Stein M, et al. Gunshot and explosion injuries: characteristics, outcomes, and implications for care of terror-related injuries in Israel. Ann Surg. 2004;239:311–8.
73. Buduhan G, McRitchie DI. Missed injuries in patients with multiple trauma. J Trauma. 2000;49:600–5.
74. Mosheiff R, Weil Y, Khoury A, et al. The use of computerized navigation in the treatment of gunshot and shrapnel injury. Comput Aided Surg. 2004;9:39–43.
75. Leibner ED, Weil Y, Gross E, et al. A broken bone without a fracture: traumatic foreign bone implantation resulting from a mass casualty bombing. J Trauma. 2005;58:388–90.
76. Wong JM, Marsh D, Abu-Sitta G, et al. Biological foreign body implantation in victims of the London July 7th suicide bombings. J Trauma. 2006;60:402–4.

Management of Traumatic Bone Defects

Richard P. Meinig

Contents

24.1	Introduction	295
24.2	**Traumatic Bone Defect Treatment Algorithm**	296
24.2.1	Phase I: Initial Patient Management	296
24.2.2	Phase II: Interim Management – Skeletal Fixation and Definitive Soft Tissue Coverage	297
24.2.3	Phase III: Final Bone Defect Reconstitution	297
24.3	Clinical Case	299
References		303

R.P. Meinig
Front Range Orthopaedics Association, 175 Union,
Suite 200, Colorado Springs, CO 80910, USA
e-mail: rmeinig@comcast.net

24.1 Introduction

Traumatic bone loss has long been a challenging clinical problem. Contemporary techniques in the management of acute bone stabilization, revascularization, and soft tissue reconstruction have led to an increase in limb salvage [1]. There are numerous options in reconstruction of bone defects. Generally, the management of bone defects can be divided into two approaches. The first approach involves reconstitution of a bone defect that has been stabilized in situ by autologous bone grafting or one of its variations. The second approach involves distraction osteogenesis. The two approaches are not mutually exclusive but have their relative indications and difficulties. Distraction osteogenesis therapy is generally more protracted, technically very challenging, and accompanied by high complication rates [2]. However, distraction osteogenesis can be spectacularly successful in the simultaneous management of soft tissue coverage, bone defect, and spatial deformity. Because of the complexity of frame construction, pin site management, patient compliance, and duration of treatment, distraction osteogenesis procedures are perhaps best reserved for specialty clinics. Management of bone defects by skeletal stabilization, early soft tissue coverage, and by autologous reconstruction utilizes implants, techniques, and resources that are widely available. This chapter presents a summary of contemporary techniques that allow for the primary therapy of complex traumatic bone loss.

24.2 Traumatic Bone Defect Treatment Algorithm

I. *Initial Patient Resuscitation*: Resuscitation, Revascularization, Bone and Soft tissue debridement, Provisional or definitive skeletal stabilization, Wound Therapy. Days 1–3.
II. *Interim Management with Skeletal Fixation*: Definitive Soft Tissue Therapy, Conversion to definitive Skeletal Stabilization + bone defect/dead space management. Days 3–28.
III. *Final Bone Defect Reconstitution*: Autologous reconstruction with cancellous bone, vascularized graft, marrow aspirate, intramedullary harvest, growth factor application, bone graft substitute augmentation. Weeks 2–6.

24.2.1 Phase I: Initial Patient Management

Trauma that produces bone defect is frequently high energy and therefore associated with mortality and morbidity of visceral or traumatic brain injury. Assessment of the long bone injury determines whether the limb is viable and should be amputated versus limb salvage. Considerations for limb salvage are obviously complex and efforts to quantitate the injury in regards to amputation such as the Mangled Extremity Severity Scale (MESS) or the Orthopaedic Trauma Association Limb Evaluation and Assessment Protocol (LEAP) are often helpful but not definitive [3, 4]. Limb salvage requires a limb in which vascularity can be reestablished, adequate neurologic function in terms of sensation and motor, viable muscle–tendon groups, and soft tissues–bone injury in which sepsis can be ultimately ablated. The actual extent of bone loss that limits limb salvage has yet to be defined regardless of reconstruction technique. In addition to the biological factors, the patient's psychosocial systems need to be evaluated as reconstruction and limb salvage is a relatively long process possibly requiring multiple surgical interventions, medical therapies, rehabilitation, and patient compliance.

The initial management of a limb deemed suitable for limb salvage will consist of emergent resuscitation of the patient. Priority for reestablishing hemodynamic stability and managing the closed head injury component will frequently preclude definitive skeletal stabilization. The concept of "damage control orthopaedics" has recently emerged in which spanning external fixation or unreamed intramedullary nailing is expediently performed to limit the anesthetic time and reduce pulmonary exposure to medullary canal contents in severely injured patients [5]. When performed under these circumstances, pin sites and implants should be chosen to allow for subsequent definitive fixation and stabilization of the bone defect. Conversion to definitive fixation should be performed as soon as feasible to minimize potential septic seeding from external fixation pin sites – generally less than 10 days. Stabilization of open fractures with intramedullary nails has been validated to be acceptable in terms of infection risk [6]. In general, locked intramedullary stabilization of a diaphyseal and some metaphyseal defects is preferred as length, rotation, and axial alignment can be reestablished and maintained in a single procedure. The intramedullary nail allows for immediate rehabilitation of the limb in near-anatomic position. In addition, the Intramedullary (IM) nail has the biomechanical advantages of strength and symmetric load sharing in comparison to plates. The locked plate is a relatively recent development which allows for improved mechanical stability in situations of poor bone quality, bone defect or comminution, and articular fracture patterns associated with metaphyseal or diaphyseal extension. Plate fixation can be performed with minimal exposure to provide stable bridging constructs for the management of bone defects. If a limb requires vascular repair, plate or IM nail fixation needs to be coordinated with the vascular reconstruction to provide a stable environment for the repair as well as utilize the surgical exposure if indicated. An essential early step in the management of a bone defect is the initial debridements of bone and soft tissue. The initial debridements are likely to reduce the septic burden and reestablish soft tissue viability in the shortest time. The principles of debridement are well established and consist of excision and removal of nonviable osseous and soft tissues. Serial debridements are frequently required to discern borderline tissues on a clinical basis. The decision of implant and technique is therefore dictated by patient hemodynamic and neurologic status, concomitant vascular repair, tissue and bone debridement, and soft tissue coverage. Initial management of the bone defect is directed at managing the dead space of the defect in preparation for soft tissue coverage and bone reconstitution. During debridements, the defect can be provisionally managed with commercially available PMMA-antibiotic beads or surgeon-fabricated PMMA-antibiotic spacers. The PMMA-antibiotic beads or PMMA-spacers can be serially exchanged during debridements to aid in reducing deep sepsis and has been well described [7].

In summary, the initial phase consists of patient resuscitation with provisional or possibly definitive fixation of the skeletal defect. This is combined with establishment of a sterile bone defect and clean wound by surgical debridement and soft tissue wound care. The time line would be days 1–3.

24.2.2 Phase II: Interim Management – Skeletal Fixation and Definitive Soft Tissue Coverage

After the patient has been resuscitated, efforts can be directed at limb reconstruction. If the limb has been treated with spanning external fixation, conversion to IM nail or plate implant can be performed – generally within 10 days. At this point, soft tissue coverage should be obtained either by wound closure, wound-vac therapy, or local/free flap coverage. Early soft tissue reconstitution aids in the prevention of deep sepsis as well as preparing an environment advantageous for bone grafting. The bone defect can be managed either primarily with early bone grafting or vascularized bone transfer. However, the cultivation of an "induced membrane" has clinical and basic science advantages for delaying definitive autologous bone transfer into segmental defects for a period of 4–6 weeks [8, 9].

Conversion from spanning external fixation or provisional stabilization to definitive implant fixation should restore the limb to near-anatomic length, axial alignment, and rotation. The definitive implant should have sufficient mechanical properties to function during the duration of bone reconstruction. With early restoration and maintenance of the limb in anatomic position, patient comfort, rehabilitation, and function are greatly enhanced – a distinct advantage over distraction osteogenesis.

The keystone step during the Interim Management Phase is perhaps the reestablishment of an environment amenable to successful bone grafting. Animal studies and clinical studies indicate that a biologically active membrane that facilitates bone regeneration can be induced by the temporary implantation of a Polymethylmethacrylate Cement (PMMA) cement spacer. Histological, immunohistochemical, and biochemical assay in animal models demonstrate that by 4–6 weeks, a fibrous, highly vascularized, growth factor–rich encapsulating membrane has encapsulated about the PMMA spacer. At 4–6 weeks postimplantation, vascular endothelial growth factor (VEGF), transforming growth factor (TGF-beta), bone morphogenetic protein-2 (BMP-2) are at peaking levels within the membrane [10]. Autologous bone techniques may therefore optimally be performed at 4–6 weeks post-PMMA spacer implantation. The technique is easily performed. PMMA cement is prepared, and a tubular or appropriately shaped spacer is fabricated to span the defect and overlap the native bone ends. Antibiotic cement can be utilized as an adjunct to around the bone defect to prevent deep sepsis. Commercial antibiotic-PMMA mixtures that are available for primary total joint arthroplasty can be utilized (Biomet, Warsaw, IN; Zimmer, Warsaw, IN; and Stryker, Mahwah, NJ). The surgeon, however, can prepare PMMA with higher amounts of added heat-stable antibiotic to produce a bactericidal spacer [11].

In summary, the interim phase consists of obtaining: (1) early definitive internal fixation to stabilize the bone defect and limb in near-anatomic alignment and (2) preparation of a sterile osteogenic defect for osseous regeneration. A stable soft tissue environment is reestablished by wound closure or flap coverage if needed. In many cases, an induced membrane is formed by the temporary implantation of bulk PMMA with planned autologous grafting at approximately 4 weeks.

24.2.3 Phase III: Final Bone Defect Reconstitution

Autologous bone grafting remains the gold standard in the reconstitution of bone defects. Autograft is the only material that provides osteogenic cells (osteocytes, osteoblasts, marrow stem cells), osteoconductive matrix (inorganic mineral), and osteoinductive molecules (BMP's, transforming growth factor-beta, vascular endothelial growth factor, and others) [12].

There are many techniques described for bone graft harvest including iliac graft harvest, local cancellous bone harvest, bone marrow aspirations and concentration, vascularized fibula, and most recently, intramedullary canal harvest (Reamed Irrigator Aspirator-Synthes, Inc., West Chester, PA) [13–17]. In addition to autologous bone harvest, there are commercially available sources for recombinant osteoinductive bone morphogenetic proteins (BMP-7/OP01 and BMP-2).

The primary limiting factor in autologous bone transplant has been reported morbidity and complications associated with the harvest site as well as adequate volume for large defects. With defects of 2 cm or less, traditional anterior iliac crest bone graft is usually sufficient as 5–72 mL can be harvested [13]. Larger defects can still be grafted with iliac crest by multiple harvest sites such as the contra lateral site or use of the posterior iliac crests with amounts of 25–90 mL being obtained [13]. In addition, the use of a small acetabular reamer may result in less donor site pain and larger volume of graft [14].

The most recent development in autologous harvest techniques is the intramedullary canal harvest. A recent review confirms that the use of the Reamed Irrigator Aspirator (RIA) in a single pass reaming of the femur produces significant amounts of bone graft (25–90 mL) with low rates of complications and postoperative pain [13]. While the rate of complication is lower than that described in conventional in iliac harvest, iatrogenic femur fracture has occurred. In addition, studies of RIA harvest material suggest that it is rich in growth factors, viable cells, and morselized trabecular bone [15]. The RIA harvest can thus be considered biologically equivalent to iliac graft. The bone marrow harvest, however, lacks any structural properties that can be achieved with tricortical iliac harvest.

In addition to autologous bone graft, bone graft substitutes can be utilized to augment the autograft harvest. Bone graft substitutes include osteoconductive materials such as synthetic tricalcium phosphates, calcium sulfates, and coral. These materials are fabricated as granules, blocks, strips, putties, and pastes. However, the efficacy of these materials as stand-alone graft in segmental defects is unknown [18]. Similarly, there are currently at least 40 commercial preparations of Demineralized Bone Matrix (DBM). Demineralized bone matrix is an acid extract of human cadaveric bone consisting largely of type I collagen and other acid-stable proteins including bone morphogenetic proteins. The osteoinductive content of the Demineralized bone matrix is low and subject to the variables of donor biological activity, processing, and carrier [16]. The osteoconductive properties of the various commercial Demineralized bone matrix's relate to carrier chemistry, adjunctive inorganic additives such as cadaveric cancellous bone or synthetic mineral. At present, there are no prospective studies proving the benefits of Demineralized bone matrix for the reconstruction of segmental bone defect. The primary use of Demineralized bone matrix may be as an extender for autologous bone harvests such as intramedullary reaming harvest, cancellous bone, or marrow aspirates and concentrates [16]. The role of recombinant bone morphogenetic proteins in bone defect reconstruction continues to evolve [19]. The high cost, carrier characteristics, biological activity, and mechanical qualities of available commercial BMP preparations limit its use at present mainly to small cortical defects and acute open tibia fractures (Infuse rhBMP-2, Medtronic, Memphis, TN; Op-1/rhBMP-7, Stryker, Mahwah, NJ).

There are numerous options for the application of the autologous bone graft. Defects up to 29 cm have been successfully grafted using the induced membrane technique as described recently by Masquelet [9]. At 4–6 weeks post-PMMA block implantation, the block is removed by longitudinally incising the encapsulating membrane. Autologous bone in the form of iliac graft or RIA bone marrow harvest, or autologous bone–bone substitute or autologous bone-allograft mixture is then used to fill the resulting cavity. A defect stabilized with an intramedullary nail will require less bone graft volume than defects stabilized with external fixation or plate constructs. A resorbable polylactide membrane can also be used to shape and contain the graft for applications such as the distal tibia and femur. In addition, resorbable membranes can be used to contain the graft in applications near the spinal cord, interosseous membrane of the forearm, or other applications where the reconstruction needs to be precisely configured [20]. The polymeric membrane may be used where bone grafting is done primarily such as the reconstruction of an unstable thoracic burst fracture where cancellous bone graft is combined with a

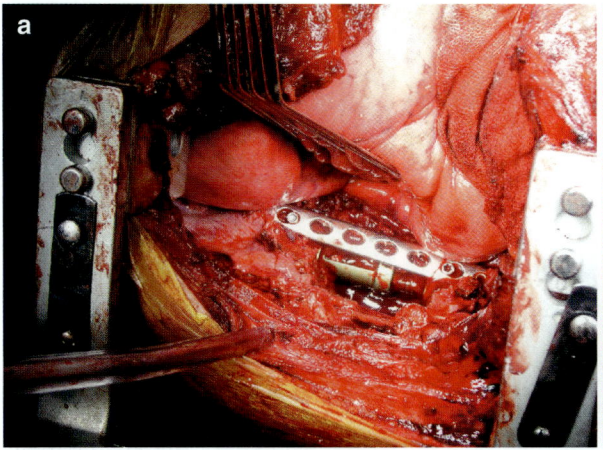

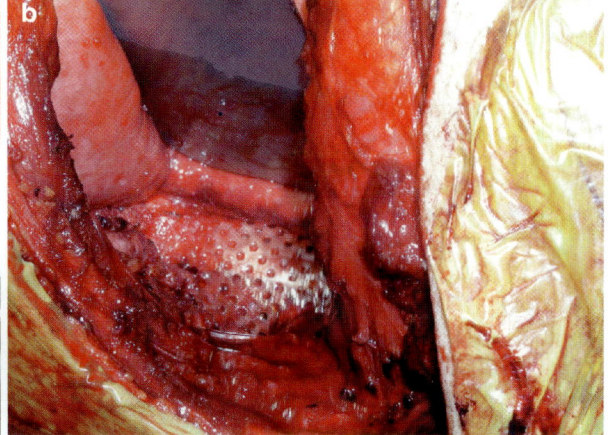

Fig. 24.1 (**a**) Thoracic spine burst fracture of T6 with corpectomy and stabilization of body with titanium mesh gauge and small fragment plate. Spinal cord is exposed. (**b**) PLA membrane is fabricated to form posterior wall following corpectomy of T6. Mixture of autologous bone from vertebral body fracture and Demineralized bone matrix putty is grafted in cage as well as anterior to the membrane which protects cord from bone graft spillage into spinal canal

titanium vertebral reconstructions cage and a posterior vertebral body wall is fabricated by molding a polymer membrane (Fig. 24.1). Another technique for applying autograft is the use of cylindrical titanium cages to form a weight bearing diaphysis. In this technique, titanium mesh cages that are typically used in spinal vertebral reconstructions are fashioned to bridge the defect which has been stabilized with an intramedullary nail. The cage is packed with cancellous bone and the cage–host bone margins are autografted to create a construct which has considerable immediate mechanical stability [21].

In summary, Phase III consists of bone reconstitution of the defect with an autologous bone graft. The autologous bone graft can consist of harvested iliac crest, intramedullary reaming harvests, or combinations of autogenous materials with synthetic bone substitutes or allograft materials. The stabilized defect can be prepared with the formation of an induced membrane, or bridged with a resorbable polylactide membrane or titanium mesh cage. Because of adequate mechanical stability from the internal fixation construct, functional rehabilitation can be instituted very early in the clinical course of limb salvage and bone defect reconstruction. The three-phase algorithm incorporates surgical techniques and implants that are widely available.

24.3 Clinical Case

Patient is a 49-year-old male involved in a motorcycle versus car accident. Patient sustains a pubic symphysis diastasis, unilateral sacroiliac joint dislocation, thumb CMC dislocation, and an open IIIa distal tibia diaphysis shaft fracture. Patient undergoes initial debridement via medial skin wound with removal of devitalized bone (Fig. 24.2a; Radiograph of tibia as splinted in ED). The fibula is plated, and the 5-cm defect is stabilized with an unreamed interlocked intramedullary nail. The wound is primarily closed and bone defect allografted with a Demineralized bone matrix putty by the index orthopaedist at 3 days postinjury (Fig. 24.2b; AP radiograph of distal diaphyseal defect with IM nail and fibula bridge plate). The patient is referred for bone defect management at approximately 8 weeks postinjury. The patient's clinical exam reveals a well-healed medial skin wound with palpable bone defect of the distal tibia. There is normal sensation, normal vascular exam, and near normal ankle motion. The AP/LAT X-rays demonstrate and anatomically aligned tibia and fibula with a persistent defect of the distal tibia which is unchanged from the postoperative films following initial IM fixation. The patient is taken to surgery where the defect is explored and cultured utilizing a new incision

Fig. 24.2 (a) Injury film of open grade IIIb tibia and fibula fracture. (b) AP radiograph at 2 months post-op following debridement of diaphyseal bone segment, IM nailing, and primary wound closure. No evidence of bone regeneration

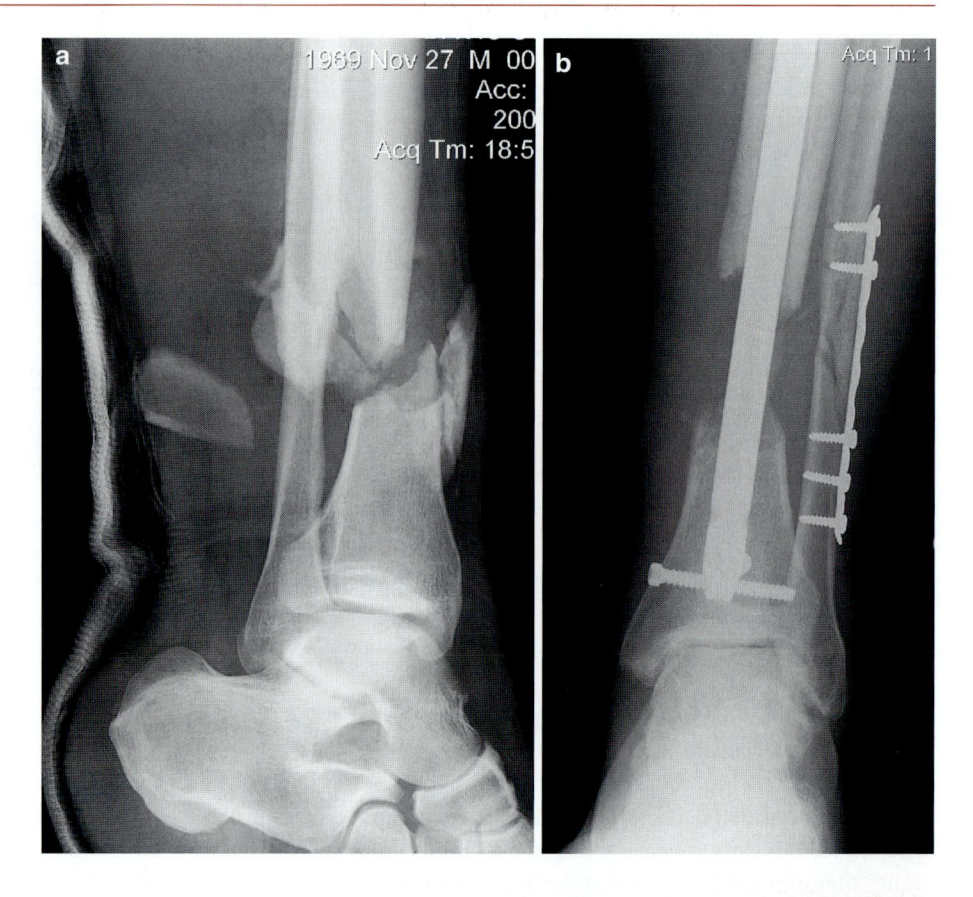

lateral to the tibia crest. There is no evidence of any bone regeneration within the defect. Cultures are obtained of the fluid and soft tissues in the defect and are negative for bacterial growth. A PMMA-antibiotic spacer (Biomet Cobalt, Warsaw, IN) is fabricated about the nail with approximately 1 cm overlap with the host bone ends (Figs. 24.3 and 24.4). Implantation of PMMA-antibiotic spacer with Biomet Cobalt polymethylmethacrylate cement cement. At 4 weeks, the encapsulating membrane is incised and the antibiotic spacer is removed (Fig. 24.5; Removal of spacer with preservation of encapsulating membrane). An intramedullary reaming harvest is made of the ipsilateral femur with the Synthes RIA (Synthes, Paoli, PA) resulting in approximately 40 mL of graft (Fig. 24.6; Intramedullary reaming from RIA). The defect is spanned with a polylactide meshed membrane (Synthes Orthomesh, Paoli, PA) and the defect cavity packed with the RIA auto graft (Figs. 24.7 and 24.8). Defect construct of IM nail, intramedullary reamings, polylactide membrane. The incision is closed over a suction drain, sutures removed at 12 days, and non-weight bearing maintained for 6 weeks. Serial radiographs are obtained at 6 and 12 weeks with partial weight bearing

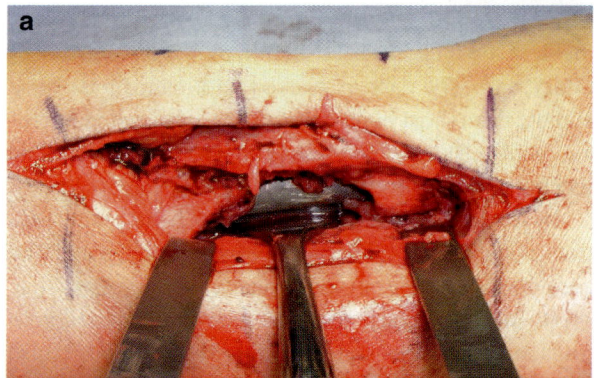

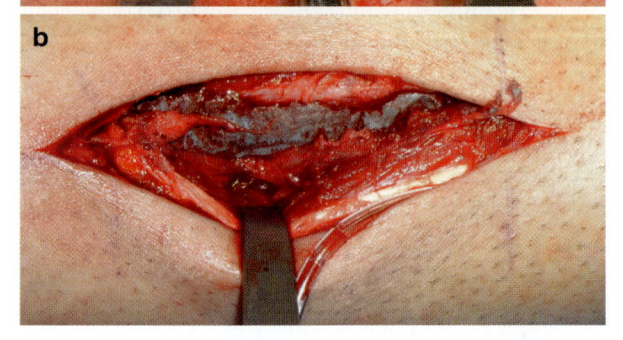

Fig. 24.3 (a) Surgical exposure of diaphyseal defect with exposed IM nail and bone ends. (b) PMMA-antibiotic spacer formed around IM nail and overlapping cortical bone ends by 1 cm

Fig. 24.4 AP and Lateral radiographs of PMMA-antibiotic spacer implant

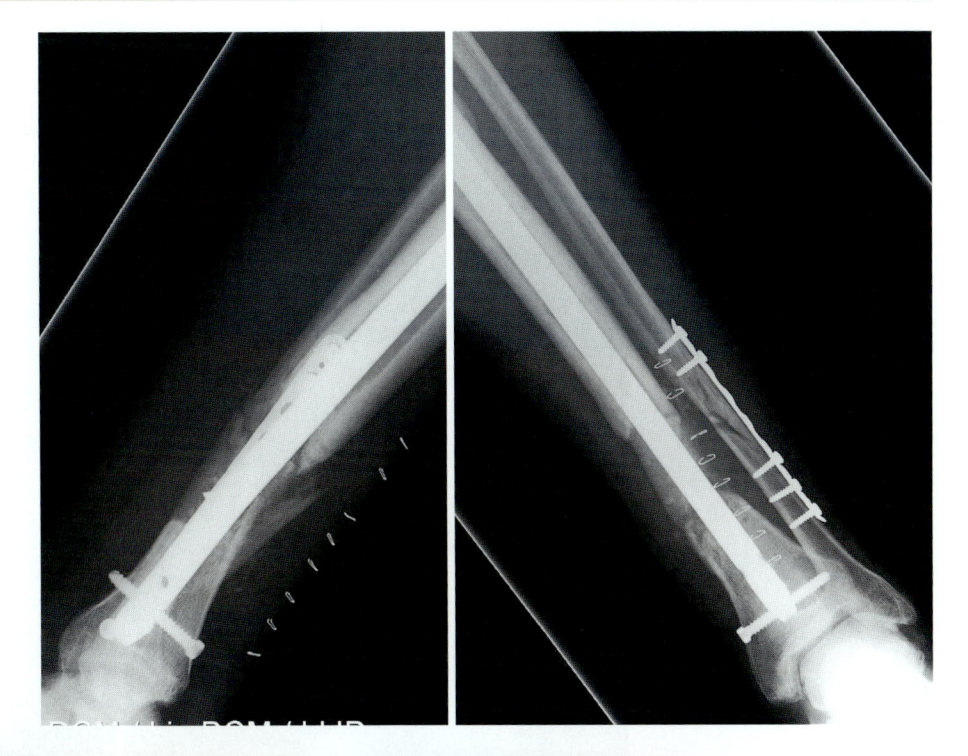

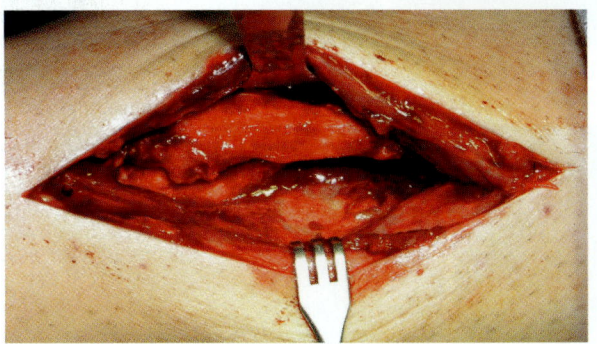

Fig. 24.5 PMMA-antibiotic spacer has been removed with reactive induced membrane lining bone defect cavity

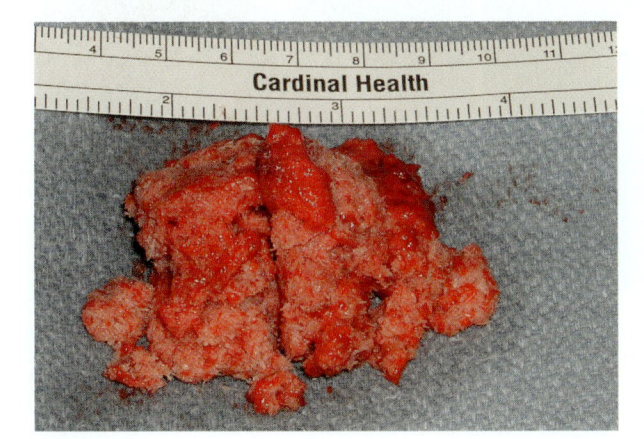

Fig. 24.6 Intramedullary bone graft harvested from ipsilateral femur using RIA device

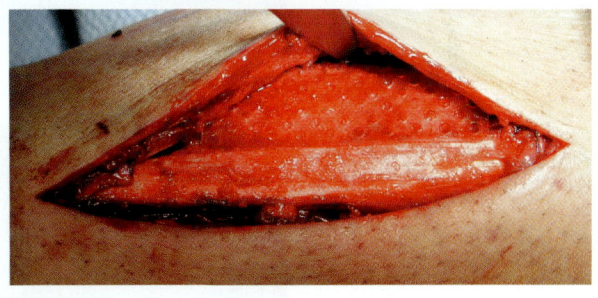

Fig. 24.7 PLA membrane applied as a tube to span defect and support the medial skin and keep graft from adhering to overlying Tibialis Anterior tendon

Fig. 24.8 Postoperative AP and Lateral radiographs of intramedullary RIA bone graft harvest and resorbable PLA membrane

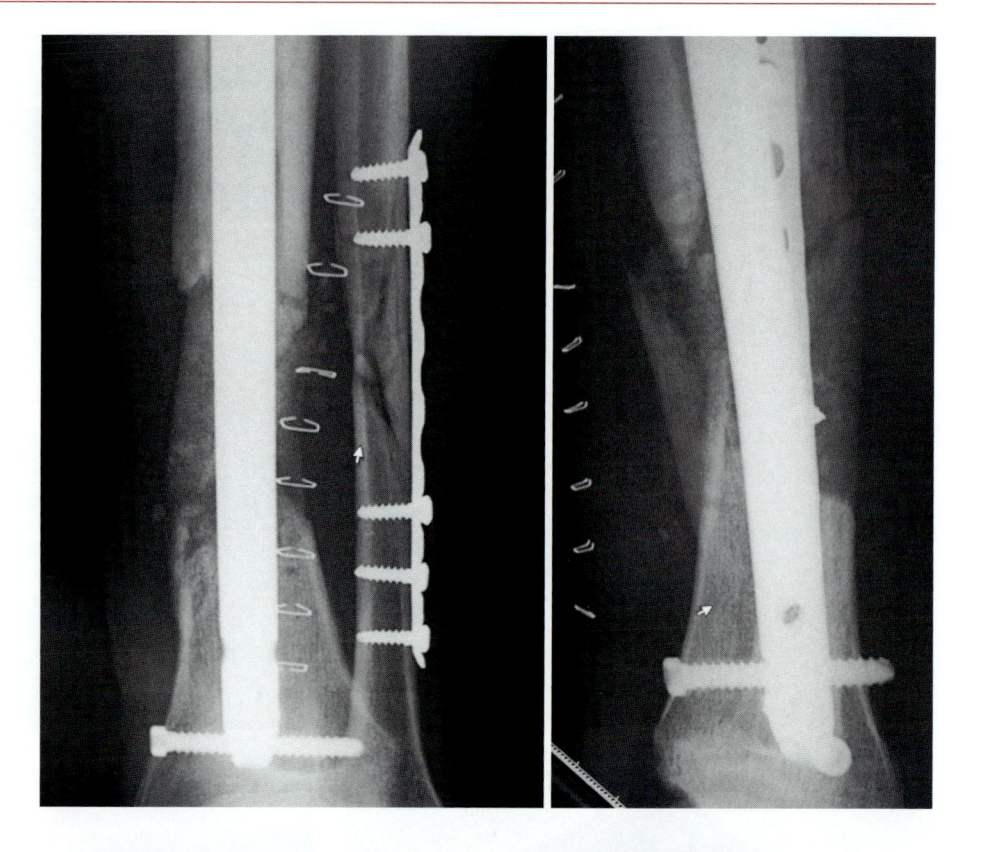

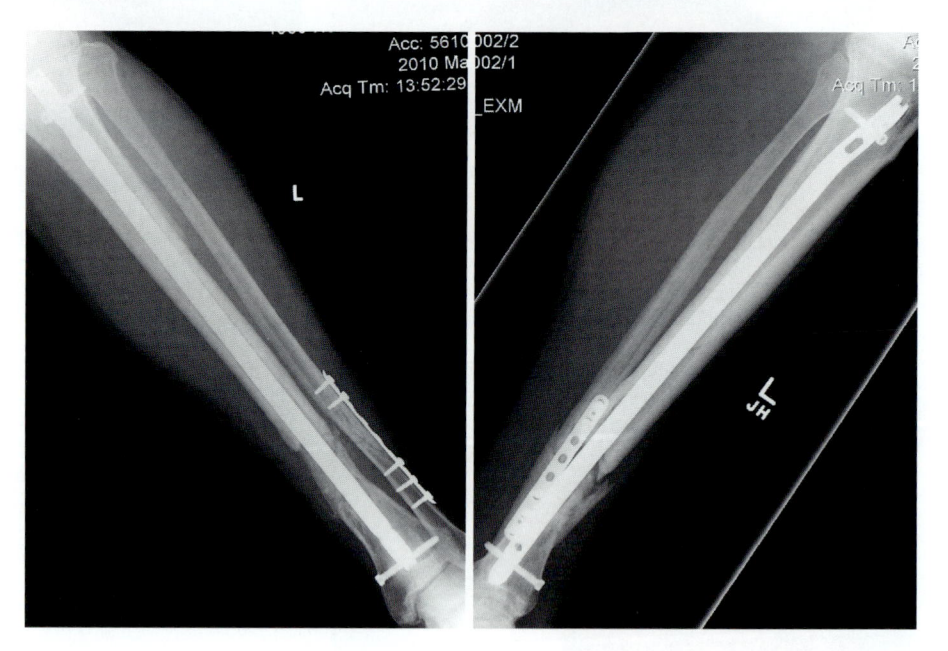

Fig. 24.9 Radiographs at 5-months post-bone grafting and membrane implantation. Patient is full weight bearing with full range of motion at knee, ankle, and foot

started at post-op week 6 and full weight bearing at 12 weeks post-autologous grafting. Patient is full weight bearing with normal gait and normal ankle and knee function at 5 months (Fig. 24.9; AP/Lateral x-ray of tubular bone regenerate).

References

1. Wiese A, Pape HC. Bone defects caused by high-energy injures, bone loss, infected nonunions, and nonunions. Orthop Clin North Am. 2010;41:1–4.
2. Abdel-Aal AM. Ilizarov bone transport for massive tibial bone defects. Orthopedics. 2006;29(1):70–4.
3. Webb LW, Bosse MJ, Castillo RC, Mackenzie EJ. Analysis of surgeon controlled variable in the type III open tibial diaphysis fracture. J Bone Joint Surg Am. 2007;89:923–8.
4. McNamara MG, Heckman JD, Corley EG. Severe open fractures of the lower extremity: a retrospective evaluation of the mangled extremity severity score. J Orthop Trauma. 1994;8:81–4.
5. Roberts CS, Pape HC, Jones AL, Malkini AL, Rodriquez JL, Giannoulis PV. Damage control orthopaedics: evolving concepts in the treatment of patients who have sustained orthopaedic trauma. J Bone Joint Surg Am. 2005;87:434–49.
6. Parekh AA, Smith W, Silva S, et al. Treatment of distal femur and proximal tibia fractures with external fixation followed by planned conversion to internal fixation. J Trauma. 2008;64(3):736–9.
7. Adams K, Crouch L, Cierney G, Calhoun J. In vitro and in vivo evaluation of antibiotic diffusion from antibiotic impregnated polymethylmethacrylate beads. Clin Orthop Relat Res. 1992;278:244–52.
8. Klaue K, Anton C, Knothe U, et al. Biological implementation of in situ induced autologous foreign body membranes in consolidation of massive cancellous bone grafts. J Bone Joint Surg Br. 1993;79:236.
9. Masquelet AC, Begue T. The concept of induced membrane for reconstruction of long bone defects. Orthop Clin North Am. 2010;41:27–37.
10. Viateau V, Bensidhoum M, Guilleman G, et al. Use of the induced membrane technique for bone tissue engineering purposes: animal studies. Orthop Clin North Am. 2010;41:49–56.
11. Ristiniemi J, Lakovaara M, Flinikkila T, et al. Staged method using antibiotic beads and subsequent autografting for large traumatic tibial bone loss: 22 of 23 fractures healed after 5–20 months. Acta Orthop. 2007;78(4):520–7.
12. Marino JT, Ziran B. Use of solid and cancellous autologous bone graft for fractures and nonunions. Orthop Clin North Am. 2010;41:15–6.
13. Conway JD. Autograft and nonunions: morbidity with intramedullary bone graft versus iliac crest bone graft. Orthop Clin North Am. 2010;41:75–84.
14. Dick W. Use of the acetabular reamer to harvest autogenic bone graft material: a simple method for producing bone paste. Arch Orthop Trauma Surg. 1986;185:225–8.
15. McCall TA, Brokaw DS, Jelen BA, et al. Treatment of large segmental bone defects with reamer-irrigator-aspirator bone graft: technique and case series. Orthop Clin North Am. 2010;41:63–73.
16. Blum B, Moseley J, Miller L, et al. Measurement of bone morphogenetic proteins and other growth factors in demineralized bone matrix. Orthopedics. 2004;27(1):161–5.
17. Hernigou P, Poignard A, Buejean F, et al. Percutaneous autologous bone-marrow grafting for nonunions. Influence of number and concentration of progenitor cells. J Bone Joint Surg Am. 2005;87(7):1490–7.
18. Janhangir AA, Nunley RM, Mehta S, et al. Bone graft substitutes in orthopaedic surgery. J Am Acad Orthop Surg. 2008;2(1):35–7.
19. Jones AL, Bucholz RW, Bosse MJ, et al. Recombinant human BMP-2 and autogenous bone graft for reconstruction of diaphyseal tibial fractures with cortical defects. A randomized, controlled trial. J Bone Joint Surg Am. 2006;88(7):1431–41.
20. Meinig RP. Clinical use of resorbable polymeric membranes in the treatment of bone defects. Orthop Clin North Am. 2010;41:39–47.
21. Gugala Z, Lindsey RW, Gogolewski S. New approaches in the treatment of critical-size segmental defects in long bones. Macromol Symp. 2007;253:147–61.

Acute Soft Tissue and Bone Infections

Lena M. Napolitano

Contents

25.1	Introduction	305
25.2	Classification of SSTIs	305
25.3	Specific Types of SSTIs	306
25.3.1	Traumatic Wound Infections	306
25.3.2	Surgical Site Infections (SSIs)	306
25.3.3	Necrotizing Soft Tissue Infections (NSTIs)	309
25.3.4	Pyomyositis	311
25.3.5	Osteomyelitis	311
25.3.6	Four Important Steps in SSTI Treatment	312
25.3.7	Epidemiology and Microbiology of SSTIs	313
25.4	Conclusion	316
References		316

25.1 Introduction

Skin and soft tissue infections (SSTIs) span a broad spectrum of clinical entities from limited cellulitis or small abscess to rapidly progressive necrotizing fasciitis, which may be associated with septic shock or toxic shock syndrome [1–5]. Severe and complicated SSTIs may result in critical illness and require management in the intensive care unit [6]. The complex interplay of environment, host, and pathogen are important to consider when evaluating SSTIs and planning therapy. The key to a successful outcome in caring for patients with severe SSTIs is (1) early diagnosis and differentiation of necrotizing vs. non-necrotizing SSTI, (2) early initiation of appropriate empiric broad-spectrum antimicrobial therapy with consideration of risk factors for specific pathogens, (3) "source control", i.e., early aggressive surgical intervention for drainage of abscesses and debridement of necrotizing soft tissue infections, and (4) pathogen identification and appropriate de-escalation of antimicrobial therapy (Table 25.1).

25.2 Classification of SSTIs

The US Food and Drug Administration (FDA) classifies SSTIs into two broad categories for the purpose of clinical trials evaluating new antimicrobials for the treatment of SSTIs: *uncomplicated* and *complicated* (Table 25.2). *Uncomplicated* SSTIs include superficial infections such as cellulitis, simple abscesses, impetigo, and furuncles. These infections can be treated by antibiotics and/or surgical incision for drainage of abscess alone. In contrast, *complicated* SSTIs include deep soft tissue infections that require significant surgical intervention, such as infected ulcers, infected

L.M. Napolitano
Department of Surgery, University of Michigan Health System, University Hospital, Room 1C421, 1500 East Medical Drive, 48109-0033 Ann Arbor, MI, USA
e-mail: lenan@umich.edu

Table 25.1 Steps in optimal management of patients with severe SSTIs

1. Early diagnosis and differentiation of necrotizing vs. non-necrotizing SSTI
2. Early initiation of appropriate empiric broad-spectrum antimicrobial therapy with anti-MRSA coverage and consideration of risk factors for specific pathogens
3. "Source control" of SSTI (i.e., early aggressive surgical intervention for drainage of abscesses and debridement of necrotizing soft tissue infections)
4. Pathogen identification and appropriate de-escalation of antimicrobial therapy

Table 25.2 Classification of SSTIs by FDA

Uncomplicated	Complicated
• Superficial infections such as:	• Deep soft tissue such as:
– Simple abscesses	– Infected ulcers
– Impetiginous lesions	– Infected burns
– Furuncles	– Major abscesses
– Cellulitis	• Significant underlying disease state that complicates response to treatment
• Can be treated by antibiotics or surgical incision alone	• Requires significant surgical intervention and antimicrobials

Source: From http://www.fda.gov/ohrms/dockets/98fr/2566dft.pdf

burns, and major abscesses, and these patients also have significant underlying comorbidities, i.e., disease states that complicate (and usually delay) response to treatment. Complicated SSTIs are a significant clinical problem, in part related to the increasing resistance of infecting bacteria to our current antibiotic therapies.

Uncomplicated SSTIs are associated with *low* risk for life- or limb-threatening infection. These patients can be treated with empiric antibiotic therapy according to likely pathogen and local resistance patterns.

Complicated SSTIs are associated with *high* risk for life- or limb-threatening infection. In these patients, it is of paramount importance to initiate appropriate and adequate broad-spectrum initial empiric antimicrobial therapy with coverage for MRSA and to consider the need for surgical intervention for abscess drainage or debridement.

Patients with complicated SSTIs require hospitalization for treatment. Specific circumstances that warrant hospitalization include the presence of tissue necrosis, sepsis, severe pain, altered mental status, immunocompromised state, and organ failure (respiratory, renal, and hepatic). SSTIs can lead to serious potentially life-threatening local and systemic complications. The infections can progress rapidly and early recognition and proper medical and surgical management is the cornerstone of therapy.

25.3 Specific Types of SSTIs

25.3.1 Traumatic Wound Infections

A recent report from the Lower Extremity Assessment Project (LEAP), a multi-institutional prospective observational study of 545 patients with limb-threatening lower extremity trauma with 2-year follow-up at eight Level-1 trauma centers, documented that wound infection (34%) was the most common complication in the primary amputation group, and that nonunion (31.5%) and wound infections (23.2%) were the most common complications in the limb salvage group. Furthermore, the late amputation group had the highest complication rate (68%), mostly due to wound infection [7]. When traumatic wound infections occur, it is recommended to initiate early empiric broad-spectrum antibiotic therapy to cover methicillin-resistant *Staphylococcus aureus* (MRSA) and all other potential pathogens, obtain wound cultures, and then tailor definitive antimicrobial therapy once the culture results return. In addition, the wound may require surgical debridement to provide adequate source control.

25.3.2 Surgical Site Infections (SSIs)

SSIs are one of the most common SSTIs that occur in orthopedic and trauma care. SSIs are defined as "superficial incisional" or "deep incisional" SSI based on the depth of the infection as defined by the Centers for Disease Control (CDC) and the National Healthcare Safety Network (NHSN) (Table 25.3).

A number of SSI prevention strategies have significantly decreased the rate of SSIs following orthopedic surgery and fracture repair in the past decade. The Surgical Care Improvement Project (SCIP) has implemented three measures for antibiotic

Table 25.3 CDC/NHSN classification of surgical site infections (SSIs)

Type of SSI	Definition
Superficial incisional	Infection occurs within 30 days after the operative procedure and involves only skin and subcutaneous tissue of the incision and patient has at least one of the following: (a) Purulent drainage from the superficial incision (b) Organisms isolated from an aseptically obtained culture of fluid or tissue from the superficial incision (c) At least one of the following signs or symptoms of infection: pain or tenderness, localized swelling, redness, or heat, and superficial incision is deliberately opened by surgeon and is culture positive or not cultured. A culture-negative finding does not meet this criterion (d) Diagnosis of superficial incisional SSI by the surgeon or attending physician
Deep incisional	Infection occurs within 30 days after the operative procedure if no implant[a] is left in place or within 1 year if implant is in place and the infection appears to be related to the operative procedure and involves deep soft tissues (e.g., fascial and muscle layers) of the incision and patient has at least one of the following: (a) Purulent drainage from the deep incision but not from the organ/space component of the surgical site (b) A deep incision spontaneously dehisces or is deliberately opened by a surgeon and is culture positive or not cultured when the patient has at least one of the following signs or symptoms: fever (38 C), or localized pain or tenderness. A culture-negative finding does not meet this criterion (c) An abscess or other evidence of infection involving the deep incision is found on direct examination, during reoperation, or by histopathologic or radiologic examination (d) Diagnosis of a deep incisional SSI by a surgeon or attending physician

Source: From Horan et al. [8]
[a]Implant: A nonhuman-derived object, material, or tissue (e.g., prosthetic heart valve, nonhuman vascular graft, mechanical heart, or hip prosthesis) that is permanently placed in a patient during an operative procedure and is not routinely manipulated for diagnostic or therapeutic purposes

Table 25.4 Antibiotics for SSI prevention in orthopedic surgery

Choice of antimicrobial agent
- Cephalosporin (cefazolin, cefuroxime)
- If β-lactam allergy, use clindamycin or vancomycin
- Consider preoperative screening for MRSA colonization
- If infected or colonized with MRSA, use vancomycin

Timing of administration
- Start up to 60 min before incision: cefazolin, cefuroxime, clindamycin
- Start up to 120 min before incision: vancomycin
- Infusion completed 10 min before tourniquet inflation

Dosing
- Cefazolin, 1–2 g (2 g for patient weighing >80 kg)
- Cefuroxime, 1.5 g
- Vancomycin (15 mg/kg) and clindamycin (600–900 mg) dosing based on patient mass
- Pediatric dosing based on patient mass

Duration of antimicrobial use
- Single preoperative dose
- Redose antimicrobial intraoperatively for prolonged procedure or significant blood loss
- When using postoperative doses, discontinue within 24 h after wound closure

Source: Adapted from Prokuski [9]

prophylaxis for SSI prevention: (1) antibiotic received within 1 h prior to surgical incision, (2) appropriate antibiotic selection based on surgical procedure performed, and (3) antibiotic discontinued within 24 h after surgery completed (Table 25.4). Additional evidence-based strategies for SSI prevention include the following: (1) appropriate hair removal (clipping, no shaving), (2) maintenance of normothermia intraoperatively and perioperatively, (3) glycemic control, (4) appropriate skin preparation, and (5) supplemental oxygen administration.

25.3.2.1 Microbiology of SSIs

S. aureus is the most common causative pathogen for all SSIs in the US data reported by the NHSN (Table 25.5), and an increasing percentage of these *S. aureus* isolates are methicillin-resistant (MRSA). Comparison of the causative pathogens for SSI in US hospitals documents that *S. aureus* increased from 22.5% (1986–2003) to 30% (2006–2007), with MRSA now the leading causative pathogen, comprising 49.2% of all isolates [10, 11]. The advent of community-associated MRSA (CA-MRSA) has impacted SSI significantly. Recent studies document that CA-MRSA is replacing traditional healthcare-associated or nosocomial MRSA strains in SSI among inpatients [12]. CA-MRSA has emerged as a leading

Table 25.5 Causative pathogens for surgical site infections (SSI) in US hospitals 2006–2007, National Healthcare Safety Network

Organism	SSIs from all types of surgeries No. (%) of SSIs Total n = 7,025	SSIs from orthopedic surgeries No. (%) of SSIs Total n = 963
Staphylococcus aureus	2,108 (30.0%)	548 (48.6%)
Methicillin-sensitive (MSSA)	1,102 (50.8%)	
Methicillin-resistant (MRSA)	1,006 (49.2%)	
Coagulase-negative staphylococci	965 (13.7%)	173 (15.3%)
Enterococcus spp.	788 (11.2%)	104 (10.8%)
Escherichia coli	671 (9.6%)	34 (3.0%)
Pseudomonas aeruginosa	390 (5.6%)	38 (3.4%)
Enterobacter spp.	293 (4.2%)	37 (3.3%)
Klebsiella spp.	213 (3.0%)	19 (2.0%)

Source: Adapted from Hidron et al. [10]

cause of healthcare-associated infections among patients with prosthetic joint SSIs [13].

In a study of 8,302 patients readmitted to US hospitals from 2003 to 2007 with culture-confirmed SSI, the proportion of infections caused by MRSA increased significantly, from 16.1% to 20.6%, and these infections were associated with higher mortality rates, longer stays, and higher hospital costs [14]. In view of this important finding, some surgeons have advocated strongly that patients be screened for nasal carriage of MRSA prior to elective surgery, with consideration of decolonization prior to surgery, and modification of antimicrobial agents for SSI prevention on the basis of the results.

Interestingly, when evaluating the microbiology of SSIs related to orthopedic surgical cases, S. aureus comprised an even greater percentage of isolates (48.6%) when compared to isolates reported for SSIs from all surgical cases (30%) (Table 25.5). Although knowledge of national microbiology of SSIs related to specific surgical procedures is important, it is of even greater importance to know the microbiology of SSIs within your own institution, and this should help to guide empiric antimicrobial management for treatment of SSIs in your local setting. Reports of resistant Gram-negative isolates, particularly multidrug-resistant Enterobacter isolates producing extended spectrum beta-lactamases (ESBLs), as the etiology of SSIs in orthopedic and trauma surgery is worrisome [15, 16]. This highlights the importance of pathogen identification, i.e., obtaining material for Gram stain and culture, in the management of all SSIs.

25.3.2.2 Closed Long Bone Fractures

A recent Cochrane Database systematic review of patients undergoing surgery for proximal femoral and other closed long bone fractures (data from 8,447 participants in 23 studies) documented that single dose antibiotic prophylaxis significantly reduced deep incisional SSI (risk ratio 0.40, 95% CI 0.24–0.67), superficial incisional SSI, urinary infections, and respiratory tract infections. Multiple dose antibiotic prophylaxis had an effect of similar size on deep incisional SSI. Therefore, appropriate antibiotic prophylaxis should be used in all patients undergoing surgical management of hip or other closed long bone fractures [17].

25.3.2.3 Open Fractures

Antibiotics reduce the incidence of early infections in open fractures of the limbs, confirmed by a Cochrane Database systematic review of 913 participants in seven studies. The use of antibiotics had a protective effect against early infection compared with no antibiotics or placebo (relative risk 0.41 [95% confidence interval (CI) 0.27–0.63]; absolute risk reduction 0.08 (95% CI 0.04–0.12); number needed to treat (NNT) 13 (95% CI 8–25). There were insufficient data in the included studies to evaluate other outcomes [18]. The Surgical Infection Society evidence-based guidelines for prophylactic antibiotic use in open fractures recommend the use of a short course of first-generation cephalosporins, begun as soon as possible after injury, in addition to modern orthopedic fracture wound management (Table 25.6) [19]. Open fracture grade (Gustilo) and the degree of associated soft tissue injury are independent determinants of infection risk. A recent single-institution review of patients with Gustilo IIIB tibial

Table 25.6 Risk of SSTI in adult trauma patients with open extremity fractures and antimicrobial prophylaxis recommendations

Grade of open fracture	Characteristics of Gustilo grade open fracture	Infection rate	Amputation rate
Grade I	Clean wound smaller than 1 cm in diameter, simple fracture pattern, no skin crushing	0–2%	0%
Grade II	A laceration larger than 1 cm but without significant soft tissue crushing, including no flaps, degloving, or contusion. Fracture pattern may be more complex	2–7%	0%
Grade III	An open segmental fracture or a single fracture with extensive soft tissue injury. Also included are injuries older than 8 h. Type III injuries are subdivided into three types:		
Grade III A	Adequate soft tissue coverage of the fracture despite high energy trauma or extensive laceration or skin flaps	5–10%	2.5%
Grade III B	Inadequate soft tissue coverage with periosteal stripping. Soft tissue reconstruction is necessary	10–50%	5.6%
Grade III C	Any open fracture that is associated with an arterial injury that requires repair	25–50%	25%
Grade of open fracture	Recommended Antibiotic		Alternate if PCN allergy
Grade I or II	Kefzol 1–2 g load then 1 g IV q8h for 48 h		Clindamycin 900 mg IV q8h for 48 h
Grade III	Ceftriaxone 1 g IV q24h for 48 h		Clindamycin 900 mg IV q8h and Aztreonam 1 g IV q8h for 48 h

Sources: Hauser et al. [19], Luchette et al. [20], Okike and Bhattachyaryya [21], Holtom [22], Gustilo and Anderson [23]

fractures (*n* = 52) determined that nosocomial bacterial pathogens (*Enterococci*, *Pseudomonas*, *Enterobacter*, and MRSA) were responsible for deep tissue infections, and advocated for tailoring antimicrobial prophylaxis against nosocomial organisms at the time of definitive wound closure [24].

25.3.3 Necrotizing Soft Tissue Infections (NSTIs)

NSTIs are aggressive soft tissue infections that cause widespread necrosis, and can include necrotizing cellulitis, fasciitis, and myositis/myonecrosis [25, 26]. Establishing the diagnosis of NSTI can be the main challenge in treating patients with NSTI, and knowledge of all available tools is key for early and accurate diagnosis [27]. There have been a number of recent advances in the definition, pathogenesis, diagnostic criteria, and treatment of necrotizing soft tissue infections [28, 29].

Patients with NSTIs require prompt aggressive surgical debridement, appropriate intravenous antibiotics, and intensive support. Despite aggressive treatment, their mortality and morbidity rates remain high, with some series reporting mortality rates of 25–35% [30]. A high index of suspicion should be used in conjunction with laboratory and imaging studies to establish the diagnosis as rapidly as possible. Successful treatment requires early, aggressive surgical debridement of all necrotic tissue, appropriate broad-spectrum systemic antibiotic therapy, and supportive care (fluid resuscitation, organ and critical care support) to maintain oxygenation and tissue perfusion. Delayed definitive debridement remains the single most important risk factor for death.

A recent single-institution series of 166 patients documented that the overall mortality rate was 16.9% and limb loss occurred in 26% of patients with extremity involvement [31]. Independent predictors of mortality included white blood cell count greater than $30,000 \times 10^3/\mu L$, creatinine level greater than 2 mg/dL (176.8 μmol/L), and heart disease at hospital admission. Independent predictors of limb loss included heart disease and shock (systolic blood pressure <90 mm Hg) at hospital admission. Clostridial infection was an independent predictor for both limb loss (odds ratio, 3.9 [95% confidence interval, 1.1–12.8]) and mortality (odds ratio, 4.1 [95% confidence interval, 1.3–12.3]) and was highly associated with intravenous drug use and a high rate of leukocytosis on hospital admission.

25.3.3.1 Aids to Diagnosis of NSTIs

Early operative debridement is a major determinant of outcome in NSTIs. However, early recognition of NSTIs is difficult clinically. A novel diagnostic scoring system for distinguishing NSTIs from other severe soft tissue infections based on laboratory tests routinely performed for the evaluation of severe SSTIs is called the Laboratory Risk Indicator for Necrotizing Fasciitis (LRINEC) score (Table 25.7) [32].

The LRINEC score was initially developed in a retrospective observational study including 145 patients with necrotizing fasciitis and 309 patients with severe cellulitis or abscesses admitted to the two tertiary care hospitals. The cutoff value for the LRINEC score was six points with a positive predictive value of 92.0% and negative predictive value of 96.0%. The LRINEC score is a robust score capable of detecting even clinically early cases of necrotizing fasciitis. The variables used are routinely measured to assess severe soft tissue infections. Patients with a LRINEC score of ≥6 should be carefully evaluated for the presence of necrotizing fasciitis.

Since the initial development of the LRINEC score, a number of other cohort studies have validated its utility in the diagnosis of NSTIs [33]. A recent multicenter study in 229 patients with NSTIs from 2002 to 2005 reported an overall mortality rate of 15.8% and amputation rate of 26.3%. This study also documented that a LRINEC score ≥6 was associated with a higher rate of both mortality and amputation [34].

25.3.3.2 Diagnostic Imaging in NSTIs

A high clinical index of suspicion is required if the diagnosis is to be made sufficiently early for successful treatment. NSTIs necessitate prompt aggressive surgical debridement for satisfactory treatment in addition to antimicrobial therapy. It is critical to remember that because of the rapidly progressive and potentially fatal outcome of this condition, if imaging cannot be performed expeditiously, delaying treatment is not justified. Plain film findings may reveal extensive soft tissue gas. CT examination can reveal asymmetric thickening of deep fascia in association with gas, and associated abscesses may also be present. MR imaging can also assist in the diagnosis of NSTIs [35]. MR imaging has been documented to effectively differentiate between necrotizing and non-necrotizing infections of the lower extremity, but should not delay prompt surgical intervention in NSTIs management [36].

Table 25.7 The laboratory risk indicator for necrotizing fasciitis (LRINEC) score

Variable, units	Score
C-reactive protein, mg/L	
<150	0
≥150	4
Total white cell count, per mm^3	
<15	0
15–25	1
>25	2
Hemoglobin, g/dL	
>13.5	0
11–13.5	1
<11	2
Sodium, mmol/L	
≥135	0
<135	2
Creatinine, μmol/L	
≤141	0
>141	2
Glucose, mmol/L	
≤10	0
>10	1

The maximum score is 13; a score ≥6 should raise the suspicion of necrotizing fasciitis and a score of ≥8 is strongly predictive of this disease

25.3.3.3 Microbiology of NSTIs

Necrotizing fasciitis and myonecrosis are typically caused by infection with Group A *Streptococcus*, *Clostridium perfringens*, or, most commonly, aerobic and anaerobic organisms as part of a polymicrobial infection that may include *S. aureus*. In case series, CA-MRSA has recently been described as a predominantly monomicrobial cause of necrotizing fasciitis [37, 38]. A retrospective review of patients presenting with necrotizing fasciitis between 2000 and 2006 indicated that MRSA was the most common pathogen, accounting for one-third of the organisms isolated [39].

NSTIs have been classified into two types, either polymicrobial (Type I) or monomicrobial (Type II). Polymicrobial infections are more common, due to both aerobic and anaerobic organisms, and commonly occur in the trunk and perineum. NSTIs that are monomicrobial in origin commonly occur in the limbs and are typically caused by infection with Group A *Streptococcus*, *C. perfringens*, or *S. aureus*. NSTIs are categorized into these two specific types based on the microbiologic etiology of the infection, and this classification does impact on the specific antimicrobial agents required for treatment of these NSTIs.

- Type 1 or polymicrobial
- Type 2 or monomicrobial

Increasingly, MRSA has been identified as the causative microbe in NSTIs, but a separate category for this NSTI does not currently exist [40–44]. Given this finding, anti-MRSA empiric antimicrobial therapy should be initiated in all patients with NSTIs and pathogen-directed antimicrobial therapy considered once tissue culture results are available.

Uncommon microbiologic causes of NSTIs and primary sepsis include *Vibrio* and *Aeromonas* spp., virulent Gram-negative bacteria, and members of the Vibrionaceae family that thrive in aquatic environments [45]. These NSTIs are likely to occur in patients with hepatic disease, diabetes, and immunocompromised conditions [46]. These organisms are found in warm sea waters and are often present in raw oysters, shellfish, and other seafood. The diagnosis of *Vibrio* NSTIs should be suspected when a patient has the appropriate clinical findings and a history of contact with seawater or raw seafood [47]. Early fasciotomy and culture-directed antimicrobial therapy should be aggressively performed in those patients with hypotensive shock, leukopenia, severe hypoalbuminemia, and underlying chronic illness, especially a combination of hepatic dysfunction and diabetes mellitus. The rate of amputation and mortality is very high in these patients, and early definitive management is of paramount importance [48–50].

25.3.4 Pyomyositis

Myositis is a rare infection that may lead to serious and potentially life-threatening local and systemic complications [51]. The infection can progress rapidly, and early recognition and proper medical and surgical management is therefore the cornerstone of therapy. With the increasing prevalence of community-associated MRSA as a pathogen in severe SSTIs, pyomyositis is more common than in past years. Myositis often occurs in muscle sites that have been compromised by injury, ischemia, malignancy, or surgery. The predominant pathogens are *S. aureus*, Group A streptococci (GAS), Gram-negative aerobic and facultative bacilli, and the indigenous aerobic and anaerobic cutaneous and mucous membranes local microflora.

CT scan imaging is a rapid and sensitive diagnostic test and commonly demonstrates diffuse enlargement of the involved muscle and may demonstrate the presence of fluid or gas collections within the muscle suggesting the presence of abscesses. MRI is more sensitive in showing early inflammatory changes prior to development of abscesses in myositis [52]. Emergency surgical exploration is warranted in order to define the nature of the infective process that is accomplished by direct examination of the involved muscles. Surgical intervention is required to perform appropriate abscess drainage and debridement and to also evaluate for necrotizing myositis. Fasciotomies and extremity amputation are sometimes necessary.

25.3.5 Osteomyelitis

Bone and joint infections are challenging to diagnose and treat [53]. The key to successful management is early diagnosis. This requires bone sampling for microbiological and pathological examination to allow targeted appropriate antimicrobial therapy. There are three types of *acute* osteomyelitis (in order of decreasing frequency):

1. Osteomyelitis secondary to a contiguous focus of infection (after trauma, surgery, or insertion of a joint prosthesis)
2. Osteomyelitis secondary to vascular insufficiency (in diabetic foot infections or peripheral vascular disease)
3. Osteomyelitis secondary to hematogenous origin

The rate of osteomyelitis following severe limb-threatening lower extremity trauma reported in the LEAP study was 9.4% in the total study cohort of 330 patients. The rates of osteomyelitis ranged from 3.1% in the primary amputation group to the highest rate of 27.3% in patients with Grade IIIC tibia fracture [54].

Acute osteomyelitis is treated with antibiotics and careful assessment of any associated wound to determine if the soft tissue and wound require infection

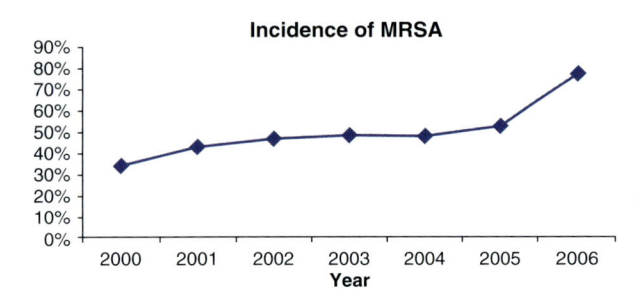

Fig. 25.1 Incidence of MRSA isolated from patients presenting with SSTI and requiring surgical intervention over 7 years (2000–2006) (From Hidayat et al. [74])

to large abscesses, severe pyomyositis, and fulminant necrotizing soft tissue infections [41, 72, 73].

MRSA has also been identified as the most common cause of severe SSTIs requiring surgical drainage and debridement in a single-center 7-year study from Houston [74]. From 2000 to 2006, 288 patients with SSTIs that required operative debridement were identified. The most common microorganism retrieved from intraoperative cultures was *S. aureus*, 70% of which were MRSA. *Streptococcus* spp. accounted only for 15% of microbes isolated. Monomicrobial etiology was identified in 67% of patients and MRSA was also the predominant microbe isolated from such cultures (68%). The frequency of MRSA isolates increased significantly during the study from 34% in the year 2000 to 77% in the year 2006, $p<0.001$, (Fig. 25.1). Interestingly, the examination of vancomycin MIC demonstrated a shift for MRSA isolates over this time period, with 38% of the isolates having an MIC$\geq$1 µg/mL, with 31% of isolates with MIC=2 µg/mL. This is concerning given recent reports documenting high treatment failure rates for MRSA infections with increased MIC [75, 76].

In a study of 12,506 patients with culture-proven skin, soft tissue, bone or joint infection in hospitalized patients, *S. aureus* caused infection in 54.6% of patients and 28.0% of the *S. aureus* isolates recovered were methicillin-resistant. Healthcare-associated infections and complicated SSTIs were associated with significantly higher mortality rates, longer and more costly length of hospital stay [77].

Based on this change in microbiologic etiology of SSTIs, all patients who present with or develop severe cSSTIs should be treated with broad-spectrum antimicrobial therapy, including mandatory coverage for MRSA. Patients who present to the hospital with severe infection or infection progressing despite antibiotic therapy should be treated aggressively. In these cases, if *S. aureus* is cultured, the clinician should assume the organism may be resistant and should treat with agents effective against MRSA, such as vancomycin, linezolid, or daptomycin [78]. Although risk factors for MRSA SSTIs have been identified, in patients with severe SSTIs one should not rely solely on the use of risk factors for MRSA in the decision making regarding whether empiric anti-MRSA antimicrobials should be used.

Choice of empiric antimicrobial therapy for SSTIs is guided by a number of factors. For patients with severe SSTIs that are surgical site infections, it is important to choose an empiric antimicrobial agent that is different from the class of antibiotics that was used for surgical site infection prophylaxis at the time of the initial surgery. In the case of surgical site infection (SSI), the type and site of operation dictate which pathogens are suspected. Infections following operations in the gastrointestinal or genitourinary tract may be monomicrobial or mixed, and may be caused by Gram-positive or Gram-negative bacteria. In contrast, infections following clean operations in other parts of the body are typically caused by Gram-positive pathogens. Immunocompromised or neutropenic patients are, of course, at increased risk of infection and are less able to control local infection and therefore should be treated with empiric, broad-spectrum antibiotics at the first clinical signs of infection, including fever.

It is important to provide anti-MRSA coverage in the empiric regimen of all patients with severe SSTIs. Four anti-MRSA antimicrobials are approved by the FDA (vancomycin, linezolid, daptomycin, tigecycline) and a number of new anti-MRSA antimicrobials are in development. A comprehensive review of SSTI antimicrobial studies has recently been published [79].

When selecting empiric antimicrobials for treatment of severe cSSTIs, selection of specific antimicrobials that inhibit toxin production may be helpful, particularly in those patients with evidence of toxic shock syndrome. This is commonly present in patients with streptococcal and staphylococcal infections. Protein cytotoxins play an important role in the pathogenesis of a variety of staphylococcal infections, and toxin production should be considered when selecting an antimicrobial agent for Gram-positive pathogens [80]. The recent identification of a class of secreted staphylococcal peptides (phenol-soluble modulin (PSM) peptides) document that they have a remarkable ability to recruit, activate, and lyse human neutrophils, thus eliminating the main cellular defense against MRSA infection [81]. The β-lactams actually enhance toxin production. In contrast, both clindamycin and linezolid have the ability to inhibit toxin production by suppression of translation, but not transcription, of toxin genes for *S. aureus* and by direct inhibition of synthesis of group A streptococcal toxins. Particularly when patients exhibit signs and symptoms of streptococcal toxic shock syndrome (shock, coagulopathy, organ failure, and NSTI), anti-toxin antimicrobials should be promptly initiated [82].

25.3.7.1 "Source control": early aggressive surgical intervention for drainage of abscesses and debridement of necrotizing soft tissue infections

"Source control" includes drainage of infected fluids, debridement of infected soft tissues, removal of infected devices or foreign bodies, and finally, definite measures to correct anatomic derangement resulting in ongoing microbial contamination and to restore optimal function [83]. Source control represents a key component of success in the therapy of sepsis, since it is the best method of prompt reduction of the bacterial inoculum at the site of infection. Source control has been best identified as an important therapeutic strategy in the treatment of complicated abdominal infections [84], but is of paramount importance in the treatment of cSSTIs as well. Appropriate and timely source control is mandatory in the treatment of severe SSTIs, particularly in the case of NSTIs. This is depicted as the main pillar of the "Treatment Triangle" of SSTIs in Fig. 25.2.

Surgical Drainage and Debulking
- Incision and drainage of abscesses
- Removal of prosthetic material (if possible)

Prevention of Transmission
- Improved hand hygiene
- Cleaning of shared equipment between uses
- Separation of infected patients; avoidance of overcrowding
- Selective decolonization

Wound Culture
- Community-associated MRSA: consider TMP-SMX, tetracycline, erythromycin, clindamycin, vancomycin
- Health care-associated MRSA: consider vancomycin, rifampin, linezolid, (and possibly daptomycin, quinupristin-dalfopristin, fusidic acid)

Antibiotic Therapy
- MSSA: antistaphylococcal penicillin, 1-CEF
- Community-associated MRSA: TMP-SMX, clindamycin, doxycycline
- Health care-associated MRSA: vancomycin, linezolid, daptomycin, rifampin plus fusidic acid

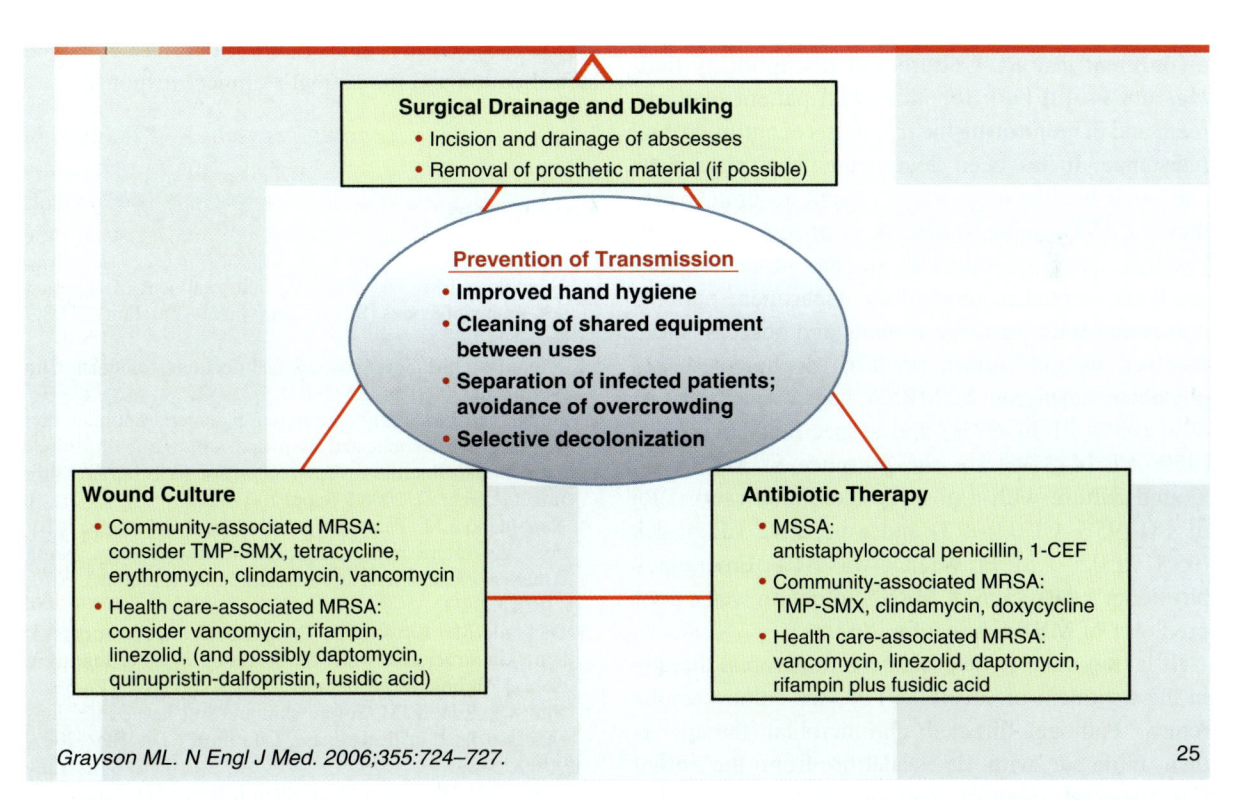

Grayson ML. N Engl J Med. 2006;355:724–727.

Fig. 25.2 Treatment triangle for *Staphylococcus aureus* infection. The three components of the treatment of presumed *S. aureus* infection include surgical drainage and debridement, obtaining a wound culture, and initiation of appropriate empiric antimicrobial therapy. If MRSA SSTI is confirmed, it is critically important to utilize all methods to prevent microbial transmission, including hand hygiene. For wound cultures that are positive for community-associated MRSA (usually not a multidrug-resistant phenotype), in vitro susceptibility to trimethoprim–sulfamethoxazole (*TMP-SMX*), tetracycline, erythromycin, clindamycin, and vancomycin should be assessed. If the isolate is resistant to erythromycin but susceptible to clindamycin, the clindamycin D-zone test should be performed if clindamycin therapy is being considered. For wound cultures that are positive for healthcare-associated MRSA (usually a multidrug-resistant phenotype), in vitro susceptibility to vancomycin, rifampin, and linezolid should be assessed. Assessment of susceptibility to daptomycin and quinupristin–dalfopristin is not necessary unless therapy with these agents is being considered. Susceptibility to fusidic acid may be assessed in countries where this agent is available. Empirical antibiotic therapy should be reviewed once susceptibility data are known. For methicillin-susceptible *S. aureus* (*MSSA*), antistaphylococcal penicillin or a first-generation cephalosporin (*1-CEF*) may be suitable. For community-associated MRSA, TMP-SMX, clindamycin, or tetracycline may be suitable. For healthcare-associated MRSA, vancomycin, linezolid, daptomycin, or rifampin plus fusidic acid may be suitable (Adapted from Grayson [85])

25.3.7.2 Pathogen identification and appropriate de-escalation of antimicrobial therapy

Given the increasing prevalence of multidrug-resistant pathogens as the etiology of severe SSTIs, pathogen identification is of paramount importance. All patients with severe SSTIs should have blood cultures obtained on admission, prior to initiation of empiric antimicrobial therapy if possible. In addition, cultures should be obtained directly from the SSTI site, either abscess fluid when incision and drainage is performed or tissue sample in the case of NSTIs when surgical debridement is performed.

Initial management of cSSTIs should include collection of specimens for culture and antimicrobial susceptibility testing from *all* patients with abscesses or purulent lesions. Culture and susceptibility findings are useful both for individual patient management and in monitoring local patterns of antimicrobial resistance. It has been documented that physicians and other healthcare workers cannot accurately predict if a SSTI is due to MRSA. A prospective observational study conducted in an urban tertiary academic center in emergency department patients presenting with purulent wounds and abscesses that received wound culture ($n = 176$) documented that physician suspicion of MRSA had a sensitivity of 80% (95% CI 71–87%) and a specificity of 23.6% (95% CI 14–37%) for the presence of MRSA on wound culture with a positive likelihood ratio (LR) of 1.0 (95% CI 0.9–1.3) and a negative LR of 0.8 (95% CI 0.5–1.3). Prevalence was 64%. Emergency physician's suspicion of MRSA infection was a poor predictor of MRSA infection [86].

It is important to de-escalate antimicrobial therapy in the treatment of severe SSTIs once culture results return. Pathogen-directed antimicrobial therapy is then initiated, with de-escalation from the initial broad-spectrum empiric antimicrobial regimen, with an attempt to decrease to monotherapy if at all possible. De-escalation of antimicrobial therapy should occur as early as possible, but is only possible if appropriate microbiologic specimens are obtained at the time of SSTI source control. De-escalation is founded on identification of the pathogen and its antibiotic susceptibilities.

25.4 Conclusion

SSTIs are associated with significant morbidity and mortality, and it is important to differentiate necrotizing vs. non-necrotizing SSTIs early in the course of treatment. MRSA is the most common cause of purulent cSSTIs. All patients who present with complicated SSTIs should be treated with broad-spectrum antimicrobial therapy, including mandatory coverage for MRSA. Source control, including abscess drainage and surgical debridement, is the mainstay of therapy in severe cSSTIs. It is of paramount importance to obtain specimens for culture and antimicrobial susceptibilities given the high prevalence of MRSA as a causative pathogen in cSSTIs. Empiric broad-spectrum antimicrobial therapy should be de-escalated to narrower-spectrum agents based on culture pathogen identification and the patient's clinical response.

References

1. Napolitano LM. The diagnosis and treatment of skin and soft tissue infections (SSTIs). Surg Infect (Larchmt). 2008;9 Suppl 1:1.
2. Napolitano LM. Severe soft tissue infections. Infect Dis Clin North Am. 2009;23(3):571–9.
3. Napolitano LM. Early appropriate parenteral antimicrobial treatment of complicated skin and soft tissue infections caused by methicillin-resistant *Staphylococcus aureus*. Surg Infect (Larchmt). 2008;9 Suppl 1:s17–27.
4. Napolitano LM. Perspectives in surgical infections: what does the future hold? Surgical Infection Society, North America, Presidential Address. Surg Infect (Larchmt). 2010; 11(2):111–23.
5. DiNubile MJ, Lipsky BA. Complicated infections of skin and skin structures: when the infection is more than skin deep. J Antimicrob Chemother. 2004;53 Suppl 2:ii37–50.
6. Vinh DC, Embil JM. Severe skin and soft tissue infections and associated critical illness. Curr Infect Dis Rep. 2007; 9(5):415–21.
7. Harris AM, Althausen PL, Kellam J, Bosse MJ, Castillo R, Lower Extremity Assessment Project (LEAP) Study Group. Complications following limb-threatening lower extremity trauma. J Orthop Trauma. 2009;23:1–6.
8. Horan TC et al. CDC/NHSN surveillance definition of healthcare-associated infection and criteria for specific types of infections in the acute care setting. Am J Infect Control. 2008;36:309–32.
9. Prokuski L. Prophylactic antibiotics in orthopaedic surgery. J Am Acad Orthop Surg. 2008;16:283–93.

10. Hidron AI, Edwards JR, Patel J, National Healthcare Safety Network Team; Participating National Healthcare Safety Network Facilities, et al. NHSN annual update: antimicrobial-resistant pathogens associated with healthcare-associated infections: annual summary of data reported to the National Healthcare Safety Network at the Centers for Disease Control and Prevention, 2006–2007. Infect Control Hosp Epidemiol. 2008;29:996–1011.
11. Gaynes R, Edwards JR. National Nosocomial Infections Surveillance System: overview of nosocomial infections caused by gram-negative bacilli. Clin Infect Dis. 2005;41: 848–54.
12. Manian FA, Griesnauer S. Community-associated MRSA is replacing traditional healthcare-associated strains in surgical site infections among inpatients. Clin Infect Dis. 2008;47: 434–5.
13. Kourbatova EV, Halvosa JS, King MD, et al. Emergence of community-associated MRSA USA 300 clone as a cause of healthcare-associated infections among patients with prosthetic joint infections. Am J Infect Control. 2005;33: 385–91.
14. Weigelt JA, Lipsky BA, Tabak YP, et al. Surgical site infections: causative pathogens and associated outcomes. Am J Infect Control. 2010;38:112–20.
15. Haenie M, Podbielski A, Mittelmeier W, et al. Infections after primary and revision total hip replacement caused by enterobacteria producing extended spectrum beta-lactamases (ESBL): a case series. Hip Int. 2010;20(2): 248–54.
16. Martinez-Pastor JC, Vilchez F, Pitart C, et al. Antibiotic resistance in orthopaedic surgery: acute knee prosthetic joint infections due to ESBL-producing Enterobacteriaceae. Eur J Clin Microbiol Infect Dis. 2010;29(8):1039–41 [Epub ahead of print].
17. Gillespie WJ, Walenkamp GH. Antibiotic prophylaxis for surgery for proximal femoral and other closed long bone fractures. Cochrane Database Syst Rev. 2010 Mar 17;3: CD000244.
18. Gosselin RA, Roberts I, Gillespie WJ. Antibiotics for preventing infections in open limb fractures. Cochrane Database Syst Rev. 2004;(1):CD003764.
19. Hauser CJ, Adams Jr CA, Eachempati SR, Council of the Surgical Infection Society. Surgical infection society guideline: prophylactic antibiotic use in open fractures: an evidence-based guideline. Surg Infect (Larchmt). 2006;7(4): 379–405.
20. Luchette FA, Bone LB, Born CT, et al. EAST Practice management guidelines for prophylactic antibiotic use in open fractures. www.east.org/tpg/openfxupdate.pdf. 2009, Accessed 2011 Feb.
21. Okike K, Bhattachyaryya T. Trends in the management of open fractures. A critical analysis. J Bone Joint Surg Am. 2006;88:2739–48.
22. Holtom PD. Antibiotic prophylaxis: current recommendations. J Am Acad Orthop Surg. 2006;14:S98–100.
23. Gustilo RB, Anderson JT. Prevention of infection in the treatment of one thousand and twenty-five open fractures of long bones: retrospective and prospective analyses. J Bone Joint Surg Am. 1976;58(4):453–8.
24. Glass GE, Barrett SP, Sanderson F, et al. The microbiological basis for a revised antibiotic regimen in high-energy tibial fractures: Preventing deep infections by nosocomial organisms. J Plast Reconstr Aesthet Surg. 2011 Mar; 64(3):375–80.
25. Sarkar B, Napolitano LM. Necrotizing soft tissue infections. Minerva Chir. 2010;65(3):347–62.
26. Sarani B, Strong M, Pascual J, Schwab CW. Necrotizing fasciitis: current concepts and review of the literature. J Am Coll Surg. 2009;208(2):279–88.
27. Anaya DA, Dellinger EP. Necrotizing soft-tissue infection: diagnosis and management. Clin Infect Dis. 2007;44(5): 705–10.
28. Cainzos M, Gonzalez-Rodriguez FJ. Necrotizing soft tissue infections. Curr Opin Crit Care. 2007;13(4):433–9.
29. Yilmazlar T, Ozturk E, Alsoy A, Ozquc H. Necrotizing soft tissue infections: APACHE II score, dissemination, and survival. World J Surg. 2007;31(9):1858–62.
30. Cuschieri J. Necrotizing soft tissue infection. Surg Infect (Larchmt). 2008;9(6):559–62.
31. Anaya DA, McMahon K, Nathens AB, et al. Predictors of mortality and limb loss in necrotizing soft tissue infections. Arch Surg. 2005;140:151–7.
32. Wong CH, Khin LW, Heng KS, et al. The LRINEC (Laboratory Risk Indicator for Necrotizing Fasciitis) score: a tool for distinguishing necrotizing fasciitis from other soft tissue infections. Crit Care Med. 2004;32(7): 1535–41.
33. Su YC, Chen HW, Hong YC, Chen CT, Hsiao CT, Chen IC. Laboratory risk indicator for necrotizing fasciitis score and the outcomes. ANZ J Surg. 2008;78(11):968–72.
34. Su YC, Chen HW, Hong YC, et al. Laboratory risk indicator for necrotizing fasciitis score and the outcomes. ANZ J Surg. 2008;78(11):968–72.
35. Struk DW, Munk PL, Lee MJ, et al. Imaging of soft tissue infections. Radiol Clin North Am. 2001;39(2):277–303.
36. Brothers TE, Tagge DU, Stutley JE, et al. Magnetic resonance imaging differentiates between necrotizing and non-necrotizing fasciitis of the lower extremity. J Am Coll Surg. 1998;187:416–21.
37. Wong CH, Chang HC, Pasupathy S, et al. Necrotizing fasciitis: clinical presentation, microbiology, and determinants of mortality. J Bone Joint Surg Am. 2003;85-A(8): 1454–60.
38. McHenry CR, Piotrowski JJ, Petrinic D, et al. Determinants of mortality for necrotizing soft-tissue infections. Ann Surg. 1995;221(5):558–65.
39. Elhabash S, Lee L, Farrow B, et al. Characteristics and microbiology of patients presenting with necrotizing fasciitis. Paper Presented at: Association of VA Surgeons 31st Annual Meeting; 2007 May 10–12; Little Rock, Arkansas.
40. Lee TC, Carrick MM, Scott BG, et al. Incidence and clinical characteristics of MRSA necrotizing fasciitis in a large urban hospital. Am J Surg. 2007;194(6):809–12.
41. Miller LG, Perdreau-Remington F, Rieg G, et al. Necrotizing fasciitis caused by community-associated MRSA in Los Angeles. N Engl J Med. 2005;352(14):1445–53.

42. Young LM, Price CS. Community-acquired MRSA emerging as an important cause of necrotizing fasciitis. Surg Infect (Larchmt). 2008;9(4):469–74.
43. Olsen RJ, Burns KM, Chen L, et al. Severe necrotizing fasciitis in a human immunodeficiency virus-positive patient caused by MRSA. J Clin Microbiol. 2008;46(3):1144–7.
44. Dehority W, Wang E, Vernon PS, et al. Community-associated MRSA necrotizing fasciitis in a neonate. Pediatr Infect Dis J. 2006;25(11):1080–1.
45. Tsai YH, Hsu RW, Huang TJ, et al. Necrotizing soft tissue infections and sepsis caused by *Vibrio vulnificus* compared with those caused by *Aeromonas* species. J Bone Joint Surg Am. 2007;89(3):631–6.
46. Tsai YH, Hsu RW, Huang KC, et al. Systemic Vibrio infection presenting as necrotizing fasciitis and sepsis. A series of 13 cases. J Bone Joint Surg Am. 2004;86(11):2497–502.
47. Minnaganti VR, Patel Pj, Iancu D, et al. Necrotizing fasciitis caused by *Aeromonas hydrophila*. Heart Lung. 2000;29(4):306–8.
48. Bross MH, Soch K, Morales R, Mitchell RB. *Vibrio vulnificus* infection: diagnosis and treatment. Am Fam Physician. 2007;76(4):539–44.
49. Tsai YH, Huang TJ, Hsu RW, et al. Necrotizing soft tissue infections and primary sepsis caused by *Vibrio vulnificus* and *Vibrio cholerae* non-O1. J Trauma. 2009;66(3):899–905.
50. Kuo YL, Shieh SJ, Chiu HY, Lee JW. Necrotizing fasciitis caused by *Vibrio vulnificus*: epidemiology, clinical findings, treatment and prevention. Eur J Clin Microbiol Infect Dis. 2007;26(11):785–92.
51. Brook I. Microbiology and management of myositis. Int Orthop. 2004;28(5):257–60.
52. Garcia J. MRI in inflammatory myopathies. Skeletal Radiol. 2000;29:425–38.
53. Lew DP, Waldvogel FA. Osteomyelitis. Lancet. 2004;364(9431):369–79.
54. Bosse MJ, MacKenzie EJ, Kellam JF, et al. An analysis of outcomes of reconstruction or amputation of leg-threatening injuries. N Engl J Med. 2002;247(24):1924–31.
55. May AK. Skin and soft tissue infections. Surg Clin North Am. 2009;89(2):403–20.
56. Chan T, Yaghoubian A, Rosing D, et al. Low sensitivity of physical examination findings in necrotizing soft tissue infection is improved with laboratory values: a prospective study. Am J Surg. 2008;196(6):926–30. Discussion 930.
57. Wall DB, deVirgilio C, Black S, Klein SR. Objective criteria may assist in distinguishing necrotizing fasciitis from non-necrotizing soft tissue infection. Am J Surg. 2000;179(11):17–21.
58. Wall DB, Klein SR, Black S, deVirgilio C. A simple model to help distinguish necrotizing fasciitis from non-necrotizing soft tissue infections. J Am Coll Surg. 2000;191(3):227–31.
59. Kollef MH, Sherman G, Ward S, Fraser VJ. Inadequate antimicrobial treatment of infections: a risk factor for hospital mortality among critically ill patients. Chest. 1999;115: 462–74.
60. Iregui M, Ward S, Sherman G, Fraser VJ, Kollef MH. Clinical importance of delays in the initiation of appropriate antibiotic treatment for ventilator-associated pneumonia. Chest. 2002;122:262–8.
61. Garnacho-Montero J. Impact of adequate empirical antibiotic therapy on the outcome of patients admitted to the intensive care unit with sepsis. Crit Care Med. 2003;31: 2742–51.
62. Alvarez-Lerma F, the ICU-Acquired Pneumonia Study Group. Modification of empiric antibiotic treatment in patients with pneumonia acquired in the intensive care unit. Intensive Care Med. 1996;22:387–94.
63. Ruhe JJ, Smith N, Bradsher RW, Menon A. Community-onset methicillin-resistant *Staphylococcus aureus* skin and soft-tissue infections: impact of antimicrobial therapy on outcome. Clin Infect Dis. 2007;44:777–84.
64. Schramm GE, Johnson JA, Doherty JA, Micek ST, Kollef MH. Methicillin-resistant *Staphylococcus aureus* sterile-site infection: the importance of appropriate initial antimicrobial treatment. Crit Care Med. 2006;34(8):2069–74.
65. Chuck EA, Frazee BW, lambert L, McCabe R. The benefit of empiric treatment for methicillin-resistant *Staphylococcus aureus*. J Emerg Med. 2010;38(5):567–71.
66. Gorwitz RJ, Jernigan DB, Powers JH, Jernigan JA, Participants in the CDC-Convened Experts' Meeting on Management of MRSA in the Community. Strategies for clinical management of MRSA in the community: Summary of an experts' meeting convened by the Centers for Disease Control and Prevention. 2006. Available at: http://198.246.98.21/ncidod/dhqp/pdf/ar/CAMRSA_ExpMtgStrategies.pdf Accessed 2011 Mar.
67. Kumar A, Roberts D, Wood KE, et al. Duration of hypotension before initiation of effective antimicrobial therapy is the critical determinant of survival in human septic shock. Crit Care Med. 2006;34(6):1589–96.
68. Brook I. Microbiology and management of soft tissue and muscle infections. Int J Surg. 2008;6(4):328–38.
69. Naimi TS, LeDell KH, Como-Sabetti K, et al. Comparison of community- and health care-associated methicillin-resistant *Staphylococcus aureus* infection. JAMA. 2003;290: 2976–84.
70. Crum NF, Lee RU, Thornton SA, et al. Fifteen year study of the changing epidemiology of methicillin-resistant *Staphylococcus aureus*. Am J Med. 2006;119:943–51.
71. Moran GJ, Krishnadasan A, Gorwitz RJ, et al. Methicillin-resistant *S. aureus* infections among patients in the emergency department. N Engl J Med. 2006;355(7):666–74.
72. Frazee BW, Lynn J, Charlebois ED, et al. High prevalence of methicillin-resistant in emergency department skin and soft tissue infection. Ann Emerg Med. 2005;45:311–20.
73. King MD, Humphrey BJ, Wang YF. Emergence of community acquired methicillin-resistant *Staphylococcus aureus* USA 300 Clone as the prdominant cause of skin and soft-tissue infections. Ann Intern Med. 2006;144:309–17.
74. Awad SS, Elhabash SI, Lee L, et al. Increasing incidence of methicillin-resistant *Staphylococcus aureus* skin and soft tissue infections: reconsideration of empiric antimicrobial therapy. Am J Surg. 2007;194:606–10.
75. Hidayat LK, Hsu DI, Quist R, et al. High-dose vancomycin for methicillin-resistant *Staphylococcus aureus* infections. Arch Intern Med. 2006;166:2138–44.
76. Howden BP, Ward PB, Charles PGP, et al. Treatment outcomes for serious infections caused by methicillin-resistant *Staphylococcus aureus* with reduced vancomycin susceptibility. Clin Infect Dis. 2004;38:521–8.
77. Lipsky BA, Weigelt JA, Gupta V, et al. Skin, soft tissue, bone and joint infections in hospitalized patients: epidemiology and microbiological, clinical and economic outcomes. Infect Control Hosp Epidemiol. 2007;28(11):1290–8.

78. Stevens DL, Bisno AL, Chambers HF, Infectious Diseases Society of America, et al. Practice guidelines for the diagnosis and management of skin and soft tissue infections. Clin Infect Dis. 2005;41(10):1373–406.
79. Napolitano LM. Early appropriate parenteral antimicrobial treatment of complicated skin and soft tissue infections caused by methicillin-resistant *Staphylococcus aureus*. Surg Infect (Larchmt). 2008;9 Suppl 1:S15–27.
80. Stevens DL, Ma Y, Salmi DB, McIndoo E, Wallace RJ, Bryant AE. Impact of antibiotics on expression of virulence-associated exotoxin genes in methicillin-sensitive and methicillin-resistant *Staphylococcus aureus*. J Infect Dis. 2007; 195:202–11.
81. Wang R et al. Identification of novel cytolytic peptides as key virulence determinants for community-associated MRSA. Nat Med. 2007;13(12):1510–4.
82. Filbin MR, Ring DC, Wessels MR, et al. Case 2-2009: A 25 year-old man with pain and swelling of the right hand and hypotension. N Engl J Med. 2009;360:281–90.
83. Marshall JC, Maier RV, Jimenez M, Dellinger EP. Source control in the management of severe sepsis and septic shock: an evidence-based review. Crit Care Med. 2004;32 Suppl 11:S513–26.
84. Laterre PF. Progress in medical management of intra-abdominal infections. Curr Opin Infect Dis. 2008;21(4): 393–8.
85. Grayson ML. The treatment triangle for staphylococcal infections. N Engl J Med. 2006;355:724–7.
86. Kuo DC, Chasm RM, Witting MD. Emergency department physician ability to predict methicillin-resistant *Staphylococcus aureus* skin and soft tissue infections. J Emerg Med. 2010;39(1):17–20.

Chronic Osteomyelitis

Suthorn Bavonratanavech and Yuan-Kun Tu

Contents

26.1 Introduction 321
26.2 Classification and Diagnosis 322
26.2.1 Classification 322
26.2.2 Clinical Assessment 322
26.2.3 Laboratory Examination and Bacterial Culture 322
26.2.4 Imaging Studies 323
26.3 Etiology and Pathogens 323
26.4 The Effect of Implant Design and Surface Topography on Infections Associated with Fracture Fixation Devices 324
26.5 Pre-op Planning and Decision Making 325
26.6 Treatment 325
26.6.1 Debridement of Bone 326
26.6.2 Bony Stabilization 326
26.6.3 Antibiotics 326
26.6.4 Wound Management 326
26.6.5 Bone Grafting 326
26.7 Summary 329
References 331

S. Bavonratanavech (✉)
Bumrungrad Hospital, 33 Soi 3 NaNa Nua, Wattana,
Bangkok 10110, Thailand
e-mail: suthorn@bumrungrad.com

Y.-K. Tu
E-DA Hospital/I-Shou University, Kaohsiung County, Taiwan
e-mail: ed100130@edah.org.tw

26.1 Introduction

Osteomyelitis is a complicated problem characterized by progressive inflammatory destruction and new apposition of bone [1]. Treatment of osteomyelitis of the lower extremity presents one of the most difficult challenges for the reconstructive surgeon [2]. The mainstay of treatment for chronic osteomyelitis is surgery. However, until recently, the disease was particularly frustrating for both the patient and surgeon because of its persistence despite multiple surgical interventions and prolonged antibiotic regimens [1, 3, 4]. Although osteomyelitis in the adult may have a hematogenous source typically as the result of intravenous drug use, the more common causes of osteomyelitis are trauma, vascular insufficiency, diabetes, and surgical wound infection [1, 5, 6]. Usually, patients that develop chronic osteomyelitis experience acute infections early after injury. Prolonged infections are often caused by a delay in diagnosis or inadequate treatment. There are systemic and local factors that increase the susceptibility of infection. To describe the physiologic status that is associated with risk of infection, people are classified as type A, B, or C hosts [5, 6]. The differentiation is based on the presence of local and systemic host factors, which play a major role in the outcome of the interaction between the microorganisms and the host:

Type A host: Strong systemic defense, a high level of local vascularity, and a normal physiologic response to infection and surgery.

Type B host: Systemic, local, or combined deficiency in wound healing and infection response. Systemic host factors, such as end-stage renal disease, malignancy, diabetes mellitus, alcoholism, malnutrition, rheumatologic diseases, HIV infection, or immunosuppressive therapy, may reduce the ability of the immune system to have an effective response to microorganisms. Local host deficiency may be caused by arterial disease, venous stasis, post radiation, scarring of soft tissue, or smoking, all of which reduce vascularity. The original trauma with severe soft tissue injury and subsequent surgery frequently result in avascular bone fragments and more damage to the soft tissue envelope. Timing of surgery and type of operative fixation should be carefully considered.

Type C host: The local and systemic factors are so severe that the anticipated morbidity of treatment exceeds that of the disease itself.

26.2 Classification and Diagnosis

26.2.1 Classification

A detailed assessment of the patient's condition and judicious choice of medical or surgical treatment are predetermined by a clinical staging system based on four factors: site of infection, extent of necrosis, host condition, and patient disability. The Cierny–Mader classification describes the extent of bone involvement as I (medullary), II (superficial), III (localized, <5 cm), and IV (intercalary defect >5 cm). This classification also delineates the physiological class of the patient as an A host (uncompromised), BL host (soft tissue, compromised locally), BS host (systemic, compromised host), BL/BS host (local and systemic compromise), and C host (high treatment morbidity, poor prognosis) [5]. It is of paramount importance to recognize and record the clinical stage of patients with chronic osteomyelitis before treatment.

The Cierny–Mader classification differentiates four different categories of osteomyelitis according to the anatomic localization (REF). (Table 26.1)

26.2.2 Clinical Assessment

Osteomyelitis is diagnosed by history, physical examination, imaging, and laboratory tests. Clinical diagnosis of an acute osseous infection is based on the symptoms of local swelling, tenderness, purulent discharge, and

Table 26.1 Classification of chronic osteomyelitis

- Type I: Medullary osteomyelitis involving the intramedullary surface.
- Type II: Superficial osteomyelitis involving the periosteal surface. It is caused by infection when the bone surface is exposed and represents an early stage.
- Type III: Localized osteomyelitis involves full thickness of bone cortex and extends into the medullary canal.
- Type IV: Diffuse osteomyelitis characterized by circumferential involvement that causes bony destruction and instability.

erythematic change over the fracture site or surgical wound. Physical signs persisting for more than 10 days correlate with the development of necrotic bone and osteomyelitis [1, 4]. Chronic osteomyelitis is defined as a bone infection persisting for over 6 months confirmed by histological, bacteriological, and radiographic analyses [7, 8]. The patient may present with varying degrees of pain, including those who are pain-free. There are also various degrees of local swelling and erythema. Some present with chronic ulcerations and sinus drainage. Soft tissue defects with surrounding scar adhesion indicate poor vascularity. This may be a result of infection, scar tissue formation by multiple surgical procedures, or by the initial soft tissue injury. In cases of foul-smelling discharge and long-term sinus drainage, malignancy should be ruled out. Fever and sepsis are uncommon in chronic osteomyelitis, likely because of inadequate soft tissue perfusion. Osseous deformity and malunion/nonunion represent common complications.

26.2.3 Laboratory Examination and Bacterial Culture

With chronic osteomyelitis, the white blood cell count is most often normal. Erythrocyte sedimentation rate and C-reactive protein levels may be elevated. If these are inconclusive, other diagnostic tests are performed to confirm the diagnosis.

Identification of the causative microorganisms is paramount for successful diagnosis, treatment, and prognosis. The definitive diagnosis can be achieved by identification of the organism by culture. However, at times, no specific organism is identified. Antibiotic treatment may preclude the growth of pathogens.

Cultures from the wound discharge are not adequate to determine the organism because contamination is frequent. Culture from ulcers or fistula swabs can often be misleading [6, 9]. Surgical sampling or needle biopsy of the infected tissue provides indispensable information. Intraoperative specimens should include sinus tract excision, discharge fluid, and soft tissue and bone tissue. All these should be sent separately for cultures.

26.2.4 Imaging Studies

Conventional radiography is necessary for both diagnosis of osseous infections and bone defects, as well as for follow-up. Plain radiographs can provide information about bony structure and quality. Bone resorption with periosteal and endosteal new bone formation indicates an inflammatory process. In long standing cases, a sequestrum and involucrum may be visualized. Both computed tomography (CT) and magnetic resonance imaging (MRI) provide excellent resolution of the periosteum.

For questionable cases, a CT scan provides a detailed analysis of bony structures for proper preoperative planning. For those with surgical implants, the evaluation of stability is necessary to decide whether it has to be retained or can be removed. MRI is a highly sensitive tool for diagnosing osteomyelitis. It can provide anatomical details required for differentiation between bone and soft tissue demarcation of infection. The usage of MRI is limited by the presence of implants, which cause artifacts and clouds the interpretation of the infected area. In these cases, scintigraphic assessment may be helpful, especially when a leukocyte scan is used. Nuclear imaging using various agents, such as Tc99m methylene diphosphonate or gallium citrate Ga 67, is highly sensitive for the early detection of osteomyelitis [10].

26.3 Etiology and Pathogens

Osteomyelitis usually develops after complex lower extremity injuries, and is associated with open fractures with severe soft tissue destruction [3, 7]. The development of ostcomyelitis following open fractures may occur as the result of an initial massive bacterial contamination, devascularization, or delay in achieving a stable, closed wound [11, 12]. Chronic osteomyelitis develops inflammatory foci, which are surrounded by sclerotic bone with poor blood supply. This is covered by a thick, relatively avascular periosteum and scarred muscle and subcutaneous tissue [6]. Antibiotics reach such infected tissue mainly through diffusion, and sensitive organisms may survive and become active again after the therapy is discontinued. Secondary infection by organisms that are more resistant to antibiotics than the primary infecting agents is common [13]. This evolving pathogenesis in chronic osteomyelitis may account for the therapeutic failures often seen despite the extensive array of antibiotics currently available.

Staphylococcus aureus, a very common organism, may adhere to bone by expressing receptors for components of the bone matrix. Additionally, the expression of collagen-binding proteins permits the attachment of the pathogen to cartilage [1, 14]. *Staphylococcus aureus* internalized by cultured osteoblasts can survive intracellularly [15]. The intracellular survival of bacteria may explain the persistence of bone infection. Once *Staphylococcus aureus* adheres to bone, phenotypic resistance to antibiotic treatment is expressed, which may also explain the high failure rate of short courses of therapy [1, 16].

In the presence of infection, cytokines (e.g., interleukin-1, interleukin-11, and tumor necrosis factor) generated locally by inflammatory and bone cells are potent osteolytic factors. Therefore, it is common to observe bone loss in osteomyelitis. Furthermore, phagocytes attempt to contain the invading microorganisms, and in the process, generate toxic oxygen radicals and release proteolytic enzymes that lyse surrounding tissues. Several components act directly or indirectly as bone-modulating factors during bacterial-induced bone destruction [17]. The ischemic necrosis of bone may also be due to purulent material spreading into vascular channels, raising the intraosseous pressure, and impairing blood flow. Thus, neutrophil infiltration and blood vessel thrombosis are the principal histological findings in acute osteomyelitis, while necrotic bone without viable osteocytes can be recognized in the chronic form [6].

26.4 The Effect of Implant Design and Surface Topography on Infections Associated with Fracture Fixation Devices

The design of a fracture fixation device, the material of which it is composed, as well as the surface topography of the device can all influence the susceptibility to infection [31].

The most significant advancement with respect to resistance to infection of internal fixation devices has come from the development of the limited contact internal fixation plates [44]. Prior to the development of limited contact devices, the dynamic compression plates (DCPs) that were commonly used provided fixation by compression of bone fragments across the fracture gap and between the plate and the underlying bone across a large footprint. This results in compression-induced restriction of blood flow through the periosteum. As the design of the internal fixation plate developed, the compression plate was succeeded by the limited contact dynamic compression plate (LCDCP), point contact fixator (PC-Fix), and finally, the locking compression plate (LCP). All of these devices reduced the contact area with the bone and caused a lower amount of damage to the periosteum. When the resistance to infection of this new locked device model was compared with the DCP, the limited contact plate (PC-Fix) was found to display a significant improvement in infection resistance by several orders of magnitude [29]. The reason for the improved infection resistance was attributed to improved viability of periosteal tissue [29]. This is a clear example of how improving implant design can significantly improve resistance to infection.

Implant design also plays a role in infections associated with intramedullary nails. For example, hollow and cannulated nails have been developed which allow insertion of a guide wire to help align fractured bone fragments and aid nail insertion. However, this design incorporates a dead space in the center of the nail, which cannot be accessed efficiently by the host vasculature and immune system. The creation of this dead space may be expected to negatively influence susceptibility to infection. In an animal study designed to test the influence hollow slotted nails, a decreased resistance to infection was indeed observed for the hollow nail in comparison with solid nails [37]. The solid nails do not create dead space where infecting bacteria can initiate and propagate an infection.

The material and the topography of any fracture fixation device are known to influence the cellular and tissue responses [33, 34, 38, 39, 41, 43], and must also be considered as a potential influence on the development of infection. Of the commonly available orthopaedic implant materials, stainless steel is associated with an increased infection rate in comparison with titanium for DCPs and intramedullary nails in animal models [30, 32], and also for external fixation pins and spinal implants in clinical trials [42, 45]. This data suggests that implant material does influence infection rates of fracture fixation devices. However, more recently, in a locked plate (LCP) model, there was found to be no large difference in infection resistance between electropolished to a smooth surface (EPSS) and cpTi, with only a small difference in ID_{50} between the cpTi and EPSS LCPs [40]. The improved biological protection of periosteum provided by the LCP is believed to be the reason why the previously observed material-related differences in infection susceptibility experienced for EPSS and cpTi DCPs in animal studies is not observed for the LCPs in the newer study. Therefore, the impact of different materials appears to be superseded by implant design characteristics that improve protection of tissue.

At this point, it is important to note that in comparing stainless steel with titanium, that stainless steel is usually electropolished to a smooth surface, whereas titanium in its standard form has a microrough surface. Therefore, when comparing stainless steel with titanium, there is a topographical difference in addition to a material difference. The exact influence of each of these parameters on the development of infection has not been determined until recently. When polished titanium was compared with polished steel LCP's (i.e., when the topography was practically identical), there was no difference in infection susceptibility [40]. When the influence of material and topography was assessed for intramedullary nails, there was again found to be no difference in infection susceptibility between smooth TAN nails and standard TAN nails (Moriarty et al. 2010, International Journal Artificial Organs, in press). Smooth titanium and titanium alloy implants have been shown in animal studies to ease implant removal complications, and are expected to have significant clinical impact in certain applications [35, 36, 40]. Based on the results of the infection models used, these polished implants are not expected to result in an increase in infection susceptibility if implemented clinically.

In the context of orthopaedic fracture fixation devices, it must be remembered that it is difficult to directly extrapolate the data from animal models of infection to the clinical situation. Animal studies involve the artificial contamination of the implant and surgical site and do not replicate the contamination occurring in real clinical situations with respect to bacterial numbers, growth phase, nutrient status, species, and tissue damage. Nevertheless, animal models are helpful in bridging the gap between laboratory studies and clinical situations. The animal data shows that minimizing dead space and protecting the viability of the tissues in contact with the implanted device are expected to have the greatest influence upon the susceptibility to infection. Implant material [34] and topography will also play a role, though experiences to date suggest that protection of viable tissues may be even more important.

26.5 Pre-op Planning and Decision Making

Surgical management of chronic osteomyelitis is demanding and requires a thorough assessment. This should include evaluation of the soft tissue status and the exact localization and degree of bony involvement. Furthermore, the personality of patient and the social background should be assessed. In certain cases, the option of amputation should be discussed as a feasible treatment option. The soft tissue condition includes the presence of infection, chronic ulcers with soft tissue defects, scarring, and avascular zones. Extensive debridement may include the soft tissues and require major soft tissue reconstructive measures such as microvascular free flaps [2, 3, 6–8]. The neurovascular and functional status of the limb is crucial to determine the operative procedure and outcome after treatment. Nerve injury, crush injury, and diabetic neuropathy, which results in poor sensation of foot, may affect treatment and functional outcome and should be included in the assessment.

The stability of the implant is usually insufficient after prolonged infection and should be removed. This evaluation helps in planning for the approach, extent of debridement, choice of stabilization, and soft tissue reconstruction.

Several factors are summarized under the definition of the "personality of the patient," such as preinjury status, profession, comorbidity, and personal expectations.

The surgeon should have a well-documented discussion with the patient and relatives. This should include the plan and the complexity of the reconstructive procedure along with the issues related to the requirement of multiple operations.

Prolonged treatment of chronic osteomyelitis is the rule and will affect the personal life of the patient, and impose a financial burden. Amputation should be openly discussed in patients with multiple comorbidities, severe bone loss with soft tissue damage, or neurovascular deficit associated with poor functional outcome.

26.6 Treatment

The mainstay of treatment for patients with osteomyelitis is a combination of surgical debridement and systemic antibiotic therapy to promote healing and eradicate infection. The treatment can be divided into separate stages as follows:

1. Surgical debridement with antibiotic therapy
2. Bony stabilization
3. Soft issue coverage
4. Bridging of bone defect to achieve bony union

Successful treatment of osteomyelitis depends on careful patient selection, adequate administration of antibiotics, and application of four essential surgical procedures [2–4, 6, 7, 18].

1. Radical debridement: removal of all contaminated hard and soft tissue until only well-vascularized healthy tissue remains.
2. Obliteration of the resultant dead space: application of the bead-pouch technique [6, 19] with local or microsurgical free flap transfer to neo-vascularize the entire involved area.
3. Bone stabilization: adequate internal or external fixation to provide skeletal stability and prevent local recurrence of infection [3, 6, 12].
4. Bridging of the bone defect: conventional bone graft for short defects, or Ilizarov bone lengthening or VBG for defects longer than 6 cm [3, 6, 11, 18, 20].

26.6.1 Debridement of Bone

The first step is radical debridement with excision of sinus tracts and all nonviable tissue from skin, soft tissue, and bone. Debridement proceeds until viable tissue with a bleeding bed is present.

Inadequate debridement will result in persistent and recurrent infection that requires multiple operations. Specimens from the affected area are sent for aerobic and anaerobic cultures. The most common organism *Staphylococcus aureus* may be cultured alone or in combination with other pathogens. The second most common organism is *Pseudomonas aeruginosa*. For immune-compromised patients, atypical mycobacterium or fungi should be considered. To rule out malignancy, the specimen should be sent for pathological examination.

26.6.2 Bony Stabilization

In most cases of chronic osteomyelitis in the presence of a surgical implant, microorganisms are protected in a biofilm adherent to the implant surface. If the fracture is healed, the implant should be removed. In principle, if the implant is stable, then it should be retained until the fracture has united. However, adequate debridement may not be possible with an implant, as with intramedullary nails within the medullary canal. It is recommended to remove the intramedullary nail as it rarely provides goods stability. After nail removal, the medullary canal is reamed to remove the infected tissue and washed out.

Plate and screws should be removed with debridement of necrotic tissue under the plate and within the screw holes with curettes. All dead bone should be removed until there is a bleeding bone bed. The choice of stabilization varies between conventional external fixation for diaphyseal fractures, and hybrid external fixation for periarticular injuries. In cases of extensive bone loss that will require distraction osteogenesis, an Ilizarov type of frame can be assembled at the time of debridement or at a later stage [20]. Another option is a locking compression plate placed outside of skin to serve as an external fixation [21]. The advantage of external fixation is to allow repeated debridement while providing stability and maintaining proper alignment of fracture.

26.6.3 Antibiotics

Antibiotic beads can be used and removed at a subsequent procedure for repeat debridement or for soft tissue coverage and bone grafting for the defect. Local antibiotic delivery gives high local concentrations and low systemic levels of antibiotics with a reduced risk of systemic adverse effects. However, there are some disadvantages to prolonged bead placement, including the development of resistant organisms.

Broad-spectrum systemic antibiotic therapy should initially be administered to cover the most common organisms. Antibiotics should then be adjusted accordingly pending cultures and sensitivities. Short duration of intravenous administration for 1 week followed by oral antibiotics for 6 weeks is recommended.

26.6.4 Wound Management

After debridement, delayed closure is considered. Primary closure is often not possible because of an inadequate soft tissue envelope and poor vascularity. Repeated debridement may be necessary and further evaluation may be necessary to choose the appropriate procedure for soft tissue coverage. Soft tissue coverage can be achieved by skin grafts, local flaps, or free vascularized flaps [22]. The decision regarding the most appropriate treatment depends on the location and size of the defect. Muscle flaps eliminate dead space, provide soft tissue coverage, and improve vascularity, which is important to resist infection and promote healing [4, 6–8, 11, 12, 22, 23]. Soft tissue coverage is usually performed at a delayed stage 3–7 days after the initial debridement. Coverage should not be considered unless the infectious process is under control and devitalized tissue is removed completely for Case Demonstration refer (Figs. 26.1–26.6).

26.6.5 Bone Grafting

Autologous iliac bone graft is the gold standard for managing bone defects of less than 6 cm [3, 6, 12, 18]. Multiple operations may be required for larger defects, while carefully assessing the bony healing process.

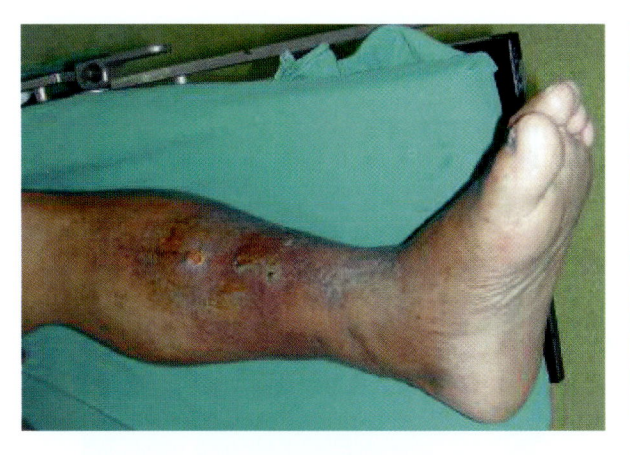

Fig. 26.1 A 68-year-old male with left tibia chronic osteomyelitis for 2 years. Acute flare of the infection is noted with erythema and purulent discharge on his affected leg

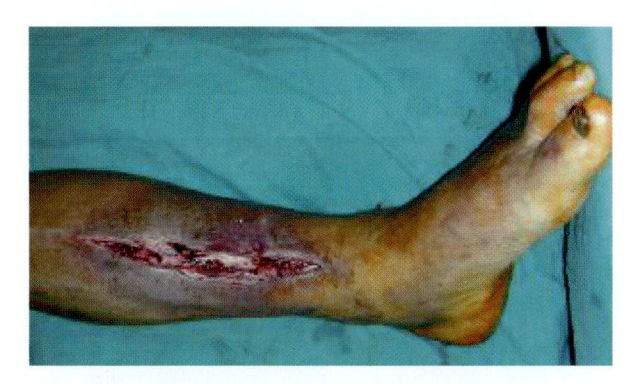

Fig. 26.2 Debridement performed with adequate soft tissue excision and curettage of necrotic bone

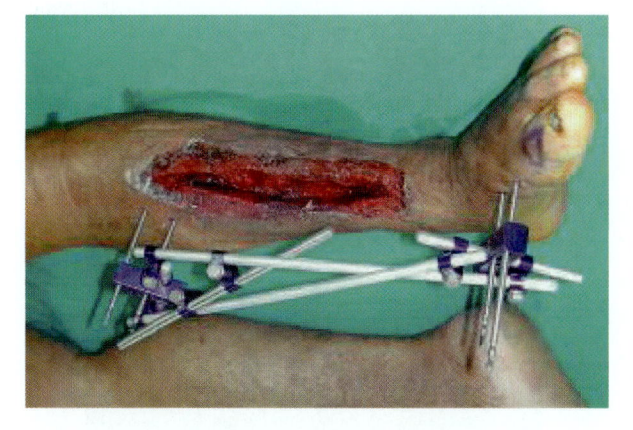

Fig. 26.3 External fixator applied after debridement for bony stability

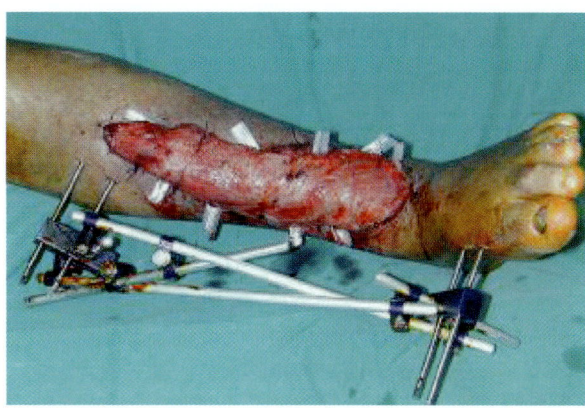

Fig. 26.4 Free latissimus dorsi (*LD*) muscle flap transferred to cover the soft tissue defect 3 days after debridement

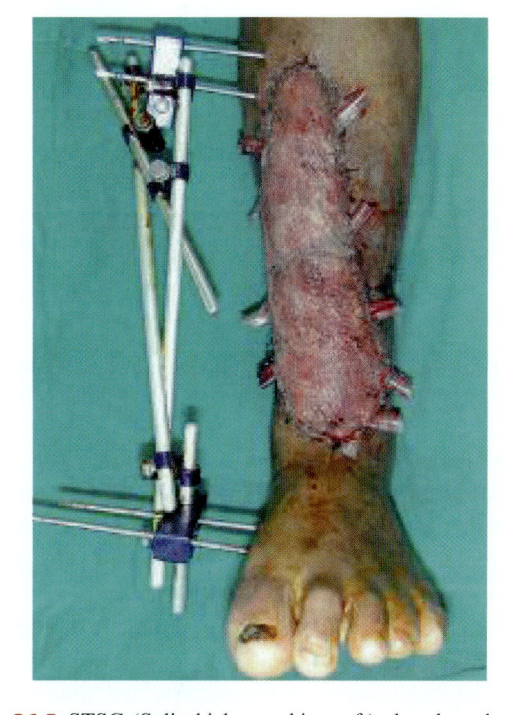

Fig. 26.5 STSG (Split thickness skin graft) placed on the surface of LD muscle flap

Correct timing is crucial in placing a graft. Bone grafting should be performed after soft tissue coverage has been accomplished, and when the infection is under control. For infected tibial nonunions, the choice of approach for the graft should be adjacent to soft tissues that have adequate vascularity.

The conventional nonvascularized cortical grafts have been utilized for the reconstruction of large segmental defects, but require at least 4–8 months for

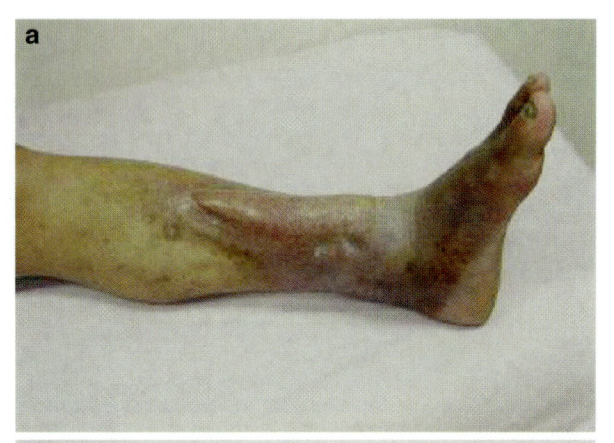

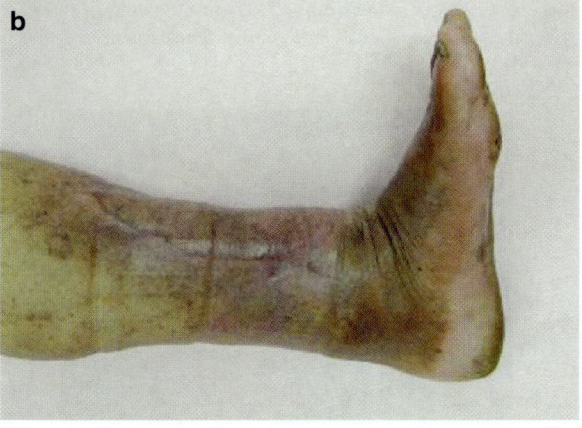

Fig. 26.6 Complete recovery from osteomyelitis, with good ankle range of motion in plantar flexion (**a**) and dorsiflexion (**b**)

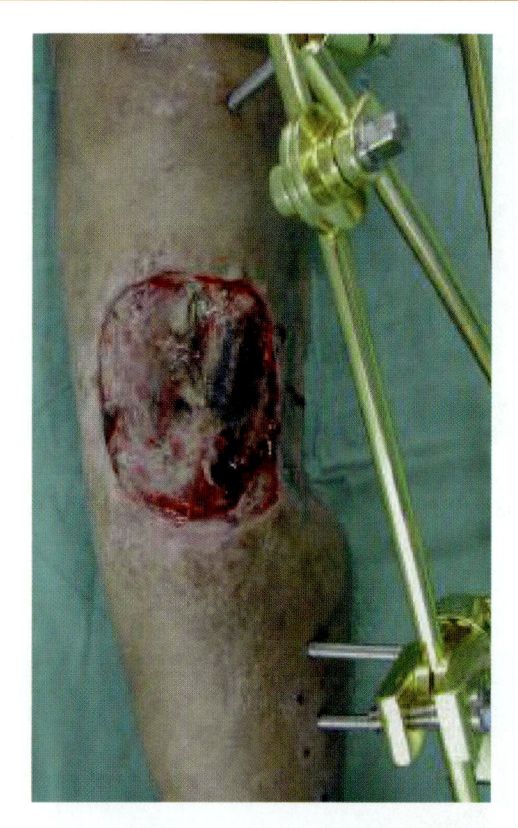

Fig. 26.7 53-year-old male with chronic osteomyelitis and combined soft tissue and bone loss of right tibia, 6 months after trauma

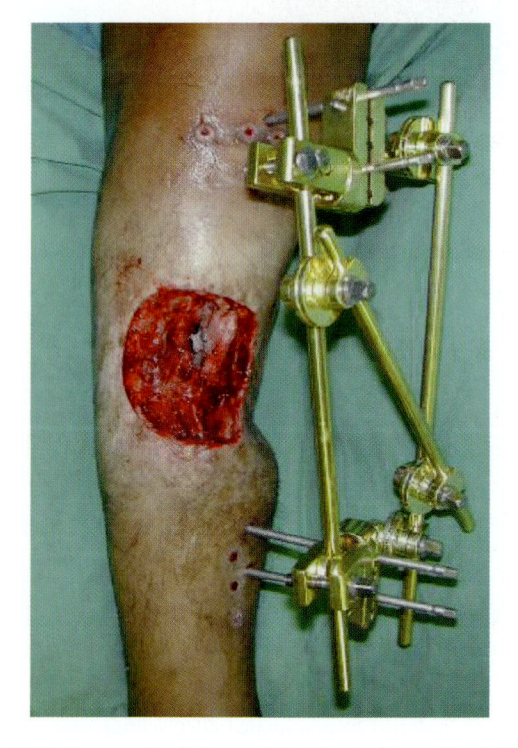

Fig. 26.8 Bone and soft tissue defect located over the right leg after debridement

revascularization. The majority of cells in autogenous grafts do not survive the transplantation and must be replaced in a process termed creeping substitution. The repair is initiated by osteoclasts, with subsequent action by osteoblasts. The graft is likely never completely replaced by healthy normal bone, existing as a mixture of necrotic and viable bone [6, 24]. Therefore, conventional autogenous nonvascularized bone graft is only indicated for filling bone defects smaller than 6 cm. Successful distraction osteogenesis in the femur and tibia for osteomyelitis has been reported in treatment of bone defects and osteomyelitis [20, 25]. The advantages of this procedure include the ability to reconstruct long bone defects, repair nonunions, correct deformities, and lengthen limbs. However, drawbacks include infection of the wire site, docking site nonunion, and prolonged course of treatment with an external fixator device [6, 26].

Vascularized bone grafts (VBG) are indicated with skeletal defects greater than 6 cm in length [3, 6, 12, 18, 24]. The vascularized bone graft is very important in

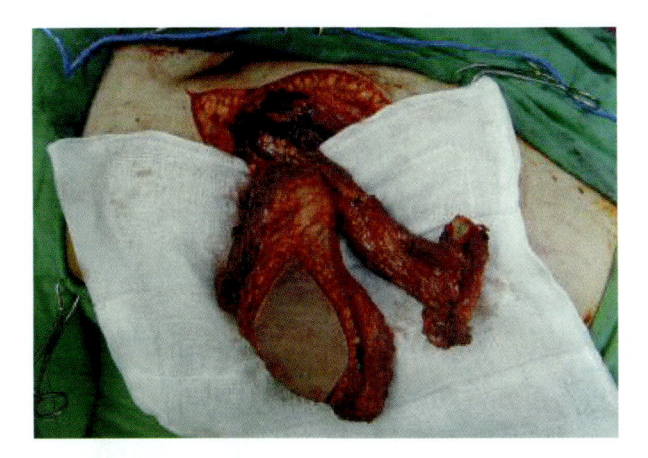

Fig. 26.9 The free latissimus dorsi, serratus anterior, ribs composite flap identified and harvested from the right upper back

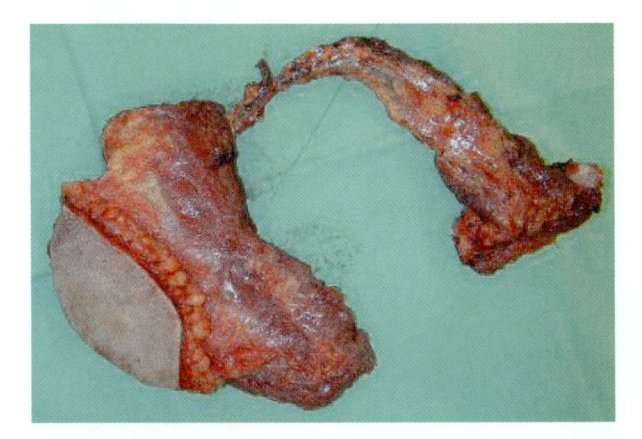

Fig. 26.10 The composite LD/SA/Ribs flap based on a single common pedicle (thoracodorsal artery and vein)

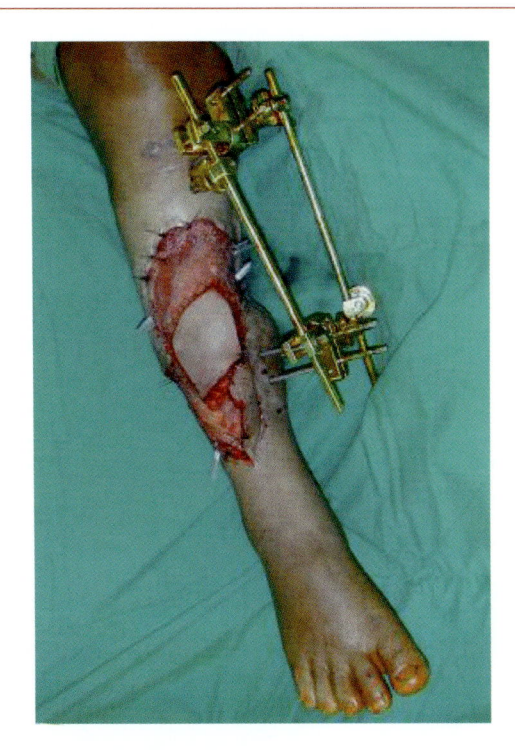

Fig. 26.11 Immediate postoperative picture demonstrating good blood supply to this composite flap

osteomyelitis treatment because of the advantages of combining the viability of cancellous grafts with the stability of cortical analogs, while leaving the nutrient blood supply intact. Furthermore, VBG is of particular utility in musculoskeletal sepsis, with selection of this procedure implying that antibiotic access to the wound and bone segment is unimpeded because of the immediate restoration of the blood supply [18]. Therefore, vascularized bone can be used to obliterate the dead space, bridge large bony defects, enhance bone healing, resist infection (with abundant blood supply), allow early rehabilitation, and ensure better clinical outcomes. The transferred vascularized bone also has the ability to hypertrophy. De Boer and Wood reported definite hypertrophy (20% width enlargement) in 43% of their cases within 1 year and 80% within 2 years [27]. Tu et al. reported that hypertrophy is more significant in the lower extremity than in the upper extremity [3]. In their study of fibular bone grafts, Tu et al. reported a mean hypertrophy index of 82.5% [6].

Another versatile free vascular composite graft is the combined ribs, serratus anterior, and latissimus dorsi muscle flap [3, 6, 28]. This muscular-osseous-cutaneous flap can be harvested by a single thoracodorsal vascular pedicle. Iliac crest vascularized tissue transfer, based on multiple nutrient perforators entering the inner cortex and arising from the deep circumflex iliac vessels, is another option for VBG [2, 6]. The curvature of the iliac crest usually limits its application to defects less than 10–12 cm in size, and is probably associated with higher donor site complication rates. The unreliability of the skin paddle of free vascularized iliac bone flap limits its clinical application, which accounts for the fact that free fibula transfer is utilized in most clinical series of lower extremity bone reconstructions [3, 6, 18, 24, 27] (Figs 26.7–26.14).

26.7 Summary

Management of chronic posttraumatic osteomyelitis poses a challenge in achieving the goals of treatment, which are control of infection, bone healing, and a

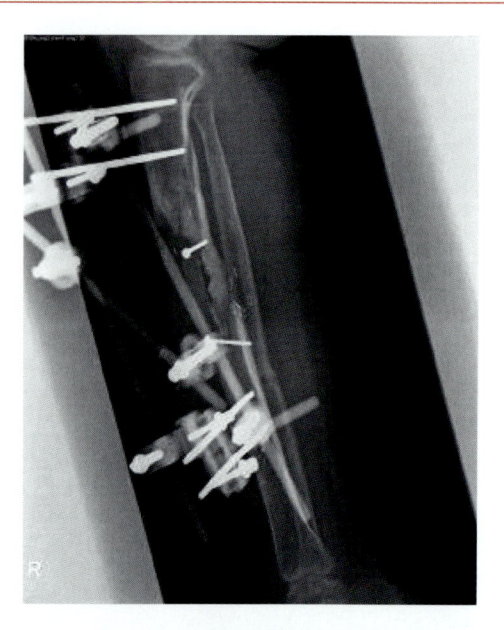

Fig. 26.12 Immediate postoperative radiography displaying ribs inserted to bridge the bone defect

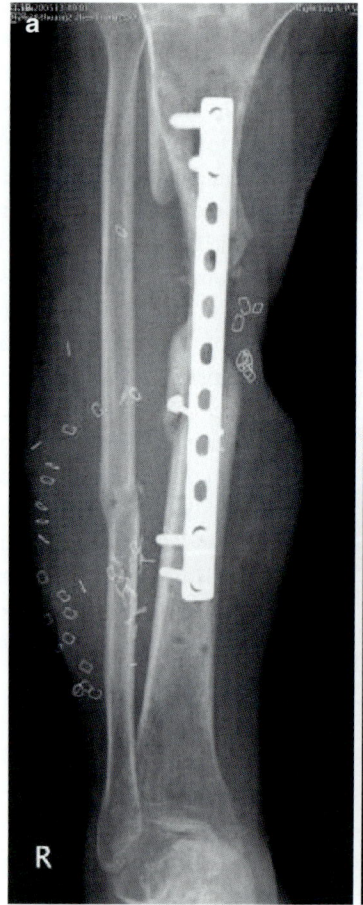

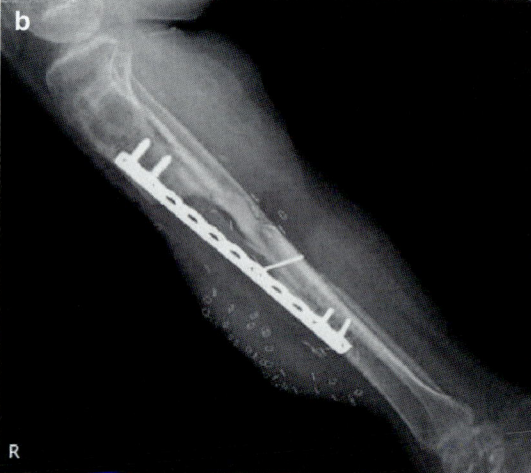

Fig. 26.13 The ESF removed and plate and screws were inserted as MIPO method 4 weeks after flap surgery, AP view (**a**) and Lateral view (**b**)

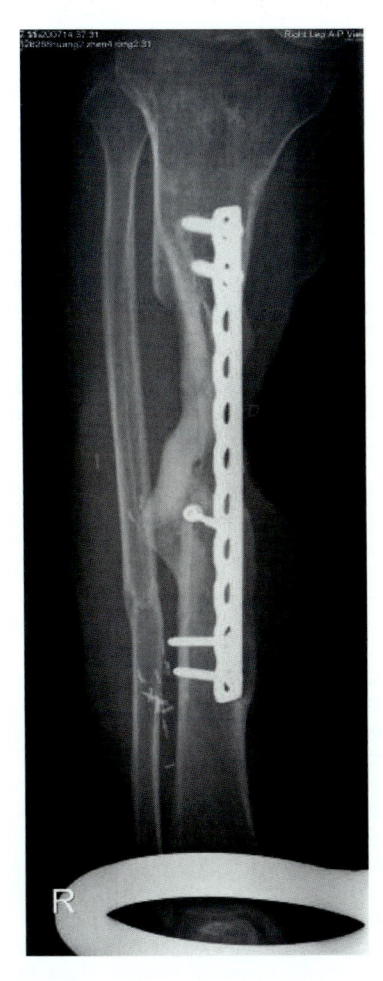

Fig. 26.14 Solid bone union and hypertrophy of the VBG (ribs) in 3 years F/U

satisfactory functional outcome. Timing and choice of fixation play a significant role to the primary surgeon treating closed or open fractures. Correct decision making and judgment will influence the incidence of postoperative infections. When an infection does occur, early aggressive debridement is required to reduce the likelihood of progressing to chronic osteomyelitis.

In the case of chronic osteomyelitis, preoperative clinical assessment and investigation of the infecting organisms, soft tissue condition, extent of infection, stability of the implant, and status of bony condition are mandatory to make a proper plan of treatment. Radical debridement of nonviable and infected tissue is necessary. Identification of organisms from infected tissue removed during debridement is recommended to identify the correct pathogens. Systemic and local antibiotics impregnated into PMMA beads are used to fill dead space and to deliver high doses of antibiotics to eradicate infection. Bony stability is usually maintained by an external fixator after debridement. Repeat debridements may be required until the infection is under control to allow early soft tissue coverage. Local or free muscle flaps may be required for reconstruction depending on the site and size of the defect. Use of autogenous bone graft or complex vascularized bone graft reconstructions depends on the length of bony defect needed to be bridged to achieve bone healing.

References

1. Lew DP, Waldvogel FA. Osteomyelitis. N Engl J Med. 1997;336:999–1007.
2. Rhomberg M, Frischhut B, Ninkovic M, et al. A single-stage operation in the treatment of chronic osteomyelitis of the lower extremity including reconstruction with free vascularized iliac bone graft and free-tissue transfer. Plast Reconstr Surg. 2003;111(7):2353–61.
3. Tu YK, Yen CY, Yeh WL. Reconstruction of posttraumatic long bone defect with free vascularized bone graft. Acta Orthop Scand. 2001;72(4):359–64.
4. Guelinckx P, Sinsel N. Refinements in the one-stage procedure for management of chronic osteomyelitis. Microsurgery. 1995;16:606–11.
5. Cierny 3rd G, Mader JT, Penninck JJ. A clinical staging system for adult osteomyelitis. Clin Orthop Relat Res. 2003;414:7–24.
6. Tu YK, Yen YC. The role of vascularized bone graft in lower extremity osteomyelitis. Orthop Clin North Am. 2007;38(1):37–49.
7. Moore JR, Weiland AJ. Vascularized tissue transfer in the treatment of osteomyelitis. Clin Plast Surg. 1986;13(4):657–62.
8. Musharafieh R, Osmani O, Musharafieh U, et al. Efficacy of microsurgical free-tissue transfer in chronic osteomyelitis of the leg and foot: review of 22 cases. J Reconstr Microsurg. 1999;15(4):239–44.
9. Mackowiak PA, Jones SR, Smith JW. Diagnostic value of sinus-tract cultures in chronic osteomyelitis. JAMA. 1978;239:2772–5.
10. Tumeh SS, Tohmeh AG. Nuclear medicine techniques in septic arthritis and osteomyelitis. Rheum Dis Clin North Am. 1991;17:559–83.
11. Gayle LB, Lineaweaver WC, Oliva A, et al. Treatment of chronic osteomyelitis of the lower extremities with debridement and microvascular muscle transfer. Clin Plast Surg. 1992;19(4):895–903.
12. Tu YK, Yen CY, Ma CH, et al. Soft tissue injury management and flap reconstruction for mangled lower extremities. Injury. 2008;39 Suppl 4:75–95.
13. Fitzgerald RH. Experimental osteomyelitis: description of a canine model and the role of depot administration of antibi-

otics in the prevention and treatment of sepsis. J Bone Joint Surg. 1983;65A(3):371–80.
14. Hermann M, Vaudaux PE, Pittet D, et al. Fibronectin, fibrinogen, and laminin act as mediators of adherence of clinical staphylococcal isolates to foreign material. J Infect Dis. 1988;158:693–701.
15. Proctor RA, van Langevelde P, Kristjansson M, et al. Persistent and relapsing infections associated with small-colony variants of *Staphylococcus aureus*. Clin Infect Dis. 1995;20:95–102.
16. Chuard C, Jucet JC, Rohner P, et al. Resistance of *Staphylococcus aureus* recovered from infected foreign body *in vivo* to killing by antimicrobials. J Infect Dis. 1991;163:1369–73.
17. Nair SP, Meghji S, Wilson M, et al. Bacterially induced bone destruction: mechanisms and misconceptions. Infect Immun. 1996;64:2371–80.
18. Wood MB, Cooney III WP. Vascularized bone segment transfers for management of chronic osteomyelitis. Orthop Clin North Am. 1984;15:461–72.
19. McKee MD, Wild LM, Schemitsch EH, et al. The use of an antibiotic impregnated, osteoconductive, bioabsorbable bone substitute in the treatment of infected long bone defects: early results of a prospective trial. J Orthop Trauma. 2002;16(9):622–7.
20. Green SA. Osteomyelitis: the Ilizarov perspective. Orthop Clin North Am. 1991;22:515–21.
21. Ma CH, Wu CH, Yu SW, Yen CY, Tu YK. Staged external and internal less invasive stabilisation system plating for open proximal tibial fractures. Injury (Int J Care Injured). 2010;41:190–6.
22. Tu YK, Tu YK, Tong GO, et al. Soft tissue injury in orthopedic trauma. Injury. 2008;39 Suppl 4:3–17.
23. Ma CH, Tu YK, Tu YK, et al. Reconstruction of upper extremity large soft tissue defect using pedicled LD flap – technique illustration and clinical outcomes. Injury. 2008;39 Suppl 4:67–74.
24. Gerwin M, Weiland AJ. Vascularized bone grafts to the upper extremity. Hand Clin. 1992;8:509–23.
25. Paley D, Catagni MA, Argnani F, et al. Ilizarov treatment of tibial nonunions with bone loss. Clin Orthop Relat Res. 1989;241:146–65.
26. Carrington NC, Smith RM, Knight SL, et al. Ilizarov bone transport over a primary tibial nail and free flap: a new technique for treating Gustilo grade 3b fractures with large segmental defects. Injury. 2000;31:112–5.
27. De Boer HH, Wood MB. Bone changes in the vascularized fibular graft. J Bone Joint Surg. 1989;71B:374–8.
28. Lin CH, Yazar S. Revisiting the serratus anterior rib flap for composite tibial defect. Plast Reconstr Surg. 2004;114(7):1871–80.
29. Arens S, Eijer H, Schlegel U, Printzen G, Perren SM, Hansis M. Influence of the design for fixation implants on local infection: experimental study of dynamic compression plates versus point contact fixators in rabbits. J Orthop Trauma. 1999;13:470–6.
30. Arens S, Schlegel U, Printzen G, Ziegler WJ, Perren SM, Hansis M. Influence of materials for fixation implants on local infection. An experimental study of steel versus titanium DCP in rabbits. J Bone Joint Surg Br. 1996;78:647–51.
31. Harris LG, Richards RG. *Staphylococci* and implant surfaces: a review. Injury. 2006;37 Suppl 2:S3–14.
32. Hauke C, Schlegel U, Melcher GA, et al. Local infection in relation to different implant materials. An experimental study using stainless steel and titanium, unlocked, intramedullary nailsin rabbits. Orthop Trans. 1997;21:835–6.
33. Hayes JS, Archer CW, Richards RG. An *in vitro* evaluation for understanding the role of surface microtopography in controlling tissue integration. World biomaterials conference. 2008.
34. Hayes JS, Richards RG. Surfaces to control tissue adhesion for osteosynthesis with metal implants: in vitro and in vivo studies to bring solutions to the patient. Expert Rev Med Devices. 2010;7:131–42.
35. Hayes JS, Seidenglanz U, Pearce AI, Pearce SG, Archer CW, Richards RG. Surface polishing positively influences ease of plate and screw removal. Eur Cell Mater. 2010;19:117–26.
36. Hayes JS, Vos DI, Hahn J, Pearce SG, Richards RG. An in vivo evaluation of surface polishing of TAN intramedullary nails for ease of removal. Eur Cell Mater. 2009;18:15–26.
37. Horn J, Schlegel U, Krettek C, Ito K. Infection resistance of unreamed solid, hollow slotted and cannulated intramedullary nails: an in-vivo experimental comparison. J Orthop Res. 2005;23:810–5.
38. Meredith DO, Eschbach L, Riehle MO, Curtis AS, Richards RG. Microtopography of metal surfaces influence fibroblast growth by modifying cell shape, cytoskeleton, and adhesion. J Orthop Res. 2007;25:1523–33.
39. Meredith DO, Eschbach L, Wood MA, Riehle MO, Curtis AS, Richards RG. Human fibroblast reactions to standard and electropolished titanium and Ti-6Al-7Nb, and electropolished stainless steel. J Biomed Mater Res A. 2005;75:541–55.
40. Moriarty TF, Debefve L, Boure L, Campoccia D, Schlegel U, Richards RG. Influence of material and microtopography on the development of local infection in vivo: experimental investigation in rabbits. Int J Artif Organs. 2009;32:663–70.
41. Pearce AI, Pearce SG, Schweiger K, Milz S, Schneider E, Archer CW, et al. Effect of surface topography on removal of cortical bone screws in a novel sheep model. J Orthop Res. 2008;26:1377–83.
42. Pieske O, Geleng P, Zaspel J, Piltz S. Titanium alloy pins versus stainless steel pins in external fixation at the wrist: a randomized prospective study. J Trauma. 2008;64:1275–80.
43. Richards RG, Perren SM. Implants and materials in fracture fixation. In: Rüedi TP, Rüedi TP, Buckley RE, Moran CG, Moran CG, editors. AO principles of fracture management. Switzerland: AO publishing; 2007.
44. Schlegel U, Perren SM. Surgical aspects of infection involving osteosynthesis implants: implant design and resistance to local infection. Injury. 2006;37 Suppl 2:S67–73.
45. Soultanis KC, Pyrovolou N, Zahos KA, Karaliotas GI, Lenti A, Liveris I, et al. Late postoperative infection following spinal instrumentation: stainless steel versus titanium implants. J Surg Orthop Adv. 2008;17:193–9.

Reconstructive Strategies for Skeletal Complications in the Polytrauma Patient

Steven Sands, Peter A. Siska, and Ivan S. Tarkin

Contents

27.1	Introduction	333
27.1.1	Nature of Bony Injury	333
27.1.2	Soft Tissue Injury	334
27.1.3	Adverse Physiology	334
27.2	Initial Surgical Tactics	334
27.2.1	Prevention of Nonunion and Deformity	335
27.2.2	Primary Fracture Treatment	335
27.2.3	Staged Fracture Care	335
27.2.4	Role of Acute Shortening	336
27.3	Secondary Reconstruction	336
27.3.1	Anticipated Nonunion	337
27.4	Established Nonunion After Polytrauma	339
27.4.1	Traditional Nonunion Reconstruction	339
27.4.2	Infected Nonunion	340
27.5	Unconventional Reconstructive Options for Periarticular Nonunions	341
27.5.1	Combined Arthrodesis and Nonunion Reconstruction	341
27.5.2	Reconstruction Using Arthroplasty Techniques	342
27.6	Conclusion	342
References		343

S. Sands, P.A. Siska, and I.S. Tarkin (✉)
Division of Orthopaedic Traumatology,
Department of Orthopaedic Surgery, University of Pittsburgh Medical Center, 3471 Fifth Avenue, Kaufmann Building, Suite 1011, Pittsburgh, PA 15213, USA
e-mail: tarkinis@upmc.edu

27.1 Introduction

Timing and prioritization of care to the multisystem trauma patient is critical for promoting survivorship. Life-threatening injuries to the head, chest, and abdomen need to be addressed first. However, the orthopaedic traumatologist serves an integral role in the temporizing and eventual definitive management of associated severe musculoskeletal injuries.

Despite appropriate musculoskeletal care, nonunion and/or deformity is a frequent consequence after high-energy fracture in this patient population. A modest percentage of fractures will develop complication as a result of the initial bony injury, adjacent soft tissue trauma, compromised host physiology, and initial stabilization tactics [1, 2]. Strategies employed for managing nonunion and deformities are of paramount importance for promoting wellness, as musculoskeletal functionality is a primary determinant on long-term outcomes in the multisystem trauma patient [3].

When planning for secondary interventions, an individualized plan of care is essential to promote physical function while minimizing surgical risk [3]. Creative solutions are sometimes necessary to solve these difficult problems. The surgeon must have a complete armamentarium of options available for the patient including traditional nonunion reconstruction as well as arthrodesis and arthroplasty solutions for periarticular injuries.

27.1.1 Nature of Bony Injury

Devastating skeletal injury is realized in the multisystem trauma patient owing to the high-energy mechanism of injury (Fig. 27.1). Energy imparted to the skeletal

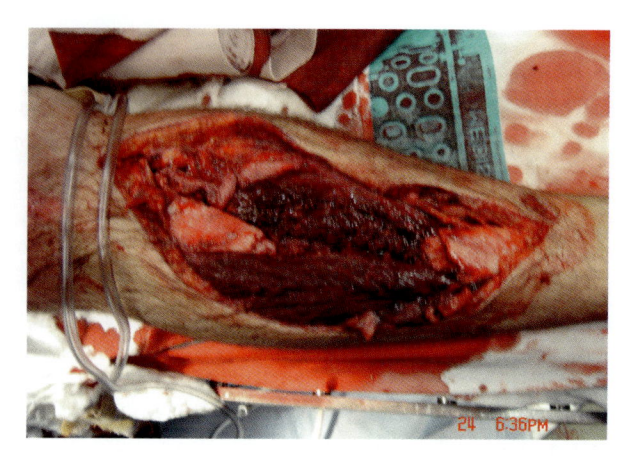

Fig. 27.1 Horrific musculoskeletal injuries are commonplace in the polytrauma patient with extensive bone and soft tissue involvement

anatomy often results in widely displaced, comminuted fracture patterns [4]. Fractures may occur in all anatomic locations including the diaphyseal, metaphyseal, and articular regions.

27.1.2 Soft Tissue Injury

Severe fractures associated with the polytrauma patient can result in delayed or frank nonunion secondary to the poor biologic potential realized by the associated compromised soft tissue sleeve. By definition, a severe high-energy fracture is associated with profound damage to the surrounding soft tissue envelope. These investing tissues are of paramount importance for uneventful fracture healing. The soft tissue sleeve through its vascular conduits brings essential factors necessary for fracture union [5–8].

Open fracture is not an uncommon finding in the polytraumatized patient. The soft tissue injury associated with open fracture portends a worse prognosis as extensive damage to the skin, muscle, and periosteum is typically evident. Further, after fracture debridement, bone loss is a frequent consequence often resulting in nonunion. Lastly, there is a heightened risk of deep infection leading to the development of septic nonunion.

27.1.3 Adverse Physiology

The overall health of the polytrauma patient impacts the success of fracture healing. A coordinated physiologic response, both local and systemic, is a requirement. Both immune dysfunction and malnutrition, frequently experienced by the polytrauma patient, adversely affect their reparative capacity.

Inflammation is part of the normal process of fracture healing. However, the multisystem trauma patient may develop hyperactivity of the immune system (Systemic Inflammatory Response Syndrome). This systemic imbalance can result in an impaired ability for the body to support organ system function (Multiple Organ Dysfunction Syndrome), ultimately affecting the body's ability to provide support for the healing of severe musculoskeletal injuries [9].

While a coordinated immune response is integral to fracture healing, optimized nutrition is another key component. During all stages of fracture healing, cellular proliferation and protein synthesis are required for the formation and remodeling of osseous tissues. Unfortunately, the polytrauma patient's nutritional reserve is constantly challenged [10]. Thereby, nonunion of fractures in this patient population is not an unexpected event.

27.2 Initial Surgical Tactics

Initial orthopaedic intervention has a profound impact on late complication after severe fracture in the polytrauma patient. Definitive treatment of these severe fractures promotes union and minimizes the possibility of deformity. Therefore, early total care is desirable when feasible and safe. However, there is select subset of critically ill polytrauma patients that cannot tolerate this surgical burden.

In this subgroup of patients, a damage control approach is instituted to provide rapid skeletal stabilization while more critical injuries are managed [1]. Closed reduction and external fixation serve as the "workhorse" strategy in this clinical setting (Fig. 27.2). External fixation is the most rigid form of provisional stabilization before definitive surgery is performed. The fixator minimizes fracture motion and stops the cycle of injury to the traumatized soft tissue sleeve. However, if the fixator is used as the definitive treatment scheme, nonunion and/or deformities are commonplace.

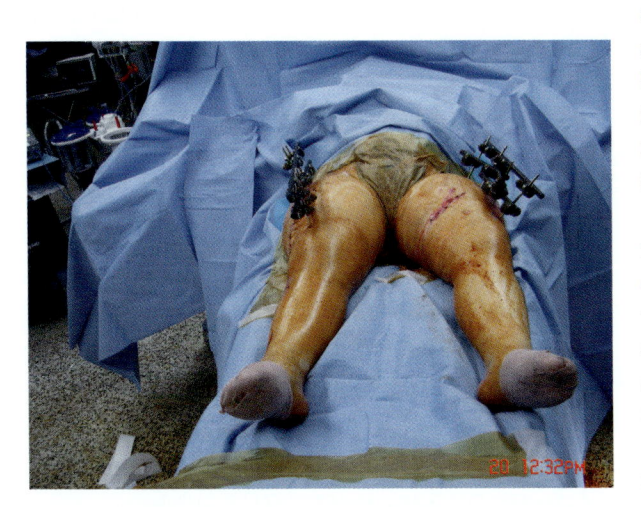

Fig. 27.2 The external fixator is an invaluable tool for rapid skeletal stabilization while awaiting definitive reconstruction efforts when the patient's overall physiology has improved

27.2.1 Prevention of Nonunion and Deformity

The orthopaedic traumatologist has an integral role in the multidisciplinary care plan for the polytrauma patient. The orthopaedic team must serve as "musculoskeletal ambassadors" for the multiply injured patient. In many cases, complications such as nonunion and deformity can be avoided if aggressive, yet safe, musculoskeletal care can be provided.

The orthopaedic team needs to be in close contact with the general surgical trauma group to coordinate the optimal timing of definitive musculoskeletal treatment. Even in the most critical patient, there is almost always a window of opportunity for efficient orthopaedic operation to optimally stabilize the skeletal injury as well as manage the associated soft tissue trauma.

27.2.2 Primary Fracture Treatment

Optimal biomechanical strategies can decrease the incidence of nonunion and/or deformity after severe fracture in the polytrauma patient. Fracture care must maximize reduction and stability while respecting the traumatized soft tissue envelope. In order to achieve uneventful union and promote physical function length, alignment and rotation of the affected extremity must be restored and anatomic alignment of intra-articular fractures is a must. However, fracture exposure and fixation must not significantly compromise the often-tenuous local biology serving to promote union.

An individualized plan of care is required for each fracture in a particular host. However, there are certainly care algorithms that have proven reliability especially with lower extremity trauma. Intramedullary nailing as a definitive strategy provides optimal fixation when feasible [11]. Rod insertion can be performed with minimal insult of the soft tissue sleeve [12]. Further, mechanical stability is optimal. Conversion from temporary external fixation to a nail is safe prior to 2 weeks [13].

Fixed angle plating is another popular strategy. This technique is warranted in cases where nail fixation is not adequate. Examples include metadiaphyseal fractures which either have a very short segment or that involve the joint. Submuscular techniques can be employed to limit soft tissue damage [14–17].

27.2.3 Staged Fracture Care

There is a subset of severe fracture cases that will not achieve uneventful union after the primary definitive intervention. These cases are treated with a staged approach with thoughtful consideration toward future interventions. For example, commonly encountered fracture patterns in the polytrauma patient are open comminuted metadiaphyseal fractures of the distal femur, proximal tibia, and distal tibia (Fig. 27.3). Often there is concomitant severe articular involvement of the adjacent joint. These fractures frequently occur as a result of motor-vehicular trauma when the affected extremity contacts the dashboard or floorboard.

The primary goal of initial fracture care is debridement to avoid septic complications. All devitalized soft and osseous tissues are excised. However, a critical size bone defect is frequently realized which will not heal primarily.

A rational initial plan of care manages the soft tissues and the horrific bone and joint injury. After all devitalized tissues are removed, soft tissue coverage is a must. Skeletal stabilization emphasizes anatomic articular reduction. The reconstructed articular block is then linked to the shaft with appropriate length, alignment, and rotation using bridge fixation technique.

Antibiotic bead application is an invaluable adjunct. Beads are installed into the bone defect site. They act as a local antibiotic delivery system to decrease the incidence of deep infection. Secondly, they serve as a "spacer" for later bone grafting strategies. Lastly, the cement incites a local inflammatory response promoting a local blood supply to encourage bone graft incorporation at the second stage of operation [18–21].

27.2.4 Role of Acute Shortening

As an alternative to staged care, fractures with bone loss may be best managed with acute shortening. The advantage of this approach is inherent in its simplicity. This technique creates an ideal biomechanical environment to promote union obviating the need for grafting procedure. Direct cortical contact and effective internal fixation encourages primary osseous union.

Acute shortening is a well-tolerated technique in the upper extremity with minimal physical dysfunction (Fig. 27.4). However, the merits of acute shortening for lower extremity trauma are more controversial. Shortening in the lower extremity can lead to gait disturbance, need for aggressive shoe lifts, eventual symptomatology in the axial skeleton, and most importantly patient dissatisfaction. Often shortened lower extremities will require subsequent complex lengthening procedures using Ilizarov methodologies.

The prime candidate for acute shortening procedure is the polytrauma patient that lacks maturity for multiple reconstructive procedures. Alternatively, this technique is warranted for the type C host that is prone to complication with more advanced techniques.

27.3 Secondary Reconstruction

Nonunion with or without deformity occurs as a result of a multitude of factors. In the polytrauma patient, most cases are expected secondary to the complex fracture, compromised soft tissue environment, and the critically ill host. However, all fractures in this patient population must be followed closely so that a proactive approach can be employed when uneventful osteosynthesis does not occur.

Fig. 27.3 Polytrauma patient with grade 3B open intra-articular fractures of the distal femur and tibia (**a**, **b**). Initial fixator applied and serial debridements performed. Once clean wound beds were evident, anatomic articular reductions were performed and bridge plating strategies were utilized. Beads were left in critical-sized tibial defect (**c**). Anticipated nonunion occurred in both fractures. Once the patient's tissues matured and overall health was maximized, uneventful bone grafting, BMP application, and supplementary internal fixation were performed (**d**)

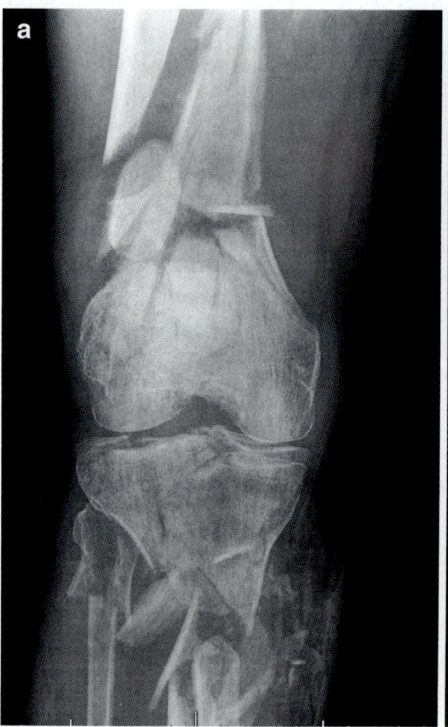

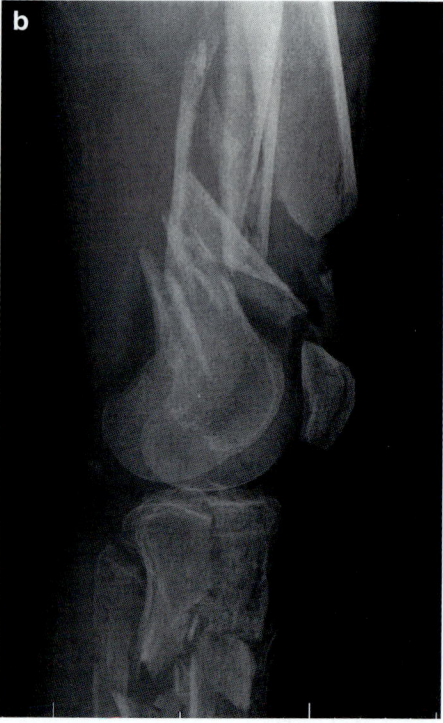

Fig. 27.3 (continued)

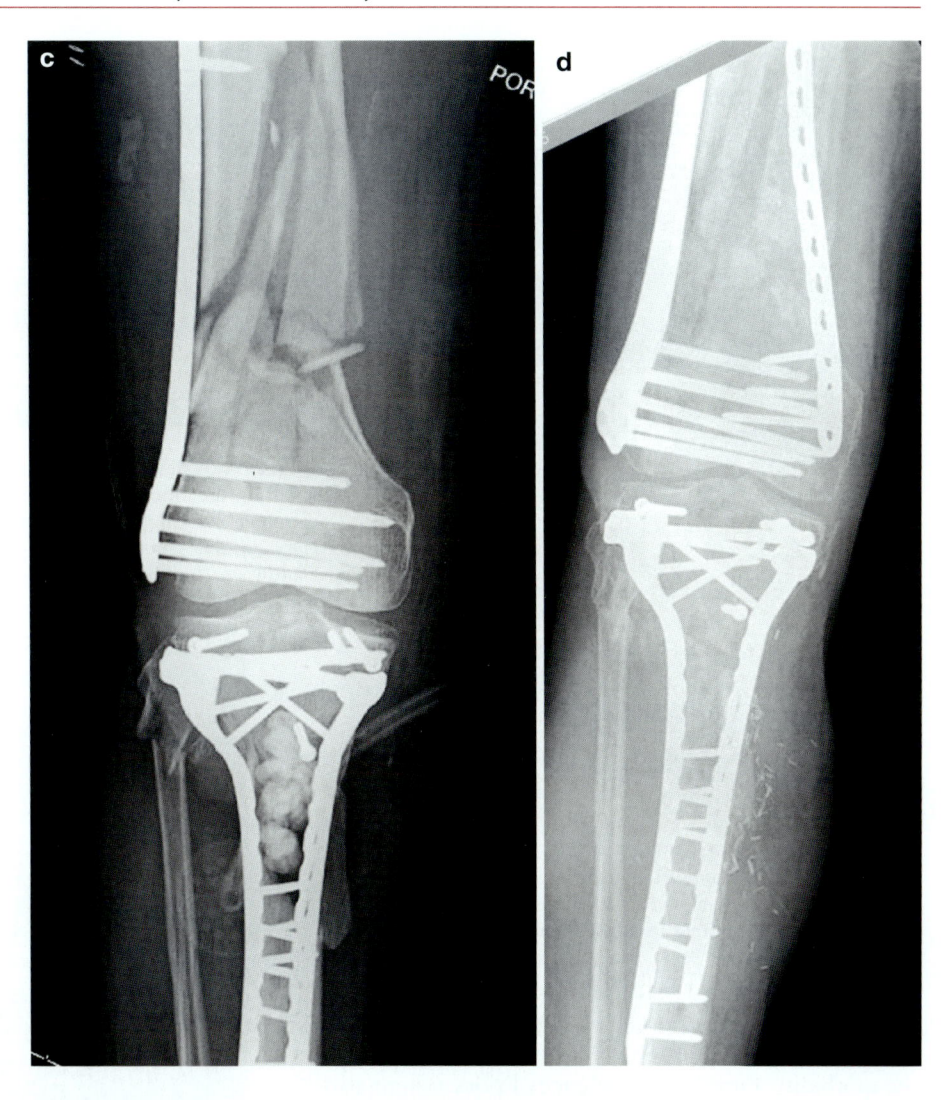

27.3.1 Anticipated Nonunion

Fractures with critical-sized bone defects will not heal without secondary intervention. The goal is to perform secondary reconstructive surgery once the host and local conditions have been optimized. Specifically, the host should be mentally and physically prepared for the reconstructive effort. Devotion to the limb salvage plan is critical. Optimizing general health including nutrition while avoidance of negative behaviors such as tobacco usage must be achieved [22]. Further, preoperative workup must exclude the possibility of local infection especially in cases of previous open fracture [23, 24]. Lastly, physical exam should reveal that the soft tissue envelope has matured implying that there are vascularized tissues to accept bone grafting procedure.

The preoperative plan should encompass both mechanical and biological strategies to promote uneventful osseous union. Biologic supplementation is critical to the success of healing bone defects. Autologous bone grafting is the gold standard. However for large defects, bone graft extenders such as cancellous allograft can be used. Further, recombinant technology has paved the way for delivery of selected bone morphogenetic proteins directly to the nonunion site [25–28].

Harvest from the iliac crest has served as the traditional site for obtaining autogenous bone [29]. Cancellous bone retrieved from this region is heralded for its osteogenic, osteoinductive, and osteoconductive

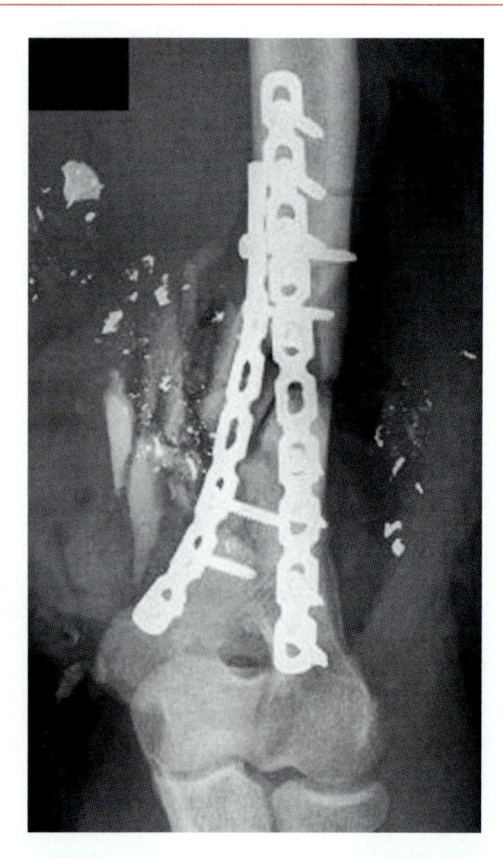

Fig. 27.4 Multiple trauma victim after assault with high-velocity weapon. Debridement and acute shortening of humerus performed to encourage primary union without the need for multiple procedures

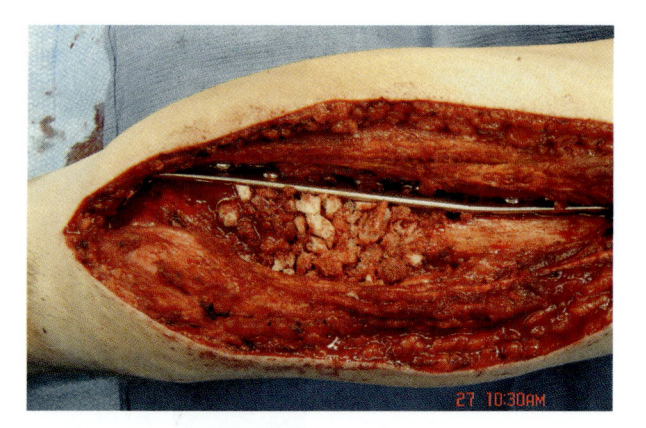

Fig. 27.5 A rigid mechanical environment and autologous bone grafting are often necessary for successful reconstruction of atrophic and oligotrophic nonunions. In this case, supplementary medial column support was added to existing lateral hardware

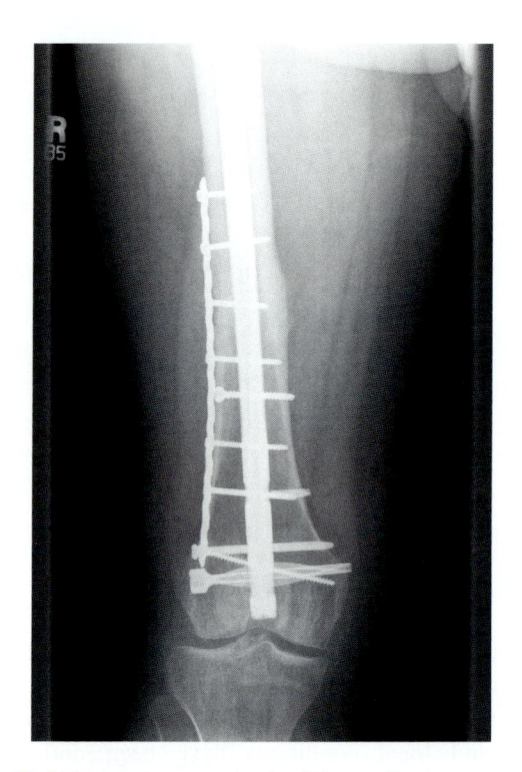

Fig. 27.6 Plating over a retained nail is an effective strategy to have in the armamentarium of nonunion reconstructive options

properties. This site, however, is infamous for donor site morbidity. Further, the presence of prior trauma to this region such as pelvic or acetabular fracture makes harvest from this region less desirable.

An alternative source of graft can come from the medullary cavity of the femur obtained using the reamer irrigator aspirator system [30]. With this technique, a large volume of cancellous bone can be retrieved with limited donor site morbidity [31]. The quality of graft material rivals iliac crest harvest with regards to its biologic activity. A learning curve, however, is notable when using this technological advance [32].

After graft harvest, the fixation strategy employed is largely dependent on the previous fixation scheme. In the controlled environment of staged treatment, the previous indwelling fixation is presumably stable holding the fracture in optimal alignment. During this stage of reconstruction, however, it is commonplace to provide supplementary internal fixation to promote rigidity. Rigid fixation will ensure continued optimal alignment of the fracture while providing the ideal biomechanical milieu for bone graft incorporation via creeping substitution.

Plating is the workhorse for supplementary internal fixation. In the case of previous plate fixation, it is typical that unicolumnar support was performed in the first stage. Thus, at the second stage experience, supplementary fixation is performed in the opposite column [33]. For example, lateral submuscular plate fixation is often performed for comminuted metadiaphyseal fracture of the distal femur. At the time of bone grafting, this plate is retained and additional support of the medial column is advantageous to avoid varus collapse (Fig. 27.5).

In the face of a retained intramedullary nail, exchange nailing is typically the performed [34–39]. Alternatively, in certain cases, a plate can be used over the nail to manipulate the local mechanical environment toward increased rigidity (Fig. 27.6). This methodology is frequently employed when open bone grafting is necessary for large bone defects [40, 41].

27.4 Established Nonunion After Polytrauma

Victims of polytrauma are at heightened risk for nonunion and deformity even after routine fracture care. Strategies employed for nonunion reconstruction depend on countless variables. Thus, a thoughtful process must be performed to marry the treatment plan to the specific nonunion, patient, and goals for physical functional.

27.4.1 Traditional Nonunion Reconstruction

Diagnosing and defining the type of nonunion is critical to the formulation of a rational treatment plan. Diagnosis is frequently made after consideration of the patient's symptoms which is correlated with objective radiographic findings notable on plain radiographs and CT scan. It is critical to distinguish nonunion "personality." Atrophic and oligotrophic variants have limited healing response, which will require both biologic and mechanical augmentation. In contrast, hypertrophic variants demonstrate an ineffective yet dramatic healing response, which frequently requires only modulation of the local mechanical environment. Further, the potential for septic nonunion must be considered.

The tactics for obtaining osseous union in the face of atrophic and oligotrophic nonunions are well

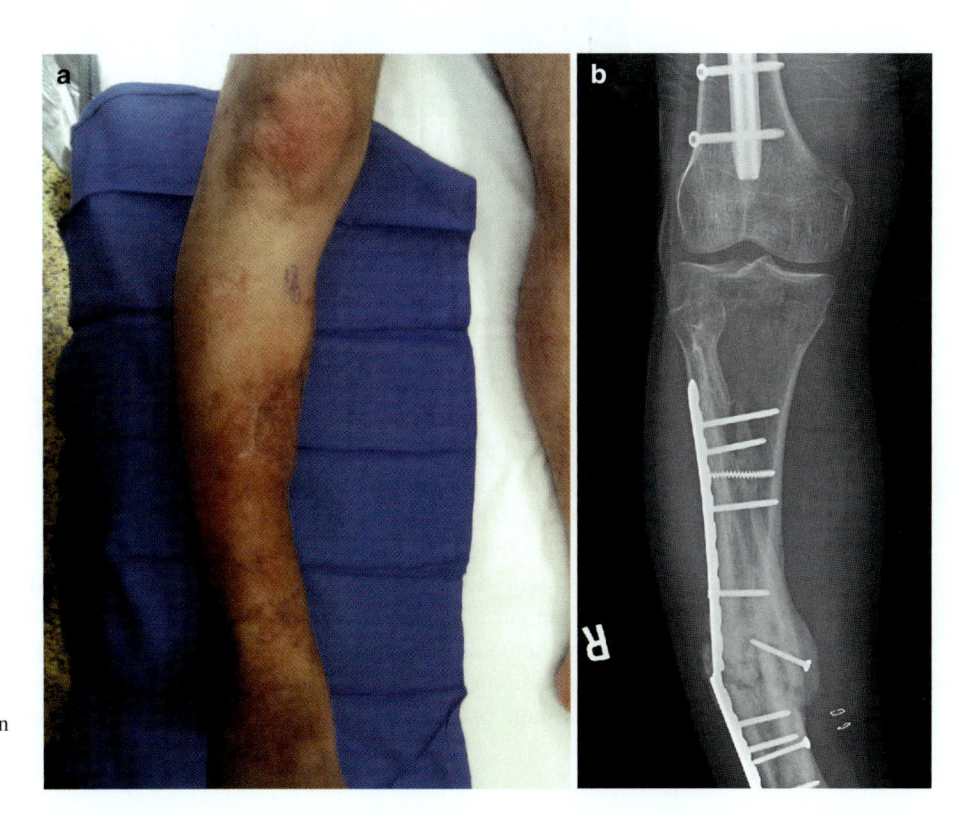

Fig. 27.7 Deformity correction is integral in the planning for nonunion reconstruction (**a**). In this hypertrophic nonunion (**b**), realignment of the mechanical axis was performed (**c**). In addition, rigid compression plating was achieved (**d**, **e**)

Fig. 27.7 (continued)

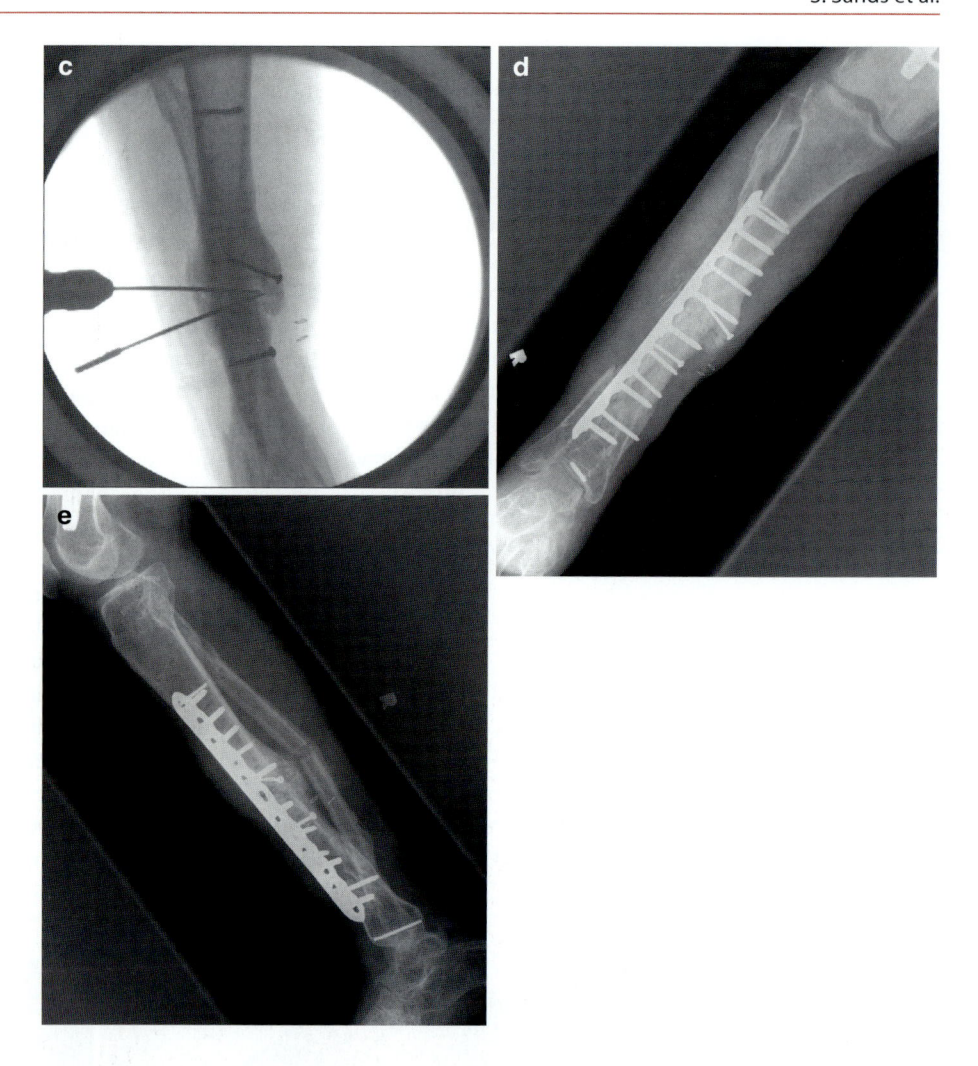

established [42]. Rigid fixation and biologic support with autogenous graft are fundamental principles of care. Deformity, when present, must also be considered in the plan to restore the anatomic and mechanical axis to promote optimal functionality (Fig. 27.7).

The paradigm for surgical care includes debridement of the fibrous scar at the site of nonunion. Further, the sclerotic medullary canal needs to be reestablished to promote endosteal healing. The nonunion site should be "stimulated" with a drilling or feathering technique to increase the surface area for healing which also causes fracture hematoma formation. Lastly, when possible, compression of the bone ends should be performed to encourage primary and/or gap healing.

27.4.2 Infected Nonunion

A staged protocol is typically employed for septic nonunion [43–45]. The patient is brought to the operative suite for hardware removal and debridement. Intraoperative cultures are obtained. Temporary fixation, most commonly with an external fixator, is applied. Organism-specific antibiotics are given both systemically and locally via beads. After at least 6 weeks, the effectiveness of treatment is judged based on clinical exam and the results of serial inflammatory markers. The patient is then withdrawn from antibiotics and taken back to the operating room for repeat debridement and culture. If inflammatory markers and biopsy specimens are favorable, then nonunion reconstruction can proceed [23, 24].

27.5 Unconventional Reconstructive Options for Periarticular Nonunions

27.5.1 Combined Arthrodesis and Nonunion Reconstruction

Preserving motion of essential joints is always a priority in promoting optimal physical functionality in the polytrauma patient. However, there is a select subset of periarticular injuries which have profound articular damage that is not recoverable despite previous attempt at anatomic reduction. In these patients, the surgical plan is designed to perform nonunion surgery in addition to selected fusion of the adjacent joint. This innovative treatment strategy is gaining popularity for the tibial plafond, calcaneous, and midfoot fractures [46, 47].

This surgical design preemptively treats posttraumatic joint dysfunction after severe high-energy periarticular trauma (Fig. 27.8). In the polytrauma patient population, this strategy prevents further operation on a multiply operated extremity. Theoretically, this aggressive treatment

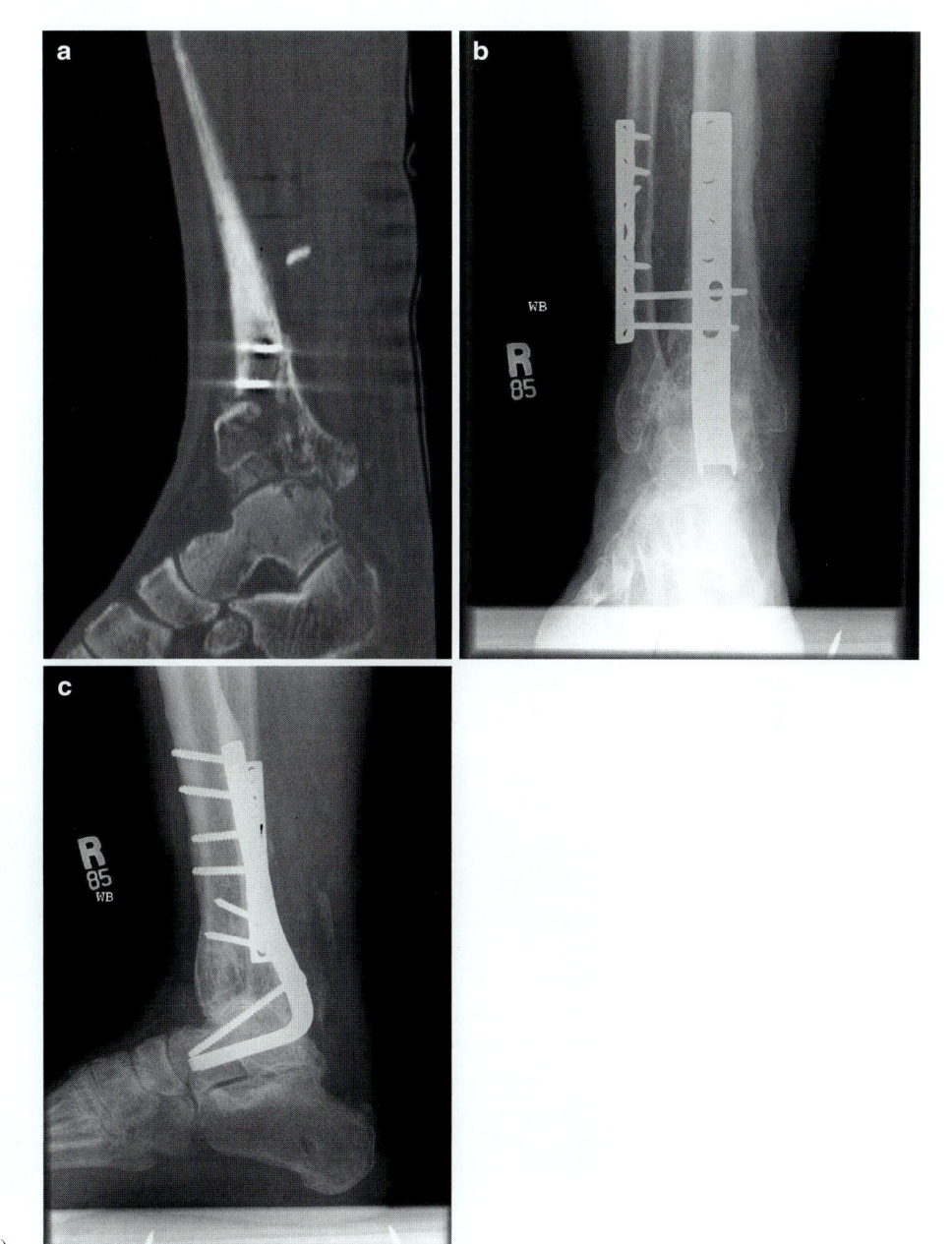

Fig. 27.8 Distal tibia nonunion with ipsilateral tibiotalar posttraumatic disease (**a**). Nonunion reconstruction with adjacent ankle fusion performed (**b, c**)

will lead to improved long-term results. However, failure of joint fusion is a potential complication. Further, gait dysfunction and adjacent joint disease can occur.

27.5.2 Reconstruction Using Arthroplasty Techniques

Arthroplasty is a suitable solution for periarticular nonunions especially involving the hip, knee, shoulder, and elbow (Fig. 27.9). This option can be used on younger patients, but it is best reserved for the middle aged or older populations as prosthetic loosening is a long-term concern. The arthroplasty option is typically in the form of a tumor type prosthesis allowing for resection of the un-united fracture. The value of this technique is unquestionable as immediate rehabilitation after operation is a favorable consequence. Weight-bearing capacity is restored in a more rapid fashion compared to other more traditional methodologies.

27.6 Conclusion

Musculoskeletal injuries occurring in the polytrauma patient present unique challenges to the orthopaedic trauma surgeon. The treatment plan must take into account multiple factors, including the personality of the fracture, the local soft tissue environment, concomitant injuries, and the patient's physiologic status. The timing

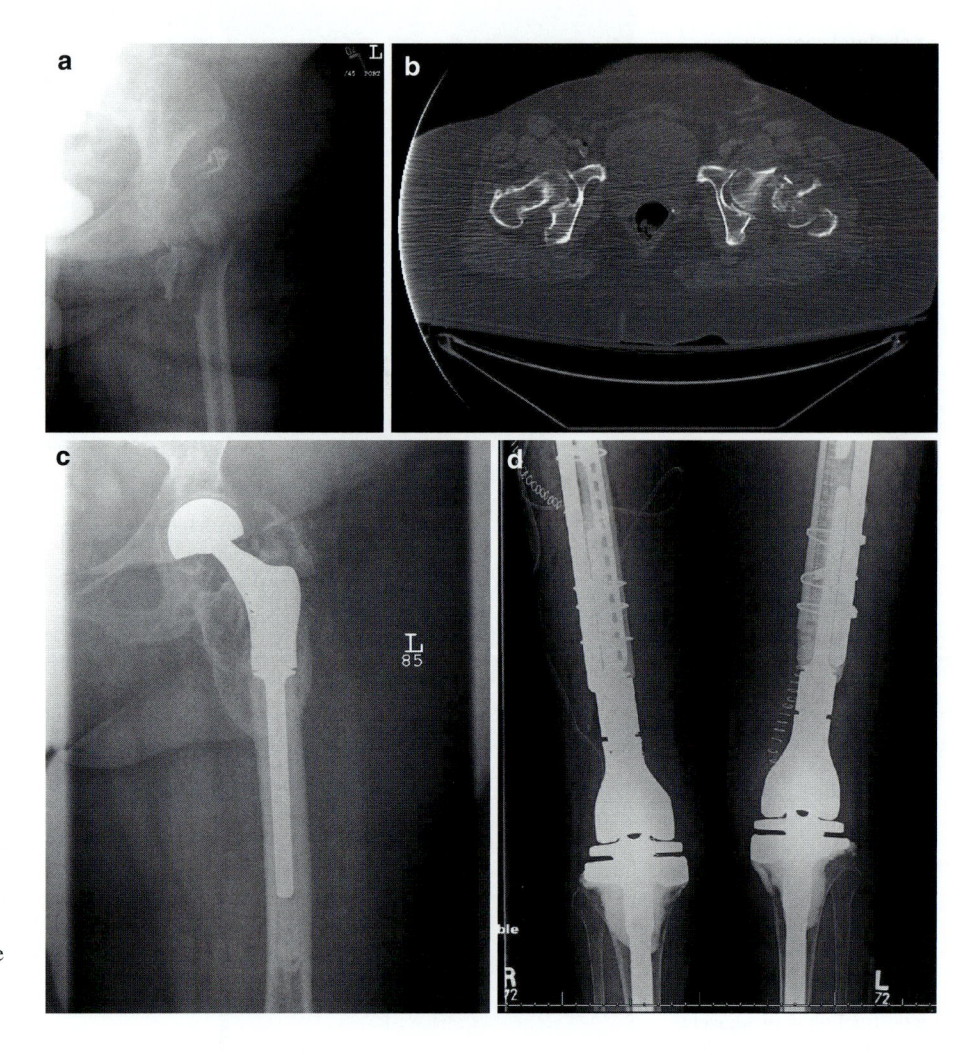

Fig. 27.9 Tumor prosthesis are effective for definitively treating non-reconstructable fractures (**a**, **b**) and periarticular nonunions around the hip (**c**), knee (**d**), and shoulder (**e**)

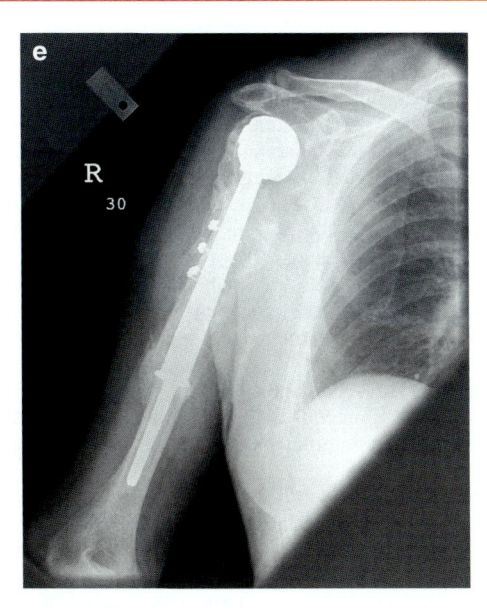

Fig. 27.9 (continued)

of skeletal reconstruction is individualized to the patient and may occur at the time of injury, or in a staged or delayed fashion. It is important to anticipate complications such as nonunion, deformity, and posttraumatic arthritis so that an organized reconstructive plan may be performed to restore physical function.

References

1. Pape HC, Tornetta 3rd P, Tarkin I, Tzioupis C, Sabeson V, Olson SA. Timing of fracture fixation in multitrauma patients: the role of early total care and damage control surgery. J Am Acad Orthop Surg. 2009;17(9):541–9.
2. Tarkin IS, Siska PA, Zelle BA. Soft tissue and biomechanical challenges encountered with the management of distal tibia nonunions. Orthop Clin North Am. 2010;41(1):119–26.
3. Tarkin IS, Sop A, Pape HC. High-energy foot and ankle trauma: principles for formulating an individualized care plan. Foot Ankle Clin. 2008;13(4):705–23.
4. Tarkin IS, Clare MP, Marcantonio A, Pape HC. An update on the management of high-energy pilon fractures. Injury. 2008;39(2):142–54.
5. Attinger CE, Evans KK, Bulan E, Blume P, Cooper P. Angiosomes of the foot and ankle and clinical implications for limb salvage: reconstruction, incisions, and revascularization. Plast Reconstr Surg. 2006;117(7 Suppl):261S–93.
6. Arany L, Baranyai T, Mândi A, Kunkli F. Arteriographic studies in delayed-union and non-union of fractures. Radiol Diagn (Berl). 1980;21(5):673–81.
7. Dickson K, Katzman S, Delgado E, Contreras D. Delayed unions and nonunions of open tibial fractures. Correlation with arteriography results. Clin Orthop Relat Res. 1994;302:189–93.
8. LeBus GF, Collinge C. Vascular abnormalities as assessed with CT angiography in high-energy tibial plafond fractures. J Orthop Trauma. 2008;22(1):16–22.
9. Pape HC, Tsukamoto T, Kobbe P, Tarkin I, Katsoulis S, Peitzman A. Assessment of the clinical course with inflammatory parameters. Injury. 2007;38(12):1358–64.
10. Biffl WL, Moore EE, Haenel JB. Nutrition support of the trauma patient. Nutrition. 2002;18:960–5.
11. Giannoudis PV, Pountos I, Morley J, Perry S, Tarkin IS, Pape HC. Growth factor release following femoral nailing. Bone. 2008;42(4):751–7.
12. Borrelli Jr J, Prickett W, Song E, Becker D, Ricci W. Extraosseous blood supply of the tibia and the effects of different plating techniques: a human cadaveric study. J Orthop Trauma. 2002;16(10):691–5.
13. Harwood PJ, Giannoudis PV, Probst C, Krettek C, Pape HC. The risk of local infective complications after damage control procedures for femoral shaft fracture. J Orthop Trauma. 2006;20:181–9.
14. Carpenter CA, Jupiter JB. Blade plate reconstruction of metaphyseal nonunion of the tibia. Clin Orthop Relat Res. 1996;332:23–8.
15. Chin KR, Nagarkatti DG, Miranda MA, Santoro VM, Baumgaertner MR, Jupiter JB. Salvage of distal tibia metaphyseal nonunions with the 90 degrees cannulated blade plate. Clin Orthop Relat Res. 2003;409:241–9.
16. Sheerin DV, Turen CH, Nascone JW. Reconstruction of distal tibia fractures using a posterolateral approach and a blade plate. J Orthop Trauma. 2006;20(4):247–52.
17. Reed LK, Mormino MA. Functional outcome after blade plate reconstruction of distal tibia metaphyseal nonunions: a study of 11 cases. J Orthop Trauma. 2004;18(2):81–6.
18. Henry SL, Ostermann PA, Seligson D. The antibiotic bead pouch technique. The management of severe compound fractures. Clin Orthop Relat Res. 1993;295:54–62.
19. Pelissier P, Martin D, Baudet J, Lepreux S, Masquelet AC. Behaviour of cancellous bone graft placed in induced membranes. Br J Plast Surg. 2002;55(7):596–8.
20. Ristiniemi J, Lakovaara M, Flinkkilä T, Jalovaara P. Staged method using antibiotic beads and subsequent autografting for large traumatic tibial bone loss: 22 of 23 fractures healed after 5–20 months. Acta Orthop. 2007;78(4):520–7.
21. Pelissier P, Masquelet AC, Bareille R, Pelissier SM, Amedee J. Induced membranes secrete growth factors including vascular and osteoinductive factors and could stimulate bone regeneration. J Orthop Res. 2004;22(1):73–9.
22. Brinker MR, O'Connor DP, Monla YT, Earthman TP. Metabolic and endocrine abnormalities in patients with nonunions. J Orthop Trauma. 2007;21(8):557–70.
23. Perry M. Erythrocyte sedimentation rate and C reactive protein in the assessment of suspected bone infection – are they reliable indices? J R Coll Surg Edinb. 1996;41(2):116–8.
24. Stucken C, et al. The preoperative diagnosis of infection in nonunions. OTA Annual Meeting, San Diego, CA 2009.
25. Johnson EE, Urist MR, Finerman GA. Distal metaphyseal tibial nonunion. Deformity and bone loss treated by open reduction, internal fixation, and human bone morphogenetic protein (hBMP). Clin Orthop Relat Res. 1990;250:234–40.
26. Giannoudis PV, Kanakaris NK, Dimitriou R, Gill I, Kolimarala V, Montgomery RJ. The synergistic effect of autograft and BMP-7 in the treatment of atrophic nonunions. Clin Orthop Relat Res. 2009;467(12):3239–48.

27. Jones AL, Bucholz RW, Bosse MJ, Mirza SK, Lyon TR, Webb LX, et al. BMP-2 Evaluation in Surgery for Tibial Trauma-Allgraft (BESTT-ALL) study group. Recombinant human BMP-2 and allograft compared with autogenous bone graft for reconstruction of diaphyseal tibial fractures with cortical defects. A randomized, controlled trial. J Bone Joint Surg Am. 2006;88(7):1431–41.
28. Dahabreh Z, Calori GM, Kanakaris NK, Nikolaou VS, Giannoudis PV. A cost analysis of treatment of tibial fracture nonunion by bone grafting or bone morphogenetic protein-7. Int Orthop. 2008;33(5):1407–14.
29. Meister K, Segal D, Whitelaw GP. The role of bone grafting in the treatment of delayed unions and nonunions of the tibia. Orthop Rev. 1990;19(3):260–71.
30. Kobbe P, Tarkin IS, Pape HC. Use of the 'reamer irrigator aspirator' system for non-infected tibial non-union after failed iliac crest grafting. Injury. 2008;39(7):796–800.
31. Kobbe P, Tarkin IS, Frink M, Pape HC. [Voluminous bone graft harvesting of the femoral marrow cavity for autologous transplantation. An indication for the"Reamer-Irrigator-Aspirator-" (RIA-)technique]. Unfallchirurg. 2008;111(6):469–72.
32. Quintero AJ, Tarkin IS, Pape HC. Technical tricks when using the reamer irrigator aspirator technique for autologous bone graft harvesting. J Orthop Trauma. 2010;24(1):42–5.
33. Chapman MW, Finkemeier CG. Treatment of supracondylar nonunions of the femur with plate fixation and bone graft. J Bone Joint Surg Am. 1999;81(9):1217–28.
34. Richmond J, Colleran K, Borens O, Kloen P, Helfet DL. Nonunions of the distal tibia treated by reamed intramedullary nailing. J Orthop Trauma. 2004;18(9):603–10.
35. Rosson JW, Simonis RB. Locked nailing for nonunion of the tibia. J Bone Joint Surg Br. 1992;74(3):358–61.
36. Court-Brown CM et al. Locked intramedullary nailing of open tibial fractures. J Bone Joint Surg Br. 1991;73(6):959–64.
37. Zelle BA, Gruen GS, Klatt B, Haemmerle MJ, Rosenblum WJ, Prayson MJ. Exchange reamed nailing for aseptic nonunion of the tibia. J Trauma. 2004;57(5):1053–9.
38. Court-Brown CM, Keating JF, Christie J, McQueen MM. Exchange intramedullary nailing. Its use in aseptic tibial nonunion. J Bone Joint Surg Br. 1995;77-B(3):407–11.
39. Hak DJ, Lee SS, Goulet JA. Success of exchange reamed intramedullary nailing for femoral shaft nonunion or delayed union. J Orthop Trauma. 2000;14(3):178–82.
40. Nadkarni B, Srivastav S, Mittal V, Agarwal S. Use of locking compression plates for long bone nonunions without removing existing intramedullary nail: review of literature and our experience. J Trauma. 2008;65(2):482–6.
41. Birjandinejad A, Ebrahimzadeh MH, Ahmadzadeh-Chabock H. Augmentation plate fixation for the treatment of femoral and tibial nonunion after intramedullary nailing. Orthopedics. 2009;32(6):409.
42. Tarkin IS Sojka JM. Biomechanical strategies for managing atrophic and oligotrophic nonunions. Oper Tech Orthop. 2008;18(2):86–94.
43. Ring D, Jupiter JB, Gan BS, Israeli R, Yaremchuk MJ. Infected nonunion of the tibia. Clin Orthop Relat Res. 1999;369:302–11.
44. Struijs PA, Poolman RW, Bhandari M. Infected nonunion of the long bones. J Orthop Trauma. 2007;21(7):507–11.
45. Shahcheraghi GH, Bayatpoor A. Infected tibial nonunion. Can J Surg. 1994;37(3):209–13.
46. Zelle BA, Gruen GS, Espiritu M, Pape HC. Posterior blade plate fusion: a salvage procedure in severe posttraumatic osteoarthritis of the tibiotalar joint. Oper Tech Orthop. 2006;16:68–75.
47. Flemister Jr AS, Infante AF, Sanders RW, Walling AK. Subtalar arthrodesis for complications of intra-articular calcaneal fractures. Foot Ankle Int. 2000;21(5):392–9.

Posttraumatic Stress Disorder and Psychological Sequelae After Severe Trauma

Adam J. Starr

Contents

28.1 Introduction 345
28.2 Magnitude of the Problem 345
28.3 Impact of the Problem 346
28.4 Addressing the Problem 347
References 347

A.J. Starr
Department of Orthopaedic Surgery,
University of Texas Southwestern Medical Center,
Dallas, TX, USA
e-mail: adam.starr@utsouthwestern.edu

28.1 Introduction

The goal of this short chapter is to introduce the reader to the topic of posttraumatic stress disorder (PTSD) after orthopaedic trauma, and to convey a few simple facts about the subject. These facts will be discussed in greater detail later, but they can be summed up as follows: First, PTSD is common after orthopaedic trauma; second, PTSD has a large effect on patients' reports of outcome after trauma; last, PTSD remains largely unrecognized and untreated among orthopaedic trauma patients.

28.2 Magnitude of the Problem

Orthopaedic surgeons are not trained to seek out, recognize, or treat psychological illness in their patients. In a way, this is surprising, because every subspecialty area of orthopaedics is impacted by the psychological makeup of the patients being treated. Every practicing surgeon knows from experience that some patients are mentally tougher than others, and that some patients deal better with pain or setbacks from injury than other patients do. Orthopaedic conditions usually cause pain, and most orthopaedists have dealt with patients who suffer from chronic pain. Helping patients deal with pain and physical impairment is a common job requirement for orthopaedic surgeons. Thus, the idea that a patient's mental state comes into play during orthopaedic treatment is not really controversial. Assessing and responding to a patient's mental state is something most orthopaedic surgeons do routinely. The patient's mental state comes into play in almost every orthopaedic condition.

Table 28.1 Prevalence of psychological distress reported by other investigators

Investigator	Population	Assessment tool	Prevalence
Feinstein and Dolan [4]	48 patients with femur, tibia, or fibula fracture	IES[a] and self-report DSM-III-R[b] checklist for PTSD	7/48 (14%) at 6 months
Shalev et al. [3]	211 trauma survivors	Clinician-administered PTSD scale, structured clinical interview for DSM-III-R	37/211 (17.5%) at 4 months
Zatzick et al. [2]	73 trauma patients	PTSD checklist	22/73 (30%) at 1 year
Michaels et al. [1]	100 trauma patients	Civilian Mississippi scale for PTSD	42/100 (42%) at 6 months
McCarthy et al. [7]	385 patients with severe lower limb injury	Brief symptom inventory to assess risk for likely psychological disorder	42% at 24 months
Crichlow et al. [6]	161 orthopaedic trauma patients	Beck depression inventory	45% 3–12 months after injury
Starr et al. [5]	580 orthopaedic trauma patients	Revised civilian Mississippi scale for PTSD	295/580 (51%) at 1 year

[a]Impact of Event Scale
[b]Diagnostic and Statistical Manual of Mental Disorders, Third Ed., Revised

However, despite the working familiarity with "mental toughness," until recently, there has been little discussion in the orthopaedic literature of the magnitude of the problem posed by psychological illness. All orthopaedists encounter patients who struggle emotionally when faced with orthopaedic illness – but do any such patients actually meet criteria for a psychiatric diagnosis? Further, how common are such patients, really? Many surgeons have memories of particular patients who became emotionally devastated by an illness or injury. On the other hand, patients with less dramatic emotional symptoms may not be noticed. If we search for psychological distress after orthopaedic trauma with diagnostic rigor, what will we find?

A brief review of the literature reveals that PTSD and psychological distress are, in fact, quite common after trauma in general, and after orthopaedic trauma in particular. Michaels et al. examined 100 trauma patients 6 months after injury and found that 42% met the criteria for PTSD [1]. Zatzick et al. followed a group of 73 trauma patients for a year after injury and found that 30% met criteria for PTSD [2]. Shalev et al. examined 211 trauma patients and found PTSD in 17.5% at 4 months [3]. In a study that examined patients with fractures of the femur, tibia, or fibula, Feinstein and Dolan found that 15% had PTSD 6 months after trauma [4]. Starr et al. found that 51% of orthopaedic trauma patients met the criteria for PTSD in a group examined 1 year after trauma, on average [5]. Crichlow et al. found the prevalence of depression after orthopaedic trauma was 45% [6]. An examination of the Lower Extremity Assessment Project patients revealed that almost one-fifth of the patients reported severe phobic anxiety and/or depression, while 42% of the patients screened positive for a likely psychological disorder at 24 months after injury [7].

Although these studies' patient populations varied, and the tools used to assess them differed, it is clear that PTSD and psychological distress after orthopaedic trauma are common. These data are presented in Table 28.1.

28.3 Impact of the Problem

The question that next arises is: if psychological distress occurs after trauma, does it have any impact on patient outcome? The impact of PTSD or psychological distress on patients' reports of outcome after trauma has not been extensively studied. In the study mentioned above, Zatzick et al. found that among the variables tested, PTSD had the strongest association with outcome as assessed using the SF-36 – stronger than Injury Severity Score, age, history of alcohol abuse, or chronic medical conditions [2]. This is a fairly remarkable finding. In their study of depression after orthopaedic trauma, Crichlow et al. found that functional outcome, assessed using the Short Musculoskeletal Functional Assessment, was strongly linked to depression, assessed using the Beck Depression Inventory [6]. Similarly, Bhandari et al. noted that in a population of orthopaedic trauma patients, patient reports of health-related quality of life, as assessed using the SF-36, were strongly associated with the intensity of the patients' psychological symptoms [8]. In a study of patients treated for fractures of the posterior wall of the acetabulum, Moed and McMichael found that, at 2 years, patients' responses to questions regarding emotional and mobility status were most strongly linked to an unsatisfactory overall outcome [9]. Moed et al. concluded, "There are important factors determining our patients' functional outcome other than how well we repair the fracture."

Thus, the literature on this area of study is clear. When patient-derived tools are used to assess results of treatment, psychological distress is strongly associated with outcome, and in fact may be the "strongest" determinant of outcome. For orthopaedists accustomed to considering bony alignment or joint range of motion as outcome measures, these findings may be surprising. However, after a moment's reflection, they are understandable. Imagine a patient who sustains a femur fracture after an automobile crash. Suppose the patient suffers from PTSD, with daily flashbacks, nightmares, intrusive memories of the accident, and anxiety. For such a patient, "outcome" after injury will not be good, even if their fracture heals in perfect alignment. The patient will rightly tie these psychological symptoms to the injury event. The patient cannot and will not divorce psychological outcome from overall outcome. The patient will consider outcome to be poor, even if physical function is good.

28.4 Addressing the Problem

As noted above, orthopaedic surgeons are not trained to seek out, recognize, or treat psychological distress after trauma. After years in practice, some surgeons may learn to recognize these symptoms and attempt to treat them. However, to date, there has been no study examining whether treatment of psychological illness after orthopaedic trauma is beneficial. Thus, for most patients, psychological distress after orthopaedic trauma remains unrecognized and untreated.

Perusal of the psychiatry and psychology literature reveals that successful treatments exist for PTSD. Two FDA-approved medications, paroxetine and sertraline, have been shown to significantly reduce PTSD symptom scores in patients suffering from the illness [10, 11]. Psychotherapy has also been shown to significantly lower symptom scores, with methods such as cognitive behavioral therapy, exposure therapy, or supportive therapy being commonly employed [12–14].

Despite the existence of successful treatments for PTSD, orthopaedic trauma surgeons may question the value of engaging in such efforts. The medications and therapies used to treat PTSD are unfamiliar to surgeons. Furthermore, the exploration of "How do you feel?" questions may slow down an already busy clinic. However, the orthopaedic surgeon's role seems likely to be limited simply to seeking out such symptoms, and asking patients about psychological problems. Definitive management of psychiatric illness will be left to mental health professionals. Besides, when one considers the potential benefits of such treatments, concerns such as these should fade away. If psychological distress is truly one of the factors to have a strong effect on outcome after trauma – and multiple studies make that conclusion – treatment of illnesses such as PTSD offers an enormous opportunity to improve outcomes. The current "standard of care" for psychological distress after orthopaedic trauma is, unfortunately, no care at all. Given the large impact psychological illness has upon outcomes, it seems clear that even small improvements in PTSD symptom scores are likely to yield significant improvements in overall patient outcome. Thus, the time seems ripe for investigating whether or not accepted treatments for PTSD, such as medication or psychotherapy, have any beneficial effect on orthopaedic trauma patients.

References

1. Michaels AJ, Michaels CE, Moon CH, Smith JS, Zimmerman MA, Taheri PA, et al. Posttraumatic stress disorder after injury: impact on general health outcome and early risk assessment. J Trauma. 1999;47:460–6.
2. Zatzick DF, Jurkovich GJ, Gentilello L, Wisner D, Rivara FP. Posttraumatic stress, problem drinking, and functional outcomes after injury. Arch Surg. 2002;137:200–5.
3. Shalev AY, Freedman S, Peri T, Brandes D, Sahar T, Orr SP, et al. Prospective study of posttraumatic stress disorder and depression following trauma. Am J Psychiatry. 1998;155:630–7.
4. Feinstein A, Dolan R. Predictors of post-traumatic stress disorder following physical trauma: an examination of the stressor criterion. Psychol Med. 1991;21:85–91.

5. Starr AJ, Smith WR, Frawley WH, Borer DS, Morgan SJ, Reinert CM, et al. Symptoms of posttraumatic stress disorder after orthopaedic trauma. J Bone Joint Surg Am. 2004;86:1115–21.
6. Crichlow RJ, Andres PL, Morrison SM, Haley SM, Vrahas MS. Depression in orthopaedic trauma patients. Prevalence and severity. J Bone Joint Surg Am. 2006;88:1927–33.
7. McCarthy ML, MacKenzie EJ, Edwin D, Bosse MJ, Castillo RC, Starr AJ, et al. Psychological distress associated with severe lower limb injury. J Bone Joint Surg Am. 2003;85:1689–97.
8. Bhandari M, Busse JW, Hanson BP, Leece P, Ayeni OR, Schemitsch EH. Psychological distress and quality of life after orthopedic trauma: an observational study. Can J Surg. 2008;51:15–22.
9. Moed BR, McMichael JC. Outcomes of posterior wall fractures of the acetabulum. J Bone Joint Surg Am. 2007;89:1170–6.
10. Brady K, Pearlstein T, Asnis GM, Baker D, Rothbaum B, Sikes CR, et al. Efficacy and safety of sertraline treatment of posttraumatic stress disorder: a randomized controlled trial. JAMA. 2000;283:1837–44.
11. Marshall RD, Beebe KL, Oldham M, Zaninelli R. Efficacy and safety of paroxetine treatment for chronic PTSD: a fixed-dose, placebo-controlled study. Am J Psychiatry. 2001;158:1982–8.
12. Bisson JI, Shepherd JP, Joy D, Probert R, Newcombe RG. Early cognitive behavioral therapy for posttraumatic stress symptoms after physical injury. Br J Psychiatry. 2004;184:63–9.
13. Blanchard EB, Hickling EJ, Devineni T, Veazey CH, Galovski TE, Mundy E, et al. A controlled evaluation of cognitive behavioral therapy for posttraumatic stress in motor vehicle accident survivors. Behav Res Ther. 2003;41(1):79–96.
14. Bryant RA, Harvey AG, Dang S, Sackville T, Basten C. Treatment of acute stress disorder: a comparison of cognitive behavioral therapy and supportive counseling. Consult Clin Psychol. 1998;66:862–6.

Late Outcome After Severe Fractures

Roman Pfeifer and Hans-Christoph Pape

Contents

29.1 General Long-Term Outcomes in Polytrauma Patients 349
29.2 Upper-Extremity Injuries 350
29.3 Pelvic Fractures 351
29.4 Lower-Extremity Fractures 352
29.5 Conclusion 353
References 353

Over the past decades, numerous improvements have been made in the delivery of trauma care and rehabilitation such as injury-prevention advancements in rescue systems, improvements in hospital diagnostics and surgical techniques, and the development of better treatment strategies. A decrease in the mortality rate (37–18%) of multiple trauma patients has been noted over the past two decades [1–6]. Thus, long-term outcome evaluation and assessment of quality of life and patient satisfaction have gained attention in polytrauma care. Severe musculoskeletal trauma is a life-altering condition leading to prolonged morbidity and numerous repetitive interventions. That it is the main contributor to work disability [7–9], impaired long-term psychosocial outcome, and persisting disabilities has been demonstrated in long-term studies, underlining the immense economic burden to society and the lasting impact on the affected individuals and their families [7–12].

29.1 General Long-Term Outcomes in Polytrauma Patients

To look beyond mortality and assess the patients' longitudinal evaluation is a helpful tool for identifying the factors that influence long-term outcome following major injuries and the appropriate beneficial interventions. Several large projects [7–9, 13–16] have recently been conducted that focus on patients long-term functional recovery following polytrauma. These studies provide evidence that not only injury-related factors, such as injury severity, injury location, and treatment methods, but also the specific characteristics of the individual, socioeconomic factors, and health habits have a strong impact on outcome [8, 13, 17]. In addition,

R. Pfeifer (✉) and H.-C. Pape
Department of Orthopaedic and Trauma Surgery,
Aachen University Medical Center, Pauwelsstr. 30,
52074 Aachen, Germany
e-mail: rpfeifer@ukaachen.de

authors have underlined the role of post-injury depression, anxiety, and chronic pain. High incidence rates of posttraumatic stress disorder (24–39%), anxiety (32–70%), and depression (35–68%) have been observed among trauma patients. Additionally, cognitive defects, such as memory impairment, difficulty with concentration, and emotional problems have been reported [7, 13, 18–20]. All these factors negatively affect a patient's functional outcome. These studies stress the need for concomitant posttraumatic psychological support. Moreover, self-efficacy has been shown to be one of the strongest predictors of the Sickness Impact Profile and return to work [7–9, 13]. It is assumed that persons with low self-efficacy are more likely to be disengaged from the physical rehabilitation and recovery process. To address this issue, it has been suggested that self-efficacy and self-management training should be introduced to polytrauma patients, especially as positive effects have been demonstrated in the treatment of patients with chronic diseases such as arthritis, diabetes, and chronic pain [21, 22].

Several groups have demonstrated evidence of gender-related differences after severe injury [16, 23]. The advantages of premenopausal women over men in the acute phase after multiple injuries have been described [16, 23]. However, long-term results demonstrate the opposite. Women showed a higher rate of posttraumatic stress disorder and psychological support, longer duration of rehabilitation, and longer sick leave time [24–27].

Blunt injuries of the trunk are acutely associated with life-threatening complications. Long-term investigations, however, demonstrate that after blunt injuries involving the chest and abdomen, substantial recovery may occur [28]. These injuries were rarely the reason for worse outcome or functional impairments in long-term follow-up studies [28–30].

The Hannover Rehab Study's goal was to evaluate functional outcome with a minimum follow-up of 10 years (mean 17.5 years) [14–16]. A total of 637 patients were identified using the electronic database. Inclusion criteria included multiple blunt injuries; Injury Severity Score (ISS) ≥ 16; treated between 1973 and 1990 in a level I trauma center; age between 3 and 60 years; and discharged alive. Two standardized scores were used: Hannover Score for Polytrauma Outcome (HASPOC) [31] and Short Form-12 (SF-12) [32]) to evaluate the long-term outcome. This study revealed that head and extremity injuries accounted for the most frequent causes of long-term disability [16]. At follow-up, 33% of patients required a medical aid for their disability, and 20.1% reported disability due to their injury. Approximately the same percent of patients (76.5%) and physicians (69.1%) reported success from rehabilitation. Extremity-related results from this study are summarized in the corresponding section.

29.2 Upper-Extremity Injuries

There is a limited number of scientific publications addressing the long-term outcome of upper extremity injuries. The available long-term studies are mainly restricted to follow-up investigations of individual fractures or treatment options [33, 34]. Isolated upper-extremity fractures are typically associated with low-energy trauma mechanisms [33]. Therefore, the results found in isolated fractures are likely to be different from those of severely injured patients who have sustained high-energy trauma and concomitant injuries. Moreover, follow-up investigations demonstrate that patients with injuries to the upper limb tend to have a better long-term outcome than patients with lower-extremity injuries [35, 36]. Nevertheless, concomitant vascular and neurological injuries (involvement of Brachial plexus and peripheral nerves) were shown to be a major determinant of worse long-term functional outcome [37]. Further, typical sequelae following upper-extremity trauma are nonunion, heterotopic ossification, and impaired range of motion [34, 38, 39].

Mkandawire and coauthors analyzed the long-term (5 years) musculoskeletal recovery in survivors of severe injuries (ISS > 15) [11]. They performed a reexamination of 158 severely injured patients (>15 years old) treated between 1989 and 1990. According to this multicenter investigation (16 hospitals), approximately 50% of patients with shoulder girdle injury were associated with functional impairments and persistent disorders. Functional disabilities were more frequently (66%) observed after fractures of the arm and forearm. Displaced and articular fractures were identified as those mainly responsible for long-term disabilities. Moreover, even after 5 years following trauma, a remarkable 45% of patients with shoulder girdle and 62% of patients with upper-extremity fractures complained of chronic pain. Multiple upper limb fractures or a combination of shoulder girdle and shaft fractures in particular were more likely to result in long-term morbidity. Furthermore, authors discussed whether associated head, facial, and thoracic injuries potentially interfere with upper limb rehabilitation, resulting in continuing disability and chronic pain.

The Hannover Rehab Study performed a functional outcome evaluation of upper-extremity fractures, focusing on the question of whether isolated articular fractures, shaft fractures, or the presence of both are significantly related to poor outcome results (Table 29.1). At time of follow-up, the physical examination showed better mobility of the affected upper limb in patients with isolated shaft fractures as measured by range of motion (ROM). Furthermore, limitations of ROM, muscle weakness (10–20%) (shoulder and elbow), and contractures of the affected region (25%) were more frequently observed following combined articular and shaft fractures. These functional results are in line with determined score outcomes as measured by HASPOC and SF-12. Patients with upper-extremity shaft fractures demonstrated significantly more favorable scores than patients with the combination of a shaft injury and an articular fracture. This might be explained by the degeneration of the affected joint following articular fractures which may lead to functional disabilities and chronic pain [40–44]. Moreover, the initial surgical reconstruction of articular and multiple fractures is more complex. A large number of these patients require additional operative treatments and reconstructions. The interference of multiple fractures in the rehabilitation process is another factor that negatively affects long-term functional results following severe injury.

29.3 Pelvic Fractures

Pelvic fractures are often associated with multiple concomitant injuries of the lower limb, spine, abdomen, and head [45, 46]. Accordingly, analysis of long-term outcomes may be difficult to interpret because the accompanying injuries may affect the results [47–49]. It has been shown that both the severity of pelvic fracture (stable vs. unstable) and the presence of associated injuries contribute to poor long-term outcome [50]. Incomplete recovery and functional impairments were observed following unstable pelvic ring fractures, while stable pelvic injuries rarely led to major long-term problems [45, 51, 52]. Others could demonstrate an association of sequelae and poor outcomes following open pelvic fractures [53]. Moreover, the clinical outcomes of patients with unstable pelvic ring trauma and associated injuries were less satisfactory than the outcomes of patients with unstable pelvic ring trauma and no associated injuries (Table 29.2) [49, 51].

Chronic pain syndromes, neurologic impairments, and nonunions have been described as determining factors that influence the long-term outcome in patients who have sustained pelvic fracture [52]. An overview of long-term (2 years) pain results was demonstrated by Pohlemann and coauthors [50, 52, 55]. Pain was observed in every fracture classification group; the rate of completely pain-free patients was 55% after A-Type fractures, 41% after B-Type, and 27% after C-Type fractures [50, 52, 55]. Nonanatomic reduction or insufficient fixation can provide poor long-term outcome results, resulting in chronic back pain, instability, and malunions or nonunions [46, 56, 57].

Moreover, authors described a close correlation between neurological and functional long-term outcome [48]. At follow-up (2.2 years), 21% of patients with B-Type and 60% with C-Type fractures had at least some neurological impairments [54]. In particular,

Table 29.1 Functional status of the upper extremities following polytrauma with fractures at different localizations

	Articular fractures N=60	Shaft fractures N=37	Combined fractures N=52
ROM >50%	88.3%	94.6%*	73.1%**
Contractures	8.3%*	10.8%	25%***
Stiffness	1.6%	2.7%	5.8%
Neurological impairment	11.7%	10.8%	13.5%
Full muscle force shoulder	90%	97.3%	88.5%
Full muscle force elbow	86.7%	100%*	80.8%**
HASPOC-total	70.2±48.9**	47±34.3*,***	69.4±44.4**
SF-12 Phy	43±11.9**	47.9±9.8*,***	43.6±9.9**

HASPOC Hannover score for polytrauma outcome, *SF-12 Psy* short-form 12 items health survey, physical component summary
*Significantly worse outcome vs. combined fractures ($p<0.05$)
**Significantly worse outcome vs. shaft fractures ($p<0.05$)
***Significantly worse outcome vs. articular fractures ($p<0.05$)

Table 29.2 Clinical examination of pelvic ring fractures following polytrauma

Study	Fracture type	Follow-up (year)	Patient[a]	Pain	Functional disability	RTW	Neurologic impairments
Pohlemann et al. [54]	Unstable fractures	2.2	58	11–66%	No data	No data	21–60%
Miranda et al. [47]	Pelvic ring fracture	5	80	16–35%	8–21%	75–81%	No data
Tornetta and Matta [46]	Unstable fracture	3.7	48	37%	37%	67%	35%
Brenneman et al. [53]	Open fracture	4	27	No data	No data	64%	18%
Kabak et al. [51]	Unstable fracture	3.8	36	31%	No data	72%	16–31%[b]
Suzuki et al. [48]	Unstable fracture	3.9	57	No data	No data	84%	28%

RTW return to work
[a]Skeletally immature patients
[b]Sexual and urinary dysfunction

vertical unstable injuries and transforaminal sacral fractures were shown to be associated with severe neurologic disabilities [58, 59]. Among the neurologic sequelae were: peripheral nerve lesions, incontinence, and sexual dysfunctions [47, 50–55, 57]. These sequelae are also the main reason for work disability [46]. Approximately 50–75% of previously employed patients with pelvic fractures were able to return to their previous occupation [47, 51, 53].

29.4 Lower-Extremity Fractures

Studies analyzing the long-term outcome of trauma patients were able to demonstrate that injuries of lower extremity especially cause significant impairments and loss of function [35, 60–62]. It could be shown that injuries of the leg are a dominant factor influencing late functional outcome [60, 61]. Patients with these injuries demonstrated low rates of full recovery and overall satisfaction [11, 12]. In particular, patients with limb-threatening lower-extremity trauma were associated with relevant complications, leading to additional operative treatments during the post-injury course [63].

A detailed investigation and description of factors influencing the long-term outcome of lower-extremity injuries was performed within the Lower Extremity Assessment Projects (LEAP) [7–9, 13]. The LEAP is a prospective multicenter (eight level I trauma centers) cohort study investigating the long-term outcome in patients with high-energy trauma below the distal femur (LEAP studies). Functional outcomes of 601 patients were assessed for patients with amputation versus reconstruction of leg-threatening injuries. Patients with open fractures, dysvascular limbs, major soft-tissue injury, and severe foot and ankle injuries were included in the study and the outcome measure performed using the Sickness Impact Profile, a multidimensional measure of self-reported health status [7–9, 13]. The results demonstrate comparable functional outcomes in both patient groups. However, regardless of the treatment option, both the limb salvage and amputation groups demonstrate severe disability as compared with general population. One half of all patients had physical subscores on the Sickness Impact Profile 10, indicative of significant disability; only 34% of patients achieved scores typical of a general population of similar age and sex. Only 58% of those working before the injury were working at 7 years post-injury; of those patients who returned to work, 20–25% were limited in their ability to match the demands of their pre-injury status. Moreover, no significant improvements were observed at the 7 year follow-up when compared to the 2-year data.

The evaluation of the Hannover Rehab Study data base [14–16] with regard to lower-extremity fractures has demonstrated the following long-term outcomes (Table 29.3): A significant percentage of patients (30–45%) with

Table 29.3 Functional status of the lower extremities following polytrauma with fractures at different localizations

	Acetabulum	Prox. femur	Femoral shaft	Knee[a]	Tibial shaft
	N=20	N=20	N=107	N=48	N=34
Persistent pain	50.0%	45.0%	32.7%	43.8%	26.5%
Abnormal gait	35.0%[*,**]	20.0%[*]	3.7%	8.3%	14.7%[*]
Work disability	27.8%[*,***,****]	10.0%	7.6%	19.8%	8.8%
Successful rehabilitation	70.0%	60.0%[*]	80.4%	56.3%[*]	67.7%
HASPOC-total	78.78[*]	70.07[*]	49.71	79.28[*]	65.73
SF-12 PCU	40.91[*]	40.95	46.05	39.81[*]	44.06

HASPOC Hannover score for polytrauma outcome, *SF-12 PCU* short-form 12 items health survey, physical component summary

[a]Knee: including fractures of the distal femur and proximal tibia

[*]Significantly worse outcome vs. femoral shaft fractures ($p<0.05$)

[**]Significantly worse outcome vs. injuries at the knee joint ($p<0.05$)

[***]Significantly worse outcome vs. fractures of the proximal femur ($p<0.05$)

[****]Significantly worse outcome vs. tibial shaft fractures ($p<0.0$)

fractures of lower limb experienced posttraumatic pain and approximately 10–30% reported limited range of motion. The rate of gait abnormalities was significantly low following femur shaft fractures. In contrast, high rates of gait abnormality were observed in patients who had sustained acetabular fractures. Moreover, outcome scores, as measured by HASPOC and SF-12, were significantly better following an isolated femur shaft fracture when compared to the scores of patients with acetabular fractures and knee-joint injuries. The observed rates of arthroplasty were 7.5% for the hip joint, 15.1% for the knee joint, and the ankle fusion rate was reported to be 12.3%. In addition, patients with lower-extremity injuries below the knee demonstrated significantly lower outcome scores than patients with lower-extremity fractures above the knee joint, as measured by the HASPOC, the SF-12, the Tegner Activity Score, and the ability to work. Authors assumed that various factors such as the thin soft tissue envelope, unfavorable blood supply, and the complex fracture patterns of many foot and ankle injuries contributed to the inferior outcomes of patients with fractures below the knee joint [15].

29.5 Conclusion

Due to the improved mortality rates of severely injured patients, long-term follow-up observation studies have gained more attention. Social reintegration of patients and return to work were defined as main long-term goals in the treatment of polytrauma patients. Large outcome studies have recently demonstrated that articular fractures, especially those with concomitant injuries, and the presence of a lower-extremity injury are associated with poor long-term functional results and unfavorable outcome scores. Moreover, studies have emphasized the importance of psychosocial variables on the long-term functional outcome. Early psychological intervention for polytrauma patients has been suggested to address this issue. Furthermore, patients with severe injuries that are associated with poor outcome should be identified earlier in order to improve their rehabilitation results.

References

1. Bardenheuer M, Obertacke U, Waydhas C, Nast-Kolb D, AG Polytrauma der DGU. Epidemiology of severe multiple trauma – a prospective registration of preclinical and clinical supply. Unfallchirurg. 2000;103:355–63.
2. Ruchholtz S, AG Polytrauma der DGU. The Trauma Registry of the German Society of Trauma Surgery as a basis for interclinical quality management. A multicenter study of the German Society of Trauma Surgery. Unfallchirurg. 2000;103:30–7.
3. Nast-Kolb D, Aufmkolk M, Rucholtz S, Obertacke U, Waydhas C. Multiple organ failure still a major cause of morbidity but not mortality in blunt multiple trauma. J Trauma. 2001;51:835–42.
4. Pape HC, Remmers D, Rice J, Ebisch M, Krettek C, Tscherne H. Appraisal of early evaluation of blunt chest trauma:

development of a standardized scoring system for initial clinical decision making. J Trauma. 2000;49(496):504.
5. Kuhne CA, Ruchholtz S, Kaiser GM, Nast-Kolb D, AG Polytrauma der DGU. Mortality in severely injured elderly trauma patients – when does age become a risk factor? World J Surg. 2005;29(1476):82.
6. Regel G, Lobenhoffer P, Grotz M, Pape HC, Lehmann U, Tscherne H. Treatment results of patients with multiple trauma: an analysis of 3406 cases treated between 1972 and 1991 at German level I trauma center. J Trauma. 1995;38(1): 70–8.
7. Bosse MJ, MacKenzie EJ, Kellam JF, et al. An analysis of outcomes of reconstruction or amputation after leg-threatening injuries. N Engl J Med. 2002;347(24):1924–31.
8. MacKenzie EJ, Bosse MJ, Pollak AN, et al. Long-term persistence of disability following severe lower-limb trauma. Results of seven-year follow-up. J Bone Joint Surg Am. 2005;87(8):1801–9.
9. MacKenzie EJ, Bosse MJ, Kellam JF, et al. Early predictors of long-term work disability after major limb trauma. J Trauma. 2006;61:688–94.
10. Braithwaite IJ, Boot DA, Patterson M, Robinson A. Disability after severe injury: five year follow up of a large cohort. Injury. 1998;29(1):55–9.
11. Mkandawire NC, Boot DA, Braithwaite IJ, Patterson M. Musculoskeletal recovery 5 years after severe injury: long term problems are common. Injury. 2002;33:111–5.
12. O'Toole RV, Castillo RC, Pollak AN, MacKenzie EJ, Bosse MJ, LEAP Study Group. Determinants of patient satisfaction after severe lower-extremity injuries. J Bone Joint Surg Am. 2008;90:1206–11.
13. MacKenzie EJ, Bosse MJ. Factors influencing outcome following limb-threatening lower limb trauma: lessons learned from the lower extremity assessment project (LEAP). J Am Acad Orthop Surg. 2006;14:S205–10.
14. Zelle BA, Panzica M, Vogt MT, Sittaro NA, Krettek C, Pape HC. Influence of workers' compensation eligibility upon functional recovery 10 to 28 years after polytrauma. Am J Surg. 2005;190(1):30–6.
15. Zelle BA, Brown SR, Panzica M, et al. The impact of injuries below the knee joint on the long-term functional outcome following polytrauma. Injury. 2005;36(1):169–77.
16. Pape HC, Zelle B, Lohse R, et al. Evaluation and outcome of patients after polytrauma: can patients be recruited for long-term follow-up? Injury. 2006;37(12):1197–203.
17. MacKenzie EJ, Rivara FP, Jurkovich GJ, et al. The impact of trauma-center care on functional outcomes following major lower-limb trauma. J Bone Joint Surg Am. 2008;90(1): 101–9.
18. Michaels AJ, Michaels CE, Smith JS, Moon CH, Peterson C, Long WB. Outcome from injury: general health, work status, and satisfaction 12 months after trauma. J Trauma. 2000;48(5):841–50.
19. Evans SA, Airey MC, Chell SM, Connelly JB, Rigby AS, Tennant A. Disability in young adults following major trauma: 5 year follow up of survivors. BMC Public Health. 2003;3(8):1–8.
20. Piccinelli M, Patterson M, Braithwaite IJ, Boot DA, Wilkinson G. Anxiety and depression disorder 5 years after severe injuries: a prospective follow-up study. J Psychosom Res. 1999;46(5):455–64.
21. Morley S, Eccleston C, Williams A. Systematic review and meta-analysis of randomized controlled trials of cognitive behavior. Pain. 1999;80:1–13.
22. Lorig KR, Sobel DS, Stewart AL, et al. Evidence suggesting that a chronic disease self-management program can improve health status while reducing hospitalisation: a randomized trial. Med Care. 1999;37:5–14.
23. Brenneman FD, Boulanger BR, McLellan BA, Culhane JP. Acute and long-term outcomes of extremely injured blunt trauma victims. J Trauma. 1995;39:320–4.
24. Probst C, Zelle B, Panzica M, et al. Clinical re-examination 10 or more years after polytrauma: is there a gender related difference? J Trauma. 2010;68(3):706–11.
25. Holbrook TL, Hoyt DB, Anderson JP. The importance of gender on outcome after major trauma: functional and psychologic outcomes in women versus men. J Trauma. 2001;50:270–3.
26. Holbrook TL, Hoyt DB, Stein MB, Siebert WJ. Gender differences in long-term posttraumatic stress disorder outcomes after major trauma: women are at higher risk of adverse outcomes than men. J Trauma. 2002;53:882–8.
27. Holbrook TL, Hoyt DB. The impact of major trauma: quality-of-life outcomes are worse in women than in men, independent of mechanism and injury severity. J Trauma. 2004; 56:284–90.
28. Holbrook TL, Anderson JP, Siebert WJ, Browner D, Hoyt DB. Outcome after major trauma: 12-month and 18-month follow-up results from the Trauma Recovery Project. J Trauma. 1999;46:765–73.
29. Amital A, Shirit D, Fox BD, et al. Long-term pulmonary function after recovery from pulmonary contusion due to blunt chest trauma. IMAJ. 2009;11:673–6.
30. Grotz M, Pape HC, Stalp M, van Griensven M, Schreiber TC, Krettek C. Long-term outcome after multiple organ failure following severe trauma. Anaesthesist. 2001;50(4): 262–70.
31. Stalp M, Koch C, Regel G, Krettek C, Pape HC. Development of a standardized instrument for quantitative and reproducible rehabilitation data assessment after polytrauma (HASPOC). Chirurg. 2001;72(3):312–8.
32. Ware JE, Kosinski M, Keller SD. A 12-item short-form-health survey. Construction of scales and preliminary tests of reliability and validity. Med Care. 1996;34(3):220–33.
33. Ekholm R, Tidermark J, Törnkvist H, Adami J, Ponzer S. Outcome after closed functional treatment of humeral shaft fractures. J Orthop Trauma. 2006;20:591–6.
34. Helfet DL, Kloen P, Anand N, Rosen HS. Open reduction and internal fixation of delayed unions and nonunions of fractures of the distal part of the humerus. J Bone Joint Surg Am. 2003;85:33–40.
35. Butcher JK, MacKenzie EJ, Cushing B, et al. Long-term outcomes after lower extremity trauma. J Trauma. 1996;41: 4–9.
36. MacKenzie EJ, Morris JA, Jurkovich GJ. Return to work following injury: the role of economic, social, and job-related factors. Am J Public Health. 1998;88:1630–7.
37. Joshi V, Harding GE, Bottoni DA. Determination of functional outcome following upper extremity arterial trauma. Vasc Endovasc Surg. 2007;41:111–4.
38. Ring D, Gulotta L, Jupiter JB. Unstable nonunions of the distal part of the humerus. J Bone Joint Surg Am. 2003;85: 1040–6.

39. Ilahi OA, Strausser DW, Gabel GT. Post-traumatic heterotopic ossification about the elbow. Orthopedics. 1998;21(3): 265–8.
40. Volpin G, Dowd GS, Stein H, Bentley G. Degenerative arthritis after intra-articular fractures of the knee. Long-term results. J Bone Joint Surg Br. 1990;72(4):634–8.
41. Harris AM, Patterson BM, Sontich JK, Vallier HA. Results and outcomes after operative treatment of high energy tibial plafond factures. Foot Ankle Int. 2006;27(4):256–65.
42. Weiss NG, Parvizi J, Trousdale RT, Bryce RD, Lewallen DG. Total knee arthroplasty in patients with a prior fracture of tibial plateau. J Bone Joint Surg Am. 2003;85-A(2): 218–21.
43. Letournel E, Judet R. Fractures of the acetabulum. 2nd ed. New York: Springer; 1993.
44. Bhandari M, Matta J, Ferguson T, Matthys G. Predictors of clinical and radiological outcome in patients with fractures of the acetabulum and concomitant posterior dislocation of the hip. J Bone Joint Surg Br. 2006;88(12):1618–24.
45. Gansslen A, Pohlemann T, Paul C, Lobenhoffer P, Tscherne H. Epidemiology of pelvic ring injuries. Injury. 1996;27 Suppl 1:S-20.
46. Tornetta III P, Matta JM. Outcome of operatively treated unstable posterior pelvic ring disruptions. Clin Orthop Relat Res. 1996;329:186–93.
47. Miranda MA, Riemer BL, Butterfield SL, Burke III CJ. Pelvic ring injuries. A long term functional outcome study. Clin Orthop Relat Res. 1996;329:152–9.
48. Suzuki T, Shindo M, Soma K, et al. Long-term functional outcome after unstable pelvic ring fracture. J Trauma. 2007;63(4):884–8.
49. Rommens PM, Hessmann MH. Staged reconstruction of pelvic ring disruption: differences in morbidity, mortality, radiologic results, and functional outcomes between B1, B2/B3, and C-type lesions. J Orthop Trauma. 2002;16(2):92–8.
50. Pohlemann T, Gansslen A, Schellwald O, Culemann U, Tscherne H. Outcome evaluation after unstable injuries of the pelvic ring. Unfallchirurg. 1996;99(4):249–59.
51. Kabak S, Halici M, Tuncel M, Avsarogullari L, Baktir A, Basturk M. Functional outcome of open reduction and internal fixation for completely unstable pelvic ring fractures (type C): a report of 40 cases. J Orthop Trauma. 2003;17(8): 555–62.
52. Pohlemann T, Tscherne H, Baumgartel F, et al. Pelvic fractures: epidemiology, therapy and long-term outcome. Overview of the multicenter study of the Pelvis Study Group. Unfallchirurg. 1996;99(3):160–7.
53. Brenneman FD, Katyal D, Boulanger BR, Tile M, Redelmeier DA. Long-term outcomes in open pelvic fractures. J Trauma. 1997;42(5):773–7.
54. Pohlemann T, Bosch U, Gansslen A, Tscherne H. The Hannover experience in management of pelvic fractures. Clin Orthop Relat Res. 1994;305:69–80.
55. Pohlemann T, Gansslen A, Schellwald O, Culemann U, Tscherne H. Outcome after pelvic ring injuries. Injury. 1996;27 Suppl 2:B31–8.
56. Kanakaris NK, Angoules AG, Nikolaou VS, Kontakis G, Giannoudis PV. Treatment and outcomes of pelvic malunions and nonunions: a systematic review. Clin Orthop Relat Res. 2009;467(8):2112–24.
57. Eid K, Keel M, Keller A, Ertel W, Trentz O. Influence of sacral fracture on the long-term outcome of pelvic ring injuries. Unfallchirurg. 2005;108(1):35–42.
58. Huittinen VM. Lumbosacral nerve injury in fracture of the pelvis. A postmortem radiographic and patho-anatomical study. Acta Chir Scand. 1972;429:3–43.
59. Majeed SA. Neurologic deficits in major pelvic injuries. Clin Orthop Relat Res. 1992;282:222–8.
60. Seekamp A, Regel G, Bauch S, Takacs J, Tscherne H. Long-term results of therapy of polytrauma patients with special reference to serial fractures of the lower extremity. Unfallchirurg. 1994;97:57–63.
61. Seekamp A, Regel G, Tscherne H. Rehabilitation and reintegration of multiply injured patients: an outcome study with special reference to multiple lower limb fractures. Injury. 1996;27:133–8.
62. Jurkovich GJ, Mock C, MacKenzie EJ, et al. The sickness impact profile as a tool to evaluate functional outcome in trauma patients. J Trauma. 1995;39:625–31.
63. Harris AM, Althausen PL, Kellam J, Bosse MJ, Castillo RC, LEAP Study Group. Complications following limb-threatening lower extremity trauma. J Orthop Trauma. 2009;23(1): 1–6.

Index

A
Abbreviated injury scale (AIS), 80, 83
Abdominal injury, 93, 99, 100
Acute phase protein (APP), 20–21
Acute respiratory distress syndrome (ARDS), 20, 22–24, 26, 27
Acute soft tissue and bone infections, 305–316
Adult respiratory distress syndrome (ARDS), 36–38
Advanced trauma life support (ATLS), 44, 45
Airway management, 82
AIS. *See* Abbreviated injury scale
American Spinal Injury Association (ASIA) motor index score and scale, 156
Amputation, 135, 136, 138–139, 145–148
Angiography, 109–112
    pelvic fracture, 109–110
Ankylosing spondylitis, 151, 152, 162
Anterior cord syndrome, 157
Anterior lateral thigh flap, 250–251
Anterior posterior compression (APC), 106–108, 110, 112
Antibiotic prophylaxis, 205
Antigen-presenting cells (APCs), 21
Anti-inflammatory cytokines, 19, 21, 23–24
APP. *See* Acute phase protein
ARDS. *See* Acute respiratory distress syndrome; Adult respiratory distress syndrome
Articular fracture, 229–241
ATLS. *See* Advanced trauma life support
ATLS management
    spine, 155, 156
Autologous nerve grafting, 51, 54, 62–65
Axonotmesis, 52, 53

B
Babysitter procedure, 62, 64–66
Bacterial translocation (BT), 27–28
BCVI. *See* Blunt cerebral vascular injuries
Bell's palsy, 58
Bell's phenomenon, 59
Bladder reconstruction, 119–121
Blast injury, 281, 285–290
Blunt cerebral vascular injuries (BCVI), 158, 159
Bone defect regeneration, 297, 299–300
Bone stabilization, 248
Brace
    for spinal injury, 159, 160
Bronchoscopy, 79
Brown-Séquard syndrome, 157
BT. *See* Bacterial translocation

C
Canadian C-spine rule, 154
Cardiac injuries, 78
CARS. *See* Counter-regulatory anti-inflammatory response syndrome
CBA. *See* Cost-benefit analysis
CEA. *See* Cost-effectiveness analysis
Central cord syndrome, 157
Central paralysis, 58, 59
Cerebral perfusion pressure (CPP), 45, 46
Cervical branches, 56, 58
CFNG. *See* Cross-facial nerve grafting
Chest radiography, 77–80, 83
Chest trauma
    in patient with spine injuries, 155
Child(ren)
    spinal injuries in, 163
Chronic fatigue, 345
Cierny–Mader classification, 322
Clinical assessment, 127–132
CM. *See* Combined mechanism
CMA. *See* Cost-minimization analysis
COI. *See* Cost of illness
Collaboration, 15–18
Combined mechanism (CM), 106, 107
Common iliac artery, 104
Complete paralysis, 59, 70
Complications, 127, 129–131
Compliment system, 21, 22, 28
Computed tomography (CT)
    of the chest, 79
    of spine, 151
Continuous axial rotational therapy, 82–83
Corticosteroid (s)
    for spinal cord injury, 159
Cost-benefit analysis (CBA), 6, 7
Cost-effectiveness analysis (CEA), 6–7
Cost-minimization analysis (CMA), 6
Cost of illness (COI), 7
Cost-utility analysis (CUA), 6, 7
Counter-regulatory anti-inflammatory response syndrome (CARS), 19

CPP. *See* Cerebral perfusion pressure
Cranial nerves, 56, 57, 59
Craniotomy, 45, 47
C-reactive protein (CRP), 20–21, 23
Cross-facial nerve grafting (CFNG), 58, 62–68, 70
CT. *See* Computed tomography
CUA. *See* Cost-utility analysis
Cutaneous flaps, 245–246

D

DALY. *See* Disability-adjusted life-years
Damage-associated molecular patterns (DAMPs), 25
Damage control orthopaedics (DCO), 34, 46, 47, 83, 84, 135, 147, 232, 296
Damage control surgery, 160, 209, 232, 289
Damage control vascular procedures, 219
DCO. *See* Damage control orthopaedics
DCPs. *See* Dynamic compression plates
Debridement, 246–249
Decompression
    for cervical vertebral injury, 158–159, 161
    for thoracolumbar injury, 161
Deep venous thrombosis (DVT)
    spine injury, 159
Deformity, 333–336, 339, 340, 343
Delayed coverage, 248, 249
Delayed responses, 3, 97, 99, 232, 248–249
Denervation, 62–66
Depression, 346–347
Devascularized, 136
Diaphragm injuries, 77
DIC. *See* Disseminated intravascular coagulation
Diffuse idiopathic skeletal hyperostosis (DISH), 152, 162
Direct cost of illness, 7
Disability-adjusted life-years (DALY), 5, 7, 9
DISH. *See* Diffuse idiopathic skeletal hyperostosis
Disseminated intravascular coagulation (DIC), 28
Dominant pedicle, 246, 247, 253, 255
Donor nerves, 54–55, 59, 62–66
DVT. *See* Deep venous thrombosis
Dynamic compression plates (DCPs), 324
Dyskinesis, 53, 59, 62, 63

E

Early total care (ETC), 46, 47, 79, 83, 84
EBM. *See* Evidence based medicine
ECMO. *See* Extracorporeal membrane oxygenation
Economic concepts, 5–7
Elastic stable intramedullary nailing (ESIN), 185
Elderly, 167–177
Elderly patients
    spinal injuries in, 151, 163
Enhanced bone grafting, 211–212, 326–329
Epidemiology, 168–169, 174, 179, 189–190, 313–315
Epineurectomy, 54
Epineurium, 53–54
Epineurotomy, 54
ESIN. *See* Elastic stable intramedullary nailing
Esophageal injuries, 77–78
ETC. *See* Early total care
Evidence based medicine (EBM), 11, 12

External fixation, 108–109, 111, 112
External iliac artery, 104
Extracorporeal membrane oxygenation (ECMO), 183
Extratemporal paralysis, 59
Extremity, 135–148

F

Facial nerve, 51–54, 56–73
    grading system, 60, 61
    grafting, 58, 62, 65
    transfer, 64–66
FAST examination, 111
Fibula flap, 253, 258
Fix and flap, 246–249
Flail chest, 76, 77, 81, 84
Floating joint injury, 230–238
Fractures, 168–177
    management, 127–134
    spine, 151–164
    temporal bone, 51, 52, 58–59, 62–63
Free flaps, 244–245, 248–250, 253, 255
Free microvascular flaps, 243, 244, 251, 253–258, 261
Free microvascular transplantation, 248, 255

G

Gardner-Wells tongs, in management of cervical spine injury, 160
Gastrocnemius flap, 249, 253, 260
GCS. *See* Glasgow coma scale
Geriatric. *See* Elderly patients
Glasgow coma scale (GCS), 44–45, 47, 181–183
Gracilis flap, 249, 251–252, 257
Gracilis muscle, 67–69
Guided bone regeneration, 297
Gunshot, 281–285, 289, 290
Gunshot wound(s)
    of spine, 162

H

Halo device, in management of cervical spine injury, 159, 160, 163
Heat shock protein (HSPs), 24–25
Hemothorax, 75–77, 79, 81
High mobility group box 1 (HMGB1), 25, 28
HSPs. *See* Heat shock protein
Hypertonic saline, 45
Hypoglossus nerve, 54, 59, 64–66
Hypovolemic shock, 180

I

ICAM-1. *See* Intercelluar adhesion molecule-1
ICP. *See* Intracranial pressure
Iliolumbar ligaments, 104
Immobilization
    of spine, 152, 154, 159, 160, 162, 163
Incidence
    spinal cord injury, 151
    spine, 151
Indirect cost of illness, 7
Infection, 206–213, 334, 336, 337, 340
Inflammation, 33–39

Intercelluar adhesion molecule-1 (ICAM-1), 22–26
Internal fixation
    anterior pelvic ring, 112–113
    posterior pelvic ring, 113
Internal iliac artery, 104
Intracranial pressure (ICP), 45–47, 182–183
Irrigation and debridement, 206–208, 211, 213

J
Jewett brace, 159, 160

K
Kallikrein-kinin system, 21, 22, 28
Knee dislocation, 238–240

L
Lagopthalmus, 59, 70, 72–73
Laminectomy
    for vertebral injury, 162
Lateral arm flap, 250
Lateral compression (LC), 106, 107, 110
Latissimus dorsi flap, 249, 255–263
Lethal triad, 46
Limb, 135–139, 145–148
Limb salvage
    associated nerve injury, 273, 277
    complications, 276
    important factors, 275
    outcomes, 274–278
    psychological distress, 276
    scoring systems, 273
Local flaps, 244–245, 248–249
Local infection, 314
Locked plate model, 324
Long-term outcome, 349–352
Lower extremity, 350, 352–353
Lower Extremity Assessment Project (LEAP) study
    inclusion criteria, 268, 269
Lung protective ventilation, 82

M
MAC. See Membrane attack complex
Magnetic resonance angiography (MRA)
    of spine, 158
Magnetic resonance imaging (MRI)
    of spine, 153
Major histocompatibility complex II (MHC II), 26
Mangled, 135–148
Mannitol, 45
MAP. See Mean arterial pressure
Marginal mandibular branches, 56–58, 63
Masseter muscle, 62, 67, 70, 72
MAST. See Military antishock trousers
Mean arterial pressure (MAP), 45, 46
Membrane attack complex (MAC), 22
Methicillin-resistant Staphylococcus aureus (MRSA), 306–316
MHC II. See Major histocompatibility complex II
Military antishock trousers (MAST), 108
Mini-hypoglossus, 62, 64–66
Minor pedicle, 246, 247, 253

MOF. See Multiple organ failure
Mortality
    spinal injury, 152, 158–160
Motor index scale
MPO. See Myeloperoxidase
MRA. See Magnetic resonance angiography
MRI. See Magnetic resonance imaging
MRSA. See Methicillin-resistant Staphylococcus aureus
Multiple injuries, 168–173
Multiple organ failure (MOF), 19–21, 23, 24, 26, 27, 39
Muscle
    flaps, 64, 66–68, 70, 246–249, 251, 253, 255, 257, 260, 262
    transfer, 62, 65–72
    transplantation, 66, 67, 70, 73
    transposition, 72
Myeloperoxidase (MPO), 26

N
Nerve
    coaptation, 53, 54, 62, 64–68, 70
    coaption, 62
    compression, 51, 53, 54
Neurapraxia, 52, 53
Neurogenic shock, 152–156
Neurologic deficit. See also Spinal cord, injury to orthosis
    cervical, 161–163
    halo-vest, 160
    thoracolumbar, 160
Neurolysis, 51, 53–54, 56, 62
Neurorrhaphy, 51, 53, 54, 62, 63
Neurotmesis, 52, 53
Nightmare, 347
Nitric oxide (NO), 20, 23, 25, 26, 28
Non-operative management (NOM), 92, 94–99
Nonunion, 333–343

O
Open fracture, 205–213, 282–283, 286, 288, 290
Operative fracture fixation, 46
Orthopaedic trauma temporary measures
Osmotic therapeutics, 45
Osteomyelitis, 311–312
Osteoporosis, 7–9
Outcome
    spinal injuries, 161, 163

P
Partial facial paralysis, 59
Pathogen-associated molecular patterns (PAMPs), 25
Pathophysiology of polytrauma, 33–39
Pattern recognition receptors (PRRs), 25, 28
PCS. See Pulmonary contusion score
PCT. See Procalcitonin
Pediatric, 180–185. See also Child(ren)
Pediatric trauma score (PTS), 181
Pelvic anatomy, 103–105
    common iliac artery
        external iliac artery, 104
        internal iliac artery, 104
    iliolumbar ligament, 104
    posterior sacroiliac ligaments, 104

sacrospinous ligament, 104
sacrotuberous ligament, 104
sciatic nerve, 105
Pelvic binders, 108
Pelvic C-clamp, 109
Pelvic fracture, 119, 121, 123, 125
Pelvic fracture classification
    Tile classification, 105, 106
    Young and Burgess classification
        anterior posterior compression (APC), 106, 107
        combined mechanism, 106, 107
        lateral compression, 106, 107
        vertical shear (VS), 106, 107
Pelvic fracture treatment
    C-clamp, 109
    external fixation, 108
    internal fixation
        anterior pelvic ring, 112–113
        posterior pelvic ring, 113
    military antishock trousers (MAST), 108
    pelvic binder, 108
    pelvic packing, 110, 111
Pelvic packing, 110, 111
Pelvis, 351–352
Penetrating trauma, 281–291
Perforator flaps, 245–247, 255, 256
Perforators, 245–247, 250, 255, 256
Perforator vessels, 245–246, 250
Pericardial injuries, 78
Perineurium, 53, 65
PMNs. *See* Polymorphonuclear cells
Pneumothorax, 75, 76, 78–79, 81
Polylactide bone grafting membrane, 298–300
Polymorphonuclear cells (PMNs), 22, 24–25
Polytrauma, 8, 168, 169, 171–173, 333–343, 349–353
Polytraumatized children, 179, 181, 183
Posterior sacroiliac ligaments, 104, 107
Posttraumatic stress disorder (PTSD) and psychological sequelae after severe trauma, 345–347
Pregnancy, 189–201
    anaesthesia, 197
    anatomic changes, 190–192
    effective doses in imaging, 194
    effects of radiation, 194–195, 197
    epidemiology, 189–190
    foetal radiation dose, 199, 200
    general assessment, 192–193
    intra-operative radiology, 197–199
    orthopaedic injuries, 199
    outcomes, 199, 201
    pelvic fracture, 199, 200
    physiologic changes, 190–192
    radiological assessment, 190, 193–197
Prehospital management
    of spine injury, 152–154
Prevention, 8–9
Primary brain injury, 43
Primary/immediate/early or secondary/delayed/late, 248
Procalcitonin (PCT), 20–21, 23
Pro-inflammatory cytokines, 19–25, 28
Prone position, 82, 83

PRRs. *See* Pattern recognition receptors
PTS. *See* Pediatric trauma score
Pulmonary contusions, 75, 77, 79–81, 84
Pulmonary contusion score (PCS), 80
Pulmonary lacerations, 76, 77

Q
Quality-adjusted life-years (QALY), 6, 7, 9

R
Radial forearm flap, 250, 251, 253
Radiography
    of spine, 157
RAGE. *See* Receptor for advanced glycation end products
Randomized controlled trial, 14
Reactive oxygen species (ROSs), 24–28
Receptor for advanced glycation end products (RAGE), 25
Reconstructive ladder, 243, 244
Reconstructive triangle, 243, 244
Rib fractures, 75–78, 80, 81
Road traffic accidents, 5, 7–8
ROSs. *See* Reactive oxygen species

S
Sacral sparing, in incomplete spinal cord injury, 156
Sacrospinous ligament, 104, 107
Sacrotuberous ligament, 104, 107
Salter Harris, 185, 186
Salvage, 135–139, 145–148
Scapular and parascapular flap, 253–255
Sciatic nerve, 105
Score according to Wagner and Jamieson, 80
Secondary brain injury, 43, 46
Secondary pedicle, 246, 247, 255
Second hit, 36–38
Septic state
Serial rib fractures, 75–77
Shotgun wound(s), 92. *See also* Gunshot wound(s)
Shunts, 220–221, 224
SIRS. *See* Systemic inflammatory response syndrome
Skin grafts, 243, 244, 250, 251, 253, 255, 257
SOD. *See* Super oxide dismutase
Soft tissue injury, 127–130, 133
Solid organ injury, 92, 94, 98
Spinal canal, decompression of, 160, 161
Spinal cord
    injury to
        incidence of, 151
        incomplete, 157
    injury to orthosis, 159
Spinal imaging. *See* Radiography
Spinal instability, 152, 154, 162
Spine
    algorithmic approach for spine injury patient, 153
    ankylosis of, fracture associated with, 151
    fracture
        non surgical treatment, 159–160
        surgical treatment, 158, 160–162

fracture management
    in hospital, 152, 154–159
    initial (emergency), 152–154
    prehospital, 152–154
gunshot wound of, 162
imaging of, 157–158
immobilization of, 152, 154, 160, 163
injury to (see Fracture)
instability, 152, 154, 158, 162
Spine board, 154
Staged approach, 130–134
Staged/delayed procedure, 248
Stif neck collar, 155, 160
Super oxide dismutase (SOD), 24
Sural nerves, 54, 55, 62
Surgery
    for vertebral injuries, 158
Surgical chest wall stabilization, 84
Synkinesis, 59, 60, 62
Systemic inflammatory response, 44
Systemic inflammatory response syndrome (SIRS), 19–21, 23, 25–27

T
Tarsorrhaphy, 72–73
Temporal bone, 52, 56
    fractures, 51, 58–59, 62–63
Temporal branches, facial nerve, 57
Temporalis muscle, 62, 70, 72
Temporalis transfer, 62, 70, 71
Temporary wound coverage, 244
TENS. See Transcutaneous electrical nerve stimulation
Tension pneumothorax, 76, 81
Thoracic trauma, 75–84
Thoracic trauma severity score (TTS), 80–81
Thoracic ultrasonography, 79
Thoracolumbosacral orthosis (TLSO), 10
Tile classification, 105, 106
Timing, 217–226, 243, 244, 248, 249
Tinel's sign, 52–53, 64, 65
Tissue necrosis, 306
Toll like receptors (TLRs), 25, 28
Tracheobronchial injuries, 77
Traction
    for cervical spine injury, 155, 158–160

Transcutaneous electrical nerve stimulation (TENS), 61
Trauma, 1–4, 11–18, 89–92, 95–100
Traumatic amputations
    amputation level, 266, 271
    completion indications, 266–268
    outcomes, 267–268, 273
    upper extremity, 267
Traumatic aortic injuries, 78
Treatment, 321–323, 325–329, 331
Trigeminal nerve, 51, 59, 63, 66, 70
TTS. See Thoracic trauma severity score
Type A host, 321
Type B host, 321–322
Type C host, 322

U
Upper extremity, 350–351
Urethral reconstruction, 117–119, 121, 125
Urological trauma, 115–125

V
VACS, 249
Vascular cell adhesion molecule (VCAM-1), 22, 25
Vascular evaluation, 217–219, 224
Vascular injury
    diagnosis of spine, 159
    treatment of spine, 159
Vascularized bone graft (VBG), 325, 328–329, 331
Vascular trauma, 218, 220
VCAM-1. See Vascular cell adhesion molecule
Vertebrae. See Spine
Vertical shear (VS), 106, 107, 110

W
Wallerian degeneration, 52–53
Wound debridement, 246–248

Y
Years lived with disability (YLD), 9
Years of life lost (YLL), 9
Young and Burgess classification, 105–107

Z
Zygomaticobuccal branches, 57–58

Printing and Binding: Stürtz GmbH, Würzburg